The
Four
Seasons
Diet

The Four Seasons Diet

Eat Right for Your Season and Lose Weight Effortlessly

Steven Capeder

Therapeutae Publishing, LLC
Duvall, Washington

THE FOUR SEASONS DIET © 2012
by Steven Capeder

For information, address: Therapeutae Publishing, LLC
P.O. Box 248, Duvall, WA, 98019

Editor: P. N. Waldygo, at Desert Sage Editorial Services
Cover Design: ACDbookcoverdesign.com
Graphics: Ken De Tore, www.detoregraphics.com

Library of Congress Cataloging-in-Publication Data
Capeder, Steven.
The four seasons diet:
Control Number: 2012947342

Contents

Part I
Four Diets for Four Unique Season-Types

Take the Quiz

Quickly learn your season-type,
Once you do, you'll discover your diet.

Take the quiz, learn your season, and discover your ideal diet. It really is that simple. Think of this book as being like an owner's manual for your make and model of automobile, except this book contains four different owners' manuals for the human body, and only one is right for you.

Have you ever driven a new car and suddenly found yourself at the gas station, trying to figure out where the gas tank release button is to open up the access to your tank? Have you ever tried to assemble a child's Christmas toy or one of those desk kits from the office supply store? Imagine trying to accomplish any of these tasks without proper instructions.

When it comes to the human body, it's not as simple as having one owner's manual or set of instructions for everyone. The task you want to accomplish when you try to lose weight is not as simple as opening up the gas tank. Successful dieting requires that you turn off the hormones that make you hungry, while you turn on the hormones that make you feel full. A food that turns off one person's hunger hormones will turn them on for somebody else, and unless you understand the rules for your season-type, dieting is about as much fun as trying to assemble that child's toy or office desk without any instructions.

This quiz is designed to help you determine which of the four "owner's manuals" or "sets of instructions" you need to follow. Once you know your season-type, I'll guide you though all of the individualized instructions, and soon you'll discover your body's secrets for losing weight effortlessly.

Many of us naturally gravitate to or away from certain

foods, based on how we feel after eating them. We often feel better after eating foods that balance out our body chemistry and help our particular season-type produce energy. We usually equate these foods with foods that we "like," but the reason we like them often has less to do with taste and more to do with how those foods make us feel. Certain foods can help balance our blood pH, give us steady energy, and provide us with mental clarity and a sense of well-being, while keeping our hunger in check between meals. Oftentimes, however, we let our preconceived thoughts undermine our instincts, because we have been told that certain foods are "bad" for us.

It's important when answering these questions that you freely choose the foods that you would prefer to eat if you had no worries or concerns based on what you have heard or read about particular types of food. For example, I've noticed that most vegetarians who gradually chose that lifestyle after realizing they felt better by eliminating meat from their diet happen to be Summers or Springs. I also know many other vegetarians who are Winters but chose to be vegetarians because they had ethical reasons for not eating meat. In cases like these, vegetarian Winters really need to think about how a meal with meat might make them feel, absent their ethical concerns. Most true Summers would not really miss giving up meat, while almost all vegetarian Winters would not feel their 100 percent best by giving up meat without the proper dietary adjustments, as I'll explain later. Similarly, I know many people who are Winters and who choose a low-fat diet because they are concerned about counting calories or have stopped eating saturated fat because they believe that it's bad for them.

Once again, you need to think about how you would really feel after eating the meals described in each question. Do not worry about calories or dwell on what people have said about certain meals being healthier for you. Simply focus on how each meal truly sounds, compared to the others, and imagine how you would feel after eating it.

A. __Favorite Breakfast__

We often have a favorite breakfast that makes us feel best and gives us the most energy in the morning. Which of the following statements would j1 apply to you?

1. A high-protein and high-fat breakfast would make me feel the best and give me the most energy. I could eat **just** a steak or six pieces of bacon for breakfast and feel great, but hearty breakfasts such as ham, eggs, sausage, and maybe a little potato with lots of butter or other similar choices would also be great.

2. I feel best eating a more balanced breakfast with a good mix of protein and carbohydrates, such as a cheese omelet and toast, but I feel best if I do not overload on too many carbohydrates.

3. I feel best eating a more balanced breakfast with a good mix of protein and carbohydrates, such as a cheese omelet and toast, but I feel best if I do not overload on too much fat.

4. I could have **just** some fruit and coffee for breakfast and feel fine, but usually I prefer plenty of carbohydrates with less protein and fat. Cereal or lots of toast with no butter, an egg or two, a glass of orange juice, and coffee would work great for me.

B. __Light Breakfast__

If all you had for breakfast was an orange, two pieces of toast with no butter or fat, one or two eggs, and a cup of black coffee, how would you feel?

1. I would feel horrible and maybe even jittery or nervous. The only way this breakfast would work for me is if I could add some sausage or bacon to it.

2. I would not feel great, and this would not be my ideal breakfast, but if I had to make it work, I probably

x

could. This breakfast would work for better for me if I could add a generous amount of butter to the toast.

3. I would probably feel alright after eating this breakfast and might prefer a small amount of butter on the toast, but I could probably get away without adding any.

4. I would feel great after eating a breakfast like this and would definitely be satisfied and would not feel the need to add any butter to the toast.

C. Heavy Breakfast
If all you had for breakfast was bacon, sausage, and a cheese omelet, how would you feel?

1. I would feel great and be able to make it to lunch with no problem.

2. I would feel alright but would probably want some carbs before lunch.

3. I would not feel great and would definitely want some carbs with that meal, or I would not feel alright.

4. I would feel horrible, sleepy, and maybe get really hungry or bloated.

D. Sweets, Protein, and Fats for Breakfast
Which of the following best describes your breakfast needs?

1. I need protein and fat for breakfast but have no need for sweets.

2. I like all three for breakfast, but I have a much greater need for fat than for sweets.

3. I like all three for breakfast but have a much greater need for sweets than for fat.

4. I really need something sweet for breakfast and do not need very much protein or fat.

E. Preferred Snacks

If you did snack, which would be your preference?

1. Salty fatty foods, such as nuts, cheese, potato chips, or a chicken leg.
2. Something like the snack above, only with some carbs and less fat, such as cheese and crackers or a peanut butter sandwich.
3. Something like the snack below, only with a little protein, such as fruit and nuts.
4. A piece of fruit or bread, with little or no fat.

F. Lunch Choices

If all that you ate for lunch was bread and a raw vegetable salad with plenty of tomatoes and onions, without any dressing, how would you feel? This question uses a numerical score of 1–10 in parentheses, with 1 being about the worst you could feel after eating a meal and 10 being about the best you could feel after eating a meal.

1. I would feel horrible (1–3) and would need to have a large piece of fatty meat with that lunch.
2. I would not feel my best (4–6) and would probably feel better if I had a large serving of cheese with that lunch.
3. I would not feel my best (5–7) and would probably feel better if I had some lean turkey breast with that lunch.
4. I would feel alright (7–10) eating this for lunch and would not necessarily have any huge need to eat more than this.

G. Dinner Choices

If all that you had for dinner was roast beef, green beans with lots of butter, and cauliflower, how would you feel? This question uses a numerical score of 1–10 in parentheses, with 1 being about the worst you could feel after eating a meal, and 10 being about the best you could feel after eating a meal.

1. I would feel great (7–10) and would not necessarily have any huge need to eat more than this.
2. I would not feel my best (5–7) and would probably feel better if I had a small serving of starch with a large serving of everything else.
3. I would not feel my best (4–6) and would probably feel better if I had a large serving of starch with a small serving of everything else.
4. I would feel horrible (1–3) if this was all ate, and I might possibly feel better if I skipped eating altogether than if I ate this for dinner.

H. **Fatty Red Meats**
Which of the following statements about consuming fatty red meat most applies to you?

1. I could easily eat fatty red meat several times a day and feel great; I could even eat it for every meal and not feel as if I were eating too much fat or meat.
2. I could eat fatty red meat at least once a day, but I might prefer leaner meat for the other meals.
3. I could eat fatty red meat 1 to 2 times a week, and still feel alright.
4. I hardly ever eat fatty red meat because I almost never feel very good after eating it.

I. **Overall**
Which of the following best describes you?

1. I feel best when I eat lots of protein and meat.
2. I feel best when I eat a mix of protein with carbohydrates, rather than just eating protein or carbohydrates alone; however, if I had to choose between eating more meat than usual with my meal or more grains and carbohydrates than usual, I would probably choose to add a little extra protein or meat to my meal.

xiii

3. I feel best when I eat a mix of protein with carbohydrates, rather than just eating protein or carbohydrates alone; however, if I had to choose between eating more meat than usual with my meal or more grains and carbohydrates than usual, I would probably choose to add a little extra carbohydrates to my meal.
4. I feel best when I eat mostly grains and vegetables, and if I do eat meat, I almost always go for lean meats.

J. Salt
How much salt in your food makes you feel best?

1. I love really salty food; in fact, I need to put a lot of salt on all of my food.
2. I usually prefer food the way it's prepared, with no overriding need to add more salt, but I prefer food that is usually more salty versus less salty.
3. I usually prefer food the way it's prepared, with no overriding need to add more salt, but I prefer food that is usually less salty versus more salty.
4. I usually prefer my food less salty than average, and I hardly ever add more salt to my food.

K. Energy from Food
Which of the following statements best describes your response to eating different types of food?

1. If I eat only foods that are high in protein and fat, I will tend to feel energized, and if I eat only foods that are high in carbohydrates, I can feel a bit too nervous or jittery, and my blood sugar may crash in thirty minutes to an hour.
2. I require a mix of protein, carbohydrates, and fat with my meals to feel energized, but if my answers were limited to #1 above or #4 below, I would pick #1.

3. I require a mix of protein, carbohydrates, and fat
   with my meals to feel energized, but if my answers
   were limited to #1 above or #4 below, I would pick
   #4.
4. If I eat only foods that are high in carbohydrates, I
   tend to feel energized, and if I eat only foods that
   are high in fat and protein I tend to feel lethargic
   and tired and may feel very heavy in the stomach.

SCORING THE QUIZ

Each question has four possible answers, which are
numbered 1–4 and also correspond to a point score for each
question as follows:

Answered #1 for a question = 1 point
Answered #2 for a question = 2 points
Answered #3 for a question = 3 points
Answered #4 for a question = 4 points

Add up your total number of points for the entire quiz. Your
season-type is determined based on your total point score as
follows:

11–16 points = Winter
17–27 points = Autumn
28–38 points = Spring
39–44 points = Summer

3-MEAL DIET TEST

When taking the quiz, many people will feel very strongly
about which answer is right, given the four choices for each
question. Other people may find it a bit more difficult to
answer, however. They may be so out of balance that their
bodies are not responding in a positive manner to any food
choices, especially if they are insulin resistant. In cases like
this, or if you are still unsure of your season-type, you can

take the following diet challenge, which should help you confirm what your season-type is.

Try the following meal plan for a day and see how you react. If you feel horrible within the first meal or two, you are probably a Winter. If you feel somewhat worse, you are probably an Autumn. If you feel somewhat better, you are probably a Spring, and if you feel great, you are probably a Summer.

Diet A

Breakfast:
Eat all three of the following items for breakfast:

1. One or two cups of black coffee.
2. One or two oranges.
3. One or two pieces of unbuttered toast.

Lunch:
Eat all three of the following items for lunch:

1. A salad consisting of lettuce greens, raw onions, 1 medium tomato, ½ of a peeled sliced cucumber, ½ of a bell pepper, with freshly squeezed lemon juice on top and two teaspoons of vegetable oil, such as olive oil, and ¼ to ½ of a minced garlic clove (optional).
2. Two egg whites, preferable hard-boiled, with the yolks thrown away.
3. One or two slices of bread, with no butter or other added fat.

Dinner:
Eat all three of the following for dinner:

1. Four ounces of chicken breast, **or,** if you are a vegetarian, four egg whites cooked in one teaspoon of oil, such as olive oil.

2. One baked or boiled potato without any added butter or toppings.
3. Steamed broccoli, with a teaspoon of vegetable oil, such as olive oil, added on top.

Diet B

Conversely, you can try the following meal plan for a day and see how you react. If you feel horrible within the first meal or two, you are probably a Summer. If you feel somewhat worse, you are probably a Spring. If you feel somewhat better, you are probably an Autumn, and if you feel great, you are probably a Winter.

Breakfast:

Eat all three of the following items for breakfast:

1. A large piece of steak, **or,** if you are a vegetarian, four eggs sunny-side up (keep the yolk runny), cooked with a teaspoon of butter. Also, if you are a vegetarian, you must consume **either** a serving of lentils or two teaspoons of brewer's yeast, which you can purchase at any health food store. This will supply you with the purines needed by Winters and Autumns, which are harder to get in a vegetarian diet.
2. Half of a potato cooked in a tablespoon of butter.
3. Fried mushrooms or asparagus.

Lunch:

Eat all three of the following items for lunch:

1. A large piece of salmon, **or,** of if you are a vegetarian, four eggs sunny-side up, cooked in at least a tablespoon of butter.
2. Green beans with 1–3 teaspoons of butter.
3. Black bean or lentil soup.

<u>Dinner:</u>
Eat all three of the following for dinner:

1. A large steak, **<u>or,</u>** of if you are a vegetarian, four eggs sunny-side up, cooked in a teaspoon of butter. Also, if you are a vegetarian, you must consume **<u>either</u>** a serving of lentils with butter (and skip the baked potato in #2, below) or two teaspoons of brewer's yeast (and include the baked potato in #2, below), which you can purchase at any health food store.
2. One baked potato with plenty of added butter and sour cream.
3. Green beans with 1–3 teaspoons of butter.

If you try both 3-meal diet tests, you should be able to tell your season-type fairly easily.

Winters will feel great on Diet B and horrible on Diet A.
Autumns will feel better on Diet B than on Diet A.
Springs will feel better on Diet A than on Diet B.
Summers will feel great on Diet A and horrible on Diet B.

Now that you have taken the quiz and know what season-type you are, it's time to learn all about your season.

Part II
Learn about Your Season

Introduction

Let's take a trip to the beach. I'll give you a road map, plus directions, and when you get there, you'll look fitter and healthier than you have in years.

All journeys begin at your current location, so let's start with where you are now. You're probably not in the kind of shape you wish you were. Perhaps years of yo-yo dieting, counting calories, and feeling hungry all the time have tempted you to give up on dieting forever. For you, the thought of dieting most likely evokes feelings of dread, similar to going to the dentist or waiting in line at the DMV. The fact that you have chosen to pick up at least one more diet book shows that you still have the resolve to go to the beach and look amazing.

Please don't blame yourself for past failures. You most likely followed the directions you were given—advice that drove you in a very large circle, right back to the same weight where you started. My directions will lead you in a straight line to your goal, taking the easiest route possible. It's a route designed for your body and your metabolism, which balances your blood sugar and turns your past diet roller-coasters into a nice gentle ride.

Let's get moving. You drive, and I'll navigate the way. You'll discover that just as there are four seasons in the year, each distinctly different from the others, there are also four distinctly different body types, each requiring its own unique diet.

Have you ever had a friend who lost a bunch of weight on a diet, which you eagerly tried, with quite different results? You see, your friend found her diet, but this was not your diet. There is no such thing as one way of eating that works for everyone, and much of what we are taught about losing weight is simply counterproductive for many people.

Amazing things can happen when you stop dieting to lose weight and instead choose a diet that kicks your metabolism into high gear, giving you a boost of energy while you lose weight. People are always amazed when I help them make simple changes to their diets that create profound changes in their lives.

My earliest such success occurred years ago, with a young lady who worked out at the same gym I did. She usually worked out around the same time as me, and during the course of a few

1

years, we became friends. I had watched her weight yo-yo up and down many times, and I could tell she struggled with weight issues. My instincts told me she had been starving herself to stay thin, and one particular day, she looked especially tired and burned out. She had finished working out early, saying that she was just too tired to go on and was waiting for her mother to pick her up. I curiously asked why she did not simply drive herself to the gym? She responded that she had been blacking out several times a day due to hypoglycemia, and that driving was far too dangerous. I suddenly realized the severity of the situation. She had been drastically limiting her food intake, because of how easily she put on weight. To her, there seemed to be only two choices: either be fat or be thin and have several hypoglycemic blackouts a day. I decided to end my workout early, too, and see whether I could help my friend in any way.

I, too, had always been sick as a teenager and had spent more than thirty years reading almost every diet book written, while dedicating myself to a healthy lifestyle at a young age. Over the years, I had learned what worked for me, and in the process of learning, I had discovered that there is no such thing as one size fits all when it comes to dieting. Even though I was in my late thirties at this point, I was still in better shape than the twenty-year-old kids in the gym, and my friend looked up to me. I felt that if anyone could get through to her, it would be me.

I asked her a few questions to help her discover what types of foods her body preferred for fuel. Years of experience had taught me that her issues with gaining weight and her lack of energy to the point of blacking out were both probably a result of the same thing: eating the wrong foods for her particular physiology. After questioning her and listening, I suggested a very different diet plan for her. I told her that if my hunch was correct, she would be able to eat more food than ever before, while actually losing weight and feeling great.

She listened, but when she heard the foods I recommended, she insisted that they would all make her fat. I finally encouraged her to try it for one day, knowing that if I was right, she would be convinced within the first two meals. Three days later, I saw my friend at the gym and could hardly recognize the transformation that had taken place. This exhausted teenager had become a radiant young woman, and with the biggest smile you can imagine, she ran over to give me a hug and thank me.

She was quite excited and explained how she had not had

a single blackout since changing her diet and was actually eating more food than she had in a long time but was losing weight in the process. After a few months, she was down to her ideal weight, all without a single blackout, and she felt great. My experience in helping her and many others through the years was the motivation behind writing this book.

I realized that people had the willpower to reach their goals and the only thing they lacked were simple instructions on how to achieve these goals. What's different about this diet book is that it recognizes you as an individual, with your own very individual diet needs. By understanding your body, you'll be able to finally take control of the powerful hormonal effects that food may be having on you. Some hormones can make you hungry and fat, while others make you feel full and burn fat.

I wrote this book for you and everyone else who wants to be and feel their best. I have faith that if you follow my simple instructions, you will learn to take control of your health and will feel better than you have in a very long time. I hope you like my easy directions, have an enjoyable journey, and, mostly, have fun at the beach!

Before making any dietary or exercise regime changes, you are advised to consult with a physician and remain under his or her supervision during any dietary or weight-loss program. Nothing in the book is intended to constitute medical advice, and no warranties are made that any diet described in this book is going to be effective. No claims are made that anything written in this book is intended to treat, cure, or prevent a specific disease or to replace the advice of your physician. Please consult with your physician if you are taking any prescription medications before making changes to your diet or exercise regime.

I
About the Four Season-Types
Why some people need a high-fat, high-protein diet,
while others need a high-carb, low-fat diet

A friend of mine owns a diesel Volkswagen Bug. She chose the Bug because it gets 50 miles per gallon and can run on either diesel or bio-diesel. My gas-powered SUV can tow an 8,000-pound trailer, and as much as I would love to get 50 miles per gallon, poor gas mileage is one of the prices you pay for being able to tow a lot of weight with a large vehicle. Imagine how silly I would be to fill up my gas tank with diesel fuel, using the logic that because my friend uses diesel and gets 50 miles per gallon, my gas-powered SUV should get 50 miles per gallon if I just put diesel in the tank.

I would be lucky if my car ran more than a few miles on diesel before dying on the side of the road. My car needs the fuel it was designed to run on. Putting the wrong fuel in the gas tank is not going to fix my mileage issue; it's just going to make my car run very poorly and then stop.

When it comes to our bodies, putting the wrong fuel in our tanks causes us to run very poorly, but instead of stopping, we simply feel bad and gain weight. Putting diesel in a gas engine to get better mileage is exactly what we do every time we try to lose weight by eating the wrong combination of foods for our engines. In the coming chapters, I'll explain why different people function best by eating certain foods. Similar to the analogy of my friend's VW Bug that was designed to run on diesel and my SUV that runs on gas, humans have four basic types of "engines," each of which needs a different type of fuel mix to maintain both a healthy weight and high energy levels. I've given the four basic types of human engines the names Winter, Spring, Summer, and Autumn to make them easy to understand and remember. You are probably already familiar with the fuels of protein, carbohydrates, and fat. What differentiates the four season-types from one another is the proportion of these different fuels that's necessary for each person to run his or her best. When you are consuming the right mix of fuels for your season-type, your blood sugar remains stable, your appetite is kept in check, and your hormones are balanced, all of which cause you to maintain a healthy weight with minimal effort.

Fuels for the Four Season-Types

Chart 1.1 shows the fuels we know as protein, carbohydrates, and fat, along with the amount preferred by each of the different season-types. Each person has a maximum rate at which he or she can burn fat for fuel. Winters have the highest fat-burning rate and burn more than three times the amount of fat per minute as Summers, who have the lowest fat-burning rate. On the other hand, Summers, who cannot burn fat for fuel very quickly, have to rely on carbohydrates for their energy needs.

CHART 1.1 MACRONUTRIENT NEEDS OF THE FOUR SEASON-TYPES

Macronutrient	Winter	Autumn	Spring	Summer
Protein Needed	High	Med High	Med Low	Low
Carbohydrates Needed	Low	Med Low	Med High	High
Fat Needed	High	Medium	Med Low	Low
Purines Needed	High	Med High	Med Low	Low

Winters function best on foods we normally consume on a cold winter's day. Their ideal foods are high in protein and fat, lower in carbohydrates, and high in a type of protein called purines, which is found in foods such as red meat, salmon, beans, and lentils. Think of eating a bowl of hearty beef chili when it's freezing outside. Winters are usually the ones who will do well on a high-protein, high-fat, low-carbohydrate diet, such as the Atkins Diet or the Paleo Diet.

At the other end of the spectrum are the Summers. Summers function best on foods we normally consume on a warm summer day: lower in protein and fat, higher in carbohydrates, and lower in purines. Think of a light salad with fresh vegetables and maybe some rice with steamed white fish. Summers are usually the ones who will do well on a high-carbohydrate, low-protein, and low-fat diet, such as the Pritikin Diet, or a low-fat vegetarian diet.

Autumns are similar to Winters but need a little less protein and fat than Winters do and a little more carbohydrates. They still run best with generous amounts of protein and fat. Springs, on the other hand, are similar to Summers but need a little more protein and fat and a little less carbohydrates. They still run best with a fair amount of carbohydrates.

Remember what happens when you put diesel fuel in a gas engine? Oftentimes, a Winter will go on a low-fat, high-carbohydrate diet to lose weight, with disastrous results, or a Summer will try a low-carb diet and feel terrible within a matter of days. The reason many diets work for some people and not for others is that sometimes people get lucky, and the diet they try just happens to have the right mix of nutrients for their season-type.

The key to effortless dieting is figuring out what type of engine you have, feeding your engine the proper fuels, and fine-tuning your mix of fuels based on your lifestyle. The most important lifestyle factors are the types of exercise you engage in and the climate you live in.

There are two basic types of engines that power our bodies, which are nearly polar opposites. I call people with these two engines either Winters or Summers, which are the two very extreme season-types. The Autumns and the Springs are simply a mix of the two engines, with Autumns being closer to Winters, and Springs being more like Summers.

White Meat vs. Dark Meat

Most of you have probably sat down to a Thanksgiving dinner and made a choice between the white meat of the turkey breast or the dark meat of the turkey's thigh. Your instinctive preference is a good clue to your season-type.

Understanding the reason for, and the difference between, white turkey meat and dark turkey meat is the key to understanding the differences between the four season-types. The analogy I am about to use is very simple, and in actuality, the way the human body produces energy is far more complex. I will elaborate on many of the complex differences later. When writing this book, however, I made the decision to keep things easy for the average reader to understand. In the interest of making it simple, I chose to take certain liberties, which may be readily apparent to people with a degree in physiology or biophysics. For example, even stating that gas engines burn gasoline is not technically correct. Technically, gasoline engines burn gasoline that has been pre-mixed with air, compressed in a cylinder, and then ignited. To drive a car, you are required to know the rules of the road and what type of fuel to put in your car at the gas station. If you want a book on advanced engine mechanics, this is not the book for you.

This book is written for people who want to get to their

ideal weight and feel fantastic, without having to learn a lot of complicated physiological terms and scientific principles. Where appropriate, I'll use the correct scientific terminology in bold type when new concepts are first introduced, along with an easier-to-remember descriptor in parentheses that will be underlined. After that, in consideration of the average reader, only the easy-to-remember descriptor will be used. In the back of this book, you will find a reverse glossary of the descriptors with their corresponding correct scientific terms, if you wish to be more technical in your understanding.

All about Your Muscles

Just as my friend's diesel Bug was designed to get 50 miles per gallon and has very little power as a result, while my SUV was designed to tow 8,000 pounds and gets really bad mileage, the difference between the white meat and the dark meat is similar.

Fat-Burning and Sugar-Burning Muscles
Turkeys spend most of their days walking around, foraging for food, and their leg muscles are adapted for great endurance, with little need for speed or power. These muscles are composed of **slow twitch muscle fibers** (fat-burning muscles), which predominately use fat to produce energy. Fat-burning muscles are very similar to the diesel engine of the VW Bug. They are efficient at producing energy but do not have a lot of power or speed. This dark meat is higher in fat, because it stores fat in the muscle fiber, since that is the fuel it prefers for producing energy. Fat-burning muscles need oxygen in order to produce energy, and the dark color is due to the presence of a protein called *myoglobin*, which contains iron and binds to oxygen, thereby giving the muscles the ready supply of oxygen they need.

Turkeys do not fly long distances but use their wings for short, quick bursts of flight, necessary to avoid predators. The wing muscles are composed of **fast twitch muscle fibers** (sugar-burning muscles), which, to get their energy, use predominately **glucose** (sugar) from carbohydrates stored in both the muscle and the liver. This glucose is called **glycogen** (note that **muscle glycogen** will be called muscle sugar, **liver glycogen** will be called liver sugar, and if talking about both, I will use the term stored sugar). Sugar-burning muscles are very similar to the big gas engine of my SUV. They can produce a lot of power, are big but not as efficient, and do not have the endurance of the fat-burning muscles. They can produce energy both with and without the need for oxygen and therefore do not need the large amounts of iron containing myoglobin, which gives dark meat its color.

Chart 1.2 highlights the basic characteristics of a turkey's fat-burning muscles vs. sugar-burning muscles.

CHART 1.2 DIFFERENCES BETWEEN FAT-BURNING MUSCLES AND SUGAR-BURNING MUSCLES

	Dark Meat (Fat-Burning Muscles)	Light Meat (Sugar-Burning Muscles)
Fuel Source	Fat	Sugar
Muscle Type	Slow Twitch	Fast Twitch
Oxygen Use	High	Low
Size	Small	Large
Speed	Slow	Fast
Endurance	High	Low

Why the Four Season-Types Excel at Different Sports

In reality, human muscles are not as clearly defined as those of the turkey. Humans have four different types of muscle fibers, one type that is like the dark meat of the turkey's fat-burning muscles, one that is like the light meat of the turkey's sugar-burning muscles, and two that are in between those two types of muscles. Furthermore, our muscle groups, such as our legs or shoulders, tend to be combinations of the various types of muscle fibers, and some people tend to have more of one type of fiber than of others. For example some people may have bodies composed predominately of fat-burning muscles, with a small amount of sugar-burning muscles, while other people's bodies consist mainly of sugar-burning muscles, with fewer fat-burning muscles. Most people have a more balanced combination of the two, allowing them to engage in a variety of activities as needed.

When you go on a long walk, you engage your fat-burning muscles, while giving your sugar-burning muscles a rest. When you run at full speed or lift something extremely heavy, you engage your sugar-burning muscles, while your fat-burning muscles often assist. Winters tend to have a very large proportion of fat-burning muscles, making them naturally gifted at endurance events, such as running long distances, while Summers tend to have a greater proportion of sugar-burning muscles, making them especially good at events that require strength and speed, such as sprinting.

Autumns and Springs have a more balanced combination of the two types of muscles, giving them an advantage in sports such as soccer, which requires the ability to run for long periods of time, while occasionally generating a great burst of speed.

Because Winters have more fat-burning muscles, it would make sense that they need more fat in their diet, since this is their primary fuel source. They also need more protein, because Winters often experience low blood sugar, which is helped by eating more protein. Summers, on the other hand, have more sugar-burning muscles, and it makes sense that they need more carbohydrates in their diet, because these get broken down and turned into stored sugar in their muscles and liver that can quickly be used for energy when needed. Summers should limit their consumption of protein, because that will assist them in burning more sugar for energy.

Autumns and Springs have a more balanced mix of the four types of muscles, so they need a more balanced diet in order to properly feed all of their muscles. One very important point worth mentioning is that these general rules do not apply for people engaged in highly competitive extreme endurance events. For example, a Winter who ran at or near his maximum capacity on a regular basis would need a vastly different diet from a Winter who was more sedentary or who engaged in moderate workouts. This will be covered in depth in the section on exercise nutrition.

We humans also derive our fat and sugar fuels from various different sources inside our bodies, depending on our activity level. For example, sugar and fat are present in the blood as **blood glucose** (blood sugar) and **free fatty acids** (blood fat). Fat is also stored inside the muscles as **intramuscular triglycerides** (muscle fat) and stored outside the muscles as **adipose tissue** (body fat). Sugar can be used from either blood sugar, stored muscle sugar, or stored liver sugar. Protein can also be converted to sugar and in some cases is used directly, without having to be converted to sugar, for very small amounts of energy. Although up to 50 to 80 percent of protein can be converted to blood sugar, the amount of protein used directly as a fuel without being converted to sugar is so small that I will not be discussing it in this book. The type of fuel used to produce energy depends on the predominant type of muscle a person has (sugar-burning vs. fat-burning) and the person's activity level, along with many other factors that I will discuss.

For all of the season-types, their muscles will be used in the order of slowest to fastest. For example, all season-types who go on a slow walk will engage their fat-burning muscles first. Because Summers have the lowest proportion of this type of muscle, they will be the first season-type to engage their mixed muscles of a high-endurance nature, as the level of intensity increases. Winters will be the last of the season-types to engage these muscles, based on level of intensity. During a moderate run, a Winter might use 90 percent fat-burning muscles, while a Summer running the same speed might use 90 percent sugar-burning muscles.

What Is Turbo Mode?

Chart 1.3 will give you a better understanding of the four main types of muscle fibers in humans. There is a third type of energy source used predominately by sugar-burning muscles, called **creatine-phosphate** (turbo mode), which is capable of providing extremely powerful and fast energy for very short periods, lasting only a matter of seconds. I call this type of energy "turbo mode," because it provides a quick boost of energy similar to a turbo-charger on an automobile.

CHART 1.3 CHARACTERISTICS OF THE FOUR TYPES OF MUSCLES

Type of Muscle Characteristics	Fat-Burning High Endurance	Mixed High Endurance	Mixed Fast/Strong	Sugar-Burning Fast/Strong
Primary Fuel Source	See Below	Mixed Muscles & Sugar-Burning Muscles Use Predominately Sugar for Energy. Sugars Come from Muscle Sugar, Liver Sugar, and Blood Sugar		
Low Intensity Fuel Source	Blood Fat & Body Fat			
Moderate Intensity Fuel Source	Muscle Fat			
High Intensity Fuel Source	Stored Sugar/Blood Sugar			
Ability to Store Muscle Fat	High	Moderate	Low	Low
Ability to Store Muscle Sugar*	Moderate	High	High	High
Ability to Use Muscle " Turbo Mode"	Low	High	High	High
Muscle Speed	Slow	Medium	Fast	Very Fast
Oxygen Use	Very High	High	Medium	Low
Muscle Size	Small	Medium	Large	Very Large
Muscle Endurance	Very High	High	Medium	Low
Sports	Endurance Running	Sprinting	Sprinting	See Below**
Recruitment Order	First	Second	Third	Fourth
Color	Red	Red to Pink	White	White

* Some sources cite that all muscle types store equal amounts of glycogen.
** Sports requiring ballistic movements, i.e., shot put, baseball swing, maximum bench press, etc.

Please do not feel overwhelmed or confused by these scientific details. If your main desire is to lose weight and be healthy, all you have to remember is that some muscles prefer to burn fat for energy, while other muscles prefer to burn sugar for energy, and most people have a mix of the two types of muscles, which correspond to the following chart:

CHART 1.4 MUSCLE COMPOSITION OF THE FOUR SEASON-TYPES

	Winter	Autumn	Spring	Summer
Fat-Burning Muscles	High	Med High	Med Low	Low
Sugar-Burning Muscles	Low	Med Low	Med High	High

The amount of fat-burning muscles vs. sugar-burning muscles in your body also tends to vary by muscle group. For example, the calf muscles of all season-types tend to have a higher proportion of fat-burning muscles than other parts of the body do, while for all of the season-types the triceps muscles, located on the backs of the upper arms, tend to have a higher density of sugar-burning muscles than other parts of the body do. The most important thing to remember is that Summers have the highest proportion of sugar-burning muscles, Winters have the highest proportion of fat-burning muscles, and Autumn and Springs have a mix of the two.

What's interesting is that even at rest, the different season-types use different proportions of fuel for energy, as measured by what is called the **respiratory quotient** (carbohydrate/fat fuel ratio). The carbohydrate/fat fuel ratio measures the percentage of fat and the percentage of carbohydrates that a person uses to produce energy. As you can see from Chart 1.5, a carbohydrate/fat fuel ratio of .7 means a person is burning 100 percent fat for energy, while a ratio of 1.0 means a person is burning 100 percent carbohydrates for energy. As the percentage of fat burned for energy decreases, the percentage of carbohydrates burned for energy increases.

This chart I created is based on the data from several studies that have looked at the resting respiratory exchange ratio (RER) of a small sample size of people. No studies have been conducted, to my knowledge, on the distribution of the RER of a large sample size of people, so my chart is intended to give you a general idea of the distribution of the RER among people, rather than exact distribution numbers, because no researcher has yet sought to determine this. This chart shows that a small percentage of people use fat for 80 to 100 percent of their energy at rest, and these people are Winters. The chart also shows that a small percentage of people burn sugar for 80 to 100 percent of their energy at rest, and these people are Summers. In the middle of these two groups are the Autumns and the Springs, who burn a more balanced mix of fat and carbohydrates at rest.

CHART 1.5 RESTING RESPIRATORY EXCHANGE RATIO (PERCENTAGE OF FAT BURNED AS FUEL AT REST)

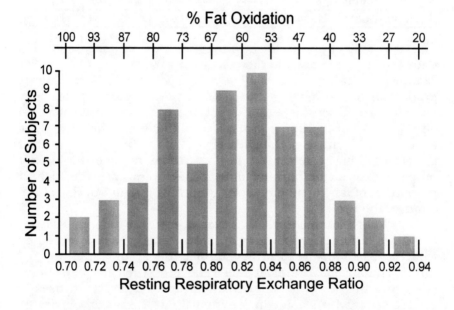

What tends to happen for all of the season-types is that the higher the level of intensity during any physical activity, the higher the proportion of sugar that is used for energy. This is because even though fat-burning muscles prefer to burn fat for energy, fat is very slow at producing energy. At higher intensity levels, fat-burning muscles are forced to switch to sugar for energy. As you can see in Chart 1.6, at lower intensity levels people tend to use more fat for energy, while at higher intensity levels people use more sugar for energy. The level of intensity is measured by "V02 max," which is the maximum amount of oxygen that an individual can use to produce energy.

CHART 1.6 EFFECT OF EXERCISE INTENSITY ON FUEL USED BY MUSCLES

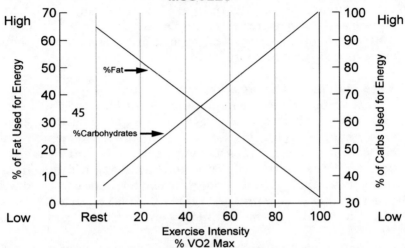

Chart 1.7 is an illustration of how all four season-types might produce energy, based on their activity level. As you can see in my simplified chart, Winters at rest are using predominantly fat for energy, while Summers are using mainly sugar for energy, with Autumns and Springs in the middle.

CHART 1.7 CARBOHYDRATE VS. FAT USE FOR ENERGY BY SEASON-TYPE AND EXERCISE INTENSITY LEVEL

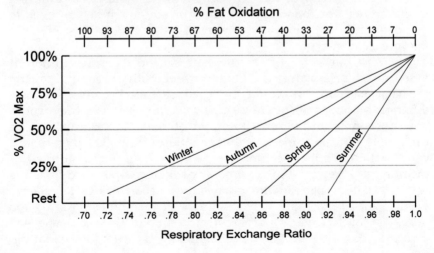

As the intensity levels rise to 50 percent of VO₂ max, Winters are
using approximately 50 percent fat and 50 percent sugar for energy,
while a Summer is using more than 90 percent sugar for energy.
Autumns and Springs are in the middle. When the intensity climbs
to 100 percent of VO₂ max, all of the season-types are using almost
100 percent sugar for energy.

How to Maintain Your Ideal Weight
This gets us to the key for maintaining your ideal weight without
effort, hunger, or loss of energy, while experiencing a general
overall feeling of well-being and mental clarity. Remember that
each season-type has a carbohydrate/fat fuel ratio that says
how much fat these types burn for energy, along with how many
carbohydrates they burn for energy, which includes carbohydrates
that are produced from ingested protein that is converted to sugar.
The key to effortlessly maintaining your weight is to make sure
that:

>*You eat fat, protein, and carbohydrates in proportion to the
amount of each that your body prefers to burn for fuel, and you eat
the right kinds of protein for your season-type.*

Eating the wrong fuel mix for your season-type, along with several
other factors you'll learn about shortly, is the cause of excessive
hunger, low energy levels, and weight gain. This is the fundamental
principle of the Four Seasons Diet. Later on, you'll learn some of
the "basic rules of the road" that will help you effortlessly control
your weight, along with some "urban myths" that may be preventing
this. Another way to look at the previous statement is: you need to
eat foods that help you burn energy in a way that is most efficient
for your season-type.

As Chart 1.7 shows, the four season-types use different
amounts of carbohydrates and fat for fuel, both at rest and during
physical exertion. It would make sense that because they use
different amounts of fuel at rest and during exercise, they would
have to consume different amounts of these macronutrients in
their diets. In the same way that the diesel Bug fills up on diesel,
people who burn more fat for energy need to fill up on more fat at
mealtimes. Likewise, in the same way that a gas-powered SUV fills
up on gasoline, people who burn more carbohydrates for energy
need to fill up on more carbohydrates at mealtimes. Eating too
much fat or too many carbohydrates for your season-type will
create a host of metabolic problems, which lead to overeating,

hunger, and low or erratic energy issues.

Studies conducted on elite runners show the great disparity between the four season-types when it comes to energy production. One study examined the differences in runners who had a high proportion of sugar-burning muscles (the Summer season-type), a high proportion of fat-burning muscles (the Winter season-type), and a mix of the two (the Autumn and Spring season-types). The study found that at rest, the people similar to those I call Summers burn nearly 70 percent carbohydrates for energy, while the people closest to those I call Winters burn nearly 80 percent fat for energy. In between were the people similar to those I call Autumns and Springs, who burned more of a mix of the two fuels. The researchers then had each group exercise at four different levels of intensity, with Level 1 being the least intense level and Level 4 being the most intense. Each level corresponded to a percentage of what is called VO_2 max, which is the maximum amount of oxygen that a person is able to transport and use for energy. Level 1 corresponded to a VO_2 max of 55 to 70 percent, and this is probably the level that most people who jog or run recreationally run at. The second level was a VO_2 max of 80 to 90 percent, the third level was 90 to 100 percent, and the fourth level was 100 percent.

At all four levels of intensity, Summers switched to burning 100 percent carbohydrates for energy. In contrast, the Winters slowly started burning more and more carbohydrates and less fat at each level of intensity. Remember that at rest, Winters were burning around 80 percent fat for energy. At the first level of intensity, Winters started to burn about 50 percent fat and 50 percent carbohydrates for energy. At the second level of intensity, they were burning about 80 percent carbohydrates for energy, and at the two highest levels of intensity, Winters were burning 100 percent carbohydrates for energy.

The Autumns and the Springs were in between the two extremes of the Summers and Winters, burning more fat than Summers and less than Winters. This is the reason low-fat diets work for some people, while low-carb diets work for others, and a balanced diet similar to the Zone Diet works for those in between. A person with mainly sugar-burning muscles will thrive on a low-fat diet, while someone with mainly fat-burning muscles will have more success on a low-carb diet, and those in between will do best on a diet that is a mix between the two. Multiple studies show that the less fat a person naturally burns for energy, the fatter he or she will tend to be later in life. This is because much of the excess fat we eat is stored for later use, and a season-type such as a Summer, who burns very little fat for energy, is always storing away fat but never really burning it off. At the opposite end of the spectrum are the Winters, who burn plenty of fat for energy but tend to overeat by consuming too many carbohydrates, which is usually the cause of their weight problem, if they have one.

Physical Characteristics of the Season-Types

You may have already guessed that the different season-types tend to have different physical characteristics, based on their proportion of fat-burning muscles vs. sugar-burning muscles. The fat-burning muscles are smaller than the sugar-burning muscles and store more fat inside the muscle fiber for use as energy. Sugar-burning muscles, on the other hand, are larger and carry more stored-sugar for energy and far less fat. Because Winters rely on fat for energy, they tend to carry more muscle fat than Summers do. Even a lean and athletic Winter, however, will look much more streamlined and have less bulky muscle mass than a lean and athletic Summer.

If you think of an elite distance runner (Winter) and an Olympic sprinter (Summer), you'll get a good mental picture of some of the differences between a Winter, who might excel at distance running, and a Summer, who might be superior at sprinting. The average elite distance runner has between 75 and 90 percent fat-burning muscles, while the average elite sprinter has between 75 and 90 percent sugar-burning muscles. Other factors besides your predominant muscle type affect your athletic performance as well, such as the size of your frame, the amount of body fat you tend to carry, your mitochondrial efficiency, and the number of enzymes in your muscles that burn fat or sugar. For example, most elite distance runners have very small muscles and frames, making them extremely efficient in their energy use. This is not to say that all Winters have small frames and muscles, but rather is an illustration of a smaller-framed Winter. Even though the distance runner may be smaller and lean, his or her muscles are usually not well defined. This is because of the large amount of fat the person tends to store inside his or her muscles for energy.

Contrast this with an elite sprinter. Sprinters tend to have larger shoulders and legs, which are very well defined because they do not store much fat in their muscles for energy. You can practically see every muscle fiber, and their tendons and ligaments are often very visible as well. Elite sprinters are usually Summers and Springs, while elite endurance athletes tend to be Winters and Autumns. This is not to say that a Summer cannot run a marathon. Summers can adapt their muscles to run long distances, but they will have to work much harder than a Winter does and will probably never win a major race. A Winter, on the other hand, will probably never put on a lot of lean and "ripped" muscle mass or have an impressive time in the 100-meter sprint. Oftentimes, large-framed Winters can get quite strong, but on a pound-for-pound of body weight basis are usually not as strong as a Summer or a Spring. Elite cyclists and swimmers usually have a balanced mix of 50 percent of each type of muscle, so these athletes will tend to be Autumns and Springs.

Our blood contains a modest amount of blood sugar and blood fat, which are used to power our muscles and brains when there is little need for energy. As our need for energy increases, our bodies begin to use the sugar and the fat stored within our muscles. In addition, we store fat outside our muscles, in body fat that is used throughout the day to keep our blood-fat levels stable and is used as energy for fat-burning muscles when there is a low demand for energy. The *adipose gene* regulates how much body fat we tend to carry in our adipose tissue.

How Genetics Determines Your Season-Type
Because humans evolved in different regions, with different climates and elevations, there are some profound variations in distinct groups of populations. For example, one factor that caused humans to slowly evolve more fat-burning muscles over many generations is living at higher elevations.

Your season-type is largely determined by your genes at birth, which is strongly influenced by where your ancestors originated. The starkest example of this contrast on the planet is between black West Africans and black East Africans. West Africa has a low average elevation, while many East African countries have a very high average elevation, and both distinct groups have adapted over thousands of years to their unique environments. Black people from West African countries tend to have a high proportion of sugar-burning muscles, and people from those counties often excel at sprinting events. In fact, 95 percent of the top records in sprinting events are held by people who can trace their ancestry back to West Africa. Black people from East African countries tend to have a high proportion of fat-burning muscles, and people from those countries frequently excel at distance-running events. Runners from Kenya, Tanzania, and Ethiopia win most long distance events at the elite races. Runners from one section of Kenya that consists of only a half-million people win about 40 percent of major international distance races, which shows the importance of genetics in determining how you produce energy and hence what types of exercise and sports you will excel at.

White people of Eurasian ancestry tend to have a mix of muscles between the two extremes of the West Africans' and the East Africans'. The harsh cold environment of their ancestors caused them to evolve larger, more muscular upper bodies, with relatively shorter arms and legs and thicker torsos, giving them on average more upper-body strength. It is not surprising that most events requiring upper-body strength, such as weight lifting and shot put, are dominated by people with Eurasian ancestry. In sports requiring sheer upper-body strength, such as the shot put, men of white Eurasian ancestry have won the gold, silver, and bronze medals in almost every Olympics held.

Asians tend to have a high proportion of fat-burning muscles and smaller frames and often excel at endurance sports, such as marathons and ultra-marathons. In fact, both the men's and the women's official IAAF world records for the 100 km (62 mile) ultra marathon are held by runners from Japan.

Although many of these statements may be considered controversial, they are based on observable data. Human beings come in all shapes and sizes, and no one type is superior to another, only different. It's far healthier to embrace the concept that one size does not fit all, and that perhaps the diet that's best for you has been to a large part determined by your ancestry. Later on, I will discuss how some season-types are more susceptible to imbalances that cause certain diseases than other season-types are, which is the reason that some diseases are far more prevalent in those season-types. The purpose of this book is to increase your understanding of your own uniqueness and help you find what works best for you. This is the reason I feel compelled to mention the role our ancestry plays in determining our season-type.

2
The Energy, Food, Hormone Connection

How the foods you eat affect the fuels your body stores and burns for energy.

Money allows us to buy goods and services in a convenient manner because it is accepted by everyone as a universal currency in exchange for items we need or want. Without a universal currency, we would be forced to barter for the things we need, and life as we know it could not continue. Imagine raising chickens for eggs and being forced to carry cartons of eggs around with you to spend as currency, rather than a small wallet full of paper money or, easier yet, a debit card that can hold thousands of dollars of universally accepted currency. It is much easier to carry a small plastic debit card in your wallet than a thousand cartons of eggs of the same value, and every merchant accepts dollars.

How Muscles Recharge Their Energy

In much the same way, our bodies convert the fuels of carbohydrates, fat, and protein into a universal energy currency that is accepted by every cell in the body and is used to carry out a multitude of metabolic functions. This energy currency consists of **two molecules of phosphate** (energy currency) joined together in a chemical bond, which releases a lot of energy when broken. This energy currency is carried in a molecule called **adenosine triphosphate** (energy debit cards), which is often called ATP for short. These energy debit cards are located throughout the body. When a cell in the body needs energy, it uses the energy currency contained in the energy debit cards, and then the card is recharged by putting more energy currency into it.

This is an extremely efficient process, which allows us to spend a lot of energy currency without having to carry it in our bodies. The human body contains about only 3 to 4 ounces of energy debit cards but recharges them at an extremely quick rate,

20

if necessary, while recycling as many of the waste products as possible into more energy currency. If our bodies were not able to recharge our energy debit cards by recycling the waste by-products of energy production, but instead were able to spend the cards only once, we would have to carry around more than 400 pounds of energy debit cards to get us through one day! Instead of carrying around an extra 400 pounds, the body simply combines the recycled waste products from energy production with about 2,500 calories' worth of food to recharge what is spent. Although this system is very efficient, it requires us to replenish our energy debit cards very quickly when we spend our currency.

Turbo Mode (Stored Muscle Energy)
The energy currency carried in our 8 ounces' worth of energy debit cards is enough to keep us moving along for about 6 seconds. Luckily for us, our bodies are able to quickly replenish our energy debit cards with more energy currency; however, the fuel we use to replenish this currency is very dependent on the type of activity we are engaged in. You probably remember that fat-burning muscles prefer to use fat for fuel during low to moderate exertion and prefer to use sugar for fuel during high exertion. When our bodies use fat or sugar for energy, it is less like burning gas in a car engine and more like replenishing a debit card with more money. Fuels such as fat and carbohydrates undergo a series of chemical reactions inside the body and are converted to the universally accepted energy currency.

The fuels that our bodies use to replenish our energy debit cards depend largely on how much energy currency we spend and how quickly we spend it, which are primarily determined by the type of activity we are engaging in, along with the predominant kind of muscle in our particular season-type. This is the reason different kinds of muscle prefer different types of fuel. The various fuels that the body converts to energy currency have different advantages and disadvantages to their use, and our bodies know how to pick the most advantageous mix of fuels for us in each moment.

Chart 2.1 highlights the various ways in which our muscles recharge their energy currency, depending on the type of muscle and the activity it is engaging in.

CHART 2.1
METHODS OF RECHARGING ENERGY DEBIT CARDS WITH ENERGY

	Method of Recharging Energy Currency			
	Turbo Mode	Fast Sugar Energy	Slow Sugar Energy	Fat
Maximum Duration of Energy Use	10-20 Seconds	30-60 Seconds	Hours	Weeks
Rate of Energy Currency Replenishment	100 *	55	23	10
Requires Oxygen	No	No	Yes	Yes
Limiting Factor Other Than Enzymes Needed	Amount Stored in Muscle	Acidic Wastes Produced by Body	Amount of Oxygen Available to Muscles	Fat Transport into Muscles
% Total Potential Energy Available In Body	0.02%	0.16%	2%	98%
Muscle Enzymes Needed Prominent in	Summers, Springs	Summers, Springs	Winters, Autumns	Winters, Autumns

*I.e., creatine phosphate, since creatine phosphate, produces energy the fastest. I give that a score of 100 and base the other scores on that.

Because our energy debit cards have enough energy currency stored in them for only about 4 to 6 seconds of use, the instant we start spending currency, our bodies get busy finding ways to replenish their energy debit cards. In addition, when we first go from rest to the start of a new activity, our bodies will use their turbo mode of energy production to help get the body going. The muscles usually store enough turbo mode fuel to replenish our energy currency for about 10 to 20 seconds. The biggest advantages to using this fuel to replenish our energy debit cards is that it's extremely fast at replacing large amounts of energy and does not require oxygen. This type of fuel is able to replenish energy at twice the rate of the next-fastest fuel. When you sprint 100 meters or lift a very heavy weight for six to ten repetitions, you are using this fuel as your predominant way to recharge your energy debit cards. Although this is the fastest way to replenish your energy debit cards, there is not very much of this turbo-mode fuel stored in your body. This is one of the many reasons you can lift a heavy weight only a limited number of times or sprint all-out for just a short duration.

Fast Sugar Energy
The next-fastest fuel for recharging our energy debit cards is from sugar that's burned for energy without using oxygen, in a process called **anaerobic glycolysis** (fast sugar energy). Fast sugar energy produces energy currency twice as fast as sugar that's burned for energy along with the use of oxygen in a process called **aerobic glycolysis** (slow sugar energy). The main drawback to fast sugar energy production is that it causes the cells to become overly acidic, which ultimately shuts down energy production until the cells' pH

can be restored. This condition is often incorrectly referred to as *lactic acidosis*; however, the acidosis is not caused by the lactate, but rather occurs alongside the increase in lactate production.

As the cells begin to get more acidic, the body loses the ability to produce energy currency in this manner. Usually, after 30 to 60 seconds of all-out exercise, the cells become so overloaded with acid that it becomes critical to remove it. Oxygen is required to remove the acid from our cells, and until we are able to do so, our ability to produce energy is greatly reduced. This is the reason why after you run at full speed for 30 to 60 seconds, you are left gasping for air and unable to move. Your body shuts down its ability to produce more energy currency and focuses all of its oxygen on removing the potentially toxic concentration of acid from inside your cells.

Slow Sugar Energy

The third-fastest way to produce energy is by using slow sugar energy, which, as I mentioned, uses both sugar and oxygen. Although this method is more than 50 percent slower than fast sugar energy at producing energy currency, it is able to produce almost twenty times as much energy currency per molecule of sugar that fast sugar energy can. The main limiting factor to producing energy this way is the availability of oxygen. Elite marathon runners running all-out will use this type of energy for their first twenty miles or so, and the expression "hitting the wall" refers to what happens when the body has been depleted of its stored sugar and begins to rely on other fuels for energy currency. As I explained in the last chapter, even though fat-burning muscles prefer to burn fat for energy, they can also burn sugar. Because slow sugar energy will recharge our energy debit cards twice as fast as fat energy will, fat-burning muscles will switch to recharging their debit cards in this manner when engaging in intense exercise. Because fat-burning muscles have the greatest ability to maintain a high level of oxygen, Winters and Autumns are most capable of producing energy using both slow sugar energy and fat energy.

The human lungs and heart can supply only so much oxygen to the body, and in well-conditioned athletes, this usually amounts to enough oxygen to power approximately 22 pounds of muscles at high-intensity levels using slow sugar energy. This is one reason elite distance runners usually have small frames and muscles. The human body simply cannot produce slow sugar energy without oxygen, and large muscles are more of a detriment than an asset in these sports, because they consume more oxygen and add more body weight that has to be moved, which also requires more oxygen.

Fat Energy Production

The last type of fuel we use to produce energy is fat, and this always requires the use of oxygen. This method is extremely slow at producing energy currency; however, our bodies have almost unlimited reserves of fat to use, when compared to stored sugar and the turbo mode. In fact, if we were to stop eating, 98 percent of the energy currency we could produce would be using this method, with slow sugar energy accounting for approximately 2 percent, and fast sugar energy and the turbo mode accounting for less than one-fifth of 1 percent.

In order to use carbohydrates or fat to replenish our energy debit cards, our bodies need to use certain enzymes that are stored inside our muscles, similar to the way you have to know your PIN code to access the currency in your bank account with your debit card. Different enzymes are needed, depending on the fuel being used, as well as on whether oxygen is being used. If you recall from the last chapter, there are four different types of muscle fibers, each with its own unique characteristics. In addition to the characteristics mentioned in that chapter, the different types of muscle fibers also carry different amounts of these various enzymes. Winters and Autumns tend to have more of the enzymes needed for producing energy currency using slow sugar energy and fat energy, while Summers and Springs tend to have more of the enzymes needed to produce energy currency using the turbo mode and fast sugar energy. Your muscles will adapt to the type of training you engage in by producing more of the type of enzymes needed; however, you cannot change your muscle fiber type, and each muscle fiber type has the ability to increase its enzymes the most for the type of activity it excels at. For example, fat-burning muscles have a greater ability to increase their concentration of the enzymes needed for fat energy and slow sugar energy, while sugar-burning muscles have a greater ability to increase their concentration of enzymes needed for fast sugar energy.

Increasing the amount of these muscle enzymes is, to a large extent, what we accomplish by engaging in different types of specialized exercise training. Contrary to popular belief, the main effect of doing traditional cardio training is not to make the heart somehow stronger or more efficient at pumping blood. The main effect of doing traditional cardio training is that the muscles respond by producing a greater concentration of the enzymes needed to replenish your energy debit cards using oxygen. Vigorous aerobic training can double the amount of these various muscle enzymes. For example, if you engage in endurance running, you can double the number of enzymes used to produce energy currency using slow sugar-energy production or fat-energy production. If, on the other hand, you engage in heavy resistance training, you will increase the number of enzymes needed for fast sugar-energy production.

Any exercise usually involves all of the methods of energy production, starting predominately with the slowest ones and moving up to the faster ones, as necessary. For example, when we walk slowly, we are primarily using fat for energy, even though we may engage the other energy systems to a small extent. As we pick up the pace to a moderate jog, we may not be able to replenish our energy debit cards quickly enough by using fat, and our slow sugar-energy system kicks in, because it is able to produce energy twice as fast as fat can. Since Winters and Autumns are far superior to Summers and Springs at producing fat energy, they will be able jog at a much faster pace before having to switch over to the slow sugar-energy system. As you pick up the pace even faster, you begin to use predominantly the fast sugar-energy system. When you reach full speed, you will have to kick into turbo mode, which is the fastest method of replenishing your energy debit cards. Because Summers and Springs have more of the muscles and the enzymes that are able to replenish energy currency in this manner, they will usually be able to run faster than Winters and Autumns can.

The opposite is also true but works a little differently. Imagine lifting a heavy weight that you can lift for only a few repetitions. All of your muscle fibers are working their hardest, using all of the different types of energy production. The weight is so heavy that your turbo mode gives out in a matter of seconds, and at this point, you have several choices, given that you still have the ability to produce energy using the other three methods. You can grab a very light weight and lift it for a lot of repetitions, using your slow sugar-energy mode and your fat-energy mode. If you choose to pick up an intermediate weight instead, which uses your fast sugar energy, you can lift that for a few more repetitions; however, once you do your maximum number, you will have to rest before being able to lift a lighter weight. This is because in choosing to engage the fast sugar-energy mode to your maximum ability, you have managed to saturate your cells with acid, and when your cells reach maximum saturation, you will have to use much of your oxygen to remove the acid from your cells and will therefore be unable to engage in an activity that requires slow sugar energy or fat energy, because both of these modes require oxygen.

Food and Hormones

Whether we are exercising or resting, our bodies must maintain a stable level of blood sugar in order to keep our brains and vital organs supplied with fuel. This process is carried out with the help of two hormones that are produced by the pancreas and have almost opposite actions. These two hormones are called *insulin* and *glucagon*. When our blood sugar is high, usually as a result of eating foods that contain carbohydrates and sugar, our bodies respond by producing insulin, which brings our blood-sugar levels back down to normal by storing away the excess sugar. When our blood-sugar levels get low, or we eat a high-protein meal, our bodies respond by producing glucagon, which raises our blood sugar and converts protein into sugar. Chart 2.2 will highlight some of the main actions of insulin and glucagon.

CHART 2.2 EFFECTS OF INSULIN AND GLUCAGON

	Insulin	Glucagon
Blood Sugar	Lowers High Blood Sugar	Raises Low Blood Sugar
Secreted in Response to	High Blood Sugar, Ingestion of Carbs or Protein	Low Blood Sugar, Ingestion of Protein
Storage of Nutrients	Shifts Metabolism into Storage Mode	Causes Release of Stored Nutrients
Effect on Stored Sugar	Encourages Storage of Excess Sugar in the Liver and Muscles	Encourages Release of Stored Sugar from Liver and Muscles
Effect on Stored Fat	Converts Some Sugar, Protein, and Blood Fat into Stored Fat	Converts Stored Fat into Blood Fat and Blood Sugar
Effect on Blood Sugar Energy	Increases Sugar Energy from Excess Blood Sugar	Decreases Sugar Energy from Blood Sugar
Effect on Stored Sugar Energy Production	Decreases	Increases
Effect on Fat Energy Production	Decreases	Increases
Effect on Conversion of Protein to Sugar	Decreases	Increases
Cholesterol	Increases Body's Production of Cholesterol	Decreases Body's Production of Cholesterol
Misc.	Decreases Secretion of Sodium, which Causes Kidneys to Retain Excess Fluids and Increases Blood Pressure	Causes Kidneys to Release Excess Fluid

What Happens When . . .

We Eat a High-Carb, Low-Protein Meal?

When we eat a meal of mainly carbohydrates and sugar, blood-sugar levels rise, and the body responds by producing a large amount of insulin to bring blood-sugar levels back to normal. Insulin shifts the body into storage mode, and most of the excess sugar is stored in the muscles and the liver as stored sugar. If there is a large amount of excess sugar or if stored-sugar levels are already full, the body goes into what is called *thermogenesis* and burns off a lot of the excess sugar as body heat. A small amount of the excess sugar is stored as body fat, depending on a person's season-type and other factors. When blood-sugar levels are high, and the body produces insulin, the body will also stop burning fat for energy. It will instead take some of the excess sugar and switch the body to using slow sugar energy and fast sugar energy as its main forms of energy production. For a Summer and a Spring, this would be an overall very beneficial experience. The excess sugar is converted to stored sugar, which is the preferred fuel source of Summers and Springs, and while this is happening, their bodies are forced to burn sugar as energy, which is their preferred source of energy anyway.

Eating a high-carbohydrate and low-protein meal has quite the opposite effect on Winters and Autumns. The high blood-sugar levels create an insulin response, which takes the Winter and the Autumn out of fat-burning mode and forces them to burn sugar as energy, which is not their preferred fuel source. The other major problem for Winters and Autumns, but especially for Winters, is their tendency to get hypoglycemia (low blood sugar) when eating excessive amounts of carbohydrates, due to how overly sensitive fat-burning muscles are to insulin, when compared with sugar-burning muscles. This is partly due to the fact that fat-burning muscles have a greater blood supply going to them than sugar-burning muscles do, so both insulin and sugar have an easier time getting into fat-burning muscles. This state of super-low blood sugar typically creates severe cravings for more sugar, and the typical response is to eat more sugar, thereby repeating the process. What Winters and Autumns really need is a way to keep their bodies in fat-burning mode, while they keep their blood sugar stable. This is accomplished by eating protein.

We Eat a Meal of Mostly Protein?

Protein eaten by itself will cause the body to secrete both glucagon and insulin. When very low amounts of carbohydrates are eaten, the body will turn roughly half of the protein eaten into sugar to help keep the body fueled. When protein is converted to sugar by the body, the effect on spiking blood sugar is much less than when carbohydrates are eaten, and much less of the sugar from protein gets stored as muscle sugar, both of which help keep the body in fat-burning mode. For Winters and Autumns, following a high-protein diet works quite well, because it keeps their bodies in fat-burning mode, which is their preferred source of energy production, and also keeps their blood-sugar levels stable by converting much of the excess protein to sugar in a way that does not upset the Winter and Autumn physiologies. The exceptions to this are Winters and Autumns who engage in super-intense endurance aerobic exercise, which burns predominantly sugar for energy. They will need to eat more carbohydrates, especially after engaging in exercise. When Winters burn more sugar for energy, they can eat more carbohydrates, because one of the keys to stable energy and blood sugar is eating the same mix of protein, carbohydrates, and fat as what your body burns.

Eating a meal consisting of only protein can be a disaster for Summers or Springs. It does not replenish their stored muscle sugar the same way that eating carbohydrates does, and as a result, they are not able to produce optimal amounts of energy. While fat-burning muscles can burn both fat and sugar for energy, sugar-burning muscles burn only sugar and rely on stored muscle sugar for much of their fuel source, especially during rigorous activity.

We Combine Protein with Carbs in a Meal?

For all of the season-types, combining protein with carbohydrates will actually produce higher levels of insulin than will eating a meal consisting only of carbohydrates. The higher the level of insulin, the more fat burning is shut down. The amount of insulin produced will be determined by the quantity of carbohydrates consumed, the glycemic index of that form of carbohydrate, and an individual's level of insulin sensitivity, along with many other factors. I will talk about glycemic index in a later chapter. If a small quantity of carbohydrates is eaten, only a little insulin will be secreted for a very short period of time, perhaps an hour or so. If a lot of carbohydrates are eaten, a large amount of insulin will be secreted, for a much longer period of time, perhaps lasting several hours.

Right now, I am simply explaining some of the basic effects

of ingesting varying amounts of protein and carbohydrates. Later, I'll give you more information and tie it together with how it all affects the four season-types. For now, the most important things to remember are that even though a large proportion of ingested protein can be converted to blood sugar, eating carbohydrates will raise blood-sugar levels to much higher levels than will eating the same number of calories from protein. There is a direct relationship between the blood-sugar level and the amount of fat a person burns for energy. When blood-sugar levels are high, the body burns less fat for energy, and when blood-sugar levels are lower, the body burns more fat for energy. This is one of many relationships between the foods we eat and the way we produce energy; however, it is an important relationship to keep in mind when choosing what foods you eat.

Keeping the body in sugar-burning mode is great for Summers because they have mainly sugar-burning muscles. Following a diet that is high in carbohydrates and lower in protein and fat will also refuel their bodies in the same way that they burn energy, which is the key to easily maintaining a stable weight. The large amount of carbohydrates will be converted to stored sugar for later use and will also be burned for sugar energy while blood-sugar levels are high. When the blood sugar drops, the body will produce glucagon, but in the absence of high amounts of protein, the glucagon will have the effect of converting stored sugar back into blood sugar, which is used by the body's muscles and organs. Summers will also burn body fat if they are resting or engaging in very moderate activity, but because they do not have the ability to produce much fat energy, they do not need very much fat in their diet. The Summers' high-carb, low-fat diet will replenish their stored sugar, and when they produce glucagon, they will either burn fat under a very low energy demand or will convert stored sugar back into blood sugar under a moderate-to-high energy demand, which is exactly what their bodies prefer. Summers still need a small amount of fat and protein, because they do have some fat-burning muscles, but the proportion of fat-burning muscles is less than in the other season-types. Springs have more fat-burning muscles than Summers do, and they will need a little more protein and fat in their diets to replenish what they use and also to keep their bodies slightly in fat-burning mode.

At the other end of the spectrum are Winters, who have mainly fat-burning muscles. Unless they are engaging in high-intensity endurance exercise, Winters are burning mainly fat for energy. If they are trying to lose weight, a high-protein, low-carb, moderate-fat diet is ideal, because it keeps their blood-sugar levels lower, which puts their bodies in the fat-burning mode for a much greater part of the day. It will also help prevent them from experiencing the low blood-sugar problems they often suffer from when eating high-carbohydrate meals. Once their ideal body weight is reached, Winters need to add significantly more fat to their diets. This, combined with high levels of protein and lower levels of carbohydrates, will keep their bodies in fat-burning mode most of the day. Eating a meal that is high in carbohydrates and high in protein will actually cause a greater release of insulin than will a diet with the same amount of carbohydrates and lower protein, which is the reason Winters need to moderate their carbohydrate intake in order to control their insulin response.

Winters need a high-protein diet and also a lower-insulin diet, and the best way to accomplish this is by keeping carbohydrate intake low and making sure it is the right type of carbohydrates for Winters. Insulin will turn off the body's ability to produce an enzyme called hormone-sensitive lipase, which is needed to burn body fat, and Winters rely on fat for much of their energy. They still have some need for carbohydrates to help fuel their brains and what sugar-burning muscles they do have; they simply need much smaller quantities of carbs than the other season-types do. By eating fewer carbohydrates, they prevent their blood-sugar levels from getting too high, which helps keep them in fat-burning mode. This will give them a steady supply of energy from fat, as well as an even supply of sugar to help fuel their brains. The excess protein will also be converted to blood sugar in a way that is beneficial to Winters, because it does not make their blood-sugar levels spike. This diet will replenish their muscle fat and keep them in fat-burning mode during the day in most situations, which is exactly what their bodies prefer. Autumns have more sugar-burning muscles than Winters do, so they need to eat more carbohydrates to replenish the stored sugar they burn. They just need to make sure they do not eat excessive amounts of carbohydrates.

Balancing Your Blood-Sugar and Insulin Levels
Your blood-sugar levels and insulin levels play the two dominant roles in this process, because high levels of either one will put you in sugar-burning mode and will prevent you from going into fat-burning mode. The composition of your meals plays the main role in how you store and produce energy. Remember, the key to

effortlessly maintaining your weight while having high energy is to eat foods with the same levels of protein, carbohydrates, and fat that your body prefers to use for fuel.

By understanding your season-type, you can begin to eat in a way that is most beneficial for you. The Four Seasons Diet will allow you store away the nutrients you use for maximum energy when there is a surplus, while secreting hormones that let you draw on those energy reserves between meals in a way that also produces maximum energy for you. When you eat according to your season-type, you keep your energy high, eliminate hunger between meals, remain emotionally balanced, and maintain high mental clarity throughout the day.

Now that you understand the basic principles behind the Four Seasons Diet, it's time to examine some of the "urban myths" and the "rules of the road" when it comes to food and dieting.

Urban Myths

Myth #1: Carbohydrates cause us to release large amounts of insulin, while protein causes us to release glucagon but not insulin.

This is one of the biggest dietary myths out there right now, especially among those who advocate a low-carbohydrate diet. The truth is that both carbohydrates and protein cause the body to secrete insulin. The amount of insulin secreted by a particular food is measured by the *insulin index*. Although a food's *glycemic index*, which measures the rate that sugars in a food enter the blood, is an important factor in a food's insulin index, the glycemic index accounts for only around 25 percent of the insulin response from a given food. The insulin index is also affected by many other factors, such as the protein and fat content of a particular food and the type of protein and the type of fat. For example, on a caloric basis, beef actually causes a higher insulin response than white pasta does, while yogurt causes a higher insulin response than white bread does, due to how quickly the proteins from fermented milk products are digested and enter into circulation.

Having high levels of insulin is only one of many factors that will get you into sugar-burning mode and out of fat burning mode. Once you understand some of the other influences besides insulin, you'll see how the Four Seasons Diet is designed to take advantage of these in a way that works best for each season-type. Another important factor that affects insulin levels, which I'll talk about later, is "insulin resistance." When people are insulin resistant, their bodies produce extremely large amounts of insulin in response to a given food. The Four Seasons Diet is designed to keep a person from becoming insulin resistant.

Myth #2: Protein causes the body to secrete glucagon, which puts the body into fat-burning mode.
This is another myth among those who advocate a low-carbohydrate diet. The first part of the statement is true, which is that eating a high-protein meal does cause the body to produce large amounts of glucagon. It's the second part of the statement that is in error. If you look at most physiology books, they specifically state that glucagon causes the body to go into what is called *lipolysis*, which is when stored fats in the body are broken down and turned into blood fats that the body can convert into energy. Although glucagon by itself can cause the conversion of stored fat into blood fat, insulin inhibits this process. In fact, the ability of insulin to inhibit this process is far stronger than glucagon's ability to initiate it. In order for glucagon to be able to cause the conversion of stored fat into blood fat in our bodies, its concentration needs to be about five to eight times higher than the concentration of insulin. Another way of saying this is that in order for insulin not to inhibit glucagon's ability to convert stored fat into blood fat for energy, insulin's concentration needs to be no higher than around 12.5 to 20 percent of the concentration of glucagon.

The food that causes the body to secrete glucagon is protein, and as you learned in Myth #1, protein also causes the body to secrete insulin. The level of insulin secreted in response to eating protein is usually well above the 12.5 to 20 percent threshold that will inhibit glucagon's ability to convert stored fat into blood fat. In addition, when the body makes its own glucagon in response to low blood sugar, it will also produce insulin in response to the glucagon. Even in this case, the level of insulin produced is usually at least 20 percent of the level of glucagon produced, so glucagon's ability to convert body fat into blood fat for energy would be inhibited. You will soon learn some of the ways that protein does help the body use more fat for energy; however, the notion that once you eat protein, you produce glucagon, which makes you burn fat, is a low-carb diet myth.

Myth #3: All of the excess carbohydrates you eat are converted to body fat.

This is another myth that has been largely perpetrated by those advocating a low-carbohydrate diet. Although excess carbohydrates can be converted into body fat, research studies show that only about 1 percent of carbohydrates get converted to fat when a person is consuming foods that make up the average diet. Excess carbohydrates are also used in thermogenesis, which is when the body converts extra calories into body heat. The amount of excess carbohydrates converted to body fat and body heat depends on the type of diet a person is following on a regular basis. This is because a person who normally has a high-carbohydrate diet usually has a high level of stored sugar, while a person who normally has a high-fat and lower-carbohydrate diet usually has lower levels of stored sugar. The result is that the person who normally has a high-carbohydrate diet and then overeats carbohydrates for a meal will tend to store more of those carbohydrates as body fat and burn more of them off as body heat than will a person who normally follows a low-carbohydrate diet. The reality is that even when someone who regularly has a high-carbohydrate diet overeats carbohydrates, the amount of those excess carbohydrates that gets converted to body fat is usually very minimal.

Studies show that even when people were put on a high-carbohydrate diet and then fed an extreme amount of carbohydrates during a five-hour period (2,000 calories of pure carbohydrates), less than 2 percent of the carbohydrates were actually converted to body fat in a 14-hour period of time. Interestingly, this same group of people actually ended up burning more body fat during a 24-hour period than they gained, for a net loss of body fat. This is because they consumed no fat; however, they still had a need to burn some fat for energy, and the amount they burned was higher than the 2 percent of carbohydrates that were converted to fat.

Remember that the key to effortlessly maintaining your weight is to consume protein, carbohydrates, and fat in the same proportion that your body prefers to burn them as fuel. If you eat what you burn and burn what you eat, you will easily maintain both high levels of energy and a stable body weight. The previous example illustrates what happens to Summers who are eating their recommended high-carbohydrate foods. They will convert around 1 to 2 percent of their carbohydrates to body fat, but as long as they are following a low-fat diet, they will burn the fat off that they gained from the carbohydrates during the day and will maintain their body weight. If Summers were to consume primarily high-fat foods in their diet, they would put on most of the excess fat calories as body fat, and because they do not burn a lot of fat for energy, they would quickly gain body fat if they continued to eat more fat than they burned. Conversely, a Summer who wanted to lose weight while maintaining high energy levels could choose a high-carb, no-fat diet for a week or two. The less fat a Summer consumes, the quicker he or she will lose weight; the more fat a Summer consumes, the faster this person will gain weight.

Winters gain weight not because their excess carbohydrates are converted to body fat, but because they tend to suffer from low blood sugar when consuming more carbohydrates than they burn for energy. This low blood sugar has them quickly turning to more food in between meals, and it's ultimately this overeating prompted by their erratic blood sugar that causes them to gain weight. In addition, by eating carbohydrates every 2 to 3 hours in an attempt to maintain their blood-sugar levels, Winters will not properly go into fat-burning mode, so they will tend to get fat, not because the carbohydrates are converted to fat, but because the fat they eat is stored as body fat, while the excessive dietary carbohydrates keep them from burning fat. Later, I will discuss some other reasons that a high-carb diet causes Winters to gain fat; however, the idea that eating 100 calories' worth of extra carbohydrates means you gain an extra 100 calories' worth of body fat is simply a myth.

When you eat according to your season-type, you should have stable blood sugar and energy throughout the day, which helps prevent you from overeating.

Rules of the Road

The Four Seasons Diet is designed to help each season-type maintain his or her ideal weight effortlessly, without hunger or the drop in energy that often accompanies dieting. Now that you know that the glucagon response produced from consuming protein does not get you into "fat-burning mode," and that both carbohydrates and protein cause the body to produce insulin, many of you may be wondering what are the exact metabolic mechanisms that make the Four Seasons Diet work for your season-type?

Carbohydrate/Fat Fuel Mix Ratio
Each season-type has a different carbohydrate/fat fuel ratio that he or she prefers to use to produce energy. Winters use the most fat for energy of any of the season-types, while Summers use the

most carbohydrates. Autumns are similar to Winters but use a little less fat and a little more carbohydrates to produce energy. Springs are similar to Summers but use a little more fat and little fewer carbohydrates to produce energy. Although each season-type has a preferred way of producing energy, following the wrong diet can upset this process and lead to erratic blood sugar, low energy, and weight gain.

Remember that the key to the Four Seasons Diet is that, ideally, you will eat foods with the same proportion of protein, carbohydrates, and fat that your body prefers to use for energy. Although we do not produce a lot of energy directly from protein, a large amount of protein can be converted to sugar and ultimately gets counted as carbohydrates in the carbohydrate/fat fuel mix ratio.

What Happens When Our Fuel Mix Ratio Is Off?
The most common problem for many season-types is eating the wrong mix of protein, carbohydrates, and fat. When this happens consistently, you will begin to burn fuel in a way that's somewhere between what your body prefers and the diet you have been following for the previous three to six days.
1. A Summer on a high-fat diet:
Summers who eat too much fat will begin to produce energy by using more fat and fewer carbohydrates than are ideal for their season-type. Although Summers can get away with eating too much fat in one meal, many problems begin to occur when Summers continually consume more fat that their bodies prefer to use for energy. Because Summers are not good at producing energy by using fat, when they eat too much fat and their bodies try to burn more fat from energy, the usual result for Summers is a really low level of energy, almost bordering on exhaustion.

One other problem that occurs with Summers on a high-fat diet is that they begin to drastically overeat in response to the low levels of carbohydrates in their diet. Studies show that we tend to feel full from a meal when the level of carbohydrates we consume is sufficient to satisfy our carbohydrate needs. When a Summer eats a high-fat meal, this person can easily consume 50 percent more calories than if he or she had eaten a low-fat meal. This is because Summers' bodies are looking for a certain amount of carbohydrates from a meal, not a certain number of calories, and Summers will continue to eat until their carbohydrate needs are met. The human body is not nearly as sensitive to consuming too little fat, because we usually have plenty of stored fat to keep us fueled. Our bodies are very sensitive to how many carbohydrates we are consuming, however, and if it's less than our bodies prefer, we will feel hungry until we get our stored carbohydrates to a level that works for our bodies. As a result of Summers overeating a high-fat meal in an attempt to get enough carbohydrates, they will tend to store the excess fat from each meal as body fat.

2. A Winter on a high-carb diet:

Winters have quite a different response when they eat the wrong meal for their season-type. The typical Winter's reaction to overeating carbohydrates is a quick rise in blood sugar, followed by a quick drop, which leads to low blood sugar and serious food cravings. While a Summer following a Winter diet usually experiences low energy levels and weight gain, a Winter following a Summer diet often gets a nice quick boost of energy from eating too many carbohydrates, followed by a sudden and severe crash that needs to be fed with more carbohydrates before the next meal. The Winter's weight gain is usually caused by constantly eating every time his or her blood sugar crashes. This overeating results in too many calories being consumed, and the nonstop ingestion of carbohydrates prevents the Winter from ever fully going into fat-burning mode.

The Futility of Most Weight-Loss Diets

One of the many reasons most weight-loss diets do not work is because we don't eat right for our season-type. Although we can voluntarily modulate our food intake in the short term, in the long term unless we are eating the right mix of fuels for our season-type we will eventually be overwhelmed and give in to our feelings of hunger and our desire for increased energy. The foods we eat affect our levels of blood sugar, blood fats, ketone bodies, and hormones that control hunger, such as ghrelin, leptin, insulin, cholecystokinin, and glucagon-like peptide. Although we can still produce energy from eating the wrong foods, doing so will upset many of these variables, causing the hunger and low energy associated with most weight-loss diets.

When we eat one wrong meal for our season-type, our bodies will usually continue to produce energy the way they prefer. For example, a Summer who follows a high-carb, low-fat diet all week and then binges on one high-fat, low-carb meal will still produce energy using mainly carbohydrates for energy during the next eight hours. Because the Summer's high-fat meal was low in carbs, he or she will draw on reserves of stored sugar for fuel, and the excess fat that was eaten will be stored as body fat for future use. Problems arise, however, if one "cheat-meal" a week becomes a weekend of bingeing or a way of life. In these cases, the Summer will continually store excess fat and will always be low on stored carbohydrates, and the Summer's weight will begin to increase, while his or her energy level plummets.

Each season-type has a unique set of metabolic disorders that occurs from eating the wrong meal, but the results are usually the same for all of the season-types: weight gain and either low or erratic energy production. Studies conducted on mice show that some strains get fat on a high-fat diet, while others get fat on a high-carbohydrate diet, which is very similar to what happens to Summers and Winters, respectively. Studies done on humans show that we tend to overeat whenever we don't consume either enough carbohydrates or enough fat to fulfill our energy needs. Studies have shown that when we do not eat enough carbohydrates for our season-type, we will consume an extra 3.5 percent calories for every 2 percent carbohydrate deficit. Similarly, it has been found that we will consume an extra .5 percent in calories for every 2 percent dietary fat deficit. The key to losing weight effortlessly is simply to eat in a way that does not make you hungry, and eating the right fuel mix for your season-type is one of the keys to controlling hunger.

Although each season-type has a preferred carbohydrate/ fat fuel mix, eating the wrong fuel mix will force the body to attempt to produce energy using a less-than-optimal proportion of macronutrients. This is ultimately the underlying cause of many health problems as the season-types begin to age.

What Happens When We Store the Wrong Nutrients for Our Season-Type?

The Four Seasons Diet is designed to take advantage of many metabolic principles that pertain to energy production. In Chapter 1, I explained how the body can store fat in the muscles as muscle fat and can store carbohydrates as either muscle sugar or liver sugar, referred to collectively as stored sugar.

The amount of stored muscle fat and stored sugar plays a role in the way that we produce energy. When our stored-sugar levels get low, our bodies will begin to use fewer carbohydrates and more fat for fuel. When we fill up our stored-sugar reserves, our bodies will use more sugar and less fat for fuel. This is one of the many reasons studies show that carbohydrate oxidation can double when people follow a high-carbohydrate diet. When we eat foods high in carbohydrates and low in fat, our stored-sugar reserves will tend to be full, while our muscle-fat reserves tend to be low, and the body responds by burning more sugar for energy.

Similarly, multiple studies show that a high-fat (more than 40 percent fat) diet increases our reserves of muscle fat by between 37 percent and 130 percent, which was found to speed up fat oxidation by greater than 70 percent when people are bicycling at 50 percent of their VO_2 max. Conversely, a high-carbohydrate diet increases our reserves of stored sugar by up to 500 percent. One study fed three groups of people three different diets. One diet was low-carb and high-fat, one diet was high-carb and low-fat, and the third diet was a mix of the two. After following these diets for three days, people on the high-carb diet had nearly five times as much stored muscle sugar when compared to those on the high-fat diet. When all three groups cycled to exhaustion, the high-carb dieters burned mainly carbohydrates for energy, while the high-fat dieters burned mainly fat for energy.

When we begin to follow a high-fat diet and store a large amount of muscle fat, our bodies start to retool the way they burn energy. A high-fat diet causes our bodies to increase the number of transporter proteins, which facilitates fat intake into the muscles, while reducing glucose tolerance, increasing fat oxidation, and decreasing carbohydrate oxidation during exercise. Although these may be beneficial changes for the average Winter, they are disastrous for the average Summer, because Summers' bodies are not designed to burn large amounts of fat. Many of a Winter's low-blood-sugar problems are caused by cells that are too sensitive to insulin, so a high-fat diet helps correct this issue for Winters.

When stored-sugar reserves begin to get low, our bodies reduce the rate at which we convert stored sugar into blood sugar, in an attempt to conserve our stored-sugar reserves. This is because our level of stored sugar is a key regulator of an enzyme called *adenosine monophosphate kinase* (AMPk), which increases the rate that our muscles burn fat for energy. Studies show that as our stored-sugar reserves get depleted, our levels of AMPk increase by approximately 150 percent, causing the muscles to burn more fat for energy.

In addition, an increase in muscle fat speeds up the rate that we burn fat for energy, especially during exercise. Studies show that although following a high-fat vs. a high-carb diet will slightly change the way that we produce energy at rest, those changes will be quite dramatic during exercise. For example, one study done on the general population (which would include all four season-types) found that on average, the high-carb dieters got 52 percent of their energy at rest from sugar, while the high-fat dieters got 41 percent of their energy at rest from sugar. When both groups exercised, however, the high-carb dieters got 79 percent of their energy from sugar, while the high-fat dieters got only 10 percent of their energy from sugar.

This is one reason Summers will experience such low energy levels on a high-fat diet, especially if they attempt to exercise. Their muscles cannot burn fat for energy the same way that a Winter's muscles can, which leaves the Summer with moderate energy at rest but very little capacity for energy at higher levels of exertion. A Winter's muscles can burn both fat and sugar for energy; however, these muscles prefer to burn fat unless they are engaging in super-strenuous activity. So while a Winter may not experience the same low-energy problems from eating the wrong foods that a Summer will, fueling a Winter on sugar during moderate activity is a bit like throwing gasoline onto a fire, which ultimately contributes to the Winter's low-blood-sugar issues.

The glycemic index of the carbohydrates that are eaten also dramatically affects how much muscle sugar the muscles will store. For example, one study examined the effect of feeding low-glycemic vs. high-glycemic carbohydrates to people after exercise. They found that feeding people higher-glycemic carbohydrates for the 24 hours following exercise resulted in the muscles storing nearly 50 percent more sugar, when compared to feeding the same amount of low-glycemic carbohydrates. This is one reason that higher-glycemic carbs are usually bad for Winters but can often be beneficial for Summers, if consumed as part of a healthy Summer diet and lifestyle plan.

Protein's Effect on the Carbohydrate/Fat Fuel Mix Ratio

The Winter diet is higher in protein because a higher-protein and lower-carbohydrate diet will help keep a person in fat-burning mode. You already learned in the section on "myths" that protein causes the body to secrete insulin and glucagon, and that the insulin prevents the glucagon from being able to put the body into fat-burning mode. Following a high-protein, lower-carbohydrate diet does have benefits for Winters and Autumns, however.

First, a large amount of the protein a person eats can be

converted to blood sugar as needed by the body. Most proteins do not cause the rapid rise in blood sugar that eating carbohydrates can cause. As a result, the blood sugar created from protein will not fill up the muscles with stored sugar the same way that eating carbohydrates will. This causes the levels of stored muscle sugar to remain lower, which helps keep the body in fat-burning mode. The lower the body's levels of stored sugar get, the more the body switches to burning fat for energy. Although protein supplies the blood sugar that's necessary to fuel the brain, it does not fuel the muscles the way that eating carbohydrates does.

Because a high-protein, lower-carbohydrate diet does not cause the blood-sugar spikes that a diet higher in carbohydrates will, it will not cause Winters and Autumns to experience the low-blood-sugar problems they tend to have from eating carbohydrates. When a person eats a meal that's high in carbohydrates, blood sugar will increase above the fasting level of blood sugar, called the *baseline*, and then a few hours later the blood sugar will actually fall below this baseline level, creating a state of low blood sugar. Eating protein will cause blood sugar to rise above the baseline value, but it does not cause blood sugar to drop below this value. Winters and Autumns tend to experience a more severe drop in blood-sugar levels below this baseline level than Summers and Springs do, so by following a diet that's higher in protein, they are able to avoid these low-blood-sugar episodes.

When Winters or Autumns experience severe low blood sugar from eating carbohydrates, they tend to self-medicate by simply eating more carbohydrates to raise their blood sugar again. They then get stuck in a vicious cycle of eating carbohydrates every few hours to avoid getting low blood sugar, which is usually the root cause of their weight-gain issues.

Because a high-protein diet does not raise blood-sugar levels as high as a high-carbohydrate diet does, the lower blood-sugar levels will help a person burn more fat for energy as well. This is because our levels of blood sugar and blood fats also influence the way that we produce energy. The lower our blood sugar, the more fat we tend to burn, and the higher our blood fat, the more fat we tend to burn. Following a high-protein diet helps keep blood sugar from getting too high, which means it will help us burn more fat for a longer period of time.

Eating larger quantities of protein also raises the body's level of a hormone called *catecholamines*. An amino acid called *tyrosine*, which is contained in most sources of protein, helps stimulate the release of catecholamines. The more protein we eat, the higher our blood level of tyrosine and the more catecholamines we produce. One of the many effects of catecholamines is that they help turn body fat into blood fat, which the body can use for energy.

The glucagon released from eating protein will cause the liver to burn fat and form *ketone bodies*. Ketone bodies can be used by the brain for fuel in place of sugar and also help decrease a person's appetite. Winters often benefit greatly from this, because they tend to have lower blood sugar and bigger appetites than Summers do. By both fueling the brain and keeping the appetite in check, protein will help a Winter's overall sense of well-being, while making it much easier for him or her to maintain the correct body weight.

Protein also affects the blood-sugar response when varying amounts are added to a meal that contains carbohydrates. The more protein you add to a set amount of carbohydrates at a meal, the lower the overall blood-glucose response will be. In one study, for example, test subjects were fed various meals containing either 100 percent carbohydrates or the same amount of carbohydrates with added protein, which amounted to either 28, 43, 59, or 86 percent of the level of carbohydrates. I will refer to this as the protein-to-carbohydrate ratio; for example, a ratio of 28 percent means there is 28 percent as much protein as carbohydrates. When compared to the pure carbohydrate meal, the more protein that was added to each meal, the lower the overall blood-sugar response was (measured as the area under the glucose curve). For example, the meal containing a 28 percent protein-to-carbohydrate ratio elicited only 60 percent of the glucose response, when compared to the same amount of carbohydrates without the added protein. The meal with a 43 percent protein-to-carbohydrate ratio elicited only 50 percent of the blood-sugar response, while the response for the meals with the 59 percent and 86 percent protein-to-carbohydrate ratios were 30 percent and 24 percent of the blood-sugar response, respectively. In addition, the more protein that was added to a meal, the sooner elevated blood sugar was able to return back to its baseline value, with the highest amount of protein causing elevated blood sugar to return back to normal nearly twice as quickly as when no protein was eaten.

When you look at the protein-to-carbohydrate ratios of the four season-types, you will see that the Summer ratio is the lowest at 30 percent, while the Winter ratio is the highest at 133 percent. When taking into account the study mentioned previously, you could reasonably expect the Winter diet to increase blood sugar only about 30 percent as much as the Summer diet does. This is great for Winters, because it helps prevent them from having the low-blood-sugar issues they often suffer from as a result of blood-sugar spikes. The lower-protein diet of the Summer and the Spring will cause a higher blood-sugar spike. This high blood sugar is beneficial for Summers and Springs, because it drives more stored sugar into their muscles, which helps keep them in sugar-burning mode.

So, for Winters and Autumns, following a higher-protein and higher-fat diet causes their blood sugar to remain low and stable, while their bodies maintain low levels of stored muscle sugar, which makes their muscles burn fat for energy. In addition, the protein produces higher levels of catecholamines, which help turn body fat into blood fat for a steady supply of fuel throughout the day. Finally, protein aids the body in producing ketone bodies, which fuel the brain and keep the appetite in check. These factors induce Winters and Autumns to stay predominately in fat-burning mode, because the levels of protein, carbohydrates, and fat in each season-type's diet determine what fuels ultimately get burned for energy.

This is also the reason the Summer and Spring diets are lower in protein. Maintaining lower levels of protein and higher levels of carbohydrates will produce higher levels of blood sugar and stored muscle sugar, which helps keep Summers and Springs in sugar-burning mode. The lower-protein diet also reduces the amount of blood fat for Summers and Springs by minimizing the release of catecholamines.

How Blood Fat Affects the Carbohydrate/Fat Fuel Mix Ratio

The level of blood fat also affects the ways that our bodies produce energy. The more fat we consume in our diet, the higher our blood-fat level will tend to be. Studies show that a person with a high-fat diet will have levels of blood fat that are about 50 percent higher than a person on a high-carbohydrate diet. Blood-fat levels are one of the regulators of energy production. High levels of blood fat will inhibit the effects normally caused by insulin, which include

1. Inhibiting the uptake of sugar into the muscles, which means you will store significantly less muscle sugar when you have a high-fat diet.
2. Inhibiting the effect that insulin normally has on the synthesis of stored sugar.

3. Inhibiting the effect that insulin usually has on making the body burn sugar for fuel.
4. Inhibiting the *phosphorylation* of glucose, which is the first step in the burning of sugar for energy and prepares it so that it can be broken down by the body.

Having higher levels of blood fats creates a type of temporary insulin resistance. When blood-fat levels are high, insulin will not be able to do its job effectively, even if the cells are not insulin resistant. Studies show that when you feed people high-fat foods instead high-carbohydrate foods, the synthesis of stored sugar and the amount of sugar burned for energy are reduced by about 50 percent. Hopefully, you are starting to see the importance of eating foods in the same proportion that your body prefers to burn for fuel. There are many reasons that eating more fat helps you burn more fat for energy, while eating more carbohydrates helps you burn more carbohydrates. Because each season-type has his or her own preferred carbohydrate/fat fuel ratio, eating according to that ratio both replenishes fuel in the same proportion to what is burned and helps your body burn the fuel mix it prefers. For example, Summers on a high-fat diet will be forced to attempt to burn far more fat than their bodies are capable of, while limiting the amount of carbohydrates they can both store and burn for energy. This leads to overeating, in an attempt to get more sugar into the body, while a large part of the excess fat that they cannot burn is simply stored as body fat. In the same way that a high level of blood fat helps Winters burn fat for energy, a high level of blood sugar helps Summers burn sugar for energy.

How Blood Sugar and Insulin Affect the Carbohydrate/Fat Fuel Mix Ratio

As mentioned earlier, insulin rises when we eat carbohydrates or protein. As insulin levels rise, we begin to burn more carbohydrates and less fat for energy. Insulin stops the body from turning body fat into blood fat. This causes the level of blood fats to decline, and we begin to burn more blood sugar for energy. Insulin also affects the key enzymes involved in energy production. For example, insulin activates three enzymes that help produce energy from sugar: *phosphoenolpyrurate carboxykinase, fructose bisphosphate,* and *glucose 6-phosphatase.* Insulin also inhibits three enzymes that help produce energy from fat: *pyruvate kinase, phosphofructokinase,* and *glucokinase.*

There is an inverse relationship between our level of blood

sugar and how much fat we burn for energy. The higher the blood sugar, the less fat we burn. There is also an inverse relationship between our level of blood fat and how much sugar we burn for energy. The higher the blood fat, the less sugar we burn. This is one of the many reasons each season-type has his or her own carbohydrate/fat fuel mix. The Winter diet is high in fat and low in carbs, which keeps Winters burning fat most of the time, as this is their preferred source of energy. The Autumn diet has less fat and more carbohydrates than the Winter diet, because Autumns prefer to burn a little more carbohydrates and a little less fat than Winters do. At the opposite end of the spectrum is the low-fat, high-carb Summer diet, which helps Summers burn mainly sugar for energy. The Spring diet is a little higher in fat and a little lower in sugar than the Summer diet because Springs use a little more fat and fewer carbohydrates for energy than Summers do.

The insulin response that occurs from eating food also affects our bodies' ability to store sugar as energy. The higher the insulin response, the more sugar our bodies will store. Even though excessive amounts of insulin are extremely unhealthy, high insulin levels occur when a person is insulin resistant. The high insulin response that results from eating high-glycemic carbohydrates will actually cause a person to store more of those carbohydrates as stored sugar than would eating an equal amount of lower-glycemic carbohydrates. You have already learned that the level of stored sugar in a person's muscles is one of many factors that determines whether the body will burn sugar or fat for energy. The higher the level of stored sugar, the more sugar a person will tend to burn for energy. This is one reason Summers are encouraged to eat medium- to high-glycemic carbohydrates, while Winters are encouraged to eat low- to medium-glycemic carbohydrates. If people are not insulin resistant, their bodies can handle the insulin response from eating high-glycemic carbohydrates, as long as they are eating according to their season-type. More than 50 percent of Americans over forty are probably insulin resistant to some degree, and the Four Seasons Diet is designed to restore the proper level of insulin sensitivity to all of the season-types. Remember that Summers are the most prone to being insulin resistant, and the primary culprit for this in Summers is eating too much fat, especially saturated fat. After Summers have restored their insulin sensitivity, they will find that eating medium- to higher-glycemic healthy carbohydrates will help them fill up on more stored sugar and will boost their energy throughout the day. Winters, on the other hand, will find that eating lower-glycemic carbohydrates helps prevent the low-blood-sugar issues they are so prone to, while keeping them from filling up on too much stored sugar and helping them stay in fat-burning mode.

Miscellaneous Rules and Tricks

Although each season-type has a preferred carbohydrate/fat fuel mix ratio, you have just learned about many of the factors that will cause each season-type to burn fuel differently from the way his or her body prefers. You can use many other little rules and tricks to maintain high levels of energy and lose weight effortlessly.

Carbs versus Calories: Which Villain Makes You Fat?

Carbohydrate consumption and calorie consumption are the two dominant factors that can influence your energy production. For example, let's say a Winter has a requirement of 2,000 calories a day to maintain his or her body weight, with 30 percent or 600 of those calories coming from carbohydrates. If Winters were to consume an extra 200 calories of carbohydrates, for a total of 2,2000 calories in a given day, they would be consuming 36 percent of their calories from carbohydrates and would then burn a little more sugar for energy than what they prefer; however, the ultimate metabolic consequences would be moderate. If, instead, Winters consumed 4,000 calories in one day and stuck to their recommended 30 percent of carbohydrates for energy, they would now be consuming 1,200 calories from carbohydrates, or double what their bodies prefer. Because carbohydrates are one of the main factors in energy production, and these Winters have just consumed an extra 600 calories of carbohydrates, the effect is that they will burn most of those extra 600 calories for energy and store the extra fat they ate as body fat. The Winters will say to themselves that "eating carbohydrates makes me fat," but this is not the truth. The truth is that the excess carbohydrates put them into sugar-burning mode, and the extra calories allowed them to store excess fat as body fat. The excess carbohydrates will probably have a negative effect on the Winters' energy production, because they prefer to burn fat, and they may experience low blood sugar and feel hungrier than if they had simply eaten half of the calories with the proper amount of carbohydrates.

Eating Excess Fat Makes Summers Insulin Resistant

Eating too much fat does not work as quickly as excess

carbohydrates to change a person's metabolism; however, in some respects the effects are far more severe. You see, Winters who overeat carbs for a few days can quickly go back into fat-burning mode and feel good while they lose the extra weight they put on by following their proper diet. Summers who overeat fat but eat the proper amount of carbohydrates will store the fat and use the carbohydrates. The problem is that most Summers have consumed far more fat during their entire lives than they can ever hope to use for energy, and because eating excess fat tends to make Summers insulin resistant, many, if not most, Summers are insulin resistant. As a result, when Summers stop eating excess fat and follow a high-carbohydrate diet, they are not able to produce optimum energy levels until their cells become 100 percent responsive to insulin again. In a later chapter, you will learn more about this; for now, however, it's worth mentioning that this can take weeks or many months to accomplish. During this period, Summers are producing very little energy from fat or carbohydrates, and they feel horrible. About the only thing that makes them feel good is eating a lot of sugar, because this has a high glycemic response and can often get them to produce enough insulin to force some of the sugar into their cells. Later on, you'll learn why this is one of the worst things a person can do, however. Once Summers have begun to follow the proper Summer diet and have lost some of their stored fat, their cells will eventually become responsive to insulin again, and in many cases, they will experience the most energy they have in years. The quickest way for Summers to achieve this is often by simply eliminating all or most fat from their diet for a few weeks.

Eating Lower-Glycemic Foods Will Help You Lose Weight

Another fact worth noting is that the higher a person's insulin response, the more food he or she tends to eat. So people who are insulin resistant will feel hungry even when they are stuffed. Later, you will learn more about the glycemic index, which measures how quickly sugars from carbohydrates enter the bloodstream. There is a correlation between a food's glycemic index and its insulin index. When you are trying to lose weight, eating foods with a lower glycemic index will produce less overall insulin and will make you tend to eat less. Some people actually have the opposite problem: they have a low appetite and have trouble eating enough food. If these people choose foods with a higher glycemic index, they usually find that their appetites increase, and they can eat more food.

Low-Fat Diets Work for Summers and Springs

For all season-types, excess dietary fat tends to get stored as body fat. Similarly, if you eat too little fat, your body will use some of your stored fat for energy. This is one reason many people experience success with weight loss on a low-fat diet, although usually it's the Summers and the Springs who find an extremely low-fat diet easy to follow and conducive to weight loss. One of the great things about the Four Seasons Diet is that you do not have to worry about what foods to eat to gain or lose weight. All you have to do is follow the diet for your season-type, watch your calories a little, and you should find it relatively easy to lose the weight you desire, with one caveat. Later on, I will talk about fructose and the need to do a two-week fructose fast and limit your fructose consumption after that. If your desire is to lose weight effortlessly and not feel hungry or not have a hard time controlling your appetite, it is imperative that you follow the fructose fast and fructose limitations you will learn about later in the book.

3
Insulin, the Master Hormone

*How eating the wrong foods for your season-type
leads to insulin resistance and disease.*

When it comes to energy production, insulin is definitely the master hormone that decides how we produce energy. In addition, insulin has a role in many other metabolic processes, and too much or too little of it can have drastic consequences, truly making insulin the master hormone.

Insulin Levels and Longevity

Many longevity studies have been conducted over the years on centenarians, people who have lived to be at least a hundred years old. New groundbreaking research is showing that elevated insulin levels are the leading cause of premature aging and premature death. Two things that most centenarians have in common are low insulin levels and high insulin sensitivity. High insulin sensitivity means that it takes a small amount of insulin to do the job of getting sugar into our cells. When the cells no longer respond to a normal amount of insulin, they are said to be *insulin resistant.* When the body becomes resistant to insulin, it responds by producing even more insulin, which ultimately makes the cells even more insulin resistant. Eventually, the pancreas loses its ability to produce insulin, due to utter exhaustion, and a person goes from being insulin resistant to being diabetic. In fact, the rate at which you age can be largely controlled by controlling your insulin levels. New research shows insulin can turn on genes that cause us to age rapidly, and low insulin levels turn on a different gene that acts like the fountain of youth.

One key to health at any age is to devise a strategy that keeps insulin levels low and makes the body highly sensitive to insulin, while maintaining a high level of energy. Although the answer may seem as simple as limiting your consumption of carbohydrates and sugar in order to keep your insulin levels low, the solution is far more complex. To fully understand how to keep your cells sensitive to insulin, which will keep your insulin levels low, you need to understand a little more about what causes insulin resistance in the first place.

Preventing Insulin Resistance

Insulin resistance can be caused a number of factors, including the overconsumption of fats for some season-types and overeating carbohydrates for other season-types, as well as having an excess of what is called intra-abdominal fat, or **visceral fat** (belly fat). Belly fat has long been known to be a marker for cardiovascular disease. People with belly fat tend to carry their body fat above their waistlines and are said to have an apple shape, while those who carry it below their waistlines are said to have a pear shape. The way that you carry your body fat can have a profound effect on how susceptible you are to both insulin resistance and cardiovascular disease. In fact, studies of obese people show that those with an apple shape are likely to suffer from insulin resistance and cardiovascular issues, while those who are equally obese but with a pear shape are often spared from both. Whether a person gains his or her fat in an apple shape or a pear shape depends primarily on the amount of a protein called 11Beta-HSD1 that individual produces, which is influenced by diet, gender, and individual physiology. Trans fats cause a large increase in this protein, saturated fats a moderate increase, and polyunsaturated fats keep it low.

The Dangers of Belly Fat
Belly fat is fat that forms inside the abdominal cavity and gets packed between the organs, such as the liver, the kidneys, the intestines, and the stomach. If you have ever gained 10 to 25 pounds of weight and found that most of it accumulated around the waistline and your waist got bigger by at least several inches, chances are you gained belly fat. Belly fat has a couple of unique properties that make it especially dangerous, due to its ability to cause cardiovascular disease and insulin resistance. The first unique property of belly fat is that it releases stored fat much more easily than other forms of stored fat are released. In fact, belly fat releases a large steady supply of fat into our bodies throughout the day, which creates an excess of blood fat. This is especially detrimental to Summers and Springs because it shuts

down production of sugar energy. Excessive blood fat is one of the main contributors to insulin resistance and leads to high levels of blood sugar, which cannot be properly stored and used by the body. The second factor that makes belly fat so dangerous is that it releases much of its fat directly into the portal vein of the liver, which overloads the liver with fat and hinders its ability to get rid of excess fat and cholesterol from the body.

Belly Fat Prevents the Liver from Eliminating Excess Cholesterol

The liver is the only organ that is able to process and dispose of excess cholesterol. Cholesterol, along with *triglycerides*, is carried in our bloodstream by substances called *lipoproteins*. Triglycerides are simply three fatty acids that have been joined together into one unit, and this is the way most fats are stored in plants and animals. Various lipoproteins have different functions; for example, LDL, often called "bad cholesterol," carries cholesterol to the body's cells, and under the right circumstances, that cholesterol can get deposited on the walls of your arteries. HDL, often called "good cholesterol," carries cholesterol from the body back to the liver, where it can be eliminated, if necessary. An easy way to remember which is the good one is to think of the "H" in HDL as standing for "healthy." HDL can also remove cholesterol from the walls of our arteries and help them remain healthy and free of plaque deposits.

Although both types of cholesterol are needed to maintain health, it's important that we maintain the proper ratio of LDL to HDL. The right level of LDL will allow our bodies to deliver just the right amount of cholesterol to the areas of our body that need it, and the right level of HDL will take any excess cholesterol back to the liver so that it cannot cause us any harm. Cholesterol is needed by every cell in our bodies, so it's not that cholesterol is bad; it's that excess cholesterol is bad. In fact, having a deficiency of cholesterol is also bad, although far more Americans suffer from an excess of cholesterol than a deficit, due to our modern diet and lifestyle. Ideally, your LDL level divided by your HDL level should be below 3. When you are in a healthy state, which includes having proper insulin sensitivity and not having excess belly fat, your body has a fairly easy time keeping your LDL and HDL at proper levels.

When you have excess belly fat, however, your body loses its ability to maintain this healthy balance. As mentioned earlier, belly fat can overload both the bloodstream and the liver with fat. The level of fat in the blood is largely determined by the rate of output from your body's fatty tissues, and because belly fat tends to produce large amounts of blood fat, having a lot of belly fat means your blood is constantly overloaded with fat, creating a state called *hypertriglyceridemia*, which means your blood contains excessive amounts of triglycerides, a form of blood fat.

Belly Fat Contributes to Insulin Resistance

Belly fat dumps large amounts of fat into the liver, where it gets converted into triglycerides and packaged into a lipoprotein called VLDL; it is then secreted for circulation into the body, raising our blood triglycerides even further. VLDL is also secreted from the liver when we eat large amounts of saturated or trans fats. Most people with too much belly fat are already in an insulin-resistant state, and it's the insulin resistance that works in concert with the belly fat to produce this excess of VLDL. After VLDL releases its triglycerides into the areas of the body that need it, such as the muscles or the adipose tissue, it is now mostly empty and is called a VLDL remnant. These VLDL remnants can be either eliminated by the liver or converted into unhealthy LDL. Normally, the liver is able to process most of these remnants and keep them from turning into the bad LDL. Because belly fat creates a state of excess VLDL, however, the liver gets overloaded, and much more LDL is produced as a result.

Insulin resistance also reduces the availability of enzymes that normally break down VLDL particles, which lengthens the amount of time they spend in our bodies. Much of this excess VLDL gets converted into the unhealthy LDL, which contains higher-than-normal levels of triglycerides. This chain of events creates the potentially deadly combination of

1. A higher than normal level of triglycerides.
2. A reduction in the enzymes that break down triglycerides, which is caused by insulin resistance.
3. An increase in the amount of time these particles stay in our bodies, which allows a different group of enzymes more time to convert LDL into the much more harmful small LDL.

Small LDL is the especially dangerous kind that leads to potentially serious arterial plaque and heart problems. These small LDL particles do not bind very easily to the normal LDL receptors of the cells that are responsible for bringing needed cholesterol into the cells, so this increases the amount of time they spend in our blood, allowing them to be deposited on our arterial walls. Insulin resistance makes the problem worse because it reduces the small

LDL, which doesn't like the LDL receptors very much to begin with the number of LDL receptors contained in each cell, meaning that, makes even fewer to attempts to attach to them, which keeps the small LDL in our blood even longer, giving it more of a chance to damage our arteries.

Remember, it's the ratio of LDL to HDL that's important; the more LDL rises and the more HDL falls, the higher the risk for cardiovascular problems. As explained previously, belly fat combined with insulin resistance dramatically increases the amount of LDL in the blood, especially the most dangerous kind to the arteries, the small LDL. Belly fat and insulin resistance also combine to wreak havoc with the good HDL. They make the good HDL become smaller than normal, which means it can carry far less cholesterol for elimination into the liver. This small HDL is also removed from the blood quicker than the normal-size HDL, which reduces the amount of beneficial HDL, and what little HDL is left is composed of the small kind, which does not have the ability to carry very much cholesterol back to the liver for elimination.

The excess insulin caused by insulin resistance plays a central role in this whole process. Normally, the presence of glucose and insulin in the bloodstream keeps the body's fat deposits from releasing fat into the bloodstream. When the body becomes resistant to insulin, the body's fat cells continue to dump fat into the blood, even when blood-sugar levels are high, and if the body has high levels of belly fat, it dumps an even greater amount of fat into the blood and directly into the liver. This keeps the blood and the liver in a constant state of fat overload, which prevents the body from being able to get the fat in the blood and the liver back to normal levels. Insulin resistance also reduces the number of enzymes that help break down the fats in lipoproteins. At the same time, it increases the amount of VLDL secreted by the liver, while keeping it in the bloodstream for a prolonged time.

Belly Fat Triggers Inflammation, Contributing to CVD

Belly fat and insulin resistance also disrupt the normal function of another lipoprotein called the *chylomicron remnant*, causing constriction of the arteries and blood vessels, while at the same time triggering inflammation in the delicate cells that line the interior of the arteries and the blood vessels. This inflammation is a major contributor to cardiovascular disease (CVD). Belly fat also causes another type of inflammation by producing large amounts of proteins called *cytokines*, which can prompt both the liver and the adipose tissue to become insulin resistant.

One of the strongest predictors of who will ultimately suffer from both cardiovascular disease and diabetes is the *lipid triad*. The lipid triad consists of higher-than-normal levels of blood triglycerides and small dense LDL, with lower-than-normal levels of HDL. Belly fat causes all three of these things, which is the reason it is such a good predictor of someone being more prone to cardiovascular disease and a heart attack. The easiest way to eliminate the lipid triad is to get rid of the belly fat that caused it in the first place.

Belly Fat and the Four Season-Types

The cause of belly fat is often different for the various season-types, and the way to reduce it is different as well. As many of you have probably figured out, excess belly fat is far more detrimental to Summers and Springs than to Winters and Autumns. Winters can often deal with the excess blood fat produced by belly fat by using it to produce energy. Summers, on the other hand, who are usually already overloaded with fat from their diets, have no way to even begin to deal with the additional fat released from belly fat. Normally, it's the Summers and the Springs who have the greatest chance of developing belly fat in the first place, because they usually eat more fat than their bodies need. Much of this excess dietary fat can end up being deposited as belly fat, and when this happens, Summers begin to produce amounts of blood fat far in excess of what they can ever hope to burn as energy or eliminate in a healthy manner.

The solution for any season-type with excess belly fat is simply to lose weight. This will often be far easier for Winters and Autumns, because they can usually keep their energy levels high while burning the fat off. Summers and Springs have a slightly harder time; however, by eating for their season-type, they can normally keep their energy at a high-enough level to make the dieting easier. One of the easiest ways for all season-types to avoid gaining belly fat in the first place is to switch from eating refined grain products to whole grain products. The other way to avoid belly fat is by not consuming excess calories, and the best way to do this is to eat according to your season-type. Remember, we tend to overeat when we do not eat foods with the same carbohydrate/ fat fuel mix ratio that our bodies prefer to burn for fuel. Eating the wrong foods for your season-type can cause your levels of stored sugar, muscle fat, blood fat, or blood sugar to become either higher or lower than your season-type prefers. This will ultimately lead to low or erratic energy production and weight gain.

Insulin Resistance Makes Us Feel Hungry and Slows Our Metabolism

I cannot stress how important it is for all of the season-types to keep their insulin levels low and insulin sensitivity at the right level. In addition to everything just mentioned, insulin resistance reduces our sensitivity to *leptin*, the hormone that makes us feel full, while at the same time causing an increase in the "reward" effect, or the feeling of pleasure we get from eating food. Many people in this state eat excessive amounts, even when their stomachs are stretched so tight they can hardly hold any more food. This makes sense, given the fact that they are not getting the proper hormonal messages to tell them they are full, while at the same time they're getting extra "rewards" and pleasure from eating more food. For anyone reading this who has a weight problem and who has been told repeatedly that you are fat simply because you are lazy, I hope you'll take some comfort in the fact that laziness is not your problem. Your problem is most likely that your body's own hormones are working against you, causing you to get fat for a number of different reasons, far beyond the control of most people in your situation. In addition to all of these effects, high insulin levels also result in a decreased metabolism, which means your body burns less energy when at rest, making you tired and even more apt to gain weight.

Some people are able to store large amounts of fat under their skin, while others have very little ability to store this type of fat, called *subcutaneous fat*. People who are not able to store much fat under their skin are the ones who are most prone to accumulating belly fat, because this is where their bodies will store fat once what little reserves they have under their skin are full. Some people can easily gain 30 to 40 pounds of extra fat under their skin and still be relatively healthy. In contrast, others who gain only 10 pounds of fat under their skin and then gain another 10 pounds of belly fat will usually be extremely unhealthy.

Just as some people's bodies prefer to be what our society considers a little on the chunky side, other people's bodies prefer to maintain a level of body fat that might be considered bordering on anorexic. If you are either of these extreme cases, I recommend that you do your best not to listen to the pressure society puts on you to be "normal"; listen to your own body, and make the choice to be "healthy" instead. For some people, this may mean they look slightly chunky, and for others, they might appear borderline anorexic, and that is alright. Although many high school and college-age girls diet, trying to attain an unrealistic ideal of what skinny means, an equal number of high school and college-age boys suck down countless weight-gainer shakes, trying to be bigger and conform to some idealized picture of what society tells them they should look like. If you eat according to your season-type, your body will naturally get to the weight it prefers, which is usually the weight at which you will also feel the best, in terms of both mood and energy.

If you follow the Four Seasons Diet, you will reach your ideal weight with very little effort and will probably feel better than you have in a long time. I hope you can learn to be happy with feeling great, even if you don't look like the women or the men in the glamour and fitness magazines.

Cell Permeability

The human body contains more than 100 trillion cells, and each cell maintains a level of autonomy from the other cells by wrapping itself in a protective coating. The job of this protective coating is not to keep everything from passing through it, but rather to be very selective about what can enter and exit the cell. Nutrients have to be allowed to enter, along with oxygen, so that the cell can produce energy, and then the waste products need to be allowed to exit. In addition, many substances need to be denied entry into and exit out of the cell. This protective coating has to maintain just the right level of permeability in order to accomplish this task. To maintain the proper level of permeability, the cell incorporates many different substances into its protective coating, all of which have various degrees of permeability. By selectively choosing the proper ratio of high, moderate, and low permeable substances, the cell is able to maintain a perfect level of overall permeability. This protective coating can become either too porous or not porous enough, both of which have health consequences. Chart 3.1 shows a few examples of common symptoms that occur when cells are too porous and or not porous enough.

CHART 3.1 CELL PERMEABILITY IMBALANCES

Cell Too Nonporous (Most Often Summers)	Cell Too Porous (Most Often Winters)
Lack of Energy	Nervous Energy
Constant Drowsiness	Insomnia
High Blood Pressure	Low Blood Pressure
Frequent Urination*	Infrequent Urination
Constipation	Diarrhea
Rapid Heart Rate	Slow Heart Rate
Often Feels Warmer Than Others	Often Feels Colder Than Others
Depression	Migraine Headaches

* May have to urinate several times a night as well.

How Nonporous Cells Lead to Insulin Resistance

If the cells' protective coating is not porous enough, small things may be able to pass through the coating, while larger things that should be able to pass though are unable to. One larger molecule that needs to pass through this protective coating is insulin, so one of the first things that happens when a cell's protective coating is not permeable enough is that insulin has a difficult time passing though. The body responds by producing more insulin, in the hope that if enough insulin is present, some may be able to pass through to do its job. The cell is now said to be insulin resistant. Although the process is very complicated, a simplified version can be explained in the following manner.

The cell's protective coating is made primarily of fatty acids. Most of the fat that we eat and store is in the form of triglycerides. Triglycerides are simply three fatty acids that have been joined together with one glycerol molecule. When the body needs fat for energy, it takes the triglyceride apart to separate the three fatty acids from one another and then uses the individual fatty acids for energy. To make the cells' protective coating, the body takes two of these fatty acids and joins them together at one end, forming *phospholipids*.

As you are probably aware, there are many different types of fat. Some fat is *saturated*, as in butter and cheese; some is *monosaturated*, such as in olive oil; while other fat is *unsaturated*, for example, in most vegetable oils. When the cells make their protective coatings, the types of fats that get incorporated into the coating have a great effect on how porous the cells are. Saturated fats tend to make the cells less porous, while unsaturated fats usually make the cells more porous. The cells also incorporate cholesterol into their protective coating; it is like a cement that holds the whole thing together and is highly nonporous. Anything that causes the body to incorporate more saturated fat and cholesterol into the protective coating will make the cells less porous, while anything that induces the body to include more unsaturated fat and less cholesterol in the coating will make the cells more porous.

The cells keep very tight control of the level of the various fats in their protective coating, and only a very slight change in the composition of the protective coating will have a profound effect. For example, a less than 2 percent increase in the level of saturated fat in our cells' protective coating can increase our fasting levels of insulin by approximately 30 percent, due to the saturated fats' ability to make the cells less porous and therefore insulin resistant. Similarly, an increase in monounsaturated fats, as found in olive oil, in our cells' protective coating of only 1.4 percent can lower our insulin levels by approximately 10 percent, which is one of the main reasons the Mediterranean diet, which features a lot of monounsaturated olive oil, is so healthy. Remember that low insulin levels are one key to longevity, and the way to have low insulin levels is by making sure your cells are not insulin resistant. Although diet plays a role in our cells' protective coating, our season-type is a far more important factor, given the effect that our season-type has on our cholesterol levels. Cholesterol has the greatest ability to make the cells less porous.

Cholesterol's Role in Making the Cells Nonporous
Most people think that our bodies get cholesterol from the food we eat, but in actuality, only 20 percent of our daily cholesterol comes from our food. The rest is manufactured by our bodies in a process that is regulated to a large extent by a protein called SREBP and an enzyme called HMG-CoA. The amount of SREBP and HMG-CoA in our bodies is increased by insulin, so the higher our insulin levels, the more cholesterol we produce. Insulin is the hormone associated with storage and growth, so when insulin levels are high, the body takes it as a signal that it's time to build new cells, and because this requires cholesterol, the body begins to produce the cholesterol needed for the job. Glucagon, on the other hand, is the hormone responsible for using stored energy and breaking down existing cells, so when glucagon levels are high, the body stops producing cholesterol. Excess cholesterol in our system tends to create a state where our cells incorporate the cholesterol into their protective coating, making them less porous. Foods can also make

our cells less porous, such as alcohol and foods high in amines, which are found in aged meats and cheeses. The goal of each diet for the four season-types is to both provide the necessary nutrients and balance the hormonal effects of food in way that works best for each season-type, while helping the cells maintain the proper level of cell permeability.

The way the average person eats can create a vicious cycle with disastrous health consequences, which looks something like this: A perfectly healthy person may start off with cells whose protective coating has just the right level of permeability. If this person eats in a way that produces excess insulin, then the body will make too much cholesterol, which will cause the cells to be less porous, while decreasing the number of insulin receptors. Insulin, being a large molecule, has trouble getting into the cells to do its job, so the body begins to produce even more insulin, with the hope that some will get in and, in the process, also begins to produce more cholesterol. More cholesterol means cells that are less and less porous, which means more and more insulin is needed. As the cells become less porous, other nutrients have trouble getting in, including oxygen, and the cells lose their ability to produce energy with oxygen, relying instead on fast-sugar energy without oxygen. This creates an extremely acidic state inside the cells, and because the cells are not porous enough, these acids have trouble exiting. This state of low energy, mental fog, and low oxygen levels in the tissues is a perfect environment for cancers to begin to grow. Almost 75 percent of older Americans are insulin resistant, to some degree, and one of the best indicators of whether you are insulin resistant is how you feel after a meal high in carbohydrates or sugar. If you feel drowsy and in a mental fog immediately after eating most meals high in carbohydrates, the odds are pretty good you are suffering from insulin resistance, to some extent. In the last stage of insulin resistance, the pancreas loses its ability to keep producing high levels of insulin, and a person becomes diabetic.

Signs That the Liver Is Insulin Resistant

Insulin resistance does not affect all cells in the body equally. Usually, the cells in the liver are the first to become insulin resistant, and when this happens, the liver's ability to properly convert thyroid hormones into their most active form begins to fail. One of the first signs of insulin resistance is that your energy level begins to drop. Next, the energy-producing cells, such as your muscles, become insulin resistant, and if you are a Summer or a

Spring, your energy levels really begin to fall because you rely on sugar energy. Because insulin is not as crucial for Winters and Autumns, they may not feel the same effects from this stage of insulin resistance. The last cells to become insulin resistant for all of the season-types are the fat cells. So, during the time when the liver and the muscles are insulin resistant, and our bodies are producing excess insulin, we are getting fat very quickly, because our fat cells are responding to all of the excess insulin by storing extra fat. We all have a "set point" at which even our fat cells become insulin resistant. Some people may still look relatively lean, yet have insulin-resistant fat cells, while other people can get morbidly obese before this happens. If you have ever felt worse and worse for a long time and then suddenly gained a lot of weight without consuming any more calories than normal, you probably experienced the state where your fat cells were the only ones properly responding to insulin.

Even though the effects of insulin resistance are quite horrible, in actuality it is a beautiful response that our bodies have to excess levels of insulin. It essentially forces us to start burning fat for energy, as our cells begin storing less and less sugar. We feel terrible as we become insulin resistant, and many of us instinctively respond by thinking that we feel fat and need to lose weight. Losing weight often makes our cells sensitive to insulin again. The burning of fat for energy produces *ketone bodies*, which actually makes the cells more permeable. Without our response of feeling so bad, nothing would keep us from overeating until we weighed more than 800 pounds, except for the stigma of being overweight. Given that most people don't diet to lose weight, even when they are insulin resistant and feel bad as a result, it's a pretty safe bet that were it not for insulin resistance, most of us would probably be morbidly obese. Most people feel so bad at the point when their fat cells become insulin resistant that they are compelled to lose weight. Remember, we usually experience a sudden weight gain when our fat cells are the only ones that are still responding properly to insulin, even though we are eating the same amount of food as in the past. Because this sudden weight gain is often accompanied by a loss of energy and feeling physically spent, due to the rest of our bodies' cells being insulin resistant, we usually blame the extra twenty pounds we just gained for our low energy. In actuality, the fat is not the reason we feel so bad, but rather the symptom. The reason we feel so bad is that our energy-producing cells have become insulin resistant, and our bodies have responded by producing more insulin, which has caused our fat cells to gain weight.

Insulin Resistance Accelerates the Aging Process

The effects of insulin resistance and the excess production of insulin that it causes are at the root of many diseases associated with aging. As your cells become more insulin resistant, your body begins to eliminate magnesium through urination, rather than store it. This loss of magnesium causes the blood vessels to constrict, resulting in high blood pressure. Insulin also makes us retain too much sodium, which adds to the high blood pressure problem. In addition, high levels of insulin excite the branch of our nervous system that is responsible for the "fight-or-flight" response, which raises our blood pressure even more.

Insulin has a role in producing signaling molecules called *eicosanoids*. There are good eicosanoids, which help enhance the immune system, reduce pain and inflammation, increase oxygen, and boost endurance. There are also bad eicosanoids, which have the opposite effect and suppress the immune system, increase pain and inflammation, cut down on oxygen flow, and lessen endurance. Insulin has a key role in producing the bad eicosanoids, so when your body is insulin resistant and is producing excess insulin, you tend to make a lot more of the bad eicosanoids and very few of the good ones. The bad eicosanoids cause inflammation, including arterial inflammation, which can contribute to heart attacks and strokes.

Insulin plays a role in the buildup of arterial plaque, by helping to create and sustain high levels of LDL cholesterol, the "bad cholesterol," in the blood. Excess insulin creates a state in the body where even though the cells already have too much cholesterol in their protective coatings, the body continues to produce more cholesterol, primarily LDL cholesterol, which travels around the body, looking for a home. Because the cells have too much cholesterol, a lot of the cholesterol in the LDL particles gets deposited on the linings of our arteries, causing arterial plaque, which can lead to a heart attack or a stroke. As mentioned earlier, it's the ratio of LDL to HDL cholesterol that is important in keeping our cholesterol levels healthy.

The Misguided Demonization of Saturated Fat

Many health professionals have advocated a high-carbohydrate, low-fat diet as a way to lower your cholesterol. Unfortunately, if not done correctly, this will lower your total cholesterol but will end up reducing your "good" HDL more than it decreases your bad LDL, which will increase your ratio in a less beneficial direction. This type of diet is also very unhealthy for Winters and Autumns, who need a diet higher in fat and protein. Unfortunately, the original research in the 1950s, which led to the demonization of saturated fat, was flawed in many respects. Subsequent research has shown that saturated fat is not the cause of most heart disease, but rather high insulin levels are. Even this research, however, fails to approach the problem in a way that is healthy for all four season-types. Most research simply assumes that everyone will respond the same way to all types of food, and nothing could be further from the truth. The cause of high insulin levels and even the causes of insulin resistance are often very different for the various season-types.

A Summer's Ideal Diet to Balance Insulin and Cholesterol Levels
Summers are the most prone to insulin resistance and heart disease, so first we'll examine the ideal Summer diet and why it works for them. Next, we'll look at what happens to a Summer when this person eats the wrong foods for his or her season-type. Summers burn mainly sugar for energy, so their ideal diet is high in carbohydrates and lower in fat and protein. If the protective coating of the cells is at the proper level of permeability, Summers are very sensitive to insulin, which helps keep their insulin levels low, and this means they are not producing excessive amounts of cholesterol. The high-carbohydrate meal produces an insulin response the body is able to handle, and the muscles and the liver fill up with stored sugar. A few hours after Summers eat, their blood-sugar levels begin to drop, and their bodies produce glucagon to raise their blood sugar. Because the Summer relies on stored sugar for energy, the glucagon will cause some of the stored sugar to be released into the blood, to keep the blood sugar stable. The other thing that happens is that the release of glucagon helps keep cholesterol in check, because the body will produce more of the good HDL cholesterol when glucagon levels are high.

The first few hours after a Summer eats a meal, insulin is the primary hormone being produced, which causes the production of cholesterol to rise, but because the cells are still sensitive to insulin, only a modest amount of insulin is produced. This low level of insulin causes only a modest increase in cholesterol. After a few hours, glucagon becomes the dominant hormone, the production of cholesterol falls, and now the Summer's body is able to deal with excess cholesterol and get rid of it. Assuming the Summer eats lunch at 12:00 p.m. and dinner at 6:00 p.m., from 12:00 to about 2:00 p.m. the insulin is storing sugar, creating cholesterol, and making the cells less porous. From about 2:00 until 6:00 p.m., however, glucagon is causing the release of stored sugar and the elimination of excess cholesterol and is making the cells more porous. By dinnertime, the Summer should have had six hours of relatively steady blood sugar, and his or her body should be back in balance. Part of the time, it was creating a little extra cholesterol, and the other part of the time it was getting rid of it; at the end of the process, the body is in balance and functioning properly, and the cells' permeability is back to normal. It's important to mention that the degree to which the cells' permeability changes from one meal is infinitesimally small and would not affect overall insulin sensitivity. It is the combined effects from many meals during a period of weeks and months that causes the cells to become either too porous or not porous enough.

Many things can happen to disrupt this process, however, and usually do. The first is that people often snack between meals. This is most detrimental to Summers, for various reasons. First, Summers tend to have a higher insulin response to a meal than the other season-types do, because sugar-burning muscles have a harder time storing sugar than fat-burning muscles do, due to the fact that they have fewer capillaries and therefore less blood flowing to them. Second, because Summers eat very little protein, the best way for them to produce adequate amounts of glucagon is by letting their blood sugar drop between meals by not snacking. If Summers eat correctly for their season-type, the release of glucagon at the point where their blood-sugar level drops a few hours after a meal will cause their bodies to release stored sugar, and Summers can easily make it to their next meal. When Summers eat the wrong meal for their season-type, however, the release of glucagon will often cause their bodies to go into fat-burning mode, and in this situation the Summer frequently feels compelled to reach for a sweet sugary snack in an attempt to increase blood sugar levels, along with insulin levels. Summers may believe that when this happens between meals, they are suffering from low blood sugar; however, in most cases if you tested their blood sugar, you would find that it is in the normal range. What is usually happening between meals when Summers do not eat right for their season-type is that their bodies switch from burning sugar for energy to burning fat, and because Summers cannot burn very much fat for energy, they experience a drop in energy, mood, and concentration that they assume is low blood sugar but is actually the point at which their bodies switch into fat-burning mode.

This is the reason the Summer diet is designed for the Summer to fill up on carbohydrates during each of the three meals, which will allow the liver and the muscles to store sugar, while keeping levels of stored muscle fat and blood fat low. This will keep a Summer in sugar-burning mode most of the day, while preventing insulin levels from getting out of control.

When Summers snack between meals, this tends to keep blood sugar and insulin levels high all day long, and when the body keeps producing insulin, it never gets a chance to produce glucagon. As a result, the body is producing cholesterol all day long, and the cells begin to incorporate too much of it into their protective coating. Eventually, they become too nonporous, and insulin can no longer get into the cells properly, which causes insulin levels to go up, producing even more cholesterol, which makes the cells even less porous, and the process keeps escalating out of control. Eventually, the blood sugar and the insulin levels become so erratic that people may find that the only way they can function is by eating every few hours. Unfortunately, this just serves to keep them in a bad state by elevating insulin levels during most of their waking hours.

When the cells become too nonporous, oxygen cannot get in, which means a person cannot produce energy properly. Winters and Autumns have muscles that are full of capillaries and are able to supply blood and nutrients to muscle cells much better than Summers and Springs can. Sugar-burning muscles tend to have far fewer capillaries, and they are already challenged when it comes to getting enough oxygen. Once the cells become too nonporous, the muscles get even less oxygen, and Summers begin to produce energy without oxygen all of the time, using fast-sugar energy. The problem with this is that it causes very low energy levels and creates a lot of acid in the cells, which has to be eliminated before more energy can be generated. A person in this state may feel short of breath or winded all of the time as a result. Because the cells are not porous enough, acid has a very difficult time getting out, and the cells become overly acidic and are in a state of low oxygen all of the time, which is the perfect environment for cancers to grow. The blood often responds to the overly acidic cells by becoming overly alkaline. I'll discuss this further in a later chapter, but when the blood becomes too alkaline, it creates many other health challenges.

The next thing that can go wrong for Summers occurs when they eat too much fat at their meals. Summers do not burn very much fat for energy, so the excess fat either gets stored or ends up circulating as LDL cholesterol, which is the last thing Summers need because they already produce large amounts of cholesterol. Much of the excess fat ends up getting stored around the muscles, which can create insulin resistance, even if there is no snacking between meals.

Another common issue for Summers is the consumption of too much fruit or, more specifically, fructose, which is the primary sugar usually found in fruit. An entire section will be devoted to this later; however, it is worth mentioning now that 30 percent of fructose gets converted into fat, so a high-fructose diet is a high-fat diet, which is the last thing a Summer needs. Fructose is also very hard on the liver of a Summer, who is usually struggling to get rid of excess fat, because most Summers eat way more fat than their bodies can use. As a result, the fructose ends up making the liver fatty and insulin resistant, which causes the Summer's energy to plummet even further. A Summer in this state is probably a caffeine addict, with very little energy throughout the day. I have helped many Summers completely turn their lives around in a matter of weeks by simply eliminating fruit and fructose from their diets for a short period of time.

Studies have compared people who have a greater proportion of sugar-burning muscles (Summers) to people with predominantly fat-burning muscles (Winters). All of the studies came to the same conclusion. As Summers age, they have a faster heart rate, higher blood pressure, a thicker left ventricle, a larger percentage of body fat, a lower level of physical activity, a greater prevalence of insulin resistance, and a higher rate of diabetes. Part of this is caused by eating too much fat. A Winter with a high-fat diet will tend to burn it off. Summers, on the other hand, will either have to store it or get rid of it, both of which contribute to insulin resistance. The insulin resistance is what ends up causing most of the other health issues for the Summer. If Summers would simply follow a low-fat, minimal-fruit diet and not snack between meals, they would not encounter these problems later in life.

Springs face a similar set of challenges; however, because they eat fewer carbohydrates than Summers do and burn more fat, they have a much easier time staying in balance, especially if they are not snacking between meals.

A Winter's Ideal Diet to Balance Insulin and Cholesterol Levels

Winters face a completely different set of problems from Summers and Springs. The ideal Winter diet is high in fat and protein, especially a type of protein called purines, which I'll discuss later. Because Winters burn fat for fuel, they don't need to eat a lot of carbohydrates, which helps maintain low insulin levels and keeps them in fat-burning mode. The biggest mistake Winters make is not eating enough fat, especially saturated fat. An entire section will be devoted to fat later in the book, but saturated fat, which has been demonized for more than fifty years, is actually a healthy fat for most Winters. A Winter who is following the proper Winter diet will produce very little insulin and will be producing glucagon most of the day. This will keep the Winter in fat-burning mode. The other thing the proper diet does is keep the Winter's cholesterol levels low. Remember that only 20 percent of the cholesterol in our bodies comes from our food, and the rest is made by our bodies, largely in response to insulin. Winters produce very little cholesterol and usually need to make sure they get enough in their diet. Butter and cheese can be a Winter's best friend, because they help keep a Winter's cells from becoming too porous.

Because Winters tend to produce low levels of cholesterol, their cells' protective coating tends to become too porous. In addition, Winters often over-rely on fat energy, and when people use a large amount of fat energy and a small amount of sugar energy, they begin to produce ketones. Ketones also contribute to making the cells too porous. This can add to a Winter's erratic and low-blood-sugar problems because their cells are often too sensitive to insulin. When they eat a lot of carbohydrates, their blood sugar goes up and then rapidly goes down, because their cells grab the sugar very quickly. When their blood sugar plummets, they often find themselves turning to more sugar. To make matters even worse, fat-burning muscles are actually more sensitive to insulin than sugar-burning muscles are. What Winters really need is more saturated fat and high-purine proteins. This will help keep their blood sugar stable and also prevent their cells from getting too porous.

A Winter on a low-fat diet is usually a Winter whose cells are far too porous. As a result, the person is usually suffering from severe hypoglycemia. In addition, oxygen has a very easy time getting into the Winter's cells, and oxidation begins to get out of control, especially in response to how quickly sugar and insulin are able to enter the cells. Often, oxygen will improperly combine with polyunsaturated fats to form peroxides, which are highly potent free radicals. Polyunsaturated vegetable oils can also cause other problems for Winters, such as combining improperly with chlorides, which allows sodium to freely enter inside the cells, creating a highly alkaline environment by entering into other combinations, especially with carbonate.

Usually, Winters do best eating foods high in protein with plenty of saturated fat and cholesterol. This provides Winters with enough fat for fuel, while helping them maintain proper cell permeability. Because their metabolism will tend to make their cells overly porous, a diet higher in cholesterol will help keep their cells from getting too porous, which will prevent their blood sugar from crashing after they eat carbohydrates.

Autumns can have problems similar to Winters; however, because they eat more carbohydrates, they usually have an easier time keeping themselves in balance.

Why Cell Permeability Can Vary for the Season-Types
Now that you understand the season-types' tendencies regarding cell permeability, it's important to realize that although tendencies do exist, any season-type can have cells that are too porous or too nonporous. The most common occurrence, though, is that Winters tend to have cells that are too porous, especially when they are younger, but years of bingeing on too many carbohydrates, due to erratic blood sugar issues, can often cause their cells to become too nonporous later in life. Summers, conversely, tend to have cells that are too nonporous most of their lives, especially if they eat large amounts of saturated fats. Autumns and Springs have an easier time keeping their cells at the proper level of permeability; however, if they are out of balance, Autumns tend to have cells that are too porous, and Springs tend to have cells that are too nonporous. Yet sometimes Autumns have cells that become too nonporous and Springs have cells that become too porous, so it's especially important for these two season-types to learn how to control their level of cell permeability with diet as the weather outside changes, a topic I'll cover in more detail later.

Most people in America consume far too many carbohydrates, especially in the form of a sugar known as *fructose*. For this reason, most older Americans suffer from insulin resistance to some degree, which also means they have high insulin levels. Many of the factors that contribute to arterial disease result from the excess insulin caused by insulin resistance. For example, high LDL and low HDL can both be attributed to too much insulin. Insulin and fructose both lower a substance in our body called *nitric oxide*, which helps dilate and relax our blood vessels and keeps our blood pressure low. Too much insulin will also cause excess estrogen and low testosterone in men, which contributes to arterial disease. Women, on the other hand, tend to produce excess testosterone when they become insulin resistant, which will bring about health problems as well. In addition, insulin will stimulate the fight-or-flight branch of your nervous system and increase the platelet adhesiveness and the coagulability of your blood, all of which contribute to cardiovascular disease. When you eat according to your season-type, however, your insulin levels should stay under control once you regain your insulin sensitivity. In a later chapter, you'll learn how to regain your sensitivity to insulin and regain your health as a result.

Insulin is not the only culprit when it comes to keeping your cells at the proper level of permeability. It's imperative that all season-types keep their cells' protective coating at the perfect level of permeability. Many factors influence the body's ability to maintain perfect permeability, such as diet, climate, lifestyle, and an individual's season-type. In later chapters, I'll discuss many of these factors, as well as food and supplements that will help keep each season-type in balance, which is the key to avoiding the diseases that each season-type seems to be especially susceptible to. The two extreme seasons, Summers and Winters, are especially prone to imbalances that can lead to certain diseases.

Summers are prone to their cells becoming far too nonporous and, as a result, later in life tend to develop conditions such as cancer, infections, high blood pressure, osteoarthritis, and seizures. The Summer diet is designed to help Summers get back into balance and stay in balance, especially in the summer months. Later, you'll learn how Summers are especially prone to slipping into an unhealthy state when it's hot outside and why Summers need to be extra diligent about limiting certain foods and adding specific supplements when the weather gets hotter. A discussion of the many complex interactions of various foods and supplements is beyond the scope of this book; however, at their core, these interactions mainly have to do with the fact that a Summer's physiology is constantly fighting to keep the cells from getting too nonporous and too acidic. By eliminating certain foods, such as cheese, butter, fermented foods, fructose, and sugar, Summers can greatly assist their bodies in maintaining balance.

At the other end of the spectrum are Winters, whose cells are prone to becoming far too porous, and, as a result, Winters tend to develop conditions later in life such as rheumatoid arthritis, multiple sclerosis, schizophrenia, psoriasis, low blood pressure, and gall bladder issues. The Winter diet is designed to help Winters get back into balance and stay in balance, especially in the winter months. Later, you'll learn how Winters are especially prone to going into an unhealthy state when it's cold outside and why Winters need to make an extra effort to limit certain foods and add certain supplements as it gets colder outside. A discussion of the complex interactions of various foods and supplements is beyond the scope of this book; however, at their core, these interactions mainly occur because a Winter's physiology is constantly fighting to keep the cells from getting too porous and too alkaline. Winters tend to have an excess of some electrolytes, while being deficient in others, which hinders the proper movement of nutrients into the cell and waste products out of the cell. By eliminating certain foods, such as vegetable oils and fried foods, while adding others, such as high-purine proteins, butter, and cheese, along with proper supplementation, Winters can greatly help their bodies maintain balance.

Autumns and Springs have a much easier time maintaining balance; however, they have to vary their diets a bit more as the weather outside changes, which you'll learn about later. Springs will usually be more like Summers, but when it gets really cold outside, they will have to eat a little more like an Autumn. Conversely, Autumns will usually be more like Winters; however, when it gets hot outside, they will have to eat a little more like a Spring. In the detailed diet section, you'll learn how to modify your diet based on the weather outside, so that you feel your best throughout the year.

You've already learned how insulin affects the cells' protective coating by creating excess cholesterol, which tends to make the cells too nonporous. Other foods and nutrients can also cause the cells to become more porous or less porous. Foods and nutrients that cause the cell to become more porous are often beneficial for Summers and detrimental to Winters, because Summers often have cells that are not porous enough, whereas a Winter's cells are often too porous. Conversely, many foods and nutrients cause the cells to become less porous, which is usually beneficial for Winters and detrimental to Summers. When you get to the diet section, you will notice that many of the foods listed as beneficial for Summers are to be avoided by Winters, and vice versa. Much of this has to do with the effects these foods have on the way that each season-type prefers to produce energy, while other foods are either recommended or cautioned against to help correct certain imbalances that are common in each season-type. Some foods can cause these imbalances to get better or worse for each season-type, so many of the foods listed have less to do with energy production and more to do with helping each season-type stay in balance. An example of this is pears, which should be avoided by Summers in excessive amounts and, to a lesser extent, by Springs. Pears, along with horseradish, contain *peroxidases*. These substances have the ability to make a person's cells even more nonporous and should usually be avoided in large amounts by Summers and, to a lesser extent, by Springs, because these season-types tend to have cells that are too nonporous.

Although eating pears occasionally will not cause serious harm to a Summer, they will tend to throw a Summer out of balance. As long as Summers are aware of this, they can act accordingly. It is like the thousand-pebbles-and-glass analogy. If you throw a single pebble at a pane of glass, odds are you are not going to cause any damage. If you throw a thousand pebbles at the glass at the same time, chances are you will break the glass. In the same way, Summers who are eating according to their season-type can eat an occasional pear without any adverse reaction. Yet if these Summers constantly eat foods such as pears, cheese, sugar, and red meat, while snacking all of the time, they will feel quite horrible.

In later chapters, you will learn why many foods affect your season-type. Some foods will be listed as beneficial and others are to be avoided. I didn't always provide an explanation because, although the Four Seasons Diet is scientific in nature, some of the science is too far beyond the scope of this book. You are encouraged to try a strict diet for your season-type for a while, to see how much better you feel. After that, you can begin to add in some of the "avoid" foods on occasion, but it's recommended that you take notice of how you feel when you do, so that you can begin to equate what you eat with how you feel.

The Blood Sugar and Blood Fat Connection

The Winter diet is high in fat and low in carbohydrates, and the carbohydrates that are recommended are considered low-glycemic carbohydrates. This means that they enter the bloodstream slowly and do not create large spikes in blood sugar or insulin. The Summer diet is at the opposite end of the spectrum and is low in fat and higher in carbohydrates, and the carbohydrates recommended are higher in glycemic value than the carbohydrates recommended for Winters. This is because, as explained earlier, there is a competition between blood sugar and blood fat for control over which fuel the body chooses to primarily burn, and insulin has a big role in this. Even though I spent the first part of this chapter explaining the danger of having high levels of insulin, the real culprit in creating high insulin levels is insulin resistance. People who have normal insulin sensitivity, who are eating the right types of foods, can keep their insulin at healthy levels. In fact, people who are insulin resistant and who begin to follow the right diet for their season-type will lose weight and restore balance and insulin sensitivity to their bodies. Part of the strategy of the Four Seasons Diet is to keep insulin at the right level for your season-type, and a big factor in this entails keeping your energy level and blood sugar stable, which will keep you from overeating due to food cravings.

Your body's blood-sugar plus insulin levels determine the rate at which you use fat as energy. When both blood sugar and insulin increase to a high-enough level, this shuts down the body's ability to use fat to produce energy in several ways. First, it stops your body from breaking down its stored fat and lowers your blood-fat levels. It also turns off a crucial step in the process of burning long-chain fatty acids as energy. Blood fats come in different lengths, called *short-chain fatty acids*, *medium-chain fatty acids*, and *long-chain fatty acids*, depending on the number of carbon atoms they contain. Short-chain fatty acids have fewer than 6 carbon atoms, medium-chain fatty acids have 6 to 12 carbon atoms, and long-chain fatty acids have more than 12 carbon atoms.

Most oils, nuts, dairy foods, and meats contain a variety of fats of varying length. For example, coconut oil primarily consists of medium-chain fatty acids, while dairy products have mainly medium- and long-chain fatty acids, and meat has a very large proportion of long-chain fatty acids. Humans store much of their fat as long-chain fatty acids. When we choose a diet that raises our blood sugar and insulin levels past a certain point, it inhibits our ability to break down our own body fat and to burn any long-chain fatty acids derived from our diet. This is one of the many reasons that the Winter diet promotes low blood sugar and insulin levels, while the Summer diet promotes low dietary fats, especially the long-chain variety. Winters prefer these long-chain fatty acids for energy, so keeping their blood sugar and insulin levels low will help them burn these for energy, while the Summer diet keeps Summers' blood sugar and insulin higher and keeps them from burning these long-chain fatty acids for energy.

As mentioned earlier, Summers are the ones most prone to obesity later in life, and this has a lot to do with the fact that because they do not burn a lot of fat for energy, they tend to accumulate body fat, even when their diet contains what most people would consider a normal amount of fat. Their optimal diet for maximum energy and well-being also keeps them from burning a lot of fat, including body fat, so they tend to store extra dietary fat while not burning it off, which ultimately leads to insulin resistance. This is also the reason belly fat is so bad for Summers. Belly fat completely overwhelms their bodies with a constant supply of blood fat, and, due to their higher glucose and insulin levels, they tend to have an impossible time trying to burn fat for energy, especially if they snack between meals. Yet even in the presence of high insulin, the body is still able to burn short- and medium-chain fatty acids (but not long-chain fatty acids), so these are often a good choice for Summers and are especially prevalent in coconut oil.

If a Winter and a Summer were to follow the same diet, the Winter would tend to have lower insulin and blood-sugar levels than the Summer. This is because the Winter's muscles usually have a higher density of capillaries to supply the muscles with blood, along with sugar, which helps the Winter's body lower the blood-sugar and insulin levels quickly. Most Winters, in fact, tend to have low blood-sugar and insulin levels, and if they eat carbohydrates that have a high glycemic index, they are prone to hypoglycemia as a result of their blood sugar crashing too quickly. Winters also tend to have lower blood-fat levels than Summers do, because they burn more fat for fuel, and the lower your level of blood fat is, the more sensitive your cells will be to insulin. Summers often have high blood-sugar and insulin levels for the opposite reason. Their muscles have far fewer capillaries, and this, combined with the fact that their cells are often too nonporous, works to keep their blood-sugar and insulin levels on the higher side. Summers also tend to have higher blood-fat levels than Winters do, because they burn less fat for fuel, which makes their cells even less sensitive to insulin. Summers are still better off eating medium- to higher-glycemic carbohydrates, however, as this can increase their stored-sugar energy by almost 15 percent when compared to eating lower-glycemic carbohydrates. Having higher levels of stored sugar will help Summers feel full between meals.

In addition to high blood-sugar and insulin levels inhibiting fat-energy production, high levels of blood fats also inhibit sugar-energy production in the presence of high insulin levels. Elevated levels of blood fat can decrease the entire body's glucose uptake by more than 30 percent, while reducing the body's ability to burn sugar for energy by up to 63 percent. As you have probably guessed, this would be quite disastrous for Summers; not only are they burning less sugar, but they are also storing less. This will often make Summers feel hungry, even after eating and especially between meals. High blood fats will decrease sugar-energy production that uses oxygen; however, the fats will have no effect on sugar-energy production that doesn't use oxygen. The problem with this is that only 5 percent of the available energy from each sugar molecule is produced without the need for oxygen, and high blood-fat levels help shut down the steps that make the other 95 percent of the energy possible. In addition, by over-relying on producing energy without the use of oxygen, you tend to accumulate a lot of acid in the cells, which can be very detrimental to the body in high concentrations and contributes to cancer.

Even though Winters rely on fat for energy production, their brains and blood cells often use sugar for energy; in fact, the blood cells can produce the energy they need to keep functioning only by using sugar energy. The brain and the blood cells do not rely on insulin in order to use sugar, so by eating enough protein, which can be converted to stable blood sugar, along with a generous amount of low-glycemic carbohydrates, Winters help fuel their brains and blood cells, while allowing their muscles to burn fat for energy.

Earlier, I discussed a food's insulin index and how both carbohydrates and protein cause the pancreas to secrete insulin. Even though foods such as beef may cause an increase in insulin, what's ultimately important is the overall effect each meal has on blood-sugar levels, insulin levels, and energy production until the next meal.

Remember, it's not insulin that's bad, but rather excessive levels of insulin caused by insulin resistance that are harmful for you. The effects of insulin resistance are especially pronounced when blood-sugar levels are also high and a person's muscles are insulin resistant. So although some protein foods may cause an increase in insulin, they do not result in the same rapid spike in blood sugar that foods high in carbohydrates do. This is one reason the Winter diet is higher in protein.

For example, a meal containing a generous portion of meat, such as one that a Winter might consume, will also be high in protein and fat, while being low in glucose. The ultimate effect of such a meal will be to keep blood-sugar levels stable from the large amount of protein, while supplying enough fat to keep the Winter going until his or her next meal. Also, recall that Winters tend to have muscles that store glucose too quickly in the presence of insulin. By keeping carbohydrate levels low, the Winter diet will help prevent Winters from experiencing erratic blood-sugar issues, which will keep them from snacking between meals and ultimately from consuming too many calories and gaining weight.

4
How Your Season-Type Affects Your pH

Why certain season-types are prone to different pH imbalances, and how to correct them.

When it comes to human health, the significance given to the body's acid and alkaline balance is one of the most unappreciated factors in disease, as well as one of the most overly abused excuses for poor health. On one hand, it's unappreciated by most conventional medical professionals, who choose to ignore its significance until it leads to symptoms and diseases that could have been avoided in the first place. Many physical and mental diseases are preceded by slight acid and alkaline imbalances that occur years before the onset of symptoms that doctors recognize as a "disease." On the other hand, people in the various alternative healing professions usually take things to the opposite extreme, blaming "acidosis" for every ill known to man. They believe that eating "alkaline-forming" foods is the cure for every disease.

Keeping the Body's pH Balanced

The topic of pH balance in the human body is very complex. Rather than go into all of the particulars, I will give you a basic explanation of what pH balance is, how it works, and, most important, how it relates to the four season-types. The pH of any substance is simply the measure of how acidic or alkaline that substance is. The pH scale ranges from 0 to 14, with 0 being the most acidic, 7 being neutral, and 14 being the most alkaline. For example, lemon juice has a pH of approximately 2 and is considered very acidic; distilled water has a pH of 7 and is considered neutral; and baking soda has a pH of around 9 and is considered moderately alkaline.

Just as various foods have different pH's, the many parts of the human body have different pH ranges that they prefer to stay within, in order to function properly. The stomach, for example, is very acidic and usually has a pH range of anywhere from 1.5

to 3.5. The intestines are one of the more alkaline places in the human body and usually have a pH range of around 8.5. The most essential pH that the body has to maintain, however, is the pH of the blood. Although most medical textbooks claim that arterial blood pH should be between 7.35 and 7.45, the few clinical doctors who have studied the topic most extensively as it relates to health have come to the conclusion that our arterial blood pH should be 7.46. According to their research, a deviation of just .01 off this value can result in health problems manifesting. In fact, if our blood pH were to drop down to 7.0 or go up to 8.0, it would most likely result in our quick death. When our blood pH changes from 7.46 in either direction, many of the enzymes in our bodies cease to function properly, and our nerve and muscle activity begins to weaken. Furthermore, many of the protein molecules in our bodies begin to change their shape, and when this happens, they alter the way they behave and react in our bodies, causing minor imbalances that over time can lead to major health problems. Our bodies work very hard to maintain the proper blood pH, and numerous factors can both increase and decrease our pH, many of which have to do with our season-type.

Does Food Affect Our pH?

Certain alternative health professionals believe that the food we eat most affects our bodies' pH. They claim that foods such as meat and sugar are acidic and will cause our bodies to become more acidic, while foods such as fruits and vegetables are alkaline and will cause our bodies to become more alkaline. This misguided belief has its roots in experiments conducted years ago, in which foods were burned until they became ash, and then the pH of the ash was measured. The burned ash of meats was found to be very acidic, while the ash of vegetables was found to be very alkaline. This was due mainly to the various minerals contained in different foods. Many elaborate charts are available in the alternative health world that list the various "acid" and "alkaline" foods, and the usual recommendation is to eat 80 percent alkaline-forming foods and only 20 percent acid-forming foods.

The problem with this belief is that although food does play a role in helping us maintain our blood pH, its function has far more to do with how our particular season-type reacts to the foods we eat than with whether the foods create an alkaline or acid ash when burned. Most of the highly acidic hydrogen ions in our bodies are metabolic by-products of energy production, and only a very small amount of acidic substances enter the body from the foods we eat. For example, the breakdown of protein, which is high in phosphorous, releases phosphoric acid into our bodies, whereas producing fast-sugar energy in the absence of oxygen creates excess hydrogen ions, and the metabolism of fats can yield ketone bodies, all of which are acidic and must be neutralized or eliminated by the body. The simple act of breathing produces carbon dioxide, which is also acidic, and this acid must be eliminated. Most of the carbon dioxide (CO_2) that our bodies produce is converted to carbonic acid, which then gets converted to other substances when transported in the blood. Most of these substances get reconverted back into CO_2 when they enter the lungs, in order to be eliminated. When I talk about CO_2 in this chapter, I am referring to all of the CO_2 contained in the blood in whatever form, which increases the blood's acidity.

The Role of Buffers

To help maintain the proper pH balance of its various organs and fluids, the body uses several different mechanisms. The first is the use of *buffers*. Buffers are similar to sponges that can soak up highly acidic or highly alkaline substances and in the process convert them to slightly acidic or slightly alkaline substances. Although buffers do not eliminate these substances, they do tie them up temporarily by minimizing their pH effect until the body can deal with them and eliminate them. The biggest advantage of these buffers is that they work extremely quickly, in a fraction of a second, and help maintain pH values when these change quickly, as might occur during strenuous exercise. So even though the food we eat does influence our blood pH, our metabolism of those foods has a far greater influence, which can vary by season-type. Our blood levels of CO_2 also play a very significant role in our bodies' pH and are largely influenced by the rate at which we breathe to eliminate acidic CO_2, as well as by the concentration of an alkaline substance called *bicarbonate* that is contained in our blood. One of the most important regulators of our body's pH is actually our respiration—our breathing.

Breathing and pH

When the blood is too acidic due to excess CO_2, the body simply increases its respiration rate and expels more carbon dioxide. When our blood becomes too alkaline from not enough CO_2, our breathing rate decreases to hold onto more carbon dioxide. A simple doubling or halving of our respiration rate can raise or lower our blood pH by .2 in either direction, and because ideal blood pH is 7.46, this .2 change can vary our blood pH from 7.26 to 7.66 in a matter of minutes. It is very rare that a person would ever have blood as acidic as 7.26 or as alkaline as 7.66 for a prolonged period of time; someone who had either value consistently would usually be in an extremely unhealthy state. Even though carbon dioxide is an acid in our bodies, it also has the ability to act as a buffer in conjunction with the hemoglobin in our blood. Although proper breathing is highly effective and efficient at regulating blood pH, in Chapter 9 you'll learn more about how our modern high-stress Western lifestyle has undermined our health by increasing our breathing rate, and you'll find out what you can do about it.

How the Kidneys Help Balance pH

The third way the human body deals with pH imbalances is through the help of the kidneys—the slowest of the systems the body uses to regulate acid and alkaline balance. The kidneys often take days to restore pH balance by dealing with the acids produced from cellular metabolism: phosphoric acid, lactic acid, and ketone bodies. The kidneys also assist the blood by helping to regulate the level of alkaline bicarbonate and acidic hydrogen ions in the blood. To accomplish this, the kidneys use minerals such as sodium and potassium that they obtain from the foods we eat. Our modern Western diet contains far too much sodium and is usually way too low in potassium, so, in this sense, alternative health professionals who claim that fruits and vegetables can help alkalinize our bodies are partly correct. The crucial thing lacking in the modern diet is usually potassium, especially if not enough fruits and vegetables are eaten. Yet even the need for potassium is very dependent on an individual's season-type, and potassium can actually cause the blood of some season-types to become more acidic, by boosting the rate at which they burn sugar for energy, thereby increasing the levels of acidic carbon dioxide in the blood.

Weather and Climate Affect Blood pH

Another factor that can greatly affect our blood pH is the outside temperature. Warm weather tends to make the blood more alkaline, while cold weather tends to make the blood more acidic. When I talk about acidic blood vs. alkaline blood, I mean that blood with a pH below 7.46 is acidic and blood with a pH above 7.46 is alkaline. Because any pH above 7.0 is technically alkaline, both pH's are technically alkaline; however, in this case, since the ideal blood pH is 7.46, acidic blood means blood that has a pH below 7.46. When Winters are out of balance, they tend to have blood that is too acidic, so they often feel better in warm weather and worse in colder weather. When Summers are out of balance, they usually have blood that is too alkaline, and they often feel better in cold weather and worse in hot weather. When your blood pH is out of balance, you have a hard time handling temperature extremes in any direction. Both Summers and Winters who are severely out of balance will often feel bad in any extreme temperature, whether hot or cold. Yet a Winter who is out of balance because of blood that is too acidic will usually feel better if it's slightly warm and may even prefer extreme heat. Winters usually feel worse when it's slightly cold, and most will definitely feel lousy in extreme cold unless they make proper adjustments to their diet. If you think of the foods we traditionally eat in the winter, which are the foods that Winters thrive on year-round, these are the same foods that Winters need to eat even more of when it's cold outside. Foods that are high in fat and protein are Winters' staples year round, but the colder it gets, the more they need to focus on even higher levels of fat and protein, especially the type of proteins called purines, which I'll discuss later.

A Summer who is out of balance often has blood that is too alkaline and usually feels better if it's slightly cool and may even prefer extreme cold. Summers usually feel worse when it's warm and humid and will definitely feel worse in extreme heat and humidity. If you think of the foods we traditionally eat in the summer, which are the foods that Summers thrive on year round, these are the foods that Summers will have to eat even more of when it's hot, if they are out of balance: foods that are low in fat and protein, especially low in protein with purines. It's worth mentioning that when it's cold or hot outside, the humidity can have a tremendous effect on unbalancing the season-types. The higher the humidity, the more temperature fluctuations can cause imbalances in the four season-types, and the more they will have to attempt to adjust their diets.

Adjusting the Diet for Outside Temperatures

Climate has another profound effect on the season-types, besides influencing their blood pH. In Chapter 3, I talked about cell permeability, and how Winters tend to have cells that are too porous, while Summers usually have cells that are not porous enough. Climate also has an effect on cell permeability. Our cells tend to become more permeable when we're cold. For Winters whose cells already tend to be too permeable, the cold simply makes matters worse, unless Winters make sure to eat plenty of foods that are high in saturated fats and cholesterol. When we're hot, our cells tend to become less permeable. For Summers, who usually have cells that are already not permeable enough, the heat just makes matters worse, especially if it's combined with high humidity. When Summers are too hot, they need to be extra diligent about minimizing the saturated fats and the cholesterol in their diet. In essence, cold weather tends to make several of the Winter's typical imbalances worse and the Summer's imbalances better, whereas heat tends to make several of the Summer's usual imbalances worse and the Winter's imbalances better. The good news is that each of the season-types can modify his or her diet throughout the year as the temperature changes, in order to feel 100 percent year round.

The ways that the foods we eat affect our blood pH has mostly to do with our season-type and the effects that different diets have on the four season-types. When following their ideal diet, Winters tend to burn primarily fat for energy, while Summers usually burn mainly carbohydrates. This allows both season-types to maintain adequate steady levels of energy, which greatly helps their bodies keep the proper pH. Most Winters and Summers, however, are eating foods that make up the traditional Western diet, which is far from ideal for them. In fact, due to having the wrong diet, Winters often produce way too much of their energy from carbohydrates, while Summers on the wrong diet produce too much energy from fat. This is often the cause of overly acidic blood in Winters and overly alkaline blood in Summers. Although it may seem counterintuitive, when Winters and Summers get out of balance, their bodies frequently rely on the exact opposite fuels that their bodies prefer. In essence, by eating the wrong foods, they are burning the wrong fuel mix for their season-type.

There is a relationship between our levels of blood fat and blood sugar and how our bodies produce energy. This is also greatly affected by many of the imbalances I have already mentioned. A high level of blood fat, for example, has been shown to decrease carbohydrate oxidation by almost 40 percent during exercise. The other thing that interferes with the use of carbohydrates for energy production is low levels of stored sugar in the muscles and the liver, which can be caused by a low-carbohydrate diet or by insulin resistance.

Summers often suffer from insulin resistance, for a number of reasons. Because they don't burn a lot of fat for energy, they may end up storing it to use during a possible future time of deprivation that never seems to come, which contributes to insulin resistance. Also, Summers tend to have cells that are not porous enough, which usually prevents them from storing sugar as energy, in addition to contributing directly to insulin resistance. The lack of cell permeability makes their cells overly acidic, which also prevents sugar-energy production. Furthermore, they frequently have high levels of blood fat, due to the fact that Summers eating foods on the standard Western diet will easily get triple the amount of fat that their bodies can ever hope to use for energy. These problems for Summers will be even worse if they have a lot of belly fat, which tends to dump large amounts of fat into the bloodstream throughout the day. Remember that Summers have very few fat-burning muscles. The combination of overly acidic cells, high blood-fat levels, and low stored-sugar levels puts them in a state where their bodies actually rely on fat to produce energy. This is a state of extremely low energy for a Summer, and very little fat or sugar is burned with oxygen for energy. As a result, Summers in this state have very low levels of CO_2 in their blood, which makes the blood overly alkaline.

The Ratio of CO_2 to Bicarbonate in the Blood
I have explained how the body can easily compensate for high or low levels of CO_2 by changing the rate of breathing, so in a normal person whose blood pH is balanced at 7.46 most of the time this will not be a problem. This is not the case, however, for someone who is chronically out of balance, with a high or low blood pH. I mentioned that CO_2 in the blood is acidic, while bicarbonate in the blood is alkaline. The body normally keeps the ratio of bicarbonate to CO_2 at 20 parts bicarbonate to 1 part CO_2, in order to help maintain a pH of 7.46. It's not the absolute level of bicarbonate or CO_2 that determines blood pH, but, rather, it is the ratio between the two. As long as the ratio is 20 parts bicarbonate to 1 part CO_2, our blood can easily maintain a pH close to 7.46. What happens, however, is that because Summers who are in a state of poor health produce so little CO_2, their levels of bicarbonate begin to drop, as their bodies try to keep the 20-to-1 ratio. Although this does succeed in keeping the blood pH balanced, to some extent,

there is a downside. Even though the ratio determines pH, having higher overall levels of both CO_2 and bicarbonate in a 20-to-1 ratio allows the blood to maintain a perfect pH much more easily than having low levels of both in the same ratio, as I'll discuss further in Chapter 9. As a result, the kidneys have to become more involved in maintaining our pH balance, and the kidneys take days, not minutes, to restore an imbalanced pH. Before I go any further, I'll give you some background information that will make the explanation easier to understand.

Blood pH Abnormalities in the Season-Types
In the 1970s, experiments were conducted on mentally ill people whose metabolisms were similar to the individuals I call Summers and Winters and who had abnormally high or low blood pH and suffered from mental illness. Even though they were not called Summers and Winters in this experiment, I will refer to them as such, given their similar physiologies. Although healthy blood pH should be 7.46, the average mentally ill Summer had a blood pH of 7.54, while the average mentally ill Winter had a blood pH of 7.36. In these experiments, Summers were given vitamin supplements that increased the rate that they burned carbohydrates for energy, while Winters were given vitamin supplements that increased the rate that they burned fat for energy. Burning carbohydrates for energy tends to make the blood more acidic than burning fat for energy does. As a result of the patients simply ingesting the proper vitamin and mineral supplements to help restore each season-type to his or her preferred source of energy production, the average blood pH of the Summers went from 7.54 to 7.43, while the average blood pH of the Winters went from 7.36 to 7.46. The effects on their mental illness were often miraculous. Some patients who had been confined to mental institutions for years experienced complete clinical remission of their symptoms in a matter of weeks. In one case, a patient suffering from severe anxiety, which had prevented him from driving a car and working at the beginning of the experiment, was able to drive and had obtained a job at the end of the experiment. This experiment was so successful that 55 percent of the patients were classified as showing a clinical remission of symptoms, 25 percent demonstrated a marked reduction in the intensity of their symptoms, and 20 percent showed a noticeable reduction in the severity of their symptoms.

What these experiments proved was that people with physiologies similar to Summers tend to have very low levels of CO_2

when they consume too much fat and not enough carbohydrates. In fact, the "Summers" chosen for the experiment had almost half the level of CO_2 in their bodies, compared to the people in the study whom I call "Winters." Because the blood tries to keep the bicarbonate level 20 times as high as the levels of CO_2, Summers also had lower overall bicarbonate levels than the Winters did. Rather than a 20-to-1 ratio, however, the Summers in this experiment had an average ratio of greater than 27 to 1, which was the reason for their overly alkaline blood. These low overall CO_2 and bicarbonate levels make the blood far less effective at acting like a spongelike buffer that stores excess acids until the kidneys can help eliminate them. This makes it very difficult for Summers in this state of imbalance to maintain a stable blood pH, which further contributes to their erratic energy production and the awful way they feel. To make matters worse, the low level of CO_2 in the blood means much less oxygen gets into the tissues to produce energy. This is because the blood releases oxygen much easier in the presence of higher CO_2 levels, and Summers with low blood CO_2 will have less CO_2 in their tissues, which means not enough oxygen gets into their cells in order to produce energy using oxygen. Combine this with Summers having cells that are usually not porous enough, which makes it more difficult for whatever oxygen *is* released to get into the cell, and you can see why Summers in this state would have such incredibly low levels of energy. Often, to compensate, Summers begin to consume large quantities of caffeine just to get by, which helps both boost energy and acidify the blood.

Diet Remedies to Correct Blood pH
The solution for Summers in this situation is easy but often takes time. In addition to taking the right vitamin supplements, adhering to the proper Summer diet will eventually balance out a Summer's metabolism. If Summers are overweight and insulin resistant, this could take a while; however, once they begin to burn sugar instead of fat they will produce more CO_2 and take more oxygen into their cells. By combining the Summer diet with the breathing techniques described in Chapter 9, Summers will be able to raise their bicarbonate levels and CO_2 levels much higher, which will give their blood extra buffering power and make it much easier for them to maintain pH balance.

Winters have a similar but slightly different problem when they do not follow a balanced Winter diet. Their cells tend to become too porous and are often overly sensitive to insulin, even though they have much lower insulin levels on average than Summers. Remember that fat-burning muscles can also burn sugar for energy. Winters who have a standard Western diet tend to eat far too many starchy carbohydrates for their metabolism, and as a result when their blood-sugar level goes up, it can rapidly crash, especially if they are not eating enough protein and fat. Fat-burning muscles are also much better than sugar-burning muscles at allowing stored sugar to enter them, due to the fact that they have a much better blood supply. As a result, when Winters eat too many starchy carbohydrates, their erratic blood sugar keeps them constantly bingeing on carbohydrates, which can lead to weight issues, as well as insulin resistance and diabetes later in life.

Whereas Summers often suffer from insulin resistance early in life, a Winter tends to be overly sensitive to insulin early in life, which results in years of overeating carbohydrates and often leads to insulin resistance later in life. To make matters even worse for the Winter, the first step in burning carbohydrates for energy turns off the body's ability to burn long-chain fats for energy, which is the Winter's preferred fuel source. As a result, the Winter's muscles are often burning way too much sugar too quickly and not enough fat for energy. Burning carbohydrates actually produces more CO_2 for each unit of energy currency than burning fat does. So Winters burning sugar for energy end up producing excessive amounts of CO_2, and as a result, their blood tends to become overly acidic. In the previously mentioned experiment, out-of-balance Winters had almost twice the CO_2 level as out-of-balance Summers, and Winters' bicarbonate levels were lower than the 20-to-1 ratio, which ended up making their blood overly acidic. Due to the fact that out-of-balance Winters tend have an overall higher level of both CO_2 and bicarbonate than out-of-balance Summers, however, Winters who are out of balance have an easier time buffering their blood pH than do Summers who are out of balance. The higher CO_2 level leads to a higher level of oxygen in the tissues, though, and this, combined with cells that are often too permeable, contributes to oxidation, which can get out of control. Whereas the Summer's main problem when following the standard Western diet is having low levels of energy all of the time, the Winter's main problem with the standard Western diet is energy production that is out of control, with blood-sugar highs that crash and turn into blood-sugar lows that need to be fed with more carbohydrates.

By changing to the proper diet, Winters should fairly easily get their blood sugar stable and begin to burn mainly fat for energy. This will also help balance their blood pH and will make weight loss much easier, if that is their goal.

The main factors that can upset acid and alkaline balance are genetics, food, temperature, breathing, and stress. We cannot control our genetics, but once we understand our season-type, we can work with our given genetics to stay in balance. We have much more control over the other four, especially when we understand how they affect our health and how we can manage them to our benefit. I'll briefly touch on a few of the other things that often contribute to an acid or alkaline imbalance in our bodies.

Over-Breathing and Under-Breathing Affect Blood pH
In our modern high-stress society, over-breathing is one of the main reasons our blood can become too alkaline. As I'll elaborate on in Chapter 9, many scientific studies show that during the last hundred years, the rate at which most people breathe has doubled. Stress, anxiety, and worry often cause us to breathe too much, and in the process we blow off too much CO_2, which increases the alkalinity of our blood pH. Caffeine also speeds up our breathing rate by tricking the receptors in our bodies that sense CO_2 levels into thinking we have too much CO_2 in our blood, which causes our breathing rate to accelerate. In one study, drinking large quantities of caffeinated beverages resulted in a 40 percent increase in the amount of air that was breathed every minute while the study participants were at rest, which caused a significant decrease in their blood levels of CO_2. Even though this would normally cause the blood pH to become more alkaline, studies have also shown caffeine to boost sugar energy during exercise by up to 26 percent, which would make the blood more acidic. Experiments have demonstrated that caffeine ingestion usually increases the acidity of the blood by around .04 points. This boost in sugar energy and decrease in alkalinity of the blood's pH are two reasons Summers often do well on caffeine when they are out of balance, whereas Winters may feel overly excited and jittery on caffeine when they are out of balance. Sadly for Summers, however, the short-term fix of using caffeine to boost their low energy levels and acidify their overly alkaline blood ultimately causes them to breathe more frequently, which makes their blood even more alkaline if they are stressed out and tend to over-breathe throughout the day.
Under-breathing can cause our blood to become overly acidic, and although this is not as common as over-breathing, depression

of our central nervous system from drugs such as sedatives and muscle relaxants can cause us to under-breath.

Tips to Maintain a Healthy pH

As mentioned earlier, our blood pH is largely controlled by our breathing and our kidneys. The lungs control the CO_2 levels, while the kidneys control the level of bicarbonate, so our pH is really a function of how well our lungs and kidneys keep our blood balanced. Any time the ratio of bicarbonate to CO_2 falls below 20:1, acidosis exists, and when the ratio goes above 20:1, alkalosis exists. Imbalances are often brought about by eating the wrong foods for your season-type. Summers on a high-fat diet, especially if they have belly fat, will create such a fat overload that they tend to produce very little energy at all, causing low CO_2 levels, which leads to alkaline blood. A simple correction to the diet and taking specific supplements can easily correct this problem.

Similarly, a Winter on a high-carbohydrate diet will tend to burn sugar too quickly, creating high levels of CO_2, which lead to acidic blood. Winters do need to make sure to include some carbohydrates in their diets, however, because the brain prefers sugar for fuel, and the red blood cells can use only sugar for fuel. When all carbohydrates are eliminated from the diet, the body begins to convert protein and fat into fuel for the brain and the red blood cells, which can cause the blood to become too acidic. So the key for Winters is to eat just the right amount of lower-glycemic carbohydrates. The blood can become overly acidic in several ways, including the two that follow: too many high-glycemic carbohydrates can acidify the blood by overproducing CO_2, and too few carbohydrates can acidify the blood by creating too many acidic substances in an attempt to break down fat and protein to fuel the brain and the red blood cells.

Although the lungs and the kidneys do a great job of keeping our blood pH balanced, the more we eat according to our season-type, the easier it is for the body to keep itself in balance. When we are in balance, our bodies can do a much better job of maintaining our health. When we are chronically overly acidic or alkaline, our mineral balances are often upset. Sometimes, we will retain or lose too much of one mineral, such as potassium or magnesium, which can greatly add to the problems caused by acid and alkaline imbalances. The goal is to have your blood consistently stay close to the ideal blood pH of 7.46. When you are chronically out of balance in one direction, your body has a more difficult time regulating your blood pH.

One of the best gauges of how balanced you are, and how high your buffer reserves are, is how well your body is able to handle temperature fluctuations. When someone is constantly cycling back and forth between feeling too hot or too cold or comfortable and uncomfortable, there is a good chance that the person is out of balance and has low buffer reserves. Picture the difference between a healthy child and someone who is elderly and unhealthy. The child can play out in the cold without a jacket or go out in the heat and will hardly ever complain about being too hot or cold. When some people get older and their blood pH becomes erratic and their reserve buffers get low, they may find themselves repeatedly putting on a sweater or a jacket and then taking it off again, trying to help their bodies maintain balance.

As you begin to keep your blood pH more balanced and increase your supply of buffers, you should feel far more comfortable in a variety of temperatures. An out-of-balance Winter will often feel cold, when compared to other people in the same room, while an out-of-balance Summer often feels too hot compared to others in the same room. Keeping your blood pH balanced will also heighten your overall feeling of well-being, make you more clear-headed, give you steadier energy throughout the day, and help eliminate hunger between meals. The pH imbalances caused by food, temperature, breathing, and stress may make you turn to "comfort foods" to feel better. Yet although you might feel better in the short run, in the long run eating the wrong foods for your season-type is the very thing that caused you to feel bad and turn to these foods in the first place. The more out of balance you are, the more you reach for comfort foods, causing you to become yet more imbalanced, until one day a doctor tells you have diabetes, cancer, or some other disease. All of these imbalances feed on one another, leading to even greater imbalances and ultimately diseases.

The Four Seasons Diet gives you the information you need to keep yourself balanced, combined with the perfect mechanism for gauging your results—*your feelings*! The bottom line is that the more you are in balance, the better you will feel, and the more out of balance you are, the worse you will feel. Whenever I meet new people and figure out what their season-type is, I can usually tell them what all of their favorite vegetables are. This is because some vegetables help balance Winters, while others help balance Summers. The reason Winters or Summers like certain vegetables is because these vegetables make them feel better when they eat them. People have come to associate certain vegetables with feeling good after they eat them and others with feeling bad after they eat them. This ultimately has to do with energy production and blood pH. By the end of this book, you will have all of the knowledge you need to keep yourself in balance. When you use that knowledge and learn to associate the foods you eat with the feelings that result from the food keeping you in balance or out of balance, you will become the owner of your health!

The Nervous System

Note: The following section on the autonomic nervous system is based on the observations of many clinical research scientists. Although the effect that diet has on the nervous system has been well documented, the exact causes and mechanisms are not well understood at this point. As such, the following is my attempt to explain these observations and how they relate to the four season-types, given the best available science at this time. There are many questions on this topic that science has yet to fully understand or answer.

Earlier, I mentioned the experiments conducted in the 1970s on patients whose blood pH was very out of balance and who suffered from mental illness. When they were given supplements that improved their blood pH, most of them had a significant lessening of their symptoms, and their blood pH returned very close to the ideal of 7.46, as their energy production returned to normal. In these cases, the Winters had overly acidic blood, and the Summers had overly alkaline blood. Even though this is the most common pH imbalance in Winters and Summers, oftentimes the opposite can be true.

Breathing has a great effect on pH, so a Winter who over-breathes can easily have alkaline blood, while a Summer who under-breathes can have acidic blood. Another factor that can influence blood pH in the opposite direction is the difference in CO_2 produced from burning fat for energy vs. burning sugar. Remember that burning sugar with oxygen for energy produces more CO_2 per unit of energy currency than burning fat does, and CO_2 acidifies the blood. Furthermore, Winters have a much richer supply of blood and oxygen to their muscles and are usually able to oxidize far more fuel than the average Summer can. Summers who are in very good balance and able to produce a lot of energy using sugar will produce far more CO_2 than they do when they are out of balance. Conversely, Winters who are in balance and have their blood sugar under control will produce much of their energy from fat and will produce less CO_2 than they do when they are out of balance. In these cases, it will be the Summer whose blood could become overly acidic, while the Winter's blood can become overly alkaline. In both of these cases, though, energy production will be high and blood sugar stable. This makes it much easier for the season-types to stay closer to a blood pH of 7.46. When this happens, the main problem for the season-types has to do with how their imbalances affect the autonomic nervous system, as opposed to how those imbalances affect energy production.

The Autonomic Nervous System
Our autonomic nervous system controls the bodily functions that for the most part are not under our direct mental control, such as our heart rate, digestion, breathing rate, and perspiration, along with many other similar functions. Some autonomic functions, such as our breathing rate, can also be controlled by the conscious mind, although usually breathing is handled without our consciously thinking about it. The autonomic nervous system has two branches: the sympathetic branch and the parasympathetic branch.

The sympathetic branch of the autonomic nervous system is known as the "fight or flight" branch because it's the branch that is most active when we feel threatened, frightened, or excited. When this branch takes over, you may find your heart pounding, with rapid deep breathing, skin that is sweaty and cold, and dilated pupils. If you have ever narrowly avoided a serious car accident in a split second, and afterward your heart pounded and you felt suddenly excited, this is a sign that your sympathetic branch was in full gear.

The other branch of the nervous system is the parasympathetic branch, which is often referred to as the "rest and digest" branch, because it is most active when we are resting and conserving energy. This branch takes over when we relax, especially after digesting a large meal. When this branch is in charge, your heart rate, breathing rate, and blood pressure are all in the low-normal range. Your pupils constrict when the rest-and-digest branch takes over, and your focus is accommodated for close-up vision. If you have ever eaten a large dinner and then you sat on the couch, reading a good book, while you felt very relaxed and calm, this is a sign that your parasympathetic branch was in full gear.

The two branches work together to speed you up and slow you down throughout the day. It's very much like driving a car, with the sympathetic branch being the gas pedal and the parasympathetic branch the brake. You need both to get where you are going. Similar to our nervous systems, the gas pedal tells your engine to burn more fuel, and the brake tells your engine to slow down and conserve fuel.

Many Summers Are Stuck in "High Gear"

When Summers have overly acidic blood, they are usually producing plenty of energy but often have a sympathetic nervous systems that is overstimulated. It would be like trying to stop your car by hitting the brake while still pressing down on the gas pedal. You are going to slow down, but not very quickly or completely. When Winters have overly alkaline blood, they have usually balanced out their erratic blood-sugar problems, but they often have parasympathetic nervous systems that are overstimulated. This would be like trying to get your car to go somewhere, while always keeping your foot on the brake. You may move, but not very quickly.

There are many reasons that Summers often have sympathetic nervous systems that are stuck in high gear all of the time; it has to do with some of their common imbalances. Many scientists have conducted research on factors that may cause the sympathetic nervous system to become overstimulated. A large amount of blood fat, high insulin levels, too much CO_2 in the blood, high cholesterol levels, and deficiencies of the essential fats EPA and DHA have all been shown to cause the sympathetic nervous system to get out of control. With the exception of high CO_2 levels, every single one of these factors is a common imbalance among Summers when they have an alkaline blood pH and low energy production. Their CO_2 levels begin to climb as Summers get into balance and increase their energy production, at which point all of these factors can be present in Summers for a while, until they learn to control whatever is responsible by following the diet for their season-type. When a Summer's sympathetic nervous system is stuck in high gear, the person will tend to produce *catecholamines*, which help contribute to a Summer's insulin resistance. Which of the two issues manifests as the main problem for Summers depends on how out of balance they are.

When Summers are highly insulin resistant and eat too

much fat, they produce a lot of insulin but very little energy. In this state, even though their nervous systems may be in full gear, their poor state of being is dominated by their complete lack of energy production, so they usually feel tired all of the time. They are producing so little energy and CO_2 as a result that their blood in this state is usually overly alkaline. As they begin to eat according to their season-type and slowly balance their bodies, they burn more carbohydrates for energy and in the process produce more CO_2, which drives their blood pH in the acidic direction. Energy production is no longer their problem, but if their insulin, cholesterol, and blood-fat levels are still high, they will have a revved-up nervous system, along with their higher energy production. In this state, they are not exhausted but are running on high gear all of the time.

Summers tend to be extreme "type A" high achievers early in life. A very typical pattern for Summers is that when they are young and are stuck in sympathetic mode, they are high achievers, always on the go, and then often, from their thirties through their fifties, when they get really out of balance, their energy level plummets, and they find themselves unable to function at even half of their former pace. Imbalances can be caused by the Summers' using up their supply of minerals involved in carbohydrate energy production, by insulin resistance, by belly fat, or oftentimes by a combination of all three. Anything that helps Summers restore their insulin sensitivity, such as weight loss or working out regularly, will ultimately help subdue their sympathetic nervous system and balance them out.

Many Winters Are Too Laid-Back

Winters frequently have the exact opposite problem. Their parasympathetic nervous systems are often overstimulated, so that Winters constantly have their brakes pressed down. All of the things that cause the sympathetic nervous system to be overstimulated in Summers, such as high insulin and high levels of blood fat, are often very low in Winters. This can be part of what keeps a Winter's parasympathetic nervous system dominant, although there is not a lot of research on the topic at this point.

The greatest factor for both Winters and Summers, however, in their potential nervous system imbalances is usually the minerals in their bodies. Sympathetic nervous system activity is increased by the minerals calcium and phosphorous, while parasympathetic nervous system activity is intensified by the minerals potassium and magnesium. Both season-types tend to use up more of certain minerals than others in their production of energy. Summers require more potassium and magnesium in their energy production, and this, in addition their often high levels of insulin, causes them to lose even more magnesium through urination. This frequently leaves them with higher levels of calcium and phosphorous and lower levels of potassium and magnesium, which has the effect of strengthening their sympathetic nervous system, while decreasing the strength of their parasympathetic nervous system. As a result, Summers' nervous systems are always on the go, until at some point they finally burn out and find they cannot keep on going.

Winters, conversely, require more calcium and phosphorous in their energy production and often have excess potassium and magnesium. This tends to increase the strength of their parasympathetic nervous system, while decreasing the strength of their sympathetic nervous system, leaving them oftentimes relaxed and happy-go-lucky. The problem with this is that Winters are sometimes too happy-go-lucky, and things that should concern them often do not, frequently to their detriment.

The good news is that the diet and the minerals that help each season-type balance out his or her energy production also help balance out the nervous system. One example of this is how potassium benefits Summers. Potassium helps increase the rate at which Summers burn sugar for energy. Summers can often be low in this mineral, especially on the standard Western diet, which is high in sodium but low in potassium. When Summers get really out of balance from years of following the wrong diet, they may have very alkaline blood, due to low energy production. Simply giving Summers potassium will help increase the rate at which they burn sugar for energy, and in the process they will begin to produce more CO_2, which will acidify their blood. At some point, they may be producing plenty of energy and may find themselves with acidic blood and sympathetic nervous systems that are stuck in high gear. As they continue the diet and the supplementation for their season-type, many of the other factors causing the nervous system imbalance, such as high insulin levels, will also begin to correct themselves. During this time, the potassium will increase the strength of their parasympathetic system, and in the process of balancing out the nervous system, potassium will actually cause the blood to become a little less acidic, hopefully to a perfect 7.46. So, in this case, the potassium serves a few purposes and has several effects on the Summer.

Be Strict to Give the Diet a Chance to Work

Ultimately, as each season-type begins to work with his or her body by feeding it the right foods and nutrients, the body should have a much easier time staying in balance. The Four Seasons Diet was designed to take into account many subtle effects that various foods might have on the different season-types. For this reason, it's recommended that you strictly stick to the diet for a while. Although you may feel better within the first few meals, it is very easy to plateau at a certain level of wellness for a period of time, perhaps even feel a little worse now and then, and suddenly feel better than you have in years.

Here is one common example to illustrate why it's important to be strict for a while, to give your body a chance to reach its full potential. Summers are often insulin resistant and produce very low amounts of energy. When first going on the Summer diet, they may notice an increase in energy, along with a decrease in appetite and a weight loss. This is because the Summer diet is lower in fat. If Summers have an excess of belly fat, they are often producing plenty of fat, even though they are eating way less. The diet should keep their blood sugar much more balanced, and, partly due to their increased energy and decreased appetite, they will eventually burn off their belly fat. At some point, when Summers have been on the diet long enough, they will regain their insulin sensitivity and feel better than they have in years. Often, however, right before they get to that point, they will experience a drop in energy. It's as if the body realizes it has almost burned off all of the fat it wants to, but because it has not yet regained full insulin sensitivity, it is not storing enough sugar. The body has been releasing a lot of stored fat in the process of burning off the belly fat, and often, right before full insulin sensitivity returns, the level of fat the body produces suddenly drops. This is because Summers are burning off less belly fat. The brief period between when they are burning off less fat and full restoration of insulin sensitivity is usually a time where Summers' energy levels may drop for just a bit. By keeping up the diet, however, Summers will regain their full insulin sensitivity, and at that point, they begin to store and burn sugar properly for the first time in years, and their energy skyrockets.

Later in this book, you will learn how to use food to help balance each season-type, and you'll hear about some of the challenges the season-types might expect, as they begin to balance themselves out. Just remember, it has probably taken you several years to gain weight and get unhealthy, and it may take a little time before you feel 100 percent. The main thing to keep in mind is that ideally, when you eat according to your season-type, you should begin to feel more energy, less hunger between meals, more clarity of thought, and an ever increasing mental well-being.

Part III
Discover Your Ideal Diet

5
Protein, Carbohydrates, Fat, and Minerals

Various types of proteins, carbohydrates, fats, and minerals and how they affect your season-type.

Most of you have probably read the label on a package of food that lists the amount of protein, carbohydrates, and fat in that particular item. You may also have a general understanding of what protein, carbohydrates, and fats are. Unfortunately, you were probably never told that there are different types and properties of protein, carbohydrates, and fats, which determine whether they are beneficial or detrimental to your season-type. The good news is that there is a simple and easy-to-understand explanation of how various types of protein, carbohydrates, and fats, as well as other components of foods, affect your season-type. Once you learn a few simple rules for your season-type in regard to food choices, you should have an easy time eating in a way that helps you maintain your ideal weight, with high levels of energy and mental clarity throughout the day.

Don't feel overwhelmed by all of this information. In just a bit, I will explain the various diets for each season-type, in light of everything you have learned so far. I'll also provide easy-to-read food charts that will help you focus on your ideal foods, while eliminating the worst foods for your season-type. Once you learn a few basic rules about the foods to focus on and avoid, you'll have an easy time losing weight, if that's your goal. Once you're at your ideal weight, it will be far easier for you to gauge the effects of the various foods you eat, in order to fine-tune your diet to determine what works best for you.

Protein

When people hear the word *protein*, they often think of foods that are high in protein, such as meat and cheese. In reality, most foods contain some amount of protein. Even foods normally considered carbohydrates, such as grains, contain on average between 12 and 16 percent protein, with the exception being rice, which is only about 7 to 8 percent protein. Proteins in foods are large molecules, which are composed of smaller units called amino acids. **Amino acids** (<u>protein building blocks</u>) are similar to the building blocks used to create large protein molecules, so I will refer to them as "protein building blocks." There are twenty-two different protein building blocks, twenty of which are used regularly by the human body. Of these, nine are considered "essential" because they cannot be made by our bodies from the other protein building blocks but must be obtained from the foods we eat. Proteins are considered "complete" proteins when they contain adequate levels of all of the essential protein building blocks. A single large protein molecule, such as might be found in milk, is often composed of thousands of different protein building blocks arranged in various ways, quantities, and lengths. Often, a large protein molecule may lack adequate levels of one or more of the essential protein building blocks, and these large proteins are considered "incomplete proteins."

Egg whites and milk proteins are usually considered to be among the most perfect proteins, because they contain all of the essential protein building blocks in a near perfect ratio. This is not surprising, given that egg whites are consumed by the growing chick inside the egg, and milk is consumed by a growing baby mammal. In both cases, the purpose of these large proteins is to supply all of the protein building blocks necessary for optimum growth, and this requires all of the essential protein building blocks in the proper ratio.

Other foods, such as many grains, are considered "incomplete" proteins, because they lack one or more of the essential protein building blocks. By combining certain foods that may individually be incomplete proteins, however, it's possible to create a meal with complete protein. A good example of this is combining rice and beans in one meal, which, when eaten together, create a complete protein.

The amount of protein each individual needs can vary greatly, depending on age, activity level, and season-type. Typically, younger children who are still growing need greater amounts of protein, as do people engaged in strenuous activity. For optimum health and well-being, the amount of protein consumed should be tailored to someone's season-type. Of the four season-types, Winters need the most protein, followed by Autumns, Springs, and Summers. In part, this is because a high protein level helps keep someone in fat-burning mode, as explained earlier, and each season-type prefers to burn varying amounts of fat for energy. Besides containing the essential protein building blocks, which are needed by all of the season-types, many proteins also contain *purines*, which are beneficial for some season-types and detrimental to others.

Foods high in purines include meat, especially darker meats and organ meats. Many vegetarian foods, such as most beans, peas, and certain vegetables, are also high in purines. Purines have a dramatic effect on the way we burn fuels for energy, as well as on our blood pH. They are beneficial for Winters and Autumns, because they help balance out the blood-sugar "highs and lows" that are often so common in these season-types. They assist Winters and Autumns in feeling full between meals, which is one key to weight loss. Purines also help keep Winters and Autumns in fat-burning mode, which improves their mood and general overall sense of well-being. Winters generally need high levels of dietary purines, while Autumns need adequate levels as well, but far less than Winters. For Springs and especially for Summers, however, purines can act like kryptonite by plummeting their already-low energy levels even lower and further alkalinizing what is usually overly alkaline blood. The Summer and Spring diets are low in purines, because this usually produces the most energy and mental well-being for these season-types. In the next chapter, you'll learn all about the purine content of various foods, along with which foods are best for your season-type.

Carbohydrates

When people hear the word *carbohydrates*, they usually think of foods that are high in carbohydrates, such as grains and fruits. In reality, most foods, with the exception of meats and oils, contain some level of carbohydrates. Similar to the way large protein molecules are composed of varying amounts of the 22 protein building blocks, large carbohydrates are also composed of building blocks. These building blocks consist of various different types of sugars known as **monosaccharides** (sugar building blocks). The most common sugar building blocks found in the typical diet are glucose (also called dextrose), fructose (often referred to as fruit sugar), and galactose. What we call table sugar (sucrose) is actually composed of two sugar building blocks: one block of glucose and one block of fructose. Lactose, which is found in milk, is also composed of two sugar building blocks: one block of glucose and one block of galactose. The starchy carbohydrates contained in foods such as grains and potatoes can contain from 300 to more than 1,000 sugar building blocks arranged into a single molecule, and they are referred to as *complex carbohydrates*. Most of the sugar building blocks in complex carbohydrates are blocks of glucose. In order to use the glucose and other sugars contained in complex carbohydrates, our bodies have to break down the large attached strings of sugar building blocks into individual blocks. The rate at which our bodies are able to break down the large carbohydrates into individual blocks of sugar is influenced by many things, with the amount of fiber in a given food being one of the more significant ones.

Fiber in Carbohydrates, Old and New Paradigm

Most unprocessed foods that are high in carbohydrates, such as grains, vegetables, and fruit, also contain fiber. Processing grains into white-flour products or squeezing fruit into juice removes most of the fiber. Fiber is the part of plants that is considered indigestible. Even though fiber does not add any calories to our diet, it can have many health benefits, depending on the type of fiber contained in the food. I will quickly explain the current way in which fibers are classified and then tell you why this method is outdated and what it should be replaced with. Currently, fibers are classified as being either soluble or insoluble in nature.

Soluble fibers dissolve in water, causing them to swell in volume and turn into a gel. This usually helps slow the rate of digestion in both the stomach and the intestines. Most foods high in soluble fiber will stay in the stomach longer, which keeps you feeling full longer and also slows the rate at which sugars and other nutrients enter your system. Foods high in soluble fiber include oats; fruits high in pectin, such as apples and oranges; nuts, beans, and legumes; and psyllium husks. Soluble fiber helps lower cholesterol levels, especially the unhealthy LDL cholesterol. Certain foods, such as nuts, contain both soluble and insoluble fiber.

Insoluble fiber absorbs water but does not dissolve; it is the woody type of fiber often referred to as "roughage." Insoluble fiber adds extra bulk to the foods we eat, which speeds their passage through the stomach and the intestines, helping to prevent constipation. Foods high in insoluble fiber include wheat bran, corn bran, whole grains, nuts, barley, and many vegetables.

The problem with classifying fibers as either soluble or insoluble is that it does not always accurately predict what health effects a particular fiber will have on the body. For example, soluble fibers are generally believed to be fermented by the microflora that inhabit our large intestines. Fibers such as psyllium husks, xanthan gum, and modified celluloses are all very soluble fibers; however, they do not ferment in the large intestines. It was also originally believed that insoluble fibers were responsible for improving our large bowel function, but this is not necessarily the case, either. Fibers contain many different properties, but the most important for human nutrition are those that affect human health. When all of the properties of fiber are examined, the two that have the greatest impact on our health are the viscosity or thickness of a fiber when it comes into contact with water and the degree to which a particular fiber ferments in the large intestines.

The three most important health functions of fiber are to
1. Assist in lowering our cholesterol levels.
2. Help slow the rate at which sugars from a meal enter our bloodstream, which keeps our blood sugar stable.
3. Assist in maintaining healthy functioning of the large intestine.

Rather than classifying fibers as soluble or insoluble, it would make more sense to classify them as either viscous fibers or fermentable fibers. Viscous fibers would include those such as beta-glucans in oats and barley, pectins in apples and oranges, various gums, and polysaccharides from algae, such as agar and carrageenan. Fermentable fibers include those such as beta-glucans, glucomannan, pectins, oligofructose, inulin, and gum acacia. As you can see, a fiber can be both highly viscous and highly fermentable at the same time. Chart 5.1 will give you a better understanding of the nature of the various types of fibers.

CHART 5.1 PROPERTIES OF DIFFERENT TYPES OF FIBER
Viscosity

		High	Low
Fermentability	High	Beta-Glucans (Oat Bran, Barley)	Gum Acacia
		Guar Gum	Inulin
		Glucomannan	Oligofructose
		Pectins (Apples, Oranges, etc.)	Cellulose (Plant Cell Wall)
	Low	Modified Celluloses i.e., Hydroxypropyl-Methylcellulose	Hemicelluloses
			Wheat Bran and Corn Bran
		Psyllium	

When microflora in our large intestines ferment fibers, they produce short-chain fatty acids. Some of these are used by the cells of the intestinal lining and contribute to colon health, while others are absorbed as blood fats, which can be used by the body for energy. In fact, every gram of fermentable fiber can be converted to 1.5 to 2.5 calories of blood fat by the microflora in our intestines. This is usually very beneficial for Winters and Autumns, because it helps keep them full between meals by supplying extra energy in the form of fat at just the time that the fat and the sugar from their previous meal begins to drop. The biggest benefit of fermentable fiber for Summers and Springs is that it also assists in keeping blood sugar stable, so, when eaten with a higher-carbohydrate diet, fermentable fiber may help keep blood sugar higher between meals, without spiking as high after a meal.

Earlier, I mentioned the three most important functions of fiber for human health. The first one, lowering of cholesterol levels, is accomplished when we ingest viscous fibers. These include psyllium, pectins, beta-glucans from oats and barley, modified celluloses, and various gums, such as locust bean gum and guar gum. Summers and Springs are often the season-types who need to watch their cholesterol, due to their higher insulin levels, especially if they are insulin resistant. This can often be accomplished by drinking a little psyllium husk fiber at the beginning of each meal. Once they get their insulin sensitivity restored and stabilize their blood sugar, any cholesterol issues they may have should resolve themselves. Winters or Autumns who needed to lower their cholesterol would do better with fibers that are also highly fermentable, such as beta-glucans, which are found in large amounts in foods such as oats and barley.

The second potential health benefit of fiber is to help slow down the rate at which sugars from a meal enter our bloodstream.

This is also accomplished by viscous fibers, so the same recommendations as above would apply for all four season-types if they felt that they were digesting their food too quickly.

Fiber's third health benefit is to help maintain healthy functioning of the large intestines, and this can be accomplished by ingesting several different types of fibers. That is because we have more than one way to improve the function of the large intestines. For example, increasing the stool weight and frequency can be accomplished by ingesting fibers that resist fermentation, such as wheat bran or psyllium husk fiber. Another way to improve intestinal health is by providing our bodies with fermentable fibers that help feed intestinal micro flora, which in turn produce short-chain fatty acids that nourish the cells that line our large intestines. We can often best accomplish this by eating foods such as oat bran or vegetables. In addition to fermentable fiber, a type of carbohydrate is also fermentable.

Resistant-Carbohydrates
I started this discussion about carbohydrates by explaining how large carbohydrates are broken down into their individual blocks of sugar. In addition to there being different types of fiber, there are also two main types of large carbohydrates, or starch. One is called **amylose**, which I will refer to as "resistant-carbohydrates," and the other is called **amylopectin**, which I will refer to as "regular carbohydrates." Resistant-carbohydrates have a slightly different shape than regular carbohydrates, which makes them more difficult to digest in the small intestines, the place where regular carbohydrates are usually broken down into individual sugar building blocks. As a result, large amounts of resistant-carbohydrates pass through the small intestines undigested, where they are fermented by the microflora in the large intestines. This creates short-chain fatty acids, similar to the by-products of fermentable fiber.

In addition, many other beneficial metabolic effects result from ingesting varying amounts of resistant-carbohydrates. Only very recently was the significance of resistant-carbohydrates even noticed; in fact, scientists once believed that carbohydrates were carbohydrates. This is a relatively new research topic and one that is very exciting, given all of the recent discoveries. As of the writing of this book, there are far more questions than answers about resistant-carbohydrates. After analyzing all of the available research, however, I'll give you what I believe is the best explanation at this time, along with my opinion of how resistant-carbohydrates are most likely to affect the various season-types. Resistant-carbohydrates appear to be extremely beneficial for all of the season-types but for slightly different reasons. If you have a better grasp of what they are, this should help you understand some of the benefits of consuming them.

Resistant-Carbohydrates Were Abundant in Ancient Cultures

Most foods that are high in large complex carbohydrates have a mixture of regular carbohydrates and resistant-carbohydrates. The easiest way to measure the difference is by focusing on the amount of resistant-carbohydrates in a particular food, because this is the type of carbohydrate that can affect our metabolism in the opposite way that regular carbohydrates do. Historically, humans took in large amounts of resistant-carbohydrates by eating unprocessed grains, legumes, fruits, and vegetables rich in starch. Modern food processing has made some foods more digestible and palatable; however, processing removes many of the beneficial resistant-carbohydrates, which can result in severe health consequences, especially in cultures that are not used to eating such foods. This is what has happened to the Aborigines of Australia, the Pima Indians of Arizona, and many of the Pacific Islanders. In only one generation, they went from eating large amounts of resistant-carbohydrates to eating virtually none. Genetically, they were not well adapted to this type of diet, and as a result, all three populations now suffer from extreme levels of diabetes. The adult diabetes rate is close to 50 percent for Pima Indians and American Samoans and around 30 percent for Aboriginal Australians. Studies done on Aboriginal Australians clearly show that putting them back on their native diet, which is high in resistant-carbohydrates, reverses many of their health issues.

Humankind has slowly evolved on a diet with fewer and fewer resistant-carbohydrates, and many modern diseases are a direct result of eating too few of these carbohydrates. In fact, most primates eat foods that contain large amounts of resistant-carbohydrates, and it appears as though we have an evolutionary imperative to consume some of our carbohydrates in the form of resistant-carbohydrates. Currently, most Americans get only about 5 grams of resistant-carbohydrates a day, while people in less developed countries get between 15 and 20 grams. To make matters even more confusing, there are several types of resistant-carbohydrates, all of which behave a little differently; however, you do not need to worry about this, as long as you focus on the basics and make sure you get an adequate amount of resistant-carbohydrates in your diet.

The Difference between Regular and Resistant-Carbohydrates

The easiest way to understand the difference between resistant-carbohydrates and regular carbohydrates is by comparing short-grain rice, medium-grain rice, long-grain rice, and parboiled rice. Short- and medium-grain rice are typically lower in resistant-carbohydrates and as a result are more "sticky" or gooey when cooked. Certain types of Asian rice, such as the kind used in sushi, have actually been cultivated to be low in resistant-carbohydrates, and this type of rice is referred to as "sticky-rice." Long-grain rice is higher in resistant-carbohydrates, and as a result, the grains do not stick together as much when cooked. Parboiled rice, or "instant" rice, has been processed in a way that actually increases the amount of resistant-carbohydrates, and these rice grains do not stick together at all when cooked.

Many foods are naturally high in resistant-carbohydrates. Navy beans and black-eyed peas have nearly 10 grams of resistant-carbohydrates per half cup. Unripe green bananas have around 5 grams for a medium-size banana. Other foods high in resistant-carbohydrates include yams and lentils. The resistant-carbohydrate content of many starches can be increased by cooling foods in the refrigerator after they have been cooked, which turns part of the regular carbohydrates into the resistant type. For example, by baking or boiling a potato and then putting it in the refrigerator overnight, you will increase the resistant-carbohydrate content to around 3 grams per half cup. The same can be done for other starchy carbohydrates, such as rice or pasta, with varying degrees of conversion of regular carbohydrates into resistant-carbohydrates by cooling in the refrigerator. It's important to note that once the food is cooled, it needs to be eaten cold to get the benefits of the resistant-carbohydrates. If foods such as potatoes or pasta are reheated, the resistant-carbohydrates turn back into regular carbohydrates.

Resistant-Carbohydrate Powder as a Diet Supplement

Perhaps the easiest way to ensure that you get enough resistant-carbohydrates in your diet is through the use of resistant-carbohydrate powder. This powder can be added to smoothies or baked goods. One tablespoon of resistant-carbohydrate powder adds 5 grams of resistant-carbohydrates to your diet, and it is nearly tasteless. (For more information about resistant-carbohydrates and updates on when my Resistant-Carbohydrate Powder will be on the market and available to order, see <u>resistantcarbohydrates. com</u>.)

Health Benefits of Resistant-Carbohydrates

So, what are the benefits of resistant-carbohydrates? Resistant-carbohydrates have three main effects on the human body. First is their effect on the glycemic response and on insulin sensitivity, second is their colonic impact, and finally and perhaps most important is their effect on metabolism. Resistant-carbohydrates offer several benefits for the various season-types. First is the effect that resistant-carbohydrates have on the glycemic response and on insulin sensitivity when a meal is consumed. Resistant-carbohydrates help lower the glycemic blood-sugar spikes caused by a meal in a way that is beneficial for all of the season-types. They cause a slightly lower spike in blood-sugar levels, but most important, when consumed in sufficient quantities, they keep blood sugar from crashing below baseline levels an hour or two after a meal. For Winters, this means resistant-carbohydrates will help keep their blood sugar from crashing to low levels between meals. The advantage for Summers is that although their blood-sugar levels are able to spike high enough to fill up their stored-sugar reserves, their blood sugar does not crash much below pre-meal levels, which helps Summers feel full between meals. Summers who consume an adequate amount of resistant-carbohydrates should have more sustained energy throughout the day.

Resistant-carbohydrates also have a profound metabolic effect on the next meal that is eaten after the resistant-carbohydrates are consumed. For example, if resistant-carbohydrates are eaten for breakfast, they will have a significant effect on any type of meal eaten for lunch, even if that meal does not include resistant-carbohydrates. The main effect on the second meal is that resistant-carbohydrates increase insulin sensitivity and improve glucose tolerance. The exact mechanism through which this occurs is not 100 percent clear at this time, but the best available science shows that they step up the body's production of *adiponectin*, which boosts the amount of fat the body burns between meals. This lowers blood-fat levels, which ultimately improves insulin sensitivity. For Winters who eat a high-fat meal that also contains resistant-carbohydrates, the main effect will be an increased ability to burn fat between meals, helping them to stay full longer.

For Summers who eat a low-fat meal, the slight increase in fat burning caused by resistant-carbohydrates can actually be a good thing. This is because although Summers prefer to burn carbohydrates for energy, they do need to burn some fat for energy as well. The problem is that Summers often produce high levels of insulin, which keeps them stuck in sugar-burning mode too much of the time, and this keeps their blood-fat levels too high, which contributes to their insulin resistance. Eating resistant-carbohydrates, along with smaller amounts of fat, will help Summers keep their blood-fat levels lower, which will increase their insulin sensitivity in the meal that follows the consumption of resistant-carbohydrates. One study showed that insulin sensitivity was increased 33 percent and glucose clearance improved by 44 percent when adjusted for insulin, after 30 grams of resistant-carbohydrates were eaten daily for four weeks.

Most studies show that resistant-carbohydrates slow the rate at which sugar enters the bloodstream and, in doing so, also reduce the amount of insulin produced. This is very beneficial for Winters because they tend to be extremely sensitive to a sudden rise in sugar levels, due to their highly insulin-sensitive cells. As a result, a sudden rise in sugar will cause a corresponding insulin response, which usually leads to a rapid blood-sugar crash, prompting Winters to turn to more carbohydrates to raise their blood sugar again. This is the cause of weight gain for most Winters, as well as Autumns. Winters and Autumns react similarly to the way Aboriginal Australians and Pima Indians do to regular carbohydrates, which is with a rapid weight gain that eventually leads to insulin resistance, followed by diabetes.

Summers and Springs also benefit from the reduced glucose and fewer insulin spikes, but for a slightly different reason. Remember, Summers and Springs actually need to keep their glucose and insulin levels higher for maximum energy. The main problem with this is that chronically elevated levels of insulin lead to decreased cell permeability and insulin resistance. The other problem for Summers and Springs is that if insulin levels rise too much, as is caused by too many regular carbohydrates, their blood sugar will usually fall below the pre-meal level within 1 ½ to 2 hours after eating. When this happens, the body responds by increasing the levels of blood fats, which shuts down Summers' and Springs' preferred method of energy production, and they, too, turn to more carbohydrates, usually in the form of a sweet or starchy snack between meals. This will eventually lead to insulin resistance and diabetes in Summers and Springs as well. Because Summers and Springs rely on sugar for energy, they are much more affected early on by insulin resistance than Winters or Autumns are. Winters and Autumns will have adequate energy from relying on blood fats, while Summers and Springs will feel horrible without enough sugar energy. The downside for Winters and Autumns is that they can often gain a lot of extra weight, similar to the Pima Indians, before they begin to feel bad and get diabetes. Summers will usually feel worse way sooner when they gain weight, and they often attribute their bad feeling to the weight gain and respond by dieting to lose weight.

The solution for all season-types is to eat an adequate amount of resistant-carbohydrates. Remember that the Summer and Spring diets are high in carbohydrates, while the Winter and Autumn diets are low, so adding enough resistant-carbohydrates benefits all of the season-types. By keeping carbohydrate levels low and adding enough resistant-carbohydrates, Winters and Autumns keep their blood-sugar and insulin levels low enough to stay in fat burning mode, which prevents their blood sugar from crashing. By maintaining high levels of carbohydrates, but also adding in enough resistant-carbohydrates, Summers and Springs keep their blood sugar and insulin levels slightly elevated and stable, which maximizes their energy production and stops them from crashing between meals and going into fat-burning mode.

Studies show that resistant-carbohydrates will deliver the same amount of glucose to the blood during a 4- to 6-hour period as regular carbohydrates do. The difference is that regular carbohydrates will deliver too much glucose during the first 1 to 2 hours and then not enough during the last several hours. When you add in sufficient resistant-carbohydrates, you get a sustained and steady supply of blood sugar, which keeps insulin levels stable as well. In addition, by keeping their insulin levels only slightly raised, Summers and Springs will not create the metabolic conditions that cause their cells to become nonpermeable and insulin resistant. In fact, studies show that when people eat enough resistant-carbohydrates, it actually causes the cells to become more sensitive to insulin. Although this may seem to be a negative thing for Winters and Autumns, the diet for these two season-types includes enough saturated fat to ensure that their cells retain the right level of permeability. Furthermore, by balancing out their blood sugar, Winters and Autumns will begin to use glucose energy in a healthier way, which will keep them from going into ketosis as readily. Ketosis contributes to making the cells too permeable for these two season-types.

One of the primary metabolic effects of resistant-carbohydrates is that they cause the body to produce a substance called *glucagon-like peptide*, which has many benefits. One main benefit that people experience from consuming resistant-carbohydrates is an increased sense of fullness and satisfaction from eating a meal. Many studies show that eating enough resistant-carbohydrates will make you feel fuller quicker and also feel more satisfied between meals. This is one of the chief struggles people face when dieting, and the nice thing about dieting with resistant-carbohydrates is that they actually make you feel full and satisfied, so dieting is no longer the hard work it once was.

Studies show that animals eating adequate amounts of resistant-carbohydrates have half the body fat, when compared to animals fed mainly regular carbohydrates. This is due in large part to the increased appetite that develops when there is a lack of resistant-carbohydrates in the diet. When resistant-carbohydrates are combined with the proper diet for your season-type, you will probably feel better and more energized, while actually losing weight, than you used to feel when you were not dieting. Glucagon-like peptide has many other season-type specific benefits, but rather than overload you with information, I'll simply stress that the main point is that when you eat resistant-carbohydrates, you will feel fuller, which is a sign that you are creating glucagon-like peptide and you will experience all of the other benefits that go along with it.

Many studies demonstrate that resistant-carbohydrates also help the body burn its own stored fat for energy, which is great for anyone interested in weight loss. Some studies show that the amount of fat burned varies with the amount of resistant-carbohydrates added to the diet.

The last major benefit of resistant-carbohydrates is their impact on the health of the large intestines, which includes the colon. When resistant-carbohydrates make it to the large intestines, the flora that reside there break them down and convert them into short-chain fatty acids, such as butyrate, acetate, and propionate. These are very short-chain fats, which are less than six carbons in length. Much of these short-chain fats feed the cells that line the intestines, which helps keep them healthy and functioning properly. They also lower the pH of the colon, which makes many of the minerals in the food we eat, such as calcium, easier to absorb. Calcium needs an acidic environment for optimal absorption. Studies show that resistant-carbohydrates actually help keep our bones dense, because they enable us to absorb more of the minerals from the foods we eat.

The Recommended Daily Amount of Resistant-Carbohydrates

As mentioned earlier, there is still much research to conduct on resistant-carbohydrates, especially regarding how they relate to the various season-types. My best advice, if you want to test the effects on yourself, is to either add more foods that are high in resistant-carbohydrates to your diet or simply buy some resistant-carbohydrate powder and add 1 tablespoon per meal if you are a Winter or an Autumn, and ½ tablespoon per meal if you are a Summer or a Spring. You can slowly increase or decrease the amount you add to each meal, to find the amount that makes you feel best.

Our large intestines have a limited capacity for fermenting resistant-carbohydrates, so adding large quantities could have the opposite effect, by reducing the amount of regular carbohydrates in our diet below what we require. Furthermore, resistant-carbohydrates tend to decrease the transit time of food through our digestive systems, so adding too large an amount could negatively affect the proper digestive process. Our closest primate relatives, such as the large apes and chimpanzees, have large intestines that are much bigger than ours and small intestines that are much smaller. It appears that as we have slowly grown accustomed to a diet high in dense foods, such as grains, our bodies have gradually adapted by increasing the length of the small intestine, which is responsible for digesting regular carbohydrates, while shortening our large intestine, which is responsible for fermenting resistant-carbohydrates. One thing is very clear, however; we do have a need for resistant-carbohydrates, and at this point, it's up to each person to find the amount that works best for him or her.

One problem that many people have with consuming too much fiber is that it often ferments so quickly that it can cause intestinal gas, cramping, and discomfort. Resistant-carbohydrates ferment much more slowly than most fermentable fibers do, which helps minimize all of the potential problems often caused by fermentable fiber. Besides increasing the amount of foods we eat that contain resistant-carbohydrates, we can also add resistant-carbohydrate power to our smoothies, sprinkle it on top of food that contains a little moisture, or bake with it. The powder mixes very well in smoothies or over moist food and has very little taste. One tablespoon contains 5 grams of resistant-carbohydrates, and it is recommended that you try this amount to start, before going up to 10 grams and seeing what effect that has on you. You can also bake with it by using the resistant-carbohydrate powder to replace part of the flour in your recipes. You can usually replace up to 25 percent of the flour in any recipe with resistant-carbohydrate powder. You may have to adjust the baking time, because the recipe could take a little longer than usual to bake.

I am such a big believer in the health benefits of resistant- carbohydrates that I decided to start my own website at resistantcarbohydrates.com, which will both track the new research concerning resistant-carbohydrates and offer them for sale to the consumer.

Glycemic Index

Although the term *glycemic index* has been around since 1981, many people have just become aware of it during the last few years. While it can be a useful tool in helping us choose what foods to eat, there are problems with the way many people use it. The glycemic index was created to help diabetics figure out which foods were best for them to eat, based on the rate at which the carbohydrates and the sugar in various foods are digested and absorbed. As you can probably guess, the glycemic index of a food is highly influenced by the amount of fiber, resistant-carbohydrates, and sugars it contains. Usually, the digestibility and absorption of a specific food are compared to the rate at which pure glucose enters the bloodstream after being consumed, and pure glucose is given a glycemic index of 100.

For example, here is one problem with how the glycemic index is often calculated: If you add fat to any meal with carbohydrates, it will lower the glycemic index of that meal. So a piece of white bread with butter may have a far lower overall glycemic index than a piece of whole-wheat bread without butter. Another potential problem is that oftentimes, as explained earlier, certain fibers will also lower the glycemic index of a meal. A third problem that relates to the season-types is that the glycemic response to a food can be very different for each person and in fact can vary even for an individual, based on other factors such as current blood glucose levels and level of insulin sensitivity. The Four Seasons Diet will help maintain these values at a healthy level for all season-types, which will significantly help keep an individual's glycemic index response low.

Furthermore, the glycemic index can be misleading, because consuming too many low-glycemic carbohydrates for your season-type can have far worse effects than consuming the right amount of carbohydrates of a higher glycemic value. Similarly, consuming too many overall calories, even if they have a low glycemic index, can be far worse than consuming slightly too few calories of a higher glycemic index. Perhaps the biggest problem I have with the glycemic index is that because fructose, the type of sugar most often found in fruit, has a low glycemic index, its use is often encouraged, yet it can have severe metabolic consequences when consumed in large quantities. An essential part of the goal of the glycemic index is to keep blood-sugar levels low; however, fructose can actually have consequences that, despite its low glycemic index, work against another primary goal of the glycemic index: assisting diabetics and people with insulin resistance.

Fructose

Remember that carbohydrates are composed of sugar building blocks, which consist of simple sugars, such as glucose, fructose, and galactose, plus a few other less common sugar building blocks. Table sugar, which is the sugar we normally call *sugar*, is actually sucrose. It is composed of one sugar building block of glucose plus one sugar building block of fructose. Fruits are high in sugar and usually contain a mix of the simple sugars fructose and glucose, along with a little bit of sucrose. The sugars in fruit are most often between 40 and 60 percent fructose, which is the sugar building block that has a very low glycemic index. This is the reason it is often recommended for diabetics and has been considered healthy by many in the medical profession.

The problem with fructose having a low glycemic value is that it can distort some simple metabolic effects of eating foods high in fructose, such as fruit. Most fruits are a mix of fructose, glucose, and sucrose, and all three of these sugars have different glycemic indexes. Pure glucose has a glycemic index of 100, while sucrose has an index of around 68, and pure fructose has an index of around 19. When the glycemic index of a food with fructose, such as fruit, is given, all that is looked at is the total blood sugar response over a prolonged period of time. If a fruit was consumed that was 50 percent pure fructose and 50 percent pure glucose (meaning not sucrose), it would have a relatively low glycemic index, because even though the value of glucose is 100, the value of the fructose is 19. Remember that the glycemic index looks at the total effect of a food on blood sugar, so even if the glucose is metabolized quickly, the fructose is metabolized slowly, and the combined glycemic index looks good.

In reality, however, the metabolic effect may be very different from that of a complex carbohydrate with the same glycemic value. This is because if a fruit is 50 percent glucose, it will raise blood-sugar and insulin levels very quickly at first. This will cause them to drop sharply starting about an hour later, and even though the fructose is supplying a steady load of sugar, there is still an abrupt initial spike and then a fall caused by the glucose. As a result, Winters will stop burning fat very quickly after eating fruits with a high percentage of pure glucose. Often they may get a burst of energy, because they are able to burn glucose; however, if they get a quick burst, they are far more prone to crashing their insulin and blood-sugar levels than any other season-type is. Summers, on the other hand, may stop burning sugar for energy starting around three hours after eating foods high in glucose, and five hours later they may be burning as little as one-third the amount of glucose they would have, had they eaten a complex carbohydrate, instead of glucose. Their bodies react by releasing more blood fat, which plummets their energy levels, causing them to turn to more fruit or sugar.

The simple solution seems to be to eat more foods high in fructose, which is what many doctors have recommended to diabetics for years. In the long run, however, eating large amounts of fructose may be one of the most damaging things people can do to their bodies. In order to know why, you first need to understand why fructose has such a low glycemic index. Fructose has the same chemical formula as glucose, yet the way in which the atoms are arranged is slightly different. While this may seem like a minor difference, metabolically speaking it leads to an enormous difference in the way the two sugars are metabolized. Glucose can be used by every cell in the body for energy production, and because it hits the bloodstream quickly, it has a very high glycemic index. Fructose, on the other hand, due to its slightly different structure, cannot be used by most of the cells in the body but must first be broken down by the liver to be metabolized. This is where many of the problems with ingesting too much fructose in the diet begin. The potential side effects from consuming too much fructose are so numerous that rather than try to explain them all,

I decided to list them in a numbered format, in no particular order of importance.

1. <u>Fructose can deplete the liver of energy currency.</u>
One of the first steps in the liver's metabolism of fructose is its conversion of fructose to *fructose-1 phosphate.* In order to convert fructose, the liver has to use one unit of energy currency. If excess fructose is consumed, the liver can be depleted of its supply of energy currency, which impedes its ability to perform other needed metabolic functions. For example, fructose appears to block the metabolism of glucose in the liver, including the liver's ability to store glucose as stored sugar. When this happens, the pancreas secretes more insulin in an attempt to assist in the liver's ability to store glucose. As a result of this excess insulin in the body, the muscles respond by down-regulating their sensitivity to insulin. This is part of the method by which fructose contributes to insulin resistance in the entire body.

2. <u>Fructose increases uric acid levels.</u>
Next, the liver deals with the by-products left over from converting fructose into fructose-1 phosphate and in the process produces *uric acid.* Uric acid is a naturally occurring substance in the body, but in large amounts it can cause some pretty serious health problems. Historically, it has been associated with gout caused by eating too many organ meats. In our modern society, however, fructose has arguably become the main dietary factor responsible for excess uric acid levels and therefore the number-one cause of gout. One of the most detrimental effects of uric acid is that it blocks an enzyme that makes *nitric oxide.* Nitric oxide is a compound that helps expand our blood vessels and helps keep blood pressure low.

Normally, the body does a pretty good job of eliminating uric acid, but, as I will explain later, fructose can also cause insulin resistance, which impedes the body's ability to eliminate uric acid. A few of the potential damaging effects caused by the increased uric acid levels include:

    a. <u>High blood pressure</u>. For more than fifty years, fructose has been known to contribute to high blood pressure, a phenomenon called *fructose-induced hypertension.* A study in New York of more than 8,000 people showed that every 1 mg drop in uric acid levels correlates to a 10-point drop in systolic blood pressure. Not only does uric acid block nitric oxide, which expands our blood vessels, but it also stimulates the production of *angiotensin*, which causes the blood vessels to constrict, raising blood pressure higher. Studies conducted on rodents show that fructose increases the absorption of both salt and water in the small intestines, which further contributes to high blood pressure. To make matters even worse, the same study showed that fructose decreases the excretion of salt by the kidneys. This excess salt causes the blood vessels to stiffen and contract up to 10 percent smaller, independently of the constriction caused by the uric acid, adding a fourth way that fructose causes high blood pressure.

b. Damage to the brain's capillaries. Fructose can possibly contribute to dementia later in life. Studies show that people with high levels of uric acid are more likely to score poorly on memory tests, and people over the age of sixty with high levels of uric acid are up to five times more likely to have changes in their brains that suggest possible damage to their small blood vessels.

c. Gout. High uric acid can cause gout; in fact, I know of vegetarians who ate no meat but consumed a lot of fruit and suffered from gout, which was quickly eliminated by reducing their fruit consumption. Gout is caused by high uric acid levels, which can result from consuming too much fructose or too many foods high in purines, as well as from an impairment of the body's ability to excrete uric acid. High insulin levels impair the body's ability to eliminate uric acid, so people who are insulin resistant and produce high levels of insulin often suffer from gout more than those with normal insulin sensitivity do.

d. Impedes athletic performance. Excess fructose consumption can impede athletic performance, due to many of its already mentioned effects. Eating large amounts of fructose will block nitric oxide production in the body. Nitric oxide helps expand the blood vessels, so lower levels of nitric oxide will contribute to decreased blood flow to the muscles. As a result, less oxygen and nutrients will get into the muscles. High fructose consumption also contributes to insulin resistance, which causes the muscles to store less sugar. This can severely impede athletes who rely on speed or strength for their sport.

e. Sodium retention. Uric acid can cause the kidneys to retain sodium, which, in addition to raising blood pressure, has been implicated in other diseases, such as osteoporosis, strokes, and heart disease. The increase in the risk for heart disease and stroke is due to the high level of sodium, causing long-term thickening of the vessels walls and altered production of vital structural proteins, such as collagen and elastin, that help keep our blood vessels elastic. This increased risk for stroke and heart disease from the excess sodium levels caused by fructose consumption occurs even if blood pressure is normal or controlled by medication.

3. Fructose causes fatty liver, insulin resistance, and high insulin levels.

In the liver, fructose is further metabolized, and in the process, 30 percent of it gets converted to fat in the liver. This can lead to insulin resistance in the liver, which results in increased insulin levels, but can also dramatically affect liver function. In addition, similar to the way an alcoholic's liver gets cirrhosis, there is something called NAFLD, which stands for non-alcoholic fatty liver disease. It has been estimated that 10 percent of people in America under the age of twenty and 20 percent of all Americans suffer from NAFLD. Studies have demonstrated that feeding rats fructose causes them to develop fatty liver. Other studies have shown that people suffering from NAFLD consume three times as many soft drinks high in fructose as the average American. In addition, they have high levels of *fructose enzymes*, which I will elaborate on later and which further implicates fructose as a factor in their NAFLD. Furthermore, the studies went on to show that the degree of liver damage from NAFLD increases with larger amounts of fructose consumption.

While fructose is busy contributing to NAFLD, it's also activating an enzyme called JNK-1. JNK-1 inactivates a protein in the liver called IRS-1, which stands for *insulin receptor substrate 1*. This also contributes to insulin resistance in the liver. Research on humans shows that consuming fructose-sweetened beverages can cause a person to become more insulin resistant in only ten weeks. Another study demonstrated that consuming 1,000 calories of fructose a day caused insulin to become 25 percent less effective in just one week. The same study showed that consuming 1,000 calories of glucose had no negative effect on insulin sensitivity.

A study conducted at UCLA showed that rats fed large amounts of fructose for six weeks had insulin levels that were 74 percent higher than those of rats that were not fed fructose. When the fructose-fed rats were deprived of omega-3 fats (most Americans are omega-3 fat deficient), they had insulin levels that were 125 percent higher than rats that ate no fructose but received adequate amounts of omega-3 fats. Finally, the insulin resistance caused by fructose leads to high levels of insulin, the dangers of which I have already discussed. A four-week study conducted on rats found that dietary starch and glucose had no long-term effect on raising insulin levels. By the end of the four-week study, however, the rats that were fed a high-fructose diet had insulin levels that were nearly twice as high as the rats not fed fructose.

4. Fructose tricks the brain into making you fat.

Fructose causes a number of unhealthy bodily reactions that can lead to obesity. Chronic consumption of large amounts of fructose results in insulin resistance, which prompts the body to produce too much insulin. When a person has abnormally high levels of insulin, the brain can no longer properly sense a hormone called leptin. **Leptin** (which I'll refer to as the feel-full hormone) helps regulate our appetite by telling us that we are full and no longer hungry. These high levels of insulin effectively cause "feel-full hormone resistance."

Another drawback is that fructose does not cause the production of the feel-full hormone, as normal carbohydrates do. Most carbohydrates bring about a modest insulin response, which actually makes the body produce the feel-full hormone to tell you that you're full. Fructose does not do this, so you never get the message to stop eating or, in most cases now, thanks to fructose-sweetened beverages, to stop drinking them. A hormone with the opposite effect of the feel-full hormone is **ghrelin**, often called the "hunger hormone." It's produced in the stomach and makes us feel hungry. Eating most types of carbohydrates will suppress the hunger hormone. Fructose, on the other hand, does not suppress it as other carbohydrates do, so we think we are still hungry.

In addition, fructose often alters the brain's "reward" center, by changing the way our bodies deal with the feel-good neurotransmitter *dopamine.* Essentially, excessive fructose consumption will cause us to feel increased pleasure from eating foods that are high in carbohydrates. Fructose has an effect on our brain chemistry similar in many ways to what happens to the brain chemistry of a heroin or cocaine addict. Given the dramatic way in which fructose affects our hunger hormones and brains, you would expect it to cause rapid obesity. A Princeton study fed rats either rat chow, rat chow with sucrose, or rat chow with fructose. The rats eating rat chow with fructose gained 260 percent more weight during an eight-week period than did rats eating rat chow with sucrose. This, despite the fact that the rats eating rat chow with sucrose actually consumed more calories of sucrose than the other rats consumed of fructose.

If someone could create the "perfect storm" to cause obesity, it would be a food that:

a. Did not turn off the hunger hormone, as other foods did.

b. Did not produce the feel-full hormone, as other foods did.

c. Interfered with the brain's ability to sense the feel-full hormones produced by other foods.

d. Created brain changes that increase the rewards and the pleasure we feel from eating, similar to the way drugs such as cocaine and heroin affect the brains of those who abuse such drugs.

Multiple studies show that fructose is capable of producing that "perfect storm" when it comes to obesity. Many people who have struggled with dieting for years are amazed when they get their hunger hormones working for them, instead of against them. Dieting is no longer difficult but simply a matter of eliminating a few foods that have been undermining their efforts all of these years.

5. Fructose consumption contributes to diabetes.
I have discussed how insulin resistance can lead to diabetes. Given how fructose has the ability to cause insulin resistance, we would expect to see a correlation between fructose consumption and diabetes. A large-scale study conducted by Harvard University consisting of more than 90,000 nurses during an eight-year period did just that. It found that nurses who stated that they drank one or more serving of sugar-sweetened soft drinks or fruit punch (most soft drinks are now sweetened with high-fructose corn syrup) were almost twice as likely to have developed type 2 diabetes during the study, when compared to those who rarely consumed these beverages.During World War I and World War II, England experienced a serious reduction in the amount of sugar available for consumption and was forced to resort to sugar rationing. Prior to World War II, per capita sugar consumption in England was more than a hundred pounds per person per year. During the war, sugar consumption plummeted to around sixty-five pounds

per person per year. What is interesting is that diabetes mortality lessened by the same degree as the drop in sugar consumption during both wars.

Other historical evidence is even more compelling in proving the role that fructose plays in diabetes. In 1949, for example, 50,000 Jews fled Yemen and immigrated to Israel. The Jews in Yemen has consumed almost no sugar. The 1949 Yemenite Jews were compared with Jews who had fled Yemen and arrived in Israel during the 1930s, adopting a diet that contained much greater amounts of sugar than they had consumed in Yemen. When the two groups of Jews from Yemen living in Israel were examined, the results were astounding. The Jews who had left Yemen in the 1930s and had added sugar to their diet suffered from diabetes at fifty times the rate of the Jews who had left Yemen in 1949 and had never had a diet high in sugar. In fact, the Jews who had been consuming sugar in Israel since the 1930s suffered from a significantly greater prevalence of heart disease, high blood pressure, and high cholesterol.

6. **Fructose contributes to the development of breast cancer and erectile dysfunction.**

Fructose has also been implicated in gender-specific diseases. A study by the Centers for Disease Control compared the diets of more than 500 women with breast cancer with the diets of more than 1,400 healthy women and found that women who consumed sweet beverages and foods approximately 10 times per week were more than 30 percent more likely to develop early-stage breast cancer. Fructose appears to be far worse for postmenopausal women, because the science suggests that estrogen helps the body eliminate excess uric acid. Many experts theorize that the sudden increase in high blood pressure and heart attacks that women suffer after menopause is caused by the higher uric acid levels resulting from decreased estrogen in the body.

High fructose consumption, as explained earlier, shuts down the body's ability to produce nitric oxide, which dilates the blood vessels. Low nitric oxide levels are one of the factors most responsible for erectile dysfunction. In fact, drugs such as Viagra, Levitra, and Cialis work by causing the body to release a hormone called cyclic GMP, which relaxes the smooth muscles of the penis and increases blood flow. GMP is also released in response to nitric oxide, so someone with low levels of nitric oxide would be very likely to have erectile dysfunction, to some extent. There have been many testimonials of men who eliminated fructose from their diet and shortly thereafter no longer needed their erectile dysfunction medication.

7. Fructose increases cholesterol and triglycerides.
As mentioned earlier, 30 percent of fructose gets turned into fat by the liver. Fructose also causes the liver to produce the most damaging type of cholesterol there is: VLDL. One study showed that fructose has the ability to raise blood triglycerides 36 percent in only six weeks. This dramatic result was obtained simply by supplying 17 percent of an individual's daily calories in the form of fructose, which is an amount consumed by many people.

Another UCLA study fed rats a diet containing either fructose or no fructose for six weeks. Both groups were further divided into two groups, with one group getting omega-3 fats, while the other group did not receive omega-3 fats. The rats that were fed fructose and omega-3 fats had triglyceride levels that were 84 percent higher than the rats fed omega-3 fats without the fructose. Even more shocking was that the rats fed fructose without the added omega-3 fats had triglyceride levels that were 240 percent higher than the rats that received omega-3 fats and did not consume any fructose. Fructose also produces high levels of *advanced glycation end products*, which contribute to the cholesterol problem by promoting the formation of oxidized LDL cholesterol.

8. Advanced glycation end products lead to wrinkles and aging.
Advanced glycation end products (AGEs) are compounds that may form when proteins or fats react with sugars, either during cooking or in the human body during metabolism. AGEs are considered very unhealthy for the human body and are involved in the development of type 2 diabetes, cardiovascular disease, Alzheimer's disease, inflammation, aging, and many other diseases we normally associate with growing old. It's very fitting that the acronym for advanced glycation end products is AGEs. Foods in which sugars have been "browned" with protein are often high in AGEs. This includes brown bread crusts and meats that are basted and browned, such as meat with a barbeque sauce containing sugar that is then browned. This is one of the many reasons that boiling food or cooking it with water is so much healthier than frying food. It's the browning in the absence of water that can create these harmful compounds. AGEs are also produced inside

our bodies by reactions that occur there. While all sugars can form AGEs inside the body, fructose forms them at seven times the rate that glucose does. Part of what makes AGEs so detrimental to our health is that it takes a very long time for the body to eliminate them. This means that someone who consumes large amounts of fructose may have abnormally high levels of AGEs in his or her body at all times. Some areas of our bodies most vulnerable to damage from AGEs include collagen and elastin, two protein fibers that help keep our skin firm and elastic. When these protein are damaged by AGEs, our skin may become dry and brittle, leading to wrinkles and sagging skin. Diabetics, who may suffer from years of high blood sugar, often have levels of AGEs that are fifty times higher than nondiabetics, which is one reason they frequently show early signs of skin aging.

Besides keeping fructose consumption to a minimum, you can also eliminate major sources of AGEs in your diet, such as bread crusts, any browned or fried food, and meats browned with sauces that contain sugar. All of you parents out there who are cutting off the bread crusts for your kids would be well advised to cut off the crusts for yourselves as well, if you want to keep your skin looking young.

9. Fructose may make you stupid.
According to an article in *National Geographic Daily News* titled "Can Sugar Make You Stupid? 'High Concern' in Wake of Rat Study," "sweet drinks scrambled the memories and stunted learning in lab rats in a new study, leading to "high concern" over what sugary diets may do to people.

The article references a study conducted at UCLA that fed rats either a low-fructose or a high-fructose diet for six weeks and then tested their cognitive abilities by assessing how well they could remember an escape route on a maze. The study found that consuming large amounts of fructose hampered the brain's memory and learning abilities. Much of the cognitive impairment was linked to the increase in insulin resistance and in triglycerides caused by consuming fructose. High fructose consumption results in a dramatic increase in insulin levels, insulin resistance, and triglyceride levels, all of which have been found to have a negative impact on brain function. The study concluded that fructose affects both synaptic plasticity and cognitive function.

Here is how you can sum up the last nine points in a way that is easy to explain to your friends: studies show that if you take two animals and feed one fructose and the other one the same number of calories from glucose, it is only the fructose-fed animal that will develop a fatty liver, insulin resistance, obesity, high blood pressure, inflammation, high triglyceride levels, brain impairment, and many of the other abnormalities I have just described. So the question on your mind is probably how can you limit your fructose consumption? What is a safe level of fructose for most people? Based on the scientific and anecdotal evidence, I feel that consuming 15 grams of fructose a day is a safe level for most people, and I believe that it's imperative not to consume more than this amount on a regular basis.

Why High-Fructose Corn Syrup (HFCS) May Be Even Worse
HFCS Contains "Unbound" Fructose. As I mentioned, sucrose, or table sugar, is 50 percent fructose. So if you eat a candy bar, cake, or ice cream sweetened with "sugar," half of the calories from that sugar will be in the form of fructose. High-fructose corn syrup is often said to be composed of 55 percent fructose. Independent studies have suggested that in some cases, the actual percentage is much higher, often approaching 65 percent. Even if high-fructose corn syrup were 50 percent fructose, as table sugar is, there would still be some dramatic differences in the way it is metabolized, according to a lot of research. This is because in table sugar, each molecule of fructose is "bound" to a molecule of glucose, while in high-fructose corn syrup the fructose is considered to be "free" or "unbound."

There is still much research to conduct on the exact mechanisms that appear to make unbound fructose cause more problems for human health than fructose bound to glucose in table sugar does, but according to the experts, unbound fructose causes damage in several different ways. First, unbound fructose is able to enter the body much quicker than bound fructose can, because bound fructose has to go through an extra metabolic step before the body can use it. This makes unbound fructose hit the liver much faster, which is the place where fructose has to be metabolized. Research on rats demonstrates that when the liver is quickly "flushed" with high levels of unbound fructose in a matter of minutes, it can scar the rats' livers, making them resemble the livers of alcoholics with cirrhosis.

HFCS Produces Excess Carbonyls. According to research done at Rutgers, the manufacture of high-fructose corn syrup creates high levels of *carbonyls*, which are highly reactive compounds believed to cause tissue damage. Although these carbonyls are not present in table sugar, research shows that just a single can of HFCS-sweetened beverage contains five times the amount of carbonyls found in people with diabetes. This is relevant because diabetics are known to have higher levels of carbonyls than nondiabetics have, and this is believed to play a role in the tissue damage often suffered by diabetics.

HFCS Creates High Levels of Fructose Enzymes. Eating large quantities of HFCS has also been theorized to raise a person's levels of fructose enzymes, which are used to metabolize fructose. Many experts claim that it's the high levels of these enzymes that cause some of the problems associated with fructose. They claim that going off all foods containing fructose for a period of a few weeks will get someone's fructose enzymes back to a healthier level, and that maintaining a lower-fructose diet will keep the fructose enzymes from getting too high in the future.

Fructose Content of Various Sweeteners

Other sweeteners also contain varying levels of fructose. Honey is around 50 percent fructose, and the amount can vary from 45 percent to 55 percent, depending on the type of honey consumed. Agave syrup, which has been touted as the healthy natural sweetener, is around 80 percent fructose, so I would not recommend using that as a sweetener. Brown rice syrup does not have any fructose and can be used safely by those wishing to maintain a low-fructose diet. Brown rice syrup also digests more slowly than other sweeteners do, so it will have a much lower glycemic index than pure glucose. Interestingly, the old-fashioned type of corn syrup that people used for baking in the past does not contain any fructose, either. You can find the brand Karo at most grocery stores, and it is a healthy way to get your sweet-tooth fix without consuming any fructose. There was a period of time when Karo brand corn syrup added some fructose to its product, but as of the writing of this book, the company has removed the added fructose and hopefully will not add it back in at a later date. Another sweetener you can use is pure glucose; it has only 70 percent of the sweetness of table sugar, costs a bit more, and can be difficult to find in stores. You can find it online, and along with brown rice syrup and old-fashioned corn syrup, using glucose is a great way to reduce the amount of fructose you consume.

The Corn Refiners' Association and Its Stance on HFCS

The Corn Refiners Association attempted to change the name of high-fructose corn syrup to *corn sugar*; however, in June 2012 the federal government rejected this attempt. As part of their plan, the corn refiners had created a website to help counter some of the negative press that fructose has received. The site provides a lot of information, and if you read what the corn refiners association has to say, you may be left a bit confused, based on what I have just told you. To prevent that possibility, I will examine a few of the statements on their website and help clarify them, as well as offer my opinion.

I am not out to demonize high-fructose corn syrup or corn sugar. My main point has to do with the consumption of all sources of fructose, which includes high-fructose corn syrup, corn sugar, table sugar, fruit, honey, maple syrup, agave nectar, and several other foods.

I have cited many studies, which are included in the back of this book, and the corn syrup industry cites many studies as well. One of the main points the corn syrup industry makes is that once fructose hits the bloodstream, the body cannot tell the difference between fructose derived from high-fructose corn syrup and fructose from other sources. Technically, this is a true statement; however, I would like to look at the bigger picture. For example, when you eat fruit, which is high in fructose, you get fiber, potassium, vitamins, minerals, and antioxidants. When you consume high-fructose corn syrup, you do not get all of the other benefits that fruit has to offer. Remember that the Four Seasons Diet limits fructose consumption to 15 grams a day, so if you want to consume all of your fructose from high-fructose corn syrup and none from fruit, then that is your choice to make, although fruit is always recommended over soft drinks. Also, remember that the fructose in high-fructose corn syrup is largely "unbound," so it will hit the bloodstream faster than bound fructose. Many experts say the rapid manner in which unbound fructose enters the liver exacerbates the problems caused by excess fructose.

Many of the studies cited by the corn syrup industry show no differences between consuming corn syrup and table sugar. Most of these studies, however, are very short term in nature. For example, they may have consisted of testing the effects after only one meal or only a day's worth of meals. It should also be mentioned that one study cited by the corn syrup industry was designed by someone who serves as a science adviser to the Canadian Sugar Institute, as well as to Archer Daniels Midland, a major producer of high-fructose corn syrup. Another study was supported by the Suikerstichting Netherlands, which is basically a government agency that promotes the use of sugar in relation to health and nutrition. Table sugar, which used to be produced entirely from sugar cane, is now also produced from sugar beets. It appears that perhaps this agency is somehow affiliated with helping the sugar beet industry in the Netherlands, and this government agency takes a view of sugar that I would describe as an extremely positive position. A third study cited by the corn syrup industry was supported by a grant from the American Beverage Association, as well as by the Corn Refiners Association. Finally, the last major study cited was funded by PepsiCo. I mention this because, as someone who often reads hundreds of research studies in a single month, these studies did not seem to be like the other studies on fructose I cited, so I decided to see who helped to create and fund them. Research studies can be quite expensive and time consuming, and usually you do not see studies that test the effects of drinking just one beverage containing a certain ingredient. Normally, studies are conducted over a prolonged period of time to see what the long-term effects are.

For example, of the studies I cited concerning fructose:
- One was an eight-week experiment conducted on rabbits.
- One was a seven-day experiment done on human males.
- One was a 28-day experiment conducted on 27 patients.
- One was a nine-year study of 91,249 women.
- One was an eight-week study on mice.
- One was a two-week study on rats.
- One was a twelve-week study on rats.
- One was an analysis of 4,528 adults correlated to fructose consumption.

Compare these long-term studies with the study supported by a grant from the American Beverage Association and the Corn Refiners Association. Their study consisted of having participants eat a standard breakfast at 8:00 a.m. They arrived at the lab at 9:30, and at 10:10, they consumed one of several drinks sweetened with various sweeteners. At 12:30 p.m., they had lunch and after their post-lunch ratings were obtained, they left the lab. This study concluded that there was no evidence that commercial cola beverages sweetened with either fructose or corn syrup have significantly different effects on hunger or feelings of fullness after a meal. Basically, they are saying that drinking a soft drink sweetened with regular sugar a few hours before lunch will not affect you any differently than drinking a soft drink sweetened with high-fructose corn syrup. I am sure this is completely true; however, it has nothing do with what I have said. I have been talking about the long-term consumption of large amounts of fructose from any source, whether high-fructose corn syrup, table sugar, fruit, or honey, so I do not want anyone to get the idea that I am picking on high-fructose corn syrup. It's the effects of excess fructose consumption that I am talking about, which is what most of the studies I cited look at.

I explained that "unbound" fructose is purported by many experts to be more detrimental to a person's health when consumed long term than "bound" fructose is. One thing worth mentioning is that when table sugar is added to carbonated beverages such as sodas, the low pH of the carbonated water tends to cause a lot of the table sugar to disassociate and become "unbound" in a way that makes it more similar to corn syrup. So if you drink carbonated beverages, there may not be a lot of difference between those sweetened with high-fructose corn syrup vs. beverages sweetened with table sugar. In the case of noncarbonated beverages, experts say that the ones sweetened with high-fructose corn syrup will have more unbound "free-fructose" and that it will enter the bloodstream and the liver more quickly, which is responsible for certain negative metabolic consequences.

Once again, I am not advocating that you eliminate high-fructose corn syrup from your diet; I simply recommend limiting your fructose consumption to no more than 15 grams a day. Even the corn syrup website contains a quote from a university professor who says that rather than ban corn syrup from your diet, you would be better off cutting back on sugar from all sources, such as honey and table sugar. On this major point, I agree with what one of the experts on the corn syrup industry website is saying, that is, to cut back on sugar from all sources. I believe you would be far better off consuming 30 grams of high-fructose corn syrup that contained 15 grams of fructose in one day than you would be consuming large quantities of fruit that contained 80 grams of fructose. It's the fructose load that is most important, so limit yourself to 15 grams, as best you can.

Obviously, you know that natural foods such as fruit are much healthier than fructose-sweetened beverages, due to all of the reasons previously mentioned. Fruit is especially important to Summers and Springs as a source of potassium. Summers or Springs, for example, who ate cake sweetened with table sugar for their entire 15 grams of daily fructose would get negligible amounts of potassium. Eating the same number of grams of fructose from high-potassium fruits such as cantaloupe gives you not only the fructose, but also more than 1,000 mg of potassium. For a Summer or a Spring, this amount of extra potassium in a day can mean the difference between feeling vital and energetic or feeling lethargic, so these season-types in particular should try to consume their daily fructose in the form of fruit.

Plenty of scientific and anecdotal evidence suggests that limiting your fructose consumption may be the number-one thing you can do to improve your health. Much has been made about the miracle of the Japanese diet and Japan's low rates of cancer and heart disease or the amazing health benefits of the Mediterranean diet. I believe that the miracle behind both of these diets lies largely in the fact that historically these cultures have had low fructose consumption. In 1967, for example, Americans consumed an average of about 114 pounds of sugar per year per person, and by 2003, it had increased to 142 pounds per year. In contrast, in the 1960s, the average Japanese person consumed only 40 pounds of sugar per person per year, and in the 1980s, it was still less than 50 pounds per person per year.

The Mediterranean diet is a series of nutritional recommendations that were inspired in large part by observations made on the island of Crete and Corfu during the 1960s. It has been estimated that sugar consumption on these islands amounted to only around 10 pounds per person per year during the 1960s. In addition, the main oil used on Crete and Corfu during the study period was olive oil, and most of the breads consumed were whole grain. In effect, the Mediterranean diet is really a diet that's low in fructose, low in processed vegetable oils, and low in processed grains. As you will learn later, any time a culture has a diet that is low in fructose, processed vegetable oils, and processed grains, those people have vibrant health. Conversely, when a culture has a diet that is high in fructose, high in processed vegetable oils, and high in processed grains, that culture suffers from cancer, heart disease, and diabetes.

Fructose Fast
Before you start the Four Seasons Diet for your season-type, I highly recommend that you do a fructose fast for two weeks. This means

no fruit, no foods or beverages containing HFC or table sugar, and no other sources of fructose. Also, if you are a Summer or a Spring, you should start to consume lower-purine proteins during the two-week fructose fast. The reason for the fast is that the Four Seasons Diet is a lower-fructose diet, and many people experience symptoms when quitting fructose, such as loss of energy for a week or two and night sweats. By the end of the fast, these symptoms disappear, and people usually respond that they feel better than they have in a long time.

Going on a fructose fast can be very challenging for many people, especially for those who are used to eating desserts, drinking sweetened beverages, or eating a lot of fruit. It's best to get accustomed to a lower-fructose diet first by doing the fructose fast for a few weeks. It will also be far easier to tell if the positive or negative effects you feel once you start the Four Seasons Diet are from the diet or from the fructose fast. Although the quiz you took should have given you a general idea of what season-type you are, if you are suffering from many of the ill effects from too much fructose consumption, your quiz results could have been thrown off a bit, and you could actually be a different season-type than the quiz indicated. This is especially true if you are insulin resistant and suffer from both a fatty liver and belly fat. It's important to see how the diet makes you feel, and if you start the fructose fast at the same time that you start the diet, you may feel horrible and not know whether it's from the fructose fast or because you chose the wrong season-type for your diet.

Furthermore, some season-types, such as Summers, are far more prone to insulin resistance, and the fructose fast will help restore insulin sensitivity. Although all season-types will not feel 100 percent when they are insulin resistant, a Summer will feel the worst, and going on the high-carbohydrate Summer Diet when a person is insulin resistant will not have the desired affect. It's best to do the fructose fast for two weeks at first and give your body a chance to function the way it prefers. Then you can start the actual diet for your season-type and see what effect it has on your well-being.

Once you have done the fructose fast and started the Four Seasons Diet, the next question is, how much fructose is a safe level to consume every day? Many experts seem to agree that 15 to 25 grams would be a safe level for most people, which is the amount it's estimated that the average person consumed a hundred years ago. It has been further estimated that the average

American currently consumes around 70 grams of fructose a day, and roughly 25 percent of Americans consume more than 135 grams per day, which equates to nine days' worth of fructose each and every single day.

On the food charts in Chapter 6, I list the fructose content of the most common fruits, along with a notation for the vegetables that are high in fructose. To err on the side of caution until further scientific research determines the safest maximum amount of fructose for most people, I recommend limiting your fructose consumption to 15 grams or less per day. The important thing to keep in mind is that 15 grams is your recommended total fructose load per day from all sources of fructose. So if you were to eat a piece of cake sweetened with table sugar that had 30 grams of table sugar (half of the sugar in table sugar is fructose), you will have consumed your fructose load for the day.

A common trap that I have personally fallen into more times than I can count is to be lulled back into consuming more fructose. I have done a fructose fast many times, and I recommend that a person do one at least every six months. After doing the fast, I always feel better, and this is a state where most people can consume larger amounts of fructose and feel great. Summers are especially prone to falling into this trap when consuming fruit after a fructose fast. The high potassium and sugar content of fruit can give a Summer who has fructose-fasted a burst of energy like a five-year-old after Halloween. The trap is that you can feel so good for a week or two of doing this that you reach for fruit and sugar-sweetened products every chance you get. Inevitably, every time I have done this, I go back to feeling far worse after a period of several weeks.

By keeping your total daily fructose consumption to 15 grams or less, you will learn to habituate to a lifestyle that makes it easier to maintain that level. When you get there, be forewarned that if you decide to splurge one night on a big piece of cake or go out and get a large smoothie at the smoothie shop, you may find yourself bouncing off the walls just like that five-year-old. You may feel great, but keep in mind that it's highly advisable to be strict about the 15 grams during the next few days after splurging on that cake or large fruit smoothie, or else you may find that you are a sugar addict again. One large fruit smoothie from many popular smoothie shops can easily have five days' worth of fructose in it, so if you feel compelled to have one, opt for the small, and avoid fructose for a day or two afterward, if you can.

Similarly, many coffee drinks have large amounts of added sugar in them, which is often a hidden source of fructose most people don't think about. For example, just two ounces of the flavored shots added to most coffee drinks have more than an entire day's recommended amount of fructose. Some of the specialty coffee drinks contain more than 70 grams of sugar, meaning they have 35 grams of fructose, not to mention up to 500 calories. It's better to order just a latté without any added sugar, and add your own, if you feel compelled. Any time you feel the urge to splurge on foods containing fructose, go back and reread number 4, about how the brain gets tricked into making you fat again.

Ideally, the nutrition labels on food should be changed in a way that breaks down the amount of fructose sugar, as opposed to other sugars. This is very similar to the way nutrition labels break down the amount saturated fat from total fat. If even only half of what the scientists studying fructose say about its dangers is correct, the amount of money spent on health care due to excess fructose consumption is staggering. Given the litigious nature of our society, you have to wonder whether there could be future lawsuits against the large soft drink companies, blaming them for many of the diseases mentioned in this section. If all of the books and the research articles quoted in this chapter turn out to be accurate, then the monetary damages from such a lawsuit could dwarf the judgments against the tobacco companies.

Fats and Oils

Let me start off the section on fats by stating that as part of the Four Seasons Diet, it is strongly recommended that you limit your fat intake to fats that have been historically consumed by humans and are in their natural, minimally processed state. This includes fats from dairy products, such as milk, cream, and butter, along with extra-virgin olive oil, coconut oil, palm oil, small amounts of expeller-pressed sesame oil, and small amounts of cold-pressed refrigerated flax oil or cod liver oil for your omega-3 fats. For those who choose to eat meat, this would also include the fats from naturally pastured animals, but not meat from most factory-farmed animals. As you read about the effects of consuming excess omega-6 fats, remember that cows, pigs, and other animals that are fed diets high in grains such as corn will incorporate more of these fats into their fat. This means eating meat from animals raised on grains could contribute to some of the same possible effects as consuming polyunsaturated omega-6 fats.

Just as there are various types of proteins and carbohydrates that affect the season-types in different ways, there are also various types of fats that can have a profound impact on the health and well-being of the four season-types. Different types of fats can have a dramatic effect on our metabolism and affect the human body on many different levels. In the 1940s, cattle farmers experimented with trying to fatten their cattle with a type of fat that was cheap and abundant at the time: coconut oil. We had just won World War II and conquered the Pacific, and coconuts were in abundant supply and very affordable. Given their high fat content, it was thought that coconut oil would be the perfect way to fatten up cattle. When coconuts were fed to cattle, however, they got very lean and became more active, which was the exact opposite of the intended result.

For a short while thereafter, cattle were given drugs to slow their thyroid glands, which fattened them up, but it was discovered that the drugs were carcinogenic and posed a potentially serious risk to the people eating the meat. Not long after that, people discovered that corn could be used to fatten up the cattle. According to many experts, it's the polyunsaturated fats in most grains that cause this to happen by slowing our metabolism. These are the type of fats that remain highly liquid even when put in the refrigerator. Their technical name is polyunsaturated fatty acids, but to keep things short and simple, I'll refer to them as PUFAs.

Essential Fats
Although the body can manufacture most of the types of fats it needs to function from other dietary fats, a few fats are deemed "essential fats" because they are needed by the body but must be ingested because they cannot be manufactured. The first essential fat is called *alpha-linolenic acid*, or ALA for short, and is in the class of fats called omega-3 fats. I'll refer to this fat as omega-3 ALA. The other essential fat is called *linoleic acid*, or LA for short, and is in the class of fats called omega-6 fats. I'll refer to this fat as omega-6 LA. While these fats must be ingested from the foods we eat, the amount necessary for optimum human health is relatively small. Ideally, we should get around 2 percent of our calories from omega-6 LA, and 1 percent of our calories from omega-3 ALA. This amount of Omega-6 ALA is very easy to consume, because this type of fat is contained to some extent in many fats; however, it is especially abundant in corn oil and soybean oil. Most people

living in industrialized nations consume far more of these fats than necessary.

The omega-3 fat ALA is far less prevalent in most foods, however. Just one teaspoon of flaxseed oil provides an entire day's worth of this essential fat. Other foods with high levels of this fat include dark leafy greens and walnuts. Plankton and algae are also very high in these fats, which is why many fish, such as salmon, have a large amount of these fats in their tissues.

Although essential fats are necessary for human health, a lot of evidence strongly suggests that in high doses, similar to the amounts most American consume, they can actually be detrimental to the human body. Furthermore, these fats should be minimally processed, kept refrigerated, and consumed relatively soon after being manufactured. One of the unique properties of the essential fats is that they oxidize and go rancid very quickly when exposed to air, heat, and light. According to many natural health experts, the vegetable oils you buy on the store shelves have been overly processed, deodorized, and stabilized in a way that makes them extremely unhealthy. They advocate getting your daily small supply of these oils from either the foods you eat or else by supplementing with oils that have been minimally processed and immediately refrigerated.

PUFAs

Some health experts believe that many of our modern health problems are a result of switching from natural fats and oils to highly processed vegetable oils, such as corn oil and soybean oil, during the last hundred years. These processed oils contain polyunsaturated fatty acids (PUFAs), which recent studies show to have harmful effects on the human body.

Many people have heard of the French paradox, in which the French eat traditional high-fat foods such as cream and butter, yet have relatively low rates of cardiovascular disease. Very few people, however, know of the Israeli paradox, which is the opposite of the French situation. Israel has one of the highest rates of consumption of PUFAs in the world; these are the fats we have been told are good for our hearts since the 1950s. The Israeli paradox is that Israelis also have a high prevalence of cardiovascular disease, hypertension, non–insulin dependent diabetes mellitus, and other obesity diseases related to insulin resistance and high insulin levels. A research study on the subject suggested that it might be the high levels of omega-6 LA in the Israeli diet that were causing the high insulin levels and insulin resistance, leading to coronary heart disease and diabetes.

Just as fructose was originally sold as the healthy alternative to other sugars and was later found to be the harmful sugar, PUFAs were sold as the healthy oil for many years, and evidence is now suggesting that in amounts beyond our daily requirement they, too, are harmful. The question to ask is why cows eating large amounts of omega-6 PUFAs got fat? Also, why do the French, who eat butter and cheese, have low rates of cardiovascular disease, yet Israelis who consume a lot of omega-6 PUFAs have high rates of cardiovascular disease and insulin resistance?

Most people are now aware that artificially made trans fats and partially hydrogenated fats are believed almost universally to be unhealthy for the human body. What most people are not aware of is that a tremendous amount of scientific research showed this to be the case more than thirty years before it became universally accepted. Without going into the ugly history of the trans-fat fight in America, suffice it to say that most natural health food experts were sounding the alarm about trans fats starting back in the 1970s. Often, the mainstream medical community is slow to accept what seems obvious to many health and nutrition experts. In addition, millions of dollars are spent on lobbying by special interest groups, which includes the promotion of science that many believe to be "junk science." The research that cautioned against consuming large amounts of omega-6 PUFAs has been setting off alarms in the health and nutrition community for quite some time. Following are some of the more significant concerns raised, in light of the scientific clinical research that has been conducted during the last forty years.

PUFAs May Cause Breast, Prostate, and Other Cancers
As early as 1971, there were warning signs about the potential ability of PUFAs to cause cancer. This was the year that an eight-year study was published on men who ate large amounts of these fats versus men who followed a conventional diet for that time. This study showed that almost twice as many men who ate high levels of PUFAs had died from cancer, when compared to men who had the normal diet. Since then, many other studies have linked high dietary intake of omega-6 LA with various types of cancer, including breast, prostate, and colon. Conversely, numerous other studies show that the omega-3 fat ALA offers protection against many of these cancers. The protective effect of omega-3 fats has

been known since at least 1952, when a German chemist named Johanna Budwig created what she claimed was a miraculous cure for cancer. It involved large doses of flaxseed oil, which is high in the omega-3 fat ALA. Her cancer protocol is still quite popular in the natural health community to this day, and once again, mainstream science is finally catching up to what many health and nutrition experts have known for years.

Remember that both omega-6 LA and omega-3 ALA are needed by the body in small amounts. The research shows that excessive amounts of omega-6 LA promote cancer, especially when there is a corresponding low amount of omega-3 ALA. It has been estimated that for most of human history, we have had a diet with an omega-6 LA to omega-3 ALA ratio of approximately 1:1 to 2:1. This ratio has been increasing dramatically during the last fifty years, and now in most industrialized nations the ratio is around 16:1 to 18:1. In addition, the essential fats we do consume are often damaged by modern processing techniques. In Israel, the ratio of omega-6 LA to omega-3 ALA fats is 22:1 to 26:1, which could largely explain why Israelis are suffering from so many of the diseases associated with high omega-6 LA consumption.

The human body converts omega-3 ALA and omega-6 LA into other longer-chain fatty acids that are needed by the human body. For example, omega-3 ALA is converted to EPA and DHA, which are needed for optimal brain function. In fact, DHA, a derivative of omega-3 ALA, is one of the most abundant components of the brain's structural fat. Derivatives of both fats are found in the membranes of all of our cells, which is one reason it is so crucial to eat a small amount of these fats and to properly balance your consumption so that you maintain an ideal ratio. The body has a limited amount of the necessary enzymes to covert omega-6 LA and Omega-3 ALA into the longer-chain fats it needs. These two fats compete with each other for key enzymes that are needed to accomplish this conversion. Excess dietary omega-6 LA can hinder the conversion of omega-3 ALA by robbing all of the enzymes needed by the omega-3 fat.

Research suggests that many of the imbalances associated with excess omega-6 LA are triggered when the ideal ratio of 1:1 to 2:1 is increased by certain amounts. For example, keeping the ratio at 4:1, as opposed to the standard Western ratio of 16:1, was associated with a 70 percent decrease in total mortality from cardiovascular disease. A ratio of 2.5:1 was shown to reduce rectal cell proliferation in patients suffering from colorectal cancer.

Lower ratios were also associated with a decreased risk for breast cancer in women. In patients suffering from rheumatoid arthritis, a ratio of 2:1 to 3:1 was found to suppress inflammation. Asthma patients received a beneficial effect at a 5:1 ratio. This is one reason that fats that are high in omega-6 LA are not included in the Four Seasons Diet. Most people get adequate amounts of this fat by eating their regular foods. In addition to robbing the enzymes needed by omega-3 ALA, omega-6 LA also inhibits the body's ability to incorporate the omega-3 fat EPA into many of the body's cells. Monounsaturated fats do not have either of these effects, which is one reason extra-virgin olive oil is so healthy.

A breast cancer study conducted in Sweden that consisted of more than 61,000 women found that monounsaturated fats, such as those found in olive oil, offer protective benefits against breast cancer. Other studies have shown that olive oil protects against other forms of cancer as well. The same Swedish study showed that omega-6 LA increased the risk of breast cancer and that the higher the consumption of omega-6 LA, the greater a women's chance of developing breast cancer. Omega-6 LA appears to affect women more severely than men in many ways. The best theory on this right now is that it has to do with the effects of estrogen. There is even evidence to suggest that the risk for breast cancer may be imprinted on the fetus in the womb. This theory claims that a mother consuming large amounts of omega-6 LA while pregnant may predispose her daughter to a higher risk of breast cancer, along with an earlier onset of puberty. Girls now start puberty an average of six years earlier than they did a hundred years ago, which makes many people wonder what effects the foods we eat are having on the future health of our children.

Some studies suggest that in addition to inducing many cancers, excessive dietary omega-6 LA promotes the development of the tumors once they are induced. There also appears to be a connection between omega-6 LA and several stages involved in the development of breast cancer.

Oxidative Stress

Both omega-6 LA and omega-3 ALA can cause oxidative stress when consumed in amounts greater than the body needs. Oxidative stress is when the body produces excess *reactive oxygen species*, of which *free radicals* are probably the most well known. Oxidative stress is involved in many diseases and can cause long-term damage to our DNA. Many studies suggest that the oxidative DNA damage caused by excess PUFA consumption is one of the main contributors to increased cancer risk. Studies demonstrate that excess dietary PUFAs cause oxidative damage to the fat and the proteins of our mitochondria, which are the cells' power producers. Oxidative stress is also a major cause of rapid aging. Evidence shows that the two cellular traits associated with a long life span are the presence of a low amount of mitochondrial free radical production and cellular membranes that do not have an excessive amount of unsaturated fats in their membranes. Studies also show that free radicals generated from excess PUFAs cause the release of histamine. Excess histamine is known to trigger inflammatory and immune responses.

Cholesterol, Cardiovascular Disease, and Inflammatory/ Autoimmune Diseases

Prior to the twentieth century, heart attacks were very rare. Many natural heath experts claim that the increase in dietary processed foods and omega-6 LA during the last hundred years is a major cause of the huge increase in heart attacks in the same time period. A greater consumption of the omega-6 PUFA *arachidonic acid* may cause the body the produce excess inflammatory substances, which are known to cause spasms and constriction of the arterial walls, blood clots, and an increase in the viscosity of the blood. Omega-6 LA is believed to contribute to this by causing arterial inflammation.

Studies suggest that PUFAs also contribute to arterial plaque by impairing the body's ability to properly secrete cholesterol. One study showed a very strong association between serum plaque and dietary intake of PUFAs, and the findings implied a direct influence of dietary PUFAs on aortic plaque formation. Multiple studies have shown that PUFAs reduce the good HDL cholesterol levels more than either monounsaturated fats or saturated fats do. Many studies have also shown that saturated fats, which have been made the culprit for many years when it comes to coronary artery disease, have little to no effect in contributing to it. All of these studies suggest what many natural health experts have been saying for years, which is that the reason there were very few heart attacks until the twentieth century has to do with changing the types of fats we consume. This would also seem to be in keeping with the observations from both the French paradox and the Israeli paradox, which is that PUFAs have far more to do with cardiovascular disease than saturated fat does.

Insulin Resistance and Diabetes

It has been suggested that PUFAs contribute to insulin resistance and diabetes. One study that compared the dietary intake ratios of fats found that an omega-6 to omega-3 ratio of greater than 20:1 leads to an increase in non–insulin dependent diabetes, while a ratio of 6:1 prevented this increase. Several other studies have shown that consuming high levels of omega-6 LA leads to a deregulation of normal glucose sensitivity. Taken together, these studies suggest that there is an association between the consumption of omega-6 PUFAs and both insulin resistance and diabetes.

Energy Production and Metabolism

As I mentioned in the section on oxidative stress, studies show that excess dietary PUFAs cause damage to our mitochondria, which are the power producers inside our cells. Some studies demonstrate that PUFAs have a strong ability to interfere with the respiration of the mitochondria, which impairs normal energy production. In addition to affecting our energy production at the cellular level, PUFAs were shown in one study to affect fat metabolism in our bodies, in a way that favored more fat being deposited. Similar to the cows that ate corn and got fat, in this study rats were fed corn oil and got heavier and fatter than those fed lard. The studies clearly point to a correlation between dietary PUFAs and decreased energy at the cellular level.

Osteoporosis

Animal studies have shown that dietary intake of omega-3 fatty acids may positively influence bone health. The dietary ratios of omega-6 to omega-3 fatty acids were studied, and a significant association was found between higher levels of omega-6 LA and lower bone mineral density for men and women. Animal studies have suggested that omega-3 fatty acids may help minimize postmenopausal bone loss. One in vitro study showed a greater production of bone-formation markers, such as osteocalcin, after 48 hours of treatment with omega-3 ALA vs. omega-6 LA. From these studies, it appears that maintaining a healthy omega-6 to omega-3 fat ratio may play a crucial role in preserving our bones as we age.

Conclusion

Many of the potential negative health effects of ingesting excess omega-6 PUFAs appear to be tied to the harm they do to our immune systems and their tendency to cause an inflammatory response. In the 1970s, it was found that feeding large amounts of PUFAs to organ transplant patients could help suppress their immune systems and keep their bodies from rejecting the transplanted organs. Studies showed that PUFA supplementation was beneficial not only to kidney-transplant patients, but also to patients with certain autoimmune diseases. Autoimmune diseases occur when a person's immune system is overreactive, and the body actually ends up attacking its own cells. It was believed that PUFAs offered these patients some benefit by helping to suppress their immune systems.

Studies show that as you increase the ratio of omega-6 PUFAs in your diet, you also heighten the inflammatory response of the body, which has been implicated as a contributing factor in many diseases. Essential fatty acids are necessary for human health, but only in small amounts and preferably in their natural, unprocessed state. It would be extremely rare that a person following the Four Seasons Diet would ever be deficient in omega-6 PUFAs, because these fats are contained in grains, nuts, cheese, milk, olive oil, and, to a small extent, in most natural foods that contain fat. What is often deficient in most diets, however, are the omega-3 PUFAs, which are contained in foods such as flaxseed oil, cod-liver oil, walnuts, and many species of fish. When you supplement with omega-3 oils, the amount you need is relatively small. For most people, one teaspoon to one tablespoon of high omega-3 oil, such as flaxseed oil, per day would be all that is needed. In the section on flaxseed oil, I discuss the best way to buy and consume this valuable oil. Remember that excess amounts of all PUFAs, including excess omega-3 oils, can have health consequences. By limiting your fats and oils to those recommended as part of the Four Seasons Diet and supplementing with small amounts of omega-3 fats each day, you can be sure you are getting the minimum amounts of both omega-6 and omega-3 fats, in a healthy ratio of not greater than 4:1, from oils that are minimally processed.

Healthful Natural Oils
Natural traditional oils, such as extra-virgin olive oil, have been consumed for thousands of years, and numerous studies are finding that they offer many protective benefits against disease. One of the benefits of minimally processed oils, such as extra-virgin olive oil, is that they contain abundant healthy compounds besides

just monounsaturated fats. Monounsaturated fats were found to offer protection against a number of diseases and cancers, such as breast cancer. In addition to their healthy composition, they also contain other nutrients that are believed to offer protection against cancer, such as alpha-tocopherol, squalene, lignans, and various phenolics, which are very potent antioxidants. Monounsaturated fats have been found to increase our healthy HDL cholesterol without raising the bad LDL cholesterol.

Olive Oil

It's best to buy organic extra-virgin olive oil, which is the type that has been minimally processed. The main thing to remember about extra-virgin olive oil is that if you use it for cooking, you need to keep the temperature from getting too high, because heat will damage extra-virgin olive oil. For higher-temperature cooking, coconut oil or butter are recommended.

Coconut Oil, Palm Oil, Palm Kernel Oil, and Your Waistline

Coconut oil is one of the healthiest oils you can consume. It has been wrongly maligned as being an unhealthy oil ever since a study showed that it was bad for your health. The problem with that study is that it used hydrogenated coconut oil, rather than natural, minimally processed coconut oil. There were several other major flaws with the way that study was conducted, but based on this one inaccurate study, the vegetable oil companies were able to convince many food manufacturers to replace healthy unhydrogenated coconut oil with vegetable oils high in omega-6 PUFAs. Many studies conducted on natural coconut oil since this early flawed study show that it does not lead to high serum cholesterol or to coronary heart disease. Yet because coconut oil is high in saturated fats, which have been wrongly demonized for so many years, people often believe that it's an unhealthy oil.

So, what was the result of replacing healthy coconut oil in many foods in America with omega-6 PUFAs? Several studies are very suggestive of the effect that this switch has had on our health. In one study conducted in Sri Lanka, where coconuts are a staple food, they replaced the coconut oil in the diets of some participants with corn oil. Corn oil is very high in omega-6 fats. The result was a drop in the healthy HDL cholesterol by more than 40 percent. The bad cholesterol dropped as well, but only by around 20 percent. Remember from the section on cholesterol that it's the ratio that's important, so a drop of this nature would be expected to lead to a higher rate of arterial plaque deposits and coronary artery disease over a prolonged period.

Another study of the effects of coconut oil on women put half of the women on coconut oil and half the women on soybean oil, which is high in omega-6 fats, with both groups eating the same number of calories per day. After twelve weeks, the women consuming coconut oil had higher levels of good HDL cholesterol and a much higher ratio of good HDL vs. bad LDL cholesterol. Remember that the lower the ratio of LDL to HDL cholesterol, the less chance of heart disease. The women who consumed soybean oil had an increase in total cholesterol and unhealthy LDL cholesterol and an increase in the LDL to HDL ratio. Also, the women who consumed the coconut oil saw a reduction in their waist circumference, similar to the way cows that were fed coconut oil got skinny.

What makes coconut oil a unique fat is that approximately 65 percent of the oil consists of medium-chain triglycerides. These are metabolized quickly in the liver for energy and do not take part in either manufacturing or transporting cholesterol. Also, for anyone looking to lose weight, most of the fats in coconut oil are not deposited as body fat but are primarily used for energy relatively quickly after being consumed. In addition, medium-chain triglycerides increase the rate at which the body burns fat for fuel, so a diet higher in coconut oil may actually help you burn more body fat.

Flaxseed Oil, Cod Liver Oil, and Hemp Oil
Flaxseed oil, along with hemp oil, are two oils high in omega-3 ALA that have been historically consumed in order to obtain this essential fat. They are both extremely sensitive and will quickly go rancid if exposed to too much light, heat, and air. For this reason, the only oils of this type that you should consume are cold-pressed and purchased from the refrigerated section of the grocery or health-food store and kept refrigerated in your home. Some manufacturers sell these oils in capsule form on the store shelf; however, if you prick one of these capsules with a pin and let the oil out, you will often find that the oil is rancid and not palatable. When this type of oil becomes rancid, it can be extremely unhealthy to consume. Flaxseed oil is higher in omega-3 ALA, while hemp oil is higher in omega-6 LA. Because most of us easily consume all of the omega-6 fats we need but are deficient in omega-3 fats, it's recommended that you consume flaxseed oil or cod liver oil to get

your omega-3 fats. To get your entire daily supply of omega-3 ALA, take anywhere from a teaspoon to a tablespoon per day. Summers and Springs will usually have a higher need for these fats, while Winters and Autumns will have a lower need. The best way to consume these fats is with a little protein that is high in sulfur and lower in fat, such as low-fat cottage cheese, egg-white protein powder, or whey protein powder. This is because the sulfur in the protein will react with the oils in such a way as to make it water soluble, which helps the oil to get into all of the capillaries and cells of your body.

Cod liver oil has historically been consumed not only for its omega-3 fats, but also for its vitamins A and D. Although cod liver oil used to taste really horrible, several brands now add lemon oil essence and are palatable. In addition, manufacturers have developed a method of adding nitrogen to the bottle, which prevents oxidation even when on the store shelf. Once these oils are opened, however, they need to be immediately refrigerated in order to keep them from going rancid.

It is now even possible to purchase vegetarian algae oil, which is high in the omega-3 fats EPA and DHA. Normally, the body can convert the omega-3 fats in flaxseed oil to these two fats; however, someone with compromised health or people who consume excessive amounts of omega-6 fats may have difficulties converting enough for their needs and could benefit from adding this oil to their diet while they restore their health.

Reasons to be Cautious of Canola Oil
Canola oil is not included in the list of recommended oils in the Four Seasons Diet for several reasons. First, it contains 21 percent omega-6 LA, and I have already discussed many of the potential adverse effects from eating large amounts of this fat. Second, canola oil is a highly processed oil containing a fair amount of PUFAs, and I do not recommend consuming any highly processed oil, but most especially those that are highly processed and also contain a lot of PUFAs. Thirdly, it is a relatively new oil on the market for human consumption, having only been approved by the FDA in 1985 in a way that is still controversial and questionable to many natural health food experts. Finally, there are still a lot of concerns about its use among some of the leading experts in oils and natural traditional foods.

For years, most "medical authorities" told us that margarine, which is basically hydrogenated oil, was the healthy oil, while many "health food experts" were claiming as early as the 1970s that hydrogenated oils were dangerous. The same can be said of both fructose and PUFAs. They were sold as the healthy choice by the "medical authorities," while many "health food experts" were saying the opposite. In all three of these cases, the research has either vindicated or strongly vindicated the "health food experts," but it took years of opposition from the "medical authorities" before they finally admitted they had been wrong for decades. There are three major similarities in the introduction of hydrogenated oils, high-fructose corn syrup, and highly processed PUFAs into our food supply. First, they were never historically consumed in large amounts prior to 1900. Second, health food experts expressed major concerns about all three foods for decades, while medical experts touted all three foods as healthy for various reasons. Third, all three foods are highly processed.

Currently, natural health experts have many concerns about canola oil; two of them have to do with the presence of the compounds *thiouracil* and *euricic acid*, which are contained in canola oil. Thiouracil is known to depress thyroid function, while euricic acid is a known toxin to the human body. In addition, most canola oil is produced from canola that has been genetically modified (GM), and in the genetically modified organism (GMO) section you will learn why all GMOs should be avoided. Until more studies are done on canola oil, similar to the studies that were finally done on PUFAs, I cannot recommend this oil as part of your diet.

Dairy and Saturated Fats

While PUFAs in vegetable oils were being touted as healthy, saturated fat was being demonized as the cause of many health problems in America. Remember that the French eat plenty of butter and cheese and have relatively low rates of cardiovascular disease, while the Israelis are among the biggest consumers of PUFAs in the world and suffer from high rates of cardiovascular disease, hypertension, non–insulin dependent diabetes mellitus, and insulin resistance. There were numerous flaws in the studies that claimed saturated fat caused cardiovascular disease. As explained earlier, cardiovascular disease is caused in large part by a high ratio of the unhealthy LDL cholesterol to the healthy HDL cholesterol, which results from chronically high insulin levels. Chronically high levels of insulin are predominately caused by insulin resistance or decreased cellular insulin sensitivity.

The two foods that have been documented to cause insulin resistance in study after study are fructose and excessive omega-6 PUFAs, while omega-3 and monounsaturated fats can help improve insulin sensitivity. Another factor that can contribute to insulin resistance is excess fat consumption beyond what the body needs. This is one reason the Summer and Spring diets are lower in fat, especially the saturated fats *palmitic acid* and *stearic acid*. These two saturated fats have been implicated as one of the causes of insulin resistance. One theory suggests that they prompt the body to produce a substance called *ceramide*, which slows glucose uptake and storage. This is yet another reason saturated fats can be so beneficial for Winters and Autumns. New research shows that saturated fats activate JNK-1 (Jun N terminal kinase), which inhibits insulin signaling through c-Src activation and makes the cells less permeable by pushing c-Src into the cells' protective coating. Although JNK reduces insulin sensitivity, its action is partially blocked by the omega-3 fat EPA, as well as by the monounsaturated fat palmitoleic acid. These fats accomplish this by helping to prevent c-Src from incorporating into the cells' protective coating, which keeps JNK-1 from being able to reduce insulin sensitivity. Since Summers and Springs tend to suffer from insulin resistance, their Four Season diets are low in saturated fats, because these fats can activate JNK and reduce their insulin sensitivity.

Foods that contain animal fats, such as meat and dairy products, have large amounts of the saturated fats palmitic acid and stearic acid. As explained earlier, Winters usually have muscles that are highly sensitive to insulin, and their metabolism also tends to make their cells overly sensitive to insulin. Summers, on the other hand, normally have muscles that are not as sensitive to insulin, and their metabolism has a tendency to make their cells more resistant to insulin. Of course, Winters can become insulin resistant as well, but this is often caused by years of blood sugar spikes and crashes that result from overeating carbohydrates. This is the reason the Winter diet and, to a lesser extent, the Autumn diet are both higher in these two fats. These diets will help reduce Autumns' and Winters' insulin sensitivity and keep it at the proper level. The Summer diet and, to a lesser extent, the Spring diet are lower in these fats, because the fats would tend to reduce these two season-types' insulin sensitivity, and that is the last thing they usually need. Once all of the season-types get to their ideal weight, they will have a much easier time learning to feel what their metabolic state is and know when they need to add more of these fats into their diet. Winters will need to eat significantly larger amounts of these two fats in the winter when it's cold, while Summers will need to virtually eliminate these two fats in the summer when it's hot.

The one vegetable oil that is extremely high in palmitic acid is palm oil, which is not to be confused with palm kernel oil. Palm kernel oil is closer to coconut oil in its composition and is alright for all the season-types to consume, whereas palm oil is recommended only for Winters and Autumns and is not recommended for Summers and Springs.

Minerals

Vitamins and minerals can have profound effects on the various season-types. Later, I'll give you a detailed breakdown of the vitamins and minerals that are most beneficial for your season-type. For now, however, I'll mention a few essential minerals that have the greatest impact on the four season-types: calcium, magnesium, phosphorous, potassium, and sodium. These five minerals can tremendously affect the speed at which we burn sugar for energy, as well as influence our nervous systems and other metabolic functions of the body. Some minerals work best in conjunction with other minerals, almost as if they are partners.

Different Strokes for Different Folks
Studies show that two of the most important mineral partnerships are calcium/magnesium and sodium/potassium. Although the body needs all four of these minerals every day, their ratio in the diet can have a dramatic effect on many metabolic functions. The most relevant one that pertains to the season-types is the rate at which a person uses glucose for energy. For example, studies show that supplementing with magnesium will cause people to increase both their insulin sensitivity and their rate of sugar-energy production. In most cases, this is exactly what a Summer needs, but the last thing a Winter would need. Although everyone requires all of these minerals, it's the balance or ratio of the minerals in our bodies that can really affect us, especially Winters and Summers, the two extreme season-types. For example, nutrition experts normally recommend that people consume about twice as much calcium as they do magnesium. In actuality, this 2:1 ratio of calcium to magnesium would probably be too high for a Summer and too low

for a Winter. Essentially, Summers need extra magnesium, while Winters need extra calcium. They also need different levels of potassium, sodium, and phosphorous.

In general, higher magnesium and potassium levels will be most beneficial to Summers and, to a lesser extent, Springs, while they would be most detrimental to Winters and, to a lesser extent, Autumns. Conversely, higher levels of calcium, sodium, and phosphorous would be most beneficial to Winters and, to a lesser extent, Autumns, while they would be most detrimental to Summers and, to a lesser extent, Springs. An easier way to remember it is shown in Chart 5.2.

CHART 5.2 MINERAL NEEDS OF THE SEASON-TYPES

	Winters	Autumns	Springs	Summers
Calcium	Highest Need	Second Highest Need	Second Lowest Need	Lowest Need
Magnesium	Lowest Need	Second Lowest Need	Second Highest Need	Highest Need
Sodium	Highest Need	Second Highest Need	Second Lowest Need	Lowest Need
Potassium	Lowest Need	Second Lowest Need	Second Highest Need	Highest Need
Phosphorous	Highest Need	Second Highest Need	Second Lowest Need	Lowest Need

Winters do best with a higher-calcium diet and a lower-potassium diet. Summers do best with a higher-magnesium and higher-potassium diet. The best way to gauge whether you're getting too much or too little of one of these nutrients is to see how you feel after eating a meal. Take, for example, a Summer eating nothing but cheese pizza for a meal. This meal is high in calcium, high in sodium, low in potassium, low in magnesium, and high in phosphorous. It's basically the opposite of what would be best for most Summers. Such a meal would probably make Summers feel tired, in most cases. If Summers eat a high-calcium, low-magnesium meal such is this, it's a good time for them to add in some supplemental magnesium, with magnesium aspartate being the best form for Summers to take.

Summers can go too far in the other extreme, however, by eating nothing but high-potassium fruits and vegetables, with lots of grains, no calcium, and too little phosphorous-rich protein. They might feel fantastic eating this way for a week or two, but eventually, they will go too far in the other direction. When this happens, Summers will feel the way Winters often feel: they may have higher levels of energy, but it's often nervous energy with erratic blood-sugar swings, and they may feel cold even in warm weather. This is a sign that Summers need to add in a little more salt and calcium-rich dairy foods into their diet, along with perhaps a bit more phosphorous-rich protein. The same thing can happen to Winters. They may focus on eating high-calcium and high-phosphorous foods that are low in potassium and magnesium. They might feel great for a week or two but will eventually begin to feel more like Summers, with lower energy levels, and might actually feel hot even when it's a bit colder outside. When this happens, they will know it's time to ease up on the high-calcium foods and add in more vegetables and maybe even a piece or two fruit.

In a later chapter, I'll go over this in more detail, so don't feel overwhelmed. I'll explain each food group separately, along with listing foods that can help speed up and slow down your season-type. The Four Seasons Diet is designed in such a way that if you follow it and listen to your body, you should have a fairly easy time getting the proper level of these five important minerals. Remember that any time you feel out of balance, you have probably strayed from your beneficial foods listed on the food charts, and it's time to go back to focusing on those foods for a while. In the advanced section on supplements, I give a complete breakdown of all of the vitamins and minerals that can offer extra benefit to each season-type. This is especially helpful for people who work out or engage in competitive athletics and need an extra edge.

6
The Four Seasons Diet

Eat the proper foods for your season-type, and you can control your appetite, mood, metabolism, energy, and well-being.

Now that you know your season-type and understand many of the metabolic differences between the four season-types, you are ready to go over the Four Seasons Diet plan. The two most important things to remember are that

1. Your season-type determines the *ratio* of protein, carbohydrates, and fat that is best for you.
2. Your season-type determines the *types* of proteins, carbohydrates, and fats that are best for you.

Winters have the greatest need for protein and fat, while Summers have the lowest need for protein and fat. Also, Winters have the highest need for proteins with purines and long-chain saturated fats, while proteins with purines and long-chain saturated fats are needed least by Summers. Chart 6.1 lists the recommended percentage of calories from protein, carbohydrates, and fat for each season-type. It is designed to help you plan each meal with the optimum mix of nutrients for your season-type.

CHART 6.1 MACRONUTRIENT PERCENTAGES FOR EACH SEASON-TYPE

	Winter	Autumn	Spring	Summer
Protein	35-45%	30-35%	25-30%	20-25%
Carbohydrates	25-35%	35-50%	50-60%	60-70%
Fat	25-35%	20-30%	15-20%	10-15%

For those of you who hate doing math, I have come up with a simple chart for each season-type that should help you keep your calorie counts within the desired range, while you learn to gauge the proper amounts of protein, carbohydrates, and fat to consume for your season-type. Once you get accustomed to seeing how much of each macronutrient is appropriate for your season-type, you should no longer have to count calories and measure food portions, but you should be able to gauge how much of each to consume. You should also learn to associate each meal with how you feel during the next four to five hours after eating it. This will be a big help once you stop carefully measuring your food and counting calories, because if you don't do an adequate job of getting the proper amount of protein, carbohydrates, or fat in a particular meal, you should feel the effects during the next several hours.

On the next few pages, you'll find charts for the calorie and gram counts for the four season-types. The first column on the far left lists the total calorie count of a particular meal, from 350 calories up to 900 calories. To the right of that are the recommended calorie and gram ranges of protein, carbohydrates, and fat for your season-type. For example, a Winter who is eating a 500-calorie meal should try to keep his or her protein intake between 175 and 225 calories and the total grams of protein from 44 to 56 grams. Both calories and grams are listed because some people may find it easier to track their diets using calories, while others might prefer to use grams or even a combination of both.

CHART 6.2
A WINTER'S CALORIES/GRAMS OF PROTEIN, CARBOHYDRATES, AND FAT BASED ON TOTAL CALORIES IN A MEAL

	Winter Calorie and Gram Counts											
	PROTEIN				CARBOHYDRATES				FAT			
Total	Calories		Grams		Calories		Grams		Calories		Grams	
Calories	Low	High	Low	High	Low	High	Low	High	Low	High	Low	High
350	123	158	31	39	88	123	22	31	88	123	10	14
400	140	180	35	45	100	140	25	35	100	140	11	16
450	158	203	39	51	113	158	28	39	113	158	13	18
500	175	225	44	56	125	175	31	44	125	175	14	19
550	193	248	48	62	138	193	34	48	138	193	15	21
600	210	270	53	68	150	210	38	53	150	210	17	23
650	228	293	57	73	163	228	41	57	163	228	18	25
700	245	315	61	79	175	245	44	61	175	245	19	27
750	263	338	66	84	188	263	47	66	188	263	21	29
800	280	360	70	90	200	280	50	70	200	280	22	31
850	298	383	74	96	213	298	53	74	213	298	24	33
900	315	405	79	101	225	315	56	79	225	315	25	35

CHART 6.3
AN AUTUMN'S CALORIES/GRAMS OF PROTEIN, CARBOHYDRATES, AND FAT BASED ON TOTAL CALORIES IN A MEAL

	An Autumn's Calorie and Gram Counts											
	PROTEIN				CARBOHYDRATES				FAT			
Total	Calories		Grams		Calories		Grams		Calories		Grams	
Calories	Low	High	Low	High	Low	High	Low	High	Low	High	Low	High
350	105	123	26	31	123	175	31	44	70	105	8	12
400	120	140	30	35	140	200	35	50	80	120	9	13
450	135	158	34	39	158	225	39	56	90	135	10	15
500	150	175	38	44	175	250	44	63	100	150	11	17
550	165	193	41	48	193	275	48	69	110	165	12	18
600	180	210	45	53	210	300	53	75	120	180	13	20
650	195	228	49	57	228	325	57	81	130	195	14	22
700	210	245	53	61	245	350	61	88	140	210	16	23
750	225	263	56	66	263	375	66	94	150	225	17	25
800	240	280	60	70	280	400	70	100	160	240	18	27
850	255	298	64	74	298	425	74	106	170	255	19	28
900	270	315	68	79	315	450	79	113	180	270	20	30

CHART 6.4
A SPRING'S CALORIES/GRAMS OF PROTEIN, CARBOHYDRATES, AND FAT BASED ON TOTAL CALORIES IN A MEAL

	A Spring's Calorie and Gram Counts											
	PROTEIN				CARBOHYDRATES				FAT			
Total	Calories		Grams		Calories		Grams		Calories		Grams	
Calories	Low	High	Low	High	Low	High	Low	High	Low	High	Low	High
350	88	105	22	26	175	210	44	53	53	70	6	8
400	100	120	25	30	200	240	50	60	60	80	7	9
450	113	135	28	34	225	270	56	68	68	90	8	10
500	125	150	31	38	250	300	63	75	75	100	8	11
550	138	165	34	41	275	330	69	83	83	110	9	12
600	150	180	38	45	300	360	75	90	90	120	10	13
650	163	195	41	49	325	390	81	98	98	130	11	14
700	175	210	44	53	350	420	88	105	105	140	12	16
750	188	225	47	56	375	450	94	113	113	150	13	17
800	200	240	50	60	400	480	100	120	120	160	13	18
850	213	255	53	64	425	510	106	128	128	170	14	19
900	225	270	56	68	450	540	113	135	135	180	15	20

CHART 6.5
A SUMMER'S CALORIES/GRAMS OF PROTEIN, CARBOHYDRATES, AND FAT BASED ON TOTAL CALORIES IN A MEAL

	A Summer's Calorie and Gram Counts											
	PROTEIN				CARBOHYDRATES				FAT			
Total	Calories		Grams		Calories		Grams		Calories		Grams	
Calories	Low	High	Low	High	Low	High	Low	High	Low	High	Low	High
350	70	88	18	22	210	245	53	61	35	53	4	6
400	80	100	20	25	240	280	60	70	40	60	4	7
450	90	113	23	28	270	315	68	79	45	68	5	8
500	100	125	25	31	300	350	75	88	50	75	6	8
550	110	138	28	34	330	385	83	96	55	83	6	9
600	120	150	30	38	360	420	90	105	60	90	7	10
650	130	163	33	41	390	455	98	114	65	98	7	11
700	140	175	35	44	420	490	105	123	70	105	8	12
750	150	188	38	47	450	525	113	131	75	113	8	13
800	160	200	40	50	480	560	120	140	80	120	9	13
850	170	213	43	53	510	595	128	149	85	128	9	14
900	180	225	45	56	540	630	135	158	90	135	10	15

The food charts that list each food individually can look a little intimidating at first, but they are really quite simple to use. I have recreated a portion of a food chart below (Chart 6.6), to help you understand how to use them.

CHART 6.6 FOOD CHART SAMPLE

Calories per Serving							Recommended % of Calories			
							Winter	Autumn	Spring	Summer
		Protein				Protein:	35-45%	30-35%	25-30%	20-25%
			Carbohydrates			Carbohydrates:	25-35%	35-50%	50-60%	60-70%
				Fat		Fat:	25-35%	20-30%	15-20%	10-15%
Serving	Total	P	C	F	Pur=Purines*	Purines*:	High	Medium	Low	Very Low
Size	Cal	Cal	Cal	Cal	Pur		Winter	Autumn	Spring	Summer
						PROTEIN				
						MEAT				
4 oz.	302	122	0	180	+	Beef, 70% lean	:-)	:-|	:-(	:-(

* + = medium, ++ = high, +++ = very high

Explaining the Charts

The food charts are designed to help you easily keep track of the protein, carbohydrate, and fat content of the various foods you eat, so that you can try to stay within the guidelines for your season-type. If you look at the middle of the chart where it says "PROTEIN," this is the column where all of the various foods will be listed. The first food under this column is beef that is 70 percent lean.

If you look at the middle of the left-hand side, you'll notice where it says "Serving Size." This is simply the amount of each food for which information is given, for example, in this case the serving of beef is 4 ounces. To the right of "Serving Size" is "Total Cal," which is the total calories in that 4-ounce serving of beef. The next three columns to the right of that are "P Cal," "C Cal," and "F Cal," and these stand for the calories from protein, carbohydrates, and fat, respectively, for that 4-ounce serving of beef. The column to the right of "F Cal" labeled "Pur" is simply the purine content of that protein, and at the very bottom of the chart is an asterisk, which explains the purine ranking. This same column will be used for other purposes for various foods; for example, for fruit it will list the grams of fructose in a serving of fruit. Whenever this column is used for a purpose such as listing the purine or fructose content of a particular food group, it will be explained by noting what the column measures above the column heading. If you look at the example, this column is labeled "Pur" and above that, it states that "Pur = Purines," so you know this column shows the purine content of various foods listed on the chart.

On the far right side are separate columns for Winters, Autumns, Springs, and Summers. Each food is given a rating for each season-type, with a :-) meaning it's beneficial, a :-| meaning it's neutral, and a :-(meaning it's detrimental. If a food is especially beneficial for a particular season type, it will be noted with ":-) :-)" and if it is particularly detrimental for a particular season-type, it will be noted with a ":-(:-(."

These ratings are based on factors that can affect the season-types, many of which I have talked about at length. Ideally, people should try to consume foods that are either beneficial or neutral for their season-type, while keeping their protein, carbohydrates, and fat within their recommended ratios. I highly recommend that you try consuming mostly beneficial and neutral foods for the first few weeks on the diet to see how you respond and help get your season-type in balance. After that, you can try adding in some "avoid" foods, to see what your response is. It's generally alright to eat a small amount of "avoid" foods, with the key being only a small amount. Beneficial foods will help balance out your season-type, while "avoid" foods will tend to get your season-type out of balance, so the more beneficial foods and the fewer "avoid" foods you consume, the better.

Don't feel overwhelmed at this point. In a little while, I'll go over some sample meals that are ideal for each season-type, along with how each season-type might adapt to a typical family dinner. In later sections, I'll explain the benefits of adopting a vegetarian lifestyle and how each season-type can best make this change.

CHART 6.7 PROTEIN FOOD CHART

Calories per Serving							Recommended % of Calories			
							Winter	Autumn	Spring	Summer
		Protein				Protein:	35-45%	30-35%	25-30%	20-25%
			Carbohydrates			Carbohydrates:	25-35%	35-50%	50-60%	60-70%
				Fat		Fat:	25-35%	20-30%	15-20%	10-15%
Serving Size	Total Cal	P Cal	C Cal	F Cal	Pur=Purines*	Purines*:	High	Medium	Low	Very Low
					Pur	PROTEIN	Winter	Autumn	Spring	Summer
						MEAT				
4 oz.	302	122	0	180	+	Beef, 70% lean	:-)	:-|	:-(	:-(
4 oz.	304	129	0	175	+	Beef, 80% lean	:-)	:-|	:-(	:-(
4 oz.	228	122	0	108	+	Beef, 90% lean	:-)	:-)	:-(	:-(
4 oz.	183	123	0	60	+	Beef, 95% lean	:-)	:-)	:-|	:-(
4 oz.	286	116	0	170	+	Lamb	:-)	:-|	:-(	:-(
4 oz.	153	97.2	17	36.8	++	Liver	:-):-)	:-)	:-(	:-(:-(
1 slice	41	13	0	28	+	Pork, bacon	:-)	:-|	:-(	:-(
6 oz.	252	136	8	108	+	Pork, Canadian bacon	:-)	:-)	:-|	:-(
4 oz.	187	84	6	97	+	Pork, chop	:-)	:-)	:-(	:-(
4 oz.	123	77	8	38	+	Pork, tenderloin	:-)	:-)	:-|	:-(
1 oz.	34	22	0	12	+	Pork, extra lean ham	:-)	:-)	:-|	:-(
						POULTRY				
4 oz.	266	81	0	185	+	Chicken, dark with skin	:-)	:-|	:-(	:-(
4 oz.	123	111	0	12	+	Chicken, light no skin	:-|	:-|	:-)	:-|
4 oz.	224	82	0	142	+	Cornish hen	:-)	:-|	:-(	:-(
4 oz.	148	88	0	60	+	Duck	:-)	:-)	:-(	:-(
4 oz.	180	108	0	72	+	Goose	:-)	:-)	:-(	:-(
4 oz.	248	132	0	116	+	Turkey, dark with skin	:-)	:-)	:-(	:-(
4 oz.	128	112	0	16	+	Turkey, light, no skin	:-|	:-)	:-)	:-|
						SEAFOOD				
1 oz.	37	25	0	12	+++	Anchovies	:-):-)	:-)	:-(	:-(:-(
4 oz.	109	85	0	23.6		Bass	:-(	:-|	:-)	:-|
4 oz.	143	85	0	56	+	Carp	:-)	:-)	:-(	:-(
4 oz.	151	76	0	77		Catfish	:-(	:-|	:-(	:-(
4 oz.	83	61	12	10	+	Clams	:-)	:-)	:-(	:-(
4 oz.	92	86	0	6	+	Cod	:-|	:-|	:-)	:-|
4 oz.	94	88	0	6	+	Crab	:-)	:-)	:-(	:-(
4 oz.	103	91	0	12		Flounder	:-(	:-(	:-)	:-|
4 oz.	103	93	0	10		Grouper	:-(	:-(	:-)	:-|
4 oz.	123	100	0	23		Halibut	:-(	:-(	:-)	:-|
4 oz.	101	90	2	9	+	Lobster	:-)	:-)	:-|	:-(
4 oz.	230	89	0	141	++	Mackerel	:-):-)	:-|	:-(	:-(:-(
4 oz.	100	57	17	23	+	Mussels	:-)	:-)	:-)	:-|
4 oz.	91	45	23	23	+	Oysters	:-)	:-)	:-(	:-(
4 oz.	106	91	0	17	++	Perch	:-)	:-)	:-|	:-(

* + = medium, ++ = high, +++ = very high

Calories per Serving							Recommended % of Calories			
							Winter	Autumn	Spring	Summer
		Protein				Protein:	35-45%	30-35%	25-30%	20-25%
			Carbohydrates			Carbohydrates:	25-35%	35-50%	50-60%	60-70%
				Fat		Fat:	25-35%	20-30%	15-20%	10-15%
Serving Size	Total Cal	P Cal	C Cal	F Cal	Pur=Purines* Pur	Purines*:	High Winter	Medium Autumn	Low Spring	Very Low Summer
						PROTEIN				
						SEAFOOD CONT.				
4 oz.	85	78	0	7		Roughy	:-(	:-(	:-)	:-|
4 oz.	201	95	0	106	++	Salmon	:-):-)	:-)	:-(	:-(:-(
4 oz.	209	100	3	106	+++	Sardines	:-):-)	:-)	:-(	:-(:-(
4 oz.	98	80	11	7.6	++	Scallops	:-)	:-)	:-(	:-(
4 oz.	119	97	4	18	++	Shrimp	:-)	:-)	:-|	:-(
4 oz.	112	98	0	14		Snapper	:-(	:-(	:-)	:-|
4 oz.	104	75	15	14	+	Squid	:-|	:-|	:-)	:-(
4 oz.	136	95	0	41		Swordfish	:-(	:-|	:-(	:-(
4 oz.	166	99	0	67	+++	Trout	:-)	:-)	:-(	:-(
4 oz.	122	112	0	10	+	Tuna, yellowfin	:-|	:-)	:-)	:-|
4 oz.	150	91	0	59	+	Whitefish	:-)	:-)	:-(	:-(
						MISC. PROTEIN				
1 white	16	15	0	1		Egg whites	:-(	:-(	:-|	:-)
Per individual product						Whey protein	:-|	:-|	:-(	:-(
Per individual product						Milk (casein protein)	:-|	:-|	:-(	:-(
Per individual product						Soy protein	:-(	:-(	:-(	:-(
Per individual product					+++	Brewer's yeast	:-)	:-)	:-(	:-(
Per individual product					+++	Chlorella/blue-green algae	:-)	:-)	:-(	:-(

* + = medium, ++ = high, +++ = very high

CHART 6.8 DAIRY AND BEAN FOOD CHARTS

Calories per Serving							Recommended % of Calories			
							Winter	Autumn	Spring	Summer
		Protein				Protein:	35-45%	30-35%	25-30%	20-25%
			Carbohydrates			Carbohydrates:	25-35%	35-50%	50-60%	60-70%
				Fat		Fat:	25-35%	20-30%	15-20%	10-15%
Serving Size	Total Cal	P Cal	C Cal	F Cal	Pur =Purines* Pur	Purines*:	High Winter	Medium Autumn	Low Spring	Very Low Summer
						DAIRY				
						DAIRY				
1 oz.	99	26	3	70		Blue cheese	:-|	:-|	:-(	:-(
1 oz.	94	25	1	68		Brie	:-|	:-|	:-(	:-(
1 oz.	113	30	2	81		Cheddar cheese	:-|	:-|	:-(	:-(
1 oz.	110	28	3	79		Colby cheese	:-|	:-|	:-(	:-(
4 oz.	111	54	14	43		Cottage cheese/whole	:-|	:-|	:-(	:-(
4 oz.	81	60	11	10		Cottage cheese, 1%	:-(	:-(	:-|	:-(
1 tbsp.	50	4	2	44		Cream cheese	:-|	:-|	:-(	:-(
1 egg	71	25	1	45		Eggs, chicken	:-|	:-|	:-(	:-(
1 oz.	74	17	5	52		Feta	:-|	:-|	:-(	:-(
1 oz.	100	30	2	68		Gouda	:-|	:-|	:-(	:-(
1 cup	118	41	51	26		Milk, low fat	:-(	:-|	:-|	:-(
1 cup	101	42	54	5		Milk, nonfat	:-(	:-(	:-|	:-|
1 cup	146	31	44	71		Milk, whole	:-|	:-|	:-(	:-(
1 oz.	104	29	1	74		Monterey jack	:-|	:-|	:-(	:-(
1 oz.	71	29	3	39		Mozzarella, part skim	:-|	:-|	:-|	:-|
1 oz.	84	27	2	55		Mozzarella, whole	:-|	:-|	:-(	:-(
1 oz.	110	43	3	64		Parmesan	:-|	:-|	:-(	:-(
1 oz.	98	31	2	65		Provolone	:-|	:-|	:-(	:-(
1 oz.	39	14	6	19		Ricotta, part skim	:-|	:-|	:-(	:-(
1 oz.	49	14	3	32		Ricotta, whole	:-|	:-|	:-(	:-(
1 oz.	108	38	4	66		Romano	:-|	:-|	:-(	:-(
1 tbsp.	20	2	3	16		Sour cream, low fat	:-|	:-|	:-(	:-(
2 tbsp.	24	8	16	0		Sour cream, nonfat	:-|	:-|	:-|	:-|
1 tbsp.	23	1	1	21		Sour cream, whole	:-|	:-|	:-(	:-(
1 oz.	106	32	6	68		Swiss	:-|	:-|	:-(	:-(
1 cup	149	36	43	70		Yogurt, whole	:-|	:-|	:-(	:-(
1 cup	154	55	66	33		Yogurt, low fat	:-(	:-|	:-|	:-(
1 cup	137	60	73	4		Yogurt, fat free	:-(	:-(	:-|	:-|
1 cup	128	92	36	0		Yogurt, Greek, nonfat	:-(	:-(	:-|	:-|

* + = medium, ++ = high, +++ = very high

Calories per Serving							Recommended % of Calories			
							Winter	Autumn	Spring	Summer
	Protein					Protein:	35-45%	30-35%	25-30%	20-25%
		Carbohydrates				Carbohydrates:	25-35%	35-50%	50-60%	60-70%
			Fat			Fat:	25-35%	20-30%	15-20%	10-15%
Serving	Total	P	C	F	Pur=Purines*	Purines*:	High	Medium	Low	Very Low
Size	Cal	Cal	Cal	Cal	Pur		Winter	Autumn	Spring	Summer
						BEANS				
						LEGUMES*				
1 cup	294	60	232	2	+*	Aduki beans, cooked	:-)	:-)	:-|	:-(
1 cup	227	53	166	8	+*	Black beans, cooked	:-)	:-)	:-(	:-(
1 cup	198	46	145	8	++	Black-eyed peas, cooked	:-):-)	:-)	:-(	:-(:-(
1 cup	241	57	177	7	+	Cranberry beans, cooked	:-)	:-)	:-)	:-|
1 cup	187	45	136	6	+*	Fava beans, cooked	:-)	:-)	:-|	:-(
1 cup	269	50	183	36		Garbanzo beans, cooked	:-|	:-|	:-)	:-)
1 cup	209	51	151	7	++	Great northern, cooked	:-):-)	:-)	:-(	:-(:-(
1 cup	44	6	35	3	+	Green beans	:-):-)	:-)	:-|	:-(
1 cup	225	54	164	7	+*	Kidney beans, cooked	:-)	:-)	:-|	:-(
1 cup	230	62	161	7	++	Lentils, cooked	:-):-)	:-)	:-(	:-(:-(
1 cup	216	51	159	6	+	Lima beans, cooked	:-)	:-)	:-|	:-(
1 cup	212	49	156	7	++	Mung beans, cooked	:-):-)	:-)	:-(	:-(:-(
1 cup	255	52	193	10	+*	Navy beans, cooked	:-)	:-)	:-|	:-(
1 oz.	164	23	25	116	+*	Peanuts, dry roasted	:-)	:-)	:-|	:-(
2 tbsp.	188	28	25	135	+*	Peanut butter	:-)	:-)	:-|	:-(
1 cup	252	53	192	7	+*	Pink beans, cooked	:-)	:-)	:-|	:-(
1 cup	245	54	182	9	++	Pinto beans, cooked	:-)	:-)	:-(	:-(
1 cup	219	56	162	1	+	Red beans, cooked	:-)	:-)	:-(	:-(
1 cup	231	57	168	6	++	Split peas, cooked	:-):-)	:-)	:-(	:-(:-(
1 cup	298	100	69	129	++	Soybeans, cooked	:-(	:-(	:-(	:-(
1 oz.	54	18	11	25	++	Tempeh	:-|	:-|	:-|	:-(
1 oz.	20	8	2	10	++	Tofu	:-(	:-(	:-(	:-(
1 cup	254	56	189	9	++	White beans, cooked	:-)	:-)	:-(	:-(

If the purine value of a bean was unknown, it was assumed to have a + value. Unknown beans marked +

* + = medium, ++ = high, +++ = very high

CHART 6.9 CARBOHYDRATES FOOD CHART

Calories per Serving								Recommended % of Calories			
								Winter	Autumn	Spring	Summer
	Protein						Protein:	35-45%	30-35%	25-30%	20-25%
		Carbohydrates					Carbohydrates:	25-35%	35-50%	50-60%	60-70%
			Fat				Fat:	25-35%	20-30%	15-20%	10-15%
Serving Size	Total Cal	P Cal	C Cal	F Cal	Pur=Purines* Pur	GI	Purines*: GI=Glycemic Index	High Winter	Medium Autumn	Low Spring	Very Low Summer
							CARBS				
							GRAINS				
1 cup	251	32	186	33		High	Amaranth, cooked	:-)	:-)	:-|	:-|
1 cup	193	13	175	5	+	Low	Barley, cooked	:-):-)	:-)	:-(	:-(
1 cup	155	19	127	9		Low	Buckwheat, cooked	:-|	:-|	:-)	:-)
1 cup	176	24	150	2		Medium	Couscous, cooked	:-|	:-|	:-)	:-)
1/2 cup	208	15	175	18		Medium	Corn meal, uncooked	:-|	:-|	:-)	:-)
1 cup	251	40	198	13		Low	Kamut, cooked	:-|	:-|	:-)	:-)
1 cup	207	24	169	14		High	Millet, cooked	:-|	:-|	:-|	:-|
1/4 cup	152	23	106	23	+	Low	Oats, raw	:-)	:-)	:-(	:-(
2 oz.	200	24	168	8		Low-Med	Pasta, uncooked	:-|	:-|	:-)	:-)
1 cup	222	33	157	32		Low	Quinoa, cooked	:-|	:-|	:-)	:-)
1 cup	218	15	189	14		Medium	Rice, brown, cooked	:-|	:-|	:-)	:-)
1 cup	225	15	195	15		Low	Rice, br., parboiled, cooked				
1 cup	205	16	185	4		Medium	Rice, white, cooked	:-|	:-|	:-)	:-)
1/4 cup	141	19	115	9		Low	Rye, uncooked	:-|	:-|	:-)	:-)
1 cup	220	32	177	11		Low-Med	Spaghetti, cooked	:-|	:-|	:-)	:-)
1 cup	246	38	194	14		Medium	Spelt, cooked	:-|	:-|	:-)	:-)
1 oz.	102	13	85	4		Low	Wheat flour, white	:-|	:-|	:-)	:-)
1 cup	166	23	138	5		Low	Wild rice, cooked	:-|	:-|	:-)	:-)
							VEGETABLES				
1/2 cup	45	6	36	3	+	High	Artichoke, hearts	:-):-)	:-)	:-(	:-(:-(
4 stalks	13	4	8	1	+	Low	Asparagus, boiled	:-):-)	:-)	:-(	:-(:-(
1/2	114	5	21	88		Low	Avocado, California	:-)	:-)	:-|	:-(
1 oz.	3	1	2	0		Low	Bamboo shoots, boiled	:-(	:-|	:-)	:-)
1 cup	44	6	35	3	+	Low	Beans, green, cooked	:-):-)	:-)	:-|	:-(
1/2 cup	37	4	32	1		High	Beets, boiled*	:-|	:-|	:-)	:-)
1 cup	9	3	5	1		Low	Bok choy	:-(	:-|	:-)	:-)
1/2 cup	26	7	18	1	+	Low	Broccoli, cooked	:-(	:-(	:-)	:-)
1/2 cup	28	5	20	3		Medium	Brussels sprouts, cooked	:-(	:-(	:-)	:-)
1/2 cup	17	2	15	0		Low	Cabbage, cooked	:-(	:-|	:-)	:-)
1 med.	25	2	22	1		High	Carrot, raw	:-)	:-)	:-|	:-|
1/2 cup	14	3	9	2	+	Low	Cauliflower, cooked	:-):-)	:-)	:-(	:-(
1 stalk	6	1	5	0		Low	Celery	:-)	:-)	:-|	:-|
1 ear	124	20	104	4		High	Corn, on the cob	:-)	:-)	:-|	:-(
1 cup	177	13	146	18		High	Corn, sweet, cooked	:-)	:-)	:-|	:-(
1 cup	16	3	11	2		Low	Cucumber, peeled	:-(	:-(	:-)	:-)

* + = medium, ++ = high, +++ = very high

Serving Size	Total Cal	P Cal	C Cal	F Cal	Pur = Purines*	GI	GI=Glycemic Index	Winter	Autumn	Spring	Summer
Calories per Serving								Recommended % of Calories			
								Winter	Autumn	Spring	Summer
Protein							Protein:	35-45%	30-35%	25-30%	20-25%
Carbohydrates							Carbohydrates:	25-35%	35-50%	50-60%	60-70%
Fat							Fat:	25-35%	20-30%	15-20%	10-15%
								High	Medium	Low	Very Low
							CARBS				
							VEGETABLES CONT.				
1 cup	35	2	31	2		Low	Eggplant, cooked*	:-(	:-|	:-)	:-)
1 clove	5	1	4	0		Low	Garlic	:-(	:-(	:-)	:-):-)
1 cup	36	6	26	4		Low	Kale, cooked	:-(	:-(	:-)	:-)
1 leek	38	2	34	2		Medium	Leeks, cooked	:-(	:-(	:-)	:-)
1 cup	8	2	5	1		Low	Lettuce	:-(	:-(	:-)	:-)
1 cup	16	6	8	2	+	Low	Mushrooms, raw	:-):-)	:-)	:-(	:-(
1/2 cup	18	4	13	1		Medium	Okra, cooked	:-|	:-|	:-)	:-)
1 oz.	23	1	6	16		Low	Olives, canned	:-)	:-)	:-|	:-(
1 slice	6	1	5	0		Medium	Onion, raw	:-(	:-(	:-)	:-):-)
1/2 cup	56	51	3	2		High	Parsnip, cooked	:-(	:-(	:-)	:-)
1 cup	67	18	46	3	+	Medium	Peas, green cooked*	:-):-)	:-)	:-(	:-(
1 cup	30	3	25	2		Medium	Pepper, bell, raw*	:-(	:-(	:-)	:-)
1 pepper	18	2	15	1		Medium	Pepper, hot, raw	:-(	:-(	:-)	:-)
1 large	278	21	254	3		High	Potato, baked	:-|	:-|	:-)	:-)
1 cup	49	4	43	2		Medium	Pumpkin, cooked	:-(	:-(	:-)	:-)
1 med.	1	0	1	0		Low	Radish, raw	:-(	:-|	:-)	:-)
1 cup	66	6	57	3		High	Rutabaga, cooked	:-(	:-|	:-)	:-)
1 med.	5	1	4	0		Low	Scallion	:-(	:-(	:-)	:-):-)
1 oz.	13	2	9	2		Low	Seaweed	:-|	:-|	:-)	:-)
1 cup	41	13	24	4	+	Low	Spinach, boiled	:-):-)	:-)	:-|	:-|
1 cup	36	4	27	5		Low	Squash, summer, cooked	:-|	:-|	:-)	:-)
1 cup	115	6	107	2		High	Squash, winter, cooked	:-|	:-|	:-)	:-)
1 med.	103	7	95	1		Medium	Sweet potato, cooked*	:-|	:-|	:-)	:-)
1 med.	22	3	17	2		Low	Tomato, red, raw*	:-(	:-(	:-)	:-)
1 med.	34	3	30	1		Medium	Turnip, raw	:-|	:-|	:-)	:-)
1/2 cup	60	2	57	0		Low	Water chestnuts, raw	:-(	:-|	:-)	:-)
1 cup	158	6	151	1		Medium	Yams, cooked	:-|	:-|	:-)	:-)
1/2 cup	14	1	13	0		Low	Zucchini, sliced*	:-(	:-|	:-)	:-)

*Contains moderate amounts of fructose of approximately 2 grams, except peas, which contain approximately 4 grams.

* + = medium, ++ = high, +++ = very high

Calories per Serving								Recommended % of Calories			
								Winter	Autumn	Spring	Summer
		Protein					Protein:	35-45%	30-35%	25-30%	20-25%
			Carbohydrates				Carbohydrates:	25-35%	35-50%	50-60%	60-70%
				Fat			Fat:	25-35%	20-30%	15-20%	10-15%
Serving Size	Total Cal	P Cal	C Cal	F Cal	Pot = Potassium, Pot	Fru	Potassium: Fru = Fructose	Low Winter	Medium Autumn	Medium Spring	High Summer
							CARBS				
							FRUIT*				
1 med.	95	2	90	3	195 mg	13 g	Apple	:-|	:-|	:-)	:-|
1 med.	17	2	14	1	91 mg	1 g	Apricot	:-|	:-|	:-)	:-)
1 med.	105	4	98	3	422 mg	7 g	Banana	:-)	:-)	:-|	:-|
1 cup	62	7	49	6	233 mg	4 g	Blackberries	:-|	:-|	:-)	:-)
1 cup	84	4	76	4	114 mg	7 g	Blueberries	:-|	:-|	:-)	:-|
1/2 med.	94	8	82	5	737 mg	11 g	Cantaloupe	:-(	:-|	:-)	:-)
1 cup	87	5	80	2	306 mg	8 g	Cherries, sweet	:-|	:-|	:-)	:-)
1 oz.	99	3	17	79	100 mg	2 g	Coconut, meat, raw	:-)	:-)	:-|	:-|
1 med.	67	2	65	0	167 mg	8 g	Dates, medjool	:-(	:-(	:-)	:-)
1 med.	37	1	35	1	116 mg	4 g	Fig	:-(	:-(	:-|	:-|
1 cup	104	4	98	2	288 mg	6 g	Grapes	:-(	:-|	:-)	:-)
1/2 med.	52	3	47	1	166 mg	4 g	Grapefruit, pink/red	:-(	:-(	:-)	:-):-)
1 cup	112	14	85	13	688 mg	6 g	Guava	:-(	:-(	:-)	:-)
1/4 med.	90	5	83	3	570 mg	14 g	Honeydew	:-(	:-(	:-)	:-)
1 cup	108	7	94	7	522 mg	8 g	Kiwifruit	:-(	:-(	:-)	:-)
1 oz.	7	0	7	0	35 mg	3 g	Lemon juice	:-(:-(	:-(	:-)	:-):-)
1 oz.	7	1	6	0	33 mg	0	Lime	:-(:-(	:-(	:-)	:-):-)
1 med.	135	4	126	5	323 mg	16 g	Mango	:-(	:-(	:-)	:-)
1 med.	63	5	54	4	286 mg	5 g	Nectarine	:-|	:-|	:-)	:-|
1 med.	69	4	63	2	232 mg	6 g	Orange, navel	:-(:-(	:-(	:-)	:-):-)
1 med.	119	6	109	4	781 mg	11 g	Papaya	:-(	:-(	:-)	:-)
1 med.	59	5	51	3	285 mg	6 g	Peach	:-|	:-|	:-)	:-)
1 med.	103	2	99	2	212 mg	12 g	Pear	:-)	:-)	:-|	:-(
1 cup	83	3	78	2	180 mg	9 g	Pineapple	:-(	:-(	:-)	:-):-)
1 med.	30	2	27	1	104 mg	3 g	Plum	:-|	:-|	:-)	:-)
1 med.	234	16	191	27	666 mg	19 g	Pomegranate	:-(	:-(	:-)	:-)
1 med.	23	1	22	0	70 mg	1 g	Prune, dried	:-(	:-(	:-|	:-|
1 oz.	83	2	80	1	231 mg	10 g	Raisin	:-(	:-(	:-|	:-|
1 cup	64	5	52	7	186 mg	3 g	Raspberry	:-|	:-|	:-)	:-)
1 stalk	11	2	8	1	147 mg	1 g	Rhubarb	:-|	:-|	:-)	:-)
1 cup	46	3	39	4	220 mg	4 g	Strawberries, whole	:-|	:-|	:-)	:-)
1 med.	47	2	43	2	146 mg	5 g	Tangerine	:-(	:-(	:-)	:-)
1 cup	46	3	41	2	170 mg	6 g	Watermelon, diced	:-(	:-(	:-)	:-)

*Limit due to high fructose content. Do a two-week fructose fast twice a year.

CHART 6.95 FATS AND OILS, NUTS AND SEEDS FOOD CHARTS

	Calories per Serving						Recommended % of Calories			
							Winter	Autumn	Spring	Summer
	Protein					Protein:	35-45%	30-35%	25-30%	20-25%
		Carbohydrates				Carbohydrates:	25-35%	35-50%	50-60%	60-70%
				Fat		Fat:	25-35%	20-30%	15-20%	10-15%
Serving Size	Total **Cal**	P Cal	**C Cal**	F Cal	Pur=Purines* **Pur**	Purines*:	High Winter	Medium Autumn	Low Spring	Very Low Summer
						FATS & OILS				
1 tbsp.	119	0	0	119		Almond oil	:-|	:-|	:-|	:-|
1 tbsp.	100	0	0	100		Butter**	:-)	:-)	:-(	:-(
1 tbsp.	124	0	0	124		Canola oil	:-(	:-(	:-(	:-(
1 tbsp.	116	0	0	116		Coconut oil**	:-)	:-)	:-)	:-)
1 tbsp.	124	0	0	124		Corn oil	:-(	:-(	:-(	:-(
1 tbsp.	119	0	0	124		Cottonseed oil	:-(	:-(	:-(	:-(
1 tbsp.	52	0	0	52		Cream, heavy**	:-)	:-)	:-(	:-(
1 tbsp.	122	0	0	122		Fish oil**	:-|	:-|	:-)	:-)
1 tbsp.	120	0	0	120		Flaxseed oil**	:-(	:-(	:-)	:-)
1 tbsp.	112	0	0	112		Ghee**	:-)	:-)	:-(	:-(
1 tbsp.	119	0	0	119		Lard**	:-)	:-)	:-(	:-(
1 tbsp.	124	0	0	124		Olive oil**	:-)	:-)	:-)	:-)
1 tbsp.	116	0	0	116		Palm oil**	:-)	:-)	:-(	:-(
1 tbsp.	116	0	0	116		Palm kernel oil**	:-)	:-)	:-)	:-)
1 tbsp.	119	0	0	119		Peanut oil	:-|	:-|	:-|	:-|
1 tbsp.	119	0	0	119		Safflower oil	see *** below			
1 tbsp.	119	0	0	119		Sesame oil	:-|	:-|	:-|	:-|
1 tbsp.	119	0	0	119		Sunflower oil	see *** below			
						NUTS & SEEDS				
1 oz.	162	21	25	117		Almonds	:-|	:-|	:-)	:-)
1 oz.	185	14	14	157		Brazil nuts	:-)	:-)	:-|	:-|
1 oz.	155	18	35	103		Cashews	:-(	:-(	:-)	:-)
1 oz.	55	2	50	3		Chestnuts	:-(	:-(	:-)	:-)
1 oz.	185	7	27	151		Coconut, meat, dried	:-)	:-)	:-|	:-|
1 oz.	177	15	19	144		Filberts	:-)	:-)	:-|	:-|
1 oz.	184	12	21	151		Hickory nuts	:-)	:-)	:-|	:-|
1 oz.	203	8	16	179		Macadamia nuts	:-)	:-)	:-|	:-|
1 oz.	164	23	25	116		Peanuts, dry roasted	:-)	:-)	:-|	:-(
1 oz.	199	9	16	174		Pecans	:-)	:-)	:-|	:-|
1 oz.	190	13	15	162		Pine nuts	:-(	:-(	:-)	:-)
1 oz.	157	20	32	105		Pistachios	:-|	:-|	:-)	:-)
1 oz.	151	24	20	107		Pumpkin seeds	:-)	:-)	:-|	:-|
1 oz.	86	10	16	60		Sesame butter, tahini	:-|	:-|	:-)	:-)
1 oz.	164	20	23	121		Sunflower seeds	:-(	:-(	:-)	:-)
1 oz.	185	15	16	154		Walnuts	:-)	:-)	:-|	:-|

* + = medium, ++ = high, +++ = very high
**These are the healthiest oils and should be the primary ones consumed.
***Cold-pressed high oleic is :-|. Commercially processed or high linoleic is :-(.

The Four Seasons Diet

Start the Two-Week Fructose Fast

I know many of you may be tempted to skip this step, but I cannot stress how important it is to begin with this fast for the following reasons:

1. The Four Seasons Diet is a low-fructose diet, with a suggested limit of 15 grams of fructose per day. For many people, this will be a very difficult adjustment to get used to. Also, remember that table sugar is 50 percent fructose, so you'll need to eliminate all fruit and all foods with sugar during the two-week fructose fast. You can still consume dairy, as long as it consists of products such as milk, cottage cheese, or unsweetened yogurt. Remember that fructose can cause brain changes similar to those that happen to a drug addict. It's better to beat this addiction by consuming no fructose for two weeks, and then you can work on changing the rest of your diet.

2. You need to get your hunger hormones and feel-full hormones working properly before you can achieve the full benefits of eating for your season-type. Until you do a fructose fast, you may actually feel worse by eating for your season-type, especially if you are an insulin-resistant Summer. For all of the reasons mentioned in Chapter 5, fructose can inhibit your body from functioning well. It's better to get your body working properly first, then the foods for your season-type will have the optimal effect. Even if you eat according to your season-type, if you overeat beneficial foods, they will still have negative consequences. A combination of eating the right foods in the correct amounts will lead to weight loss, increased energy, and overall well-being. As long as your feel-full hormones and hunger hormones are being tricked by fructose, it will be very difficult for you to eat the proper amount of food. Fructose also contributes to insulin resistance, and if a Summer is insulin resistant, the Summer diet, which is high in carbohydrates, will not have the desired effect. While insulin resistance is very detrimental to anyone's health, an insulin-resistant Summer who overeats carbs might feel worse than he or she would by following an Autumn or a Spring diet, so until you restore your insulin sensitivity and proper hormone levels, you will not be able to tell what real effect the Four Seasons Diet is having on you.

3. You may feel worse during the two-week fructose fast. Remember, there is a pretty good chance you may be like a drug addict going off drugs, and your body may finally be healing itself from all of the damage caused by excessive fructose consumption. If you attempt the fast at the same time that you start the diet and you feel worse, you will have no way of knowing whether the fructose fast is to blame or the diet is. An essential part of the diet entails listening to how your body responds to food, based on the way you feel after eating. Until you restore your hunger hormones and your feel-full hormones, you really have no way of truly knowing how the various foods are affecting you.

4. Once you complete the fructose fast, you may find that you are not the season-type you thought you were. Remember that fructose can cause insulin resistance and a fatty liver. You may believe you are a Winter or an Autumn because you react badly to carbohydrates, when it's actually the insulin resistance and the fatty liver caused by fructose consumption that are prompting your bad reaction. Once you know your body is working properly, you will realize how the diet for your season-type is affecting you.

So, step one is a two-week fast to eliminate all sources of fructose, including sugar. After you complete the two-week fructose fast, you are ready to start the Four Seasons Diet. Just remember to keep your fructose consumption to less than 15 grams a day, as much as possible. This will help you fine-tune the diet and reach your full potential on the Four Seasons Diet.

Summers and Springs often eat large quantities of fruit because the high potassium content in fruit makes them feel good and gives them energy. During the fructose fast, Springs and Summers are advised to make an extra effort to consume foods that have high levels of potassium to help make up for the loss of potassium they experience from not eating fruit. Potatoes are a great source of potassium, with one potato having more than 600 mg of potassium, which is nearly equal to the amount found in three bananas. Beans are another excellent source of potassium; however, with the exception of garbanzo beans, most beans are high in purines and should be eaten only in moderation by Summers and Springs. Whole grains, such as whole wheat flour and brown rice, also typically have about triple the potassium content of processed grains, such as white flour and white rice, so you are encouraged to eat whole grains during the fructose fast. It's also important to eat plenty of vegetables to ensure that you get enough potassium—

with the exception of beets, eggplant, peas, bell pepper, and sweet potatoes, which all contain small amounts of fructose and should not be eaten in large quantities during the fructose fast. Summers and Springs may also find they do better during the fast if they make sure they do not consume too much sodium, because it's ultimately the ratio of their intake of potassium vs. sodium that is most important. Summers and Springs need a high level of potassium with a lower level of sodium to feel their best.

Winters and Autumns do not need the high levels of potassium that Summers and Springs do, and they generally do alright eating smaller amounts of this mineral. For this reason, most Winters and Autumns will not need to take the extra steps that Summers and Springs do to ensure that they get enough potassium during the two-week fructose fast. They can simply eliminate fructose, and as long as they have a balanced diet, with an adequate amount of vegetables and whole grains, they should be fine as far as potassium intake is concerned.

Protein

On the opposite page is the protein chart. You will find all of the food charts again at the end of the book; this will make it simple for you to refer to the charts in the future. Remember, the percentage of protein calories you should consume is based on your season-type, as follows:

Winters: 35–45% of total daily calories
Autumns: 30–35% of total daily calories
Springs: 25–30% of total daily calories
Summers: 20–25% of total daily calories

When most people think of protein, they think of foods that are high in protein, such as meat, eggs, and cheese. The reality is that most foods contain some level of protein, and the recommended percentage of calories from protein means protein from all sources. For example, most grains, such as wheat, contain around 12 to 13 percent protein, with the exception of rice and corn, which are only around 7 to 8 percent protein. The type of protein that the body needs also varies by season-type. Some season-types need high levels of purines, some require moderate levels, and some function best with low levels.

<u>Winters and Protein</u>

If you are a Winter, you need the highest amount of protein in your diet and are most likely the classic "meat-eater" type, who feels great after eating a high-fat meaty meal. You need to focus on the proteins that contain high levels of purines, and these are listed on the protein chart.

	Calories per Serving						Recommended % of Calories			
							Winter	Autumn	Spring	Summer
		Protein				Protein:	35-45%	30-35%	25-30%	20-25%
			Carbohydrates			Carbohydrates:	25-35%	35-50%	50-60%	60-70%
				Fat		Fat:	25-35%	20-30%	15-20%	10-15%
Serving Size	Total Cal	P Cal	C Cal	F Cal	Pur=Purines* Pur	Purines*:	High Winter	Medium Autumn	Low Spring	Very Low Summer
						PROTEIN				
						MEAT				
4 oz.	302	122	0	180	+	Beef, 70% lean	:-)	:-|	:-(	:-(
4 oz.	304	129	0	175	+	Beef, 80% lean	:-)	:-|	:-(	:-(
4 oz.	228	122	0	108	+	Beef, 90% lean	:-)	:-)	:-(	:-(
4 oz.	183	123	0	60	+	Beef, 95% lean	:-)	:-)	:-|	:-(
4 oz.	286	116	0	170	+	Lamb	:-)	:-|	:-(	:-(
4 oz.	153	97.2	17	36.8	++	Liver	:-):-)	:-)	:-(	:-(:-(
1 slice	41	13	0	28	+	Pork, bacon	:-)	:-|	:-(	:-(
6 oz.	252	136	8	108	+	Pork, Canadian bacon	:-)	:-)	:-|	:-(
4 oz.	187	84	6	97	+	Pork, chop	:-)	:-)	:-(	:-(
4 oz.	123	77	8	38	+	Pork, tenderloin	:-)	:-)	:-|	:-(
1 oz.	34	22	0	12	+	Pork, extra lean ham	:-)	:-)	:-|	:-(
						POULTRY				
4 oz.	266	81	0	185	+	Chicken, dark with skin	:-)	:-|	:-(	:-(
4 oz.	123	111	0	12	+	Chicken, light no skin	:-|	:-|	:-)	:-|
4 oz.	224	82	0	142	+	Cornish hen	:-)	:-|	:-(	:-(
4 oz.	148	88	0	60	+	Duck	:-)	:-)	:-(	:-(
4 oz.	180	108	0	72	+	Goose	:-)	:-)	:-(	:-(
4 oz.	248	132	0	116	+	Turkey, dark with skin	:-)	:-)	:-(	:-(
4 oz.	128	112	0	16	+	Turkey, light, no skin	:-|	:-)	:-)	:-|
						SEAFOOD				
1 oz.	37	25	0	12	+++	Anchovies	:-):-)	:-)	:-(	:-(:-(
4 oz.	109	85	0	23.6		Bass	:-(	:-|	:-)	:-|
4 oz.	143	85	0	56	+	Carp	:-)	:-)	:-(	:-(
4 oz.	151	76	0	77		Catfish	:-(	:-|	:-(	:-(
4 oz.	83	61	12	10	+	Clams	:-)	:-)	:-(	:-(
4 oz.	92	86	0	6	+	Cod	:-|	:-|	:-)	:-|
4 oz.	94	88	0	6	+	Crab	:-)	:-)	:-(	:-(
4 oz.	103	91	0	12		Flounder	:-(	:-(	:-)	:-|
4 oz.	103	93	0	10		Grouper	:-(	:-(	:-)	:-|
4 oz.	123	100	0	23		Halibut	:-(	:-(	:-)	:-|
4 oz.	101	90	2	9	+	Lobster	:-)	:-)	:-|	:-(
4 oz.	230	89	0	141	++	Mackerel	:-):-)	:-|	:-(	:-(:-(
4 oz.	100	57	17	23	+	Mussels	:-)	:-)	:-)	:-(
4 oz.	91	45	23	23	+	Oysters	:-)	:-)	:-(	:-(
4 oz.	106	91	0	17	++	Perch	:-)	:-)	:-|	:-(

* + = medium, ++ = high, +++ = very high

Calories per Serving							Recommended % of Calories			
							Winter	Autumn	Spring	Summer
Protein						Protein:	35-45%	30-35%	25-30%	20-25%
	Carbohydrates					Carbohydrates:	25-35%	35-50%	50-60%	60-70%
			Fat			Fat:	25-35%	20-30%	15-20%	10-15%
Serving Size	Total Cal	P Cal	C Cal	F Cal	Pur=Purines*	Purines*:	High Winter	Medium Autumn	Low Spring	Very Low Summer
						PROTEIN				
						SEAFOOD CONT.				
4 oz.	85	78	0	7		Roughy	:-(	:-(	:-)	:-|
4 oz.	201	95	0	106	++	Salmon	:-):-)	:-)	:-(	:-(:-(
4 oz.	209	100	3	106	+++	Sardines	:-):-)	:-)	:-(	:-(:-(
4 oz.	98	80	11	7.6	++	Scallops	:-)	:-)	:-(	:-(
4 oz.	119	97	4	18	++	Shrimp	:-)	:-)	:-|	:-(
4 oz.	112	98	0	14		Snapper	:-(	:-(	:-)	:-|
4 oz.	104	75	15	14	+	Squid	:-|	:-|	:-)	:-(
4 oz.	136	95	0	41		Swordfish	:-(	:-|	:-(	:-(
4 oz.	166	99	0	67	+++	Trout	:-)	:-)	:-(	:-(
4 oz.	122	112	0	10	+	Tuna, yellowfin	:-|	:-)	:-)	:-|
4 oz.	150	91	0	59	+	Whitefish	:-)	:-)	:-(	:-(
						MISC. PROTEIN				
1 white	16	15	0	1		Egg whites	:-(	:-(	:-|	:-)
Per individual product						Whey protein	:-|	:-|	:-(	:-(
Per individual product						Milk (casein protein)	:-|	:-|	:-(	:-(
Per individual product						Soy protein	:-(	:-(	:-(	:-(
Per individual product					+++	Brewer's yeast	:-)	:-)	:-(	:-(
Per individual product					+++	Chlorella/blue-green algae	:-)	:-)	:-(	:-(

* + = medium, ++ = high, +++ = very high

Purines will help balance out your usually erratic blood-sugar problems. Your need for purines will rise considerably when it's cold outside, especially when it's cold and humid. In the summer, when it's warm, you can usually switch to eating a more moderate level of purines. A good way to gauge whether you are getting enough purines is to keep track of how hungry you get between meals and how cold you feel relative other people. If you are starving two hours after eating, and you feel cold when everyone else is warm, chances are you are not consuming enough protein that is high in purines. When this happens, try to focus on eating protein foods and other foods with either a ++ or a +++ next to them, indicating their amount of purines. As you begin to recognize the effect that purines and climate have on your blood sugar and general overall well-being, you'll learn which proteins and other foods to consume with each meal throughout the year. Just remember that the colder it gets, the more purines you will need to consume.

Protein will usually be the central theme to your meals, and picking the right protein is the key to your well-being. When it's cold, you may find that you do best eating higher-purine foods, such as salmon, shrimp, beans, and lentils. In cold weather, you will probably have to make sure that every meal you consume contains a protein with at least a medium purine level; these are the foods marked with a + such as beef, lamb, and dark-meat chicken. Although it is very possible for you to do well on a vegetarian diet, you have the most challenging time of all of the season-types when it comes to not eating meat. In the section on being a vegetarian for your season-type, I'll explain ways that you can eliminate meat and still maintain your health.

Autumns and Protein

If you are an Autumn, first you should read about a Winter's protein requirements. Much of this applies to you as well. The main difference is that you have a lower need for protein and for purines than a Winter does. Rather than focusing on higher-purine proteins, you will need to choose protein foods with medium levels of purines. You may find that you have a moderate need for purines when it's cold outside and perhaps very little need for purines when it's warmer. You will need to gauge both your hunger level between meals and how cold or warm you feel relative to others. It is possible that if you consume too many high-purine foods, you may begin to feel too warm, and your energy may actually fall off a bit.

The good news is that you have a much easier time keeping yourself in balance than any of the other season-types while eating the standard American diet. You are probably one of those people who can eat just about anything and usually feel alright. By limiting yourself to 15 grams of fructose a day and eliminating processed vegetable oils from your diet, you should find it relatively simple to maintain a good state of health and energy. The biggest problem you have is that more than any other season-type, you can eat larger quantities of unhealthy food without feeling the ill effects for many years. Yet eventually it will catch up with you if you don't make the few changes I have mentioned. A typical scenario for your season-type is that you are someone who is never sick or is always in perfect health until the day you are diagnosed with cancer, diabetes, or some other debilitating disease. If you take charge of your health now, you should be blessed with a very long and healthy life.

Proteins are important to your overall well-being but are usually less crucial than they are for Winters. If you choose to get your purines from meat, you can usually get by on medium-purine foods for most meals when it's cold, and medium- to lower-purine foods when it's warm. In cold weather, you may be able to eat lower-purine proteins for a meal or two, or you may find you need to eat higher-purine proteins for a meal or two as well. Because beans are high in purines and you can usually tolerate more carbohydrates than Winters can, beans are often an excellent way for you to obtain your purines. You have a fairly easy time thriving on a vegetarian diet if you use beans and lentils as your source of purines and add in cheese and other dairy products for your fat and a little more protein, in addition to the protein in the beans.

Summers and Protein

As a Summer, you need the lowest amount of protein in your diet and are most likely the classic "vegetarian" type who feels great eating a higher-carbohydrate meal without any meat. You need to focus on the proteins that contain low levels of purines; these are indicated on the protein chart by a lack of any + symbols in the purine columns for any particular food. Purines will throw you even further out of balance and will cause what may already be low energy levels to plummet even lower. Your need to strictly limit purines will increase when it's warm outside, especially when it's warm and humid. In the winter, when it's cold, you may find that you are able to tolerate a meal with moderate to high amounts purines now and then. A good way to gauge whether you are getting too many purines is to keep track of your energy level and of how warm you feel relative to others. Summers have often learned to adopt a diet that is either vegetarian or, if they do eat meat, it's usually white meat chicken or turkey or white fish. A common problem for Summers who are vegetarians is that most beans are also very high in purines, and you will need to watch your bean consumption as well. Garbanzo beans are the lowest in purines, so if you are going to eat beans and want to watch your purine levels, choose garbanzo beans. Start by focusing on foods with low levels of purines. You can then try adding moderate-purine foods back into your diet and see how that makes you feel. Often, you will notice that your low-energy problems quickly return if you have a few meals in a row with moderate amounts of purines.

Proteins are often the toughest part of your meal selection. If you choose to eat meat and fish, focus on low-purine fish, such as halibut, flounder, grouper, roughy, and snapper, especially when it's warm outside. Other good protein choices are egg whites, which can be fried, or low-fat and nonfat dairy products. Remember that excess calcium can lower your energy level, so if you eat low-fat and nonfat dairy products, be sure not to go overboard and get too much calcium. Nonfat protein powders, such as egg-white protein and rice protein, are often excellent choices as well. Whey or casein protein in excess, due to its high calcium levels, can imbalance your system, so be careful not to rely on too much of this protein. When it's cold outside, you can usually tolerate a moderate-purine meal at least once a day. Of all of the season-types, you will find it easiest to be a vegetarian, as long as you don't eat too many high-purine beans and lentils and get a little high-quality protein with each meal. Remember that your diet is grain- and vegetable-based, and most grains contain 12 to 13 percent protein, except for rice and corn, which are only 7 to 8 percent protein. Use concentrated proteins, such as fish or egg whites, to supplement the protein you are not getting from grains and vegetables.

Springs and Protein

If you are a Spring, first you should read about a Summer's protein requirements. Much of this applies to you as well. The main difference is that you are able to tolerate a moderate amount of purines better than a Summer can. Rather than focusing on low-purine proteins, you should choose protein foods that have low or moderate levels of purines. You may find that you can tolerate low levels of purines when it's warmer outside and medium levels of purines when it's colder. You can probably handle an occasional high-purine meal as well. You will need to gauge your energy levels, as well as your blood-sugar levels, between meals, based on how many purines you consume. Usually, focusing on low- to moderate-purine foods will help keep your energy levels at their best. If you eat too few purines, however, especially when it's cold outside, you may find that you often feel "hyper" and that your blood sugar begins to crash between meals, and you may even feel cold when you normally would not. All of these are potential signs that you may need to eat some moderate-purine foods for a few meals until you start to feel higher levels of energy again.

You have a greater ability to tolerate purines than Summers do, but you should still focus on low-purine foods when it's warm outside. When it's colder, you can usually tolerate a moderate-purine meal at least once or twice a day. These include foods such as dark-meat chicken, beef, and pork. Also, beans such as cranberry, lima, and navy beans have a moderate purine level and are excellent choices when it's cold.

Protein Summary for All Season-Types
One main difference between the season-types is the level of protein they require, as well as their need for purines in relation to the temperature outside. As the temperature goes from cold to hot, keep the following in mind for all four season-types. When it's cold, a Winter needs to eat some high- to medium-purine foods for every meal, an Autumn will need to consume some moderate-purine foods for most meals, a Spring will need to eat some moderate-purine foods for usually at least one meal a day, and a Summer may or may not need to consume any foods with purines. When it's warmer outside, a Winter can usually get by with eating medium-purine foods for most meals, an Autumn may need to consume medium-purine foods for one or two meals a day, a Spring can consume moderate-purine foods for one meal a day or none, and a Summer will usually have to focus on consuming low-purine foods for every meal.

Dairy
On the opposite page is the dairy chart. You will find all of the food charts again at the end of the book, to make it easy to refer back to them in the future. Dairy foods consist of cheese, which is basically protein and fat, and milk products, which consist of protein, carbohydrates, and fat, except for nonfat milk items. All dairy products are low in purines and high in calcium. With the exception of nonfat dairy products, most dairy products are also high in long-chain saturated fats and cholesterol.

Winters and Dairy
As a Winter, you need the largest amount of saturated fat and calcium of all of the season-types, so, in that respect, dairy is an excellent choice for you. The problem is that dairy is low in purines, so if you attempt to use foods such as cheese as your primary source of protein, you are likely to have blood-sugar issues. Dairy

is an excellent way to get extra fat and calcium into your diet when you consume other proteins that are high in purines. For example, you can add cheese to any low-fat meat that also has moderate amounts of purines, such as white-meat chicken or turkey, as a way to get protein, purines, saturated fat, and calcium. Remember that your cells are often too porous, which contributes to your erratic blood-sugar issues. The longer-chain saturated fats and the cholesterol in dairy products are an excellent way for you to prevent your cells from becoming too porous. This is especially true when it's cold outside. If you are not getting enough of these fats from eating meat, then cheese, milk, and butter are excellent choices for you, as long as you find a way to consume enough high-purine foods.

Calories per Serving							Recommended % of Calories			
							Winter	Autumn	Spring	Summer
		Protein				Protein:	35-45%	30-35%	25-30%	20-25%
			Carbohydrates			Carbohydrates:	25-35%	35-50%	50-60%	60-70%
				Fat		Fat:	25-35%	20-30%	15-20%	10-15%
Serving Size	Total Cal	P Cal	C Cal	F Cal	Pur =Purines* Pur	Purines*:	High Winter	Medium Autumn	Low Spring	Very Low Summer
						DAIRY				
						DAIRY				
1 oz.	99	26	3	70		Blue cheese	:-|	:-|	:-(	:-(
1 oz.	94	25	1	68		Brie	:-|	:-|	:-(	:-(
1 oz.	113	30	2	81		Cheddar cheese	:-|	:-|	:-(	:-(
1 oz.	110	28	3	79		Colby cheese	:-|	:-|	:-(	:-(
4 oz.	111	54	14	43		Cottage cheese/whole	:-|	:-|	:-(	:-(
4 oz.	81	60	11	10		Cottage cheese, 1%	:-(	:-(	:-|	:-(
1 tbsp.	50	4	2	44		Cream cheese	:-|	:-|	:-(	:-(
1 egg	71	25	1	45		Eggs, chicken	:-|	:-|	:-(	:-(
1 oz.	74	17	5	52		Feta	:-|	:-|	:-(	:-(
1 oz.	100	30	2	68		Gouda	:-|	:-|	:-(	:-(
1 cup	118	41	51	26		Milk, low fat	:-(	:-|	:-|	:-(
1 cup	101	42	54	5		Milk, nonfat	:-(	:-(	:-|	:-|
1 cup	146	31	44	71		Milk, whole	:-|	:-|	:-(	:-(
1 oz.	104	29	1	74		Monterey jack	:-|	:-|	:-(	:-(
1 oz.	71	29	3	39		Mozzarella, part skim	:-|	:-|	:-|	:-|
1 oz.	84	27	2	55		Mozzarella, whole	:-|	:-|	:-(	:-(
1 oz.	110	43	3	64		Parmesan	:-|	:-|	:-(	:-(
1 oz.	98	31	2	65		Provolone	:-|	:-|	:-(	:-(
1 oz.	39	14	6	19		Ricotta, part skim	:-|	:-|	:-(	:-(
1 oz.	49	14	3	32		Ricotta, whole	:-|	:-|	:-(	:-(
1 oz.	108	38	4	66		Romano	:-|	:-|	:-(	:-(
1 tbsp.	20	2	3	16		Sour cream, low fat	:-|	:-|	:-(	:-(
2 tbsp.	24	8	16	0		Sour cream, nonfat	:-|	:-|	:-|	:-|
1 tbsp.	23	1	1	21		Sour cream, whole	:-|	:-|	:-(	:-(
1 oz.	106	32	6	68		Swiss	:-|	:-|	:-(	:-(
1 cup	149	36	43	70		Yogurt, whole	:-|	:-|	:-(	:-(
1 cup	154	55	66	33		Yogurt, low fat	:-(	:-|	:-|	:-(

Autumns and Dairy

If you are an Autumn, first read about a Winter's dairy requirements. Much of this applies to you as well. The main difference is that because you can tolerate a much higher level of carbohydrates than Winters can, you can make a lot of meals using cheese and beans. Bean are high in purines, but they are also high in carbohydrates.

If you think of many traditional Mexican dishes, these are often excellent choices for you.

Summers and Dairy

As a Summer, you need the lowest levels of both saturated fat and calcium of all of the season-types, so often dairy is a bad choice for you. Low-fat and nonfat dairy, while being an excellent way to get high-quality, low-purine protein, is very high in calcium. Remember that although the recommended calcium-to-magnesium ratio is often said to be 2:1, for you a lower ratio of 1:1 or even less will help increase your energy level. It's best to try to limit your dairy consumption to one to two servings per day, and make sure you get plenty of magnesium in your diet. Most whole-grain products have about three times as much magnesium in them as processed "white" grain products do. This is another reason whole grains are better for you than refined grains. Also, remember that you often suffer from cells that are too nonporous, and the cholesterol and the saturated fat—specifically, the longer-chain saturated fats—in dairy products all work to make your cells even more nonporous. This is especially true when it's warm outside. You can often tolerate small amounts of this type of fat when it's cold, but you will need to watch your dairy consumption when it's warm outside. The best dairy protein source for you is probably nonfat Greek-style yogurt, because this type of yogurt usually has twice the protein of regular milk and yogurt products, while typically having only one-third to one-half the amount of calcium. Just remember that excess calcium can slow you down more than any other vitamin or mineral will, so be careful not to eat too many dairy products.

Springs and Dairy

If you are a Spring, first you should read about a Summer's dairy requirements. Much of this applies to you as well. The main difference is that Springs can handle a little more calcium and saturated fat from dairy products than Summers can. You still need to avoid consuming too much calcium and saturated fat, especially when it's warm outside, but low-fat or nonfat dairy once or twice a day when it's cold out and once a day when it's warmer out should be alright for you, as long as you make sure to eat enough magnesium-rich foods. Remember that although normally a 2:1 ratio of calcium to magnesium is recommended, your season-type needs a lower ratio, perhaps closer to a 1.5:1 or 1:1 ratio.

Each person needs to do a little experimenting to see what works best for him or her, but if you eat too many calcium-rich foods, along with too many refined grains that have been stripped of their magnesium, your ratio will climb above 2:1, and you will most likely feel the effects as a reduced level of energy.

Dairy Summary for All Season-Types

Dairy foods can have a dramatic effect on the metabolism of the various season-types, mainly due to their high levels of calcium and long-chain saturated fats. Winters have the highest need for both, followed by Autumns, Springs, and finally Summers. The need for long-chain saturated fats rises when it's colder outside and falls when it's warmer. The amount of saturated fat a person should consume also varies greatly, depending on the amount of fat-burning energy he or she uses. For example, Summers usually have the least need for fat; however, a Summer who burns a lot of fat during exercise will have a greater need for dietary fat. Remember from the earlier chapters that people tend to use more fat for energy when they exercise at a lower intensity level, as measured by their maximum cardiovascular capability. For Summers, this could be accomplished by a brisk walk or a very slow and steady jog that does not wind them to any great degree. The key is to keep a pace that you can sustain relatively easily for hours without being winded, and this is a sure sign you are burning a high level of fat for energy. Remember that Winters and Autumns can produce more energy from burning fat, so they can have a much faster pace, while still burning mainly fat for energy. If you are struggling for air or you feel winded, chances are you are burning mainly carbohydrates for energy.

The important point is that the amount of fat people can tolerate from dairy products will increase as the energy they burn from fat increases. Once again, you will have to experiment, based on your own body. Every time I go to the gym, I see people huffing and puffing for air on treadmills or stationary bicycles, and I know they are trying to lose weight. If this sounds like you, odds are you are not burning off body fat, but rather are using stored sugar for energy. Take the pace down to where you feel that you could sustain it for hours, and then you can be certain you are actually burning fat. I mention this because I always hear these people comment on how hard they work on the treadmill, yet they never seem to lose weight. Stop working out so hard, and you will begin to burn fat, instead of sugar, and you will lose weight.

Beans and Legumes

On the opposite page is the bean and legume chart, which is simply labeled *legumes*. I will refer to all of them as legumes. Legumes are typically high in purines and high in potassium and are between 20 and 25 percent protein and from 75 to 80 percent carbohydrates. The exceptions are garbanzo beans, which are lower in purines, and soybean products such as tofu, which are usually around 30 to 40 percent protein, 10 to 20 percent carbohydrates, and 40 to 50 percent fat. For reasons explained in a later chapter, soybeans and soy products are not recommended as part of the Four Seasons Diet.

Winters and Legumes

Legumes are, in many respects, a Winter's best choice for carbohydrates. They have an extremely low glycemic index, are typically high in purines, and have a fair amount of protein. A hearty bowl of chili or a cup of lentil soup as a side dish is often an excellent choice for a Winter. Just make sure you don't rely on legumes as your only source of protein. Legumes, especially navy beans, black-eyed peas, and lentils, are also high in resistant-carbohydrates. Resistant-carbohydrates are extremely beneficial for your season-type, and consuming around 5 grams with each meal will help you feel full and stay in fat-burning mode. The one potential problem with legumes is that they are extremely high in potassium, which could cause blood-sugar problems for you, unless you add enough salt to your legume dishes. Remember, it's the ratio of potassium to sodium that's most important, so make sure you consume plenty of salt with any meals that contain legumes.

Autumns and Legumes

If you are an Autumn, first read about how legumes affect Winters. Much of this applies to you as well. The main difference is that because you need less protein and more carbohydrates than a Winter does, legumes can be a much more versatile part of your meals. For example, a chicken quesadilla with black beans and cheese is a very good option as a meal for you, whereas a Winter would probably not do very well eating the tortilla part of that dish. Legumes are high enough in purines that you can also have a traditional Mexican dish, such as white fish with beans, rice, and a little cheese, without having to worry about getting purines from meat.

Calories per Serving							Recommended % of Calories			
							Winter	Autumn	Spring	Summer
	Protein					Protein:	35-45%	30-35%	25-30%	20-25%
		Carbohydrates				Carbohydrates:	25-35%	35-50%	50-60%	60-70%
			Fat			Fat:	25-35%	20-30%	15-20%	10-15%
Serving Size	Total Cal	P Cal	C Cal	F Cal	Pur=Purines* / Pur	Purines*:	High Winter	Medium Autumn	Low Spring	Very Low Summer
						BEANS				
						LEGUMES*				
1 cup	294	60	232	2	+*	Aduki beans, cooked	:-)	:-)	:-|	:-(
1 cup	227	53	166	8	+*	Black beans, cooked	:-)	:-)	:-(	:-(
1 cup	198	46	145	8	++	Black-eyed peas, cooked	:-):-)	:-)	:-(	:-(:-(
1 cup	241	57	177	7	+	Cranberry beans, cooked	:-)	:-)	:-)	:-|
1 cup	187	45	136	6	+*	Fava beans, cooked	:-)	:-)	:-|	:-(
1 cup	269	50	183	36		Garbanzo beans, cooked	:-|	:-|	:-)	:-)
1 cup	209	51	151	7	++	Great northern, cooked	:-):-)	:-)	:-(	:-(:-(
1 cup	44	6	35	3	+	Green beans	:-):-)	:-)	:-|	:-(
1 cup	225	54	164	7	+*	Kidney beans, cooked	:-)	:-)	:-|	:-(
1 cup	230	62	161	7	++	Lentils, cooked	:-):-)	:-)	:-(	:-(:-(
1 cup	216	51	159	6	+	Lima beans, cooked	:-)	:-)	:-|	:-(
1 cup	212	49	156	7	++	Mung beans, cooked	:-):-)	:-)	:-(	:-(:-(
1 cup	255	52	193	10	+*	Navy beans, cooked	:-)	:-)	:-|	:-(
1 oz.	164	23	25	116	+*	Peanuts, dry roasted	:-)	:-)	:-|	:-(
2 tbsp.	188	28	25	135	+*	Peanut butter	:-)	:-)	:-|	:-(
1 cup	252	53	192	7	+*	Pink beans, cooked	:-)	:-)	:-|	:-(
1 cup	245	54	182	9	++	Pinto beans, cooked	:-)	:-)	:-(	:-(
1 cup	219	56	162	1	+	Red beans, cooked	:-)	:-)	:-(	:-(
1 cup	231	57	168	6	++	Split peas, cooked	:-):-)	:-)	:-(	:-(:-(
1 cup	298	100	69	129	++	Soybeans, cooked	:-(	:-(	:-(	:-(
1 oz.	54	18	11	25	++	Tempeh	:-|	:-|	:-|	:-(
1 oz.	20	8	2	10	++	Tofu	:-(	:-(	:-(	:-(
1 cup	254	56	189	9	++	White beans, cooked	:-)	:-)	:-(	:-(

If the purine value of a bean was unknown, it was assumed to have a + value. Unknown beans marked +

* + = medium, ++ = high, +++ = very high

Summers and Legumes

With the exception of garbanzo beans, legumes are usually not a very good option for you because of the high amounts of purines contained in most of them. You can often get by with a little bit of lower-purine beans, such as black beans, as a small side dish. The key is not to use higher-purine beans as a main dish, because they may lower your energy levels. Legumes are also very high in potassium, which will help increase your energy levels, as long as you do not eat too much salt with them. Because they are so high in potassium, you can usually get away with adding a little salt for flavor, but keeping the salt to a moderate level will help make up for some of the negative effects that may result from the purines. Hummus is often an excellent choice for you, when combined with foods such as nonfat pita bread, as long as the hummus is not made with too much olive oil. Also, most commercial varieties of hummus are now made with processed vegetable oils and not extra-virgin olive oil. If you buy your hummus already prepared, make sure it's made with extra-virgin olive oil, and count the fat calories in the hummus toward the 10 to 15 percent of fat that's recommended for you to have in that meal. It's also advised that you limit your consumption of peanut butter, because it can really throw your season-type out of balance, if eaten every day.

Springs and Legumes
If you are a Spring, first read about how legumes affect Summers. Much of this applies to you as well. The main difference is that Springs can tolerate more purines, so you can usually have more low-purine legumes as part of your meal plan. Low-fat Mexican food with rice and beans is often an excellent choice for you. If you cook your rice and beans without any fat, you can use a little cheese for your fat, and the cheese and the beans will be an excellent source of protein for you. Remember that your diet should still be lower in purines, especially when it's warmer outside, so try to use low-purine beans as a side dish no more than once a day when it's warm outside.

Legume Summary for All Season-Types
Legumes tend to be high in purines, with the exception of garbanzo beans. They are high in carbohydrates and have moderate levels of protein. They are also high in resistant-carbohydrates, especially navy beans, black-eyed peas, and lentils. They can be excellent for Winters when used as the only source of carbohydrates. Autumns can use them in a more versatile manner because they are allowed to eat more carbohydrates than Winters are. Summers should use caution with legumes, except for garbanzo beans. Springs can use lower-purine legumes as side dishes, with the frequency of consumption depending on the temperature outside.

Grains
On the opposite page is the grain chart. Grains are extremely concentrated sources of carbohydrates that may often cause a rapid rise in blood-sugar levels, especially when they are refined. I list the glycemic index of each grain as either low, medium, or high, to help each season-type choose the right grain products. Both barley and oats have moderate levels of purines. Whole grains are

usually better for you, due to their lower glycemic value and higher nutrient content.

Calories per Serving								Recommended % of Calories			
								Winter	Autumn	Spring	Summer
		Protein					Protein:	35-45%	30-35%	25-30%	20-25%
			Carbohydrates				Carbohydrates:	25-35%	35-50%	50-60%	60-70%
				Fat			Fat:	25-35%	20-30%	15-20%	10-15%
Serving Size	Total Cal	P Cal	C Cal	F Cal	Pur=Purines* Pur	GI	Purines*: GI=Glycemic Index	High Winter	Medium Autumn	Low Spring	Very Low Summer
							CARBS				
							GRAINS				
1 cup	251	32	186	33		High	Amaranth, cooked	:-|	:-)	:-|	:-|
1 cup	193	13	175	5	+	Low	Barley, cooked	:-):-)	:-)	:-(	:-(
1 cup	155	19	127	9		Low	Buckwheat, cooked	:-|	:-|	:-)	:-)
1 cup	176	24	150	2		Medium	Couscous, cooked	:-|	:-|	:-)	:-)
1/2 cup	208	15	175	18		Medium	Corn meal, uncooked	:-|	:-|	:-)	:-)
1 cup	251	40	198	13		Low	Kamut, cooked	:-|	:-|	:-)	:-)
1 cup	207	24	169	14		High	Millet, cooked	:-|	:-|	:-|	:-|
1/4 cup	152	23	106	23	+	Low	Oats, raw	:-)	:-)	:-(	:-(
2 oz.	200	24	168	8		Low-Med	Pasta, uncooked	:-|	:-|	:-)	:-)
1 cup	222	33	157	32		Low	Quinoa, cooked	:-|	:-|	:-)	:-)
1 cup	218	15	189	14		Medium	Rice, brown, cooked	:-|	:-|	:-)	:-)
1 cup	225	15	195	15		Low	Rice, br., parboiled, cooked				
1 cup	205	16	185	4		Medium	Rice, white, cooked	:-|	:-|	:-)	:-)
1/4 cup	141	19	115	9		Low	Rye, uncooked	:-|	:-|	:-)	:-)
1 cup	220	32	177	11		Low-Med	Spaghetti, cooked	:-|	:-|	:-)	:-)
1 cup	246	38	194	14		Medium	Spelt, cooked	:-|	:-|	:-)	:-)
1 oz.	102	13	85	4		Low	Wheat flour, white	:-|	:-|	:-)	:-)
1 cup	166	23	138	5		Low	Wild rice, cooked	:-|	:-|	:-)	:-)
							VEGETABLES				
1/2 cup	45	6	36	3	+	High	Artichoke, hearts	:-):-)	:-)	:-(	:-(:-(
4 stalks	13	4	8	1	+	Low	Asparagus, boiled	:-):-)	:-)	:-(	:-(:-(
1/2	114	5	21	88		Low	Avocado, California	:-)	:-)	:-|	:-(
1 oz.	3	1	2	0		Low	Bamboo shoots, boiled	:-(	:-|	:-)	:-)
1 cup	44	6	35	3	+	Low	Beans, green, cooked	:-):-)	:-)	:-|	:-(
1/2 cup	37	4	32	1		High	Beets, boiled*	:-|	:-|	:-)	:-)
1 cup	9	3	5	1		Low	Bok choy	:-(	:-|	:-)	:-)
1/2 cup	26	7	18	1	+	Low	Broccoli, cooked	:-(	:-(	:-)	:-)
1/2 cup	28	5	20	3		Medium	Brussels sprouts, cooked	:-(	:-(	:-)	:-)
1/2 cup	17	2	15	0		Low	Cabbage, cooked	:-(	:-|	:-)	:-)
1 med.	25	2	22	1		High	Carrot, raw	:-)	:-)	:-|	:-|
1/2 cup	14	3	9	2	+	Low	Cauliflower, cooked	:-):-)	:-)	:-(	:-(
1 stalk	6	1	5	0		Low	Celery	:-)	:-)	:-|	:-|
1 ear	124	20	104	4		High	Corn, on the cob	:-)	:-)	:-|	:-(
1 cup	177	13	146	18		High	Corn, sweet, cooked	:-)	:-)	:-|	:-(
1 cup	16	3	11	2		Low	Cucumber, peeled	:-(	:-(	:-)	:-)

* + = medium, ++ = high, +++ = very high

Winters and Grains

Grains are the one food that can throw you out of balance the fastest. Remember that it's recommended you keep your carbohydrate consumption between 25 and 35 percent of your total caloric intake. Ideally, at least when you first start the diet, you should try to keep your carbohydrate consumption closer to 25 percent of your total calories and choose only grains that have a low- or medium-glycemic index. Your season-type will do best if you consume a lot of your carbohydrates as either vegetables or legumes. If you choose grains, you can really minimize the glycemic impact by sprinkling a tablespoon of resistant-carbohydrate powder on top and mixing it into your grain dish. Barley and oats are two of the best grains for you to eat, due to their low glycemic index and moderate purine level. Try to avoid instant oats, because they have a much higher glycemic index. Steel-cut oats are your best choice; however, they require a longer cooking time. They can be cooked in large batches, poured into a cake pan, and cooled in the refrigerator. You can then cut them into squares and eat them in the morning as a way to get some low-glycemic carbohydrates with your breakfast. You can also try old-fashioned rolled oats, which have a higher glycemic index than steel-cut oats but a lower glycemic index than instant rolled oats. These can also be eaten as a cold cereal with milk, eliminating the hassle of cooking.

Rye bread is good choice for you, too, due to its low glycemic value. Rice cakes and any cereal made with a puffed grain product, such as puffed wheat or puffed corn, are some of the very worst grain products for your season-type. This is because in the process of puffing up the grain like popcorn, the glycemic index increases substantially. Your season-type should avoid all puffed grain products, including rice cakes. Grains with added sugar, such as processed cereals and granola bars, can also cause you problems. If you easily gain weight, odds are your weight problem is primarily tied to excess carbohydrate consumption. If you keep your fructose consumption to less than 15 grams a day, you should have a much easier time controlling your starch cravings.

Autumns and Grains

If you are an Autumn, first read about how grains affect Winters. Much of this applies to you as well. The main difference is that you can tolerate more carbohydrates and more grains. You should still strive for low- and medium-glycemic index grains and try not to make grains your major source of carbohydrates at every meal. A side of rice and beans is an excellent way to mix a little grain with lower-glycemic beans.

Summers and Grains

Carbohydrates are more important to your well-being than they are to any other season-type. Because fast-acting grains and sugars can make you feel so good in the short run, it's very easy for you to consistently get too many high-glycemic foods, causing elevated insulin levels and blood-sugar spikes that will ultimately lead to insulin resistance and will be your undoing. By eating medium- and high-glycemic whole grains, along with ample vegetables, you can keep your stored-sugar reserves high, which is your key to maximizing energy levels. Grain digestion begins in the mouth, not in the stomach, and it's crucial to chew your grains until they are completely liquefied before you swallow them. You can eat all of the right foods, but if you don't properly chew your grains, you will not be able to fully use the sugar energy contained in them. Of all of the season-types, it will take you by far the longest to eat your meals if you properly chew your grains. Oats and barley have moderate levels of purines, so if you are going to eat these grains, make sure you factor them in as part of your total purine intake. Yeast is also very high in purines, so yeasted breads or foods with added yeast, such as grape-nuts cereal, can throw you out of balance if you eat them regularly and in large quantities. A better choice for you is unyeasted grain products, such as tortillas. Many types of bread are also high in sodium, and with your high carbohydrate consumption, it's easy for bread to throw off your sodium/potassium balance, which will lower your energy levels.

Springs and Grains
If you are a Spring, first read about how grains affect Summers. Much of this applies to you as well. The main difference is that you have a slightly lower need for grains than Summers do.

Grain Summary for All Season-Types
Ideally, all season-types should choose whole grains, instead of processed white flour products or white rice. Remember, when choosing rice, to pick longer-grain rice, instead of short- and medium-grain rice. If you recall from the section on resistant-carbohydrates, longer-grain rice has a lower glycemic index than shorter-grain rice, and brown rice has a lower glycemic index than white rice. Parboiled, quick-cook brown rice is the one exception to this, because the process of making parboiled brown rice converts much of the starch to resistant-carbohydrates. When choosing products such as oatmeal, instant rolled oats have a much higher glycemic index than slower-cooking steel-cut oats, while old-fashioned oats that are not "instant" are somewhere between the two. Avoid products such as puffed wheat, puffed corn, puffed rice,

and rice cakes, because they also have a much higher glycemic index. Remember, your total calories from carbohydrates means carbohydrates from all sources, including legumes and vegetables. Winters and Autumns should try to avoid getting all of their carbohydrate calories from grains and should strive to eat plenty of vegetables and legumes. Summers and Springs can handle more grains but should also try to include plenty of vegetables and lower-purine legumes, such as garbanzo beans.

All season-types can benefit from resistant-carbohydrate powder added to their grains and mixed in with a little moisture. Current studies suggest that one tablespoon per meal might be optimum for helping Winters and Autumns stay in fat-burning mode as part of the Winter and Autumn diets, while either half a tablespoon or two tablespoons appear to be most conducive to staying in sugar-burning mode as part of the Summer and Spring diets. You may do a double-take at these measurements, but for some reason, studies have found that either a small amount or a large amount helps a person stay in sugar-burning mode, whereas a medium amount helps someone stay in fat-burning mode. Because research on resistant-carbohydrates is just beginning, and so much is still unknown about them, it's recommended that you experiment with them and find an amount that works best for you by starting with one tablespoon per meal if you are a Winter or an Autumn and a half tablespoon if you are a Summer or a Spring. You can experiement by adjusting this level up or down, until you find what works best for you.

Vegetables
On the opposite page is the vegetable chart. Vegetables are similar to grains, in that they have a glycemic index that can be used as a gauge to figure out how quickly the sugars contained in them will enter the bloodstream. Next to each vegetable, the glycemic index is listed as being either low, medium, or high. Some vegetables also contain purines, and those are listed as well. Vegetables are typically high in potassium, which can affect the metabolism of the various season-types. Many vegetables also have an ability to either acidify or alkalinize the blood, and that ability is taken into account when determining whether a particular vegetable is either beneficial or detrimental to a certain season-type. Commercial salad dressings are not recommended, because they usually contain processed vegetable oils that are high in omega-6 fats. A better choice for salads is to sprinkle on a little olive oil and

balsamic vinegar, or make your own dressings using yogurt or cottage cheese, flaxseed oil or olive oil, and apple cider vinegar. Summers and Springs should use vinegar very sparingly or, better yet, never at all, because it can really throw their metabolism out of balance, especially if they exercise regularly. For salad dressings, they could substitute lemon or lime juice for the vinegar.

Calories per Serving								Recommended % of Calories			
								Winter	Autumn	Spring	Summer
	Protein						Protein:	35-45%	30-35%	25-30%	20-25%
		Carbohydrates					Carbohydrates:	25-35%	35-50%	50-60%	60-70%
			Fat				Fat:	25-35%	20-30%	15-20%	10-15%
Serving	Total	P	C	F	Pur=Purines*		Purines*:	High	Medium	Low	Very Low
Size	Cal	Cal	Cal	Cal	Pur	GI	GI=Glycemic Index	Winter	Autumn	Spring	Summer
							CARBS				
							GRAINS				
1 cup	251	32	186	33		High	Amaranth, cooked	:-)	:-)	:-|	:-|
1 cup	193	13	175	5	+	Low	Barley, cooked	:-):-)	:-)	:-(	:-(
1 cup	155	19	127	9		Low	Buckwheat, cooked	:-|	:-|	:-)	:-)
1 cup	176	24	150	2		Medium	Couscous, cooked	:-|	:-|	:-)	:-)
1/2 cup	208	15	175	18		Medium	Corn meal, uncooked	:-|	:-|	:-)	:-)
1 cup	251	40	198	13		Low	Kamut, cooked	:-|	:-|	:-)	:-)
1 cup	207	24	169	14		High	Millet, cooked	:-|	:-|	:-|	:-|
1/4 cup	152	23	106	23	+	Low	Oats, raw	:-)	:-)	:-(	:-(
2 oz.	200	24	168	8		Low-Med	Pasta, uncooked	:-|	:-|	:-)	:-)
1 cup	222	33	157	32		Low	Quinoa, cooked	:-|	:-|	:-)	:-)
1 cup	218	15	189	14		Medium	Rice, brown, cooked	:-|	:-|	:-)	:-)
1 cup	225	15	195	15		Low	Rice, br., parboiled, cooked				
1 cup	205	16	185	4		Medium	Rice, white, cooked	:-|	:-|	:-)	:-)
1/4 cup	141	19	115	9		Low	Rye, uncooked	:-|	:-|	:-)	:-)
1 cup	220	32	177	11		Low-Med	Spaghetti, cooked	:-|	:-|	:-)	:-)
1 cup	246	38	194	14		Medium	Spelt, cooked	:-|	:-|	:-)	:-)
1 oz.	102	13	85	4		Low	Wheat flour, white	:-|	:-|	:-)	:-)
1 cup	166	23	138	5		Low	Wild rice, cooked	:-|	:-|	:-)	:-)
							VEGETABLES				
1/2 cup	45	6	36	3	+	High	Artichoke, hearts	:-):-)	:-)	:-(	:-(:-(
4 stalks	13	4	8	1	+	Low	Asparagus, boiled	:-):-)	:-)	:-(	:-(:-(
1/2	114	5	21	88		Low	Avocado, California	:-)	:-)	:-|	:-|
1 oz.	3	1	2	0		Low	Bamboo shoots, boiled	:-(	:-|	:-)	:-)
1 cup	44	6	35	3	+	Low	Beans, green, cooked	:-):-)	:-)	:-|	:-(
1/2 cup	37	4	32	1		High	Beets, boiled*	:-|	:-|	:-)	:-)
1 cup	9	3	5	1		Low	Bok choy	:-(	:-|	:-)	:-)
1/2 cup	26	7	18	1	+	Low	Broccoli, cooked	:-(	:-(	:-)	:-)
1/2 cup	28	5	20	3		Medium	Brussels sprouts, cooked	:-(	:-(	:-)	:-)
1/2 cup	17	2	15	0		Low	Cabbage, cooked	:-(	:-|	:-)	:-)
1 med.	25	2	22	1		High	Carrot, raw	:-)	:-)	:-|	:-|
1/2 cup	14	3	9	2	+	Low	Cauliflower, cooked	:-):-)	:-)	:-(	:-(
1 stalk	6	1	5	0		Low	Celery	:-)	:-)	:-|	:-|
1 ear	124	20	104	4		High	Corn, on the cob	:-)	:-)	:-|	:-(
1 cup	177	13	146	18		High	Corn, sweet, cooked	:-)	:-)	:-|	:-(
1 cup	16	3	11	2		Low	Cucumber, peeled	:-(	:-(	:-)	:-)

* + = medium, ++ = high, +++ = very high

Winters and Vegetables
The best vegetables for you are often the ones with moderate

							Calories per Serving	Recommended % of Calories			
								Winter	Autumn	Spring	Summer
		Protein					Protein:	35-45%	30-35%	25-30%	20-25%
			Carbohydrates				Carbohydrates:	25-35%	35-50%	50-60%	60-70%
				Fat			Fat:	25-35%	20-30%	15-20%	10-15%
Serving Size	Total Cal	P Cal	C Cal	F Cal	Pur = Purines* Pur	GI	Purines*: GI=Glycemic Index	High Winter	Medium Autumn	Low Spring	Very Low Summer
							CARBS				
							VEGETABLES CONT.				
1 cup	35	2	31	2		Low	Eggplant, cooked*	:-(	:-|	:-)	:-)
1 clove	5	1	4	0		Low	Garlic	:-(	:-(	:-)	:-):-)
1 cup	36	6	26	4		Low	Kale, cooked	:-(	:-(	:-)	:-)
1 leek	38	2	34	2		Medium	Leeks, cooked	:-(	:-(	:-)	:-)
1 cup	8	2	5	1		Low	Lettuce	:-(	:-(	:-)	:-)
1 cup	16	6	8	2	+	Low	Mushrooms, raw	:-):-)	:-)	:-(	:-(
1/2 cup	18	4	13	1		Medium	Okra, cooked	:-|	:-|	:-)	:-)
1 oz.	23	1	6	16		Low	Olives, canned	:-)	:-)	:-|	:-(
1 slice	6	1	5	0		Medium	Onion, raw	:-(	:-(	:-)	:-):-)
1/2 cup	56	51	3	2		High	Parsnip, cooked	:-(	:-(	:-)	:-)
1 cup	67	18	46	3	+	Medium	Peas, green cooked*	:-):-)	:-)	:-(	:-(
1 cup	30	3	25	2		Medium	Pepper, bell, raw*	:-(	:-(	:-)	:-)
1 pepper	18	2	15	1		Medium	Pepper, hot, raw	:-(	:-(	:-)	:-)
1 large	278	21	254	3		High	Potato, baked	:-|	:-|	:-)	:-)
1 cup	49	4	43	2		Medium	Pumpkin, cooked	:-(	:-(	:-)	:-)
1 med.	1	0	1	0		Low	Radish, raw	:-(	:-|	:-)	:-)
1 cup	66	6	57	3		High	Rutabaga, cooked	:-(	:-|	:-)	:-)
1 med.	5	1	4	0		Low	Scallion	:-(	:-(	:-)	:-):-)
1 oz.	13	2	9	2		Low	Seaweed	:-|	:-|	:-)	:-)
1 cup	41	13	24	4	+	Low	Spinach, boiled	:-):-)	:-)	:-|	:-|
1 cup	36	4	27	5		Low	Squash, summer, cooked	:-(	:-|	:-)	:-)
1 cup	115	6	107	2		High	Squash, winter, cooked	:-|	:-|	:-)	:-)
1 med.	103	7	95	1		Medium	Sweet potato, cooked*	:-|	:-|	:-)	:-)
1 med.	22	3	17	2		Low	Tomato, red, raw*	:-(	:-(	:-)	:-)
1 med.	34	3	30	1		Medium	Turnip, raw	:-|	:-|	:-)	:-)
1/2 cup	60	2	57	0		Low	Water chestnuts, raw	:-(	:-|	:-)	:-)
1 cup	158	6	151	1		Medium	Yams, cooked	:-|	:-|	:-)	:-)
1/2 cup	14	1	13	0		Low	Zucchini, sliced*	:-(	:-|	:-)	:-)

*Contains moderate amounts of fructose of approximately 2 grams, except peas, which contain approximately 4 grams.

* + = medium, ++ = high, +++ = very high

amounts of purines, such as artichoke hearts, asparagus, cauliflower, mushrooms, peas, and spinach. Winters can use low- and medium-glycemic vegetables as a great way to get a portion of their carbohydrates at every meal, which will help keep their blood-sugar issues under control. Due to the high potassium content in many vegetables, Winters usually do best by adding salt to vegetable dishes. In addition, vegetables are low in fat, and Winters can often benefit from adding a little butter as well, as long as they try to keep their total fat calories within their recommended range. Potatoes are a good example of this. Half of a potato, fried in a little butter with some added salt, can be an excellent way for you to get your carbohydrates in the morning. Similarly, half of a baked potato with butter, sour cream, and salt can be a great choice for dinner, along with a side of green beans. As with many other foods that can affect your blood pH, you will do best sticking to your "beneficial" vegetables when it's cold outside, and you can work in more "neutral and evensome "avoid" vegetables the warmer the weather gets.

Autumns and Vegetables
If you are an Autumn, first read about how vegetables affect Winters. Much of this applies to you as well. The main difference is that you can handle the blood-sugar and blood pH issues that certain vegetables may cause a little better than Winters can, so many of the vegetables that are listed as "avoid" for Winters are listed as "neutral" for you.

Summers and Vegetables
As a Summer, the best vegetables for you are often the ones with lower purine levels. Vegetables are high in potassium, which is great for helping you keep your energy levels high, as long as you do not add too much salt or fat to your vegetable side dishes. Your best choices are often foods such as fresh salads made from your beneficial and neutral vegetables; just be sure not to use commercial salad dressings. Making your own dressings is your best option; however, your diet is low in fat, so it's easy for you to get your entire allotment of fat in your dressing if you're not careful. You will be far better off if you can learn to eat your salads without any dressing, which allows you to obtain what little fat you are permitted from other foods. The other problem with most salad dressings is that they contain vinegar, and vinegar can have a significant negative effect on your season-type, especially if you work out on a regular basis. The vegetables that help acidify your usually overly alkaline blood include lettuce, tomatoes, onions, and garlic. When it's warmer outside, you will do best sticking to your "beneficial" vegetables; however, when it gets colder, you can work in more "neutral" and even a few "avoid" vegetables.

Springs and Vegetables
If you are a Spring, first read about how vegetables affect Summers. Much of this applies to you as well. The main difference is that many of the vegetables that are "avoids" for Summers are "neutral" for you, giving you a wider range of vegetable choices.

Vegetable Summary for All Season-Types

There is a good variety of vegetables for all of the season-types. The higher-purine vegetables are often ideal for Winters, while the ones that help acidify the blood are usually best for Summers. Winters need to add enough salt to their vegetables to avoid any negative reaction from getting too much potassium; salt will help counterbalance the effects.   Summers do best with salads and steamed vegetables.   All season-types, except Summers, should either use extra-virgin olive oil and balsamic vinegar for their salad dressings, or else make their own.   Summers are usually best off avoiding vinegar altogether; they can use lemon juice and extra-virgin olive oil for a salad dressing instead. Remember to avoid any dressings that contain processed vegetable oil that is high in omega-6 fats or any other processed vegetable oils, such as canola oil

Fruit

On the opposite page is the fruit chart. As explained in detail on the section on fructose (see Chapter 5), most fruits are high in fructose. It is strongly recommended that you limit your fructose consumption to no more than 15 grams per day. Next to each fruit, the grams of fructose per serving are listed to help you keep track of your daily fructose consumption. Remember that table sugar and honey are 50 percent fructose, so 50 percent of the sugar grams from anything sweetened with these sweeteners needs to be counted toward your fructose limit of 15 grams per day. One can of sugar-sweetened beverage or one small piece of cake can easily put you over your limit of fructose for the day, so it's best to eliminate all sugar-sweetened foods and get your sweet tooth fix from natural fruits. Unlike most sugar-sweetened processed foods, natural fruits contain fiber, vitamins, minerals, and antioxidants, all of which provide nutritional benefits. Excess fructose, however, can have many negative consequences, which I mentioned earlier. For anyone trying to lose weight, remember that excess fructose will turn off your feel-full hormones, turn on your hunger hormones, and cause brain changes that will increase your reward and pleasure sensations from eating food. Fruit is also very high in potassium and often in quick-acting sugars, such as glucose.

	Calories per Serving							Recommended % of Calories			
								Winter	Autumn	Spring	Summer
		Protein					Protein:	35-45%	30-35%	25-30%	20-25%
			Carbohydrates				Carbohydrates:	25-35%	35-50%	50-60%	60-70%
				Fat			Fat:	25-35%	20-30%	15-20%	10-15%
Serving Size	Total Cal	P Cal	C Cal	F Cal	Pot = Potassium, Pot	Fru	Potassium:	Low	Medium	Medium	High
							Fru = Fructose	Winter	Autumn	Spring	Summer
							CARBS				
							FRUIT*				
1 med.	95	2	90	3	195 mg	13 g	Apple	:-|	:-|	:-)	:-|
1 med.	17	2	14	1	91 mg	1 g	Apricot	:-|	:-|	:-)	:-)
1 med.	105	4	98	3	422 mg	7 g	Banana	:-)	:-)	:-|	:-|
1 cup	62	7	49	6	233 mg	4 g	Blackberries	:-|	:-|	:-)	:-)
1 cup	84	4	76	4	114 mg	7 g	Blueberries	:-|	:-|	:-)	:-|
1/2 med.	94	8	82	5	737 mg	11 g	Cantaloupe	:-(	:-|	:-)	:-)
1 cup	87	5	80	2	306 mg	8 g	Cherries, sweet	:-|	:-|	:-)	:-)
1 oz.	99	3	17	79	100 mg	2 g	Coconut, meat, raw	:-)	:-)	:-|	:-|
1 med.	67	2	65	0	167 mg	8 g	Dates, medjool	:-(	:-(	:-)	:-)
1 med.	37	1	35	1	116 mg	4 g	Fig	:-(	:-(	:-|	:-|
1 cup	104	4	98	2	288 mg	6 g	Grapes	:-(	:-|	:-)	:-)
1/2 med.	52	3	47	1	166 mg	4 g	Grapefruit, pink/red	:-(	:-(	:-)	:-):-)
1 cup	112	14	85	13	688 mg	6 g	Guava	:-(	:-(	:-)	:-)
1/4 med.	90	5	83	3	570 mg	14 g	Honeydew	:-(	:-(	:-)	:-)
1 cup	108	7	94	7	522 mg	8 g	Kiwifruit	:-(	:-(	:-)	:-)
1 oz.	7	0	7	0	35 mg	3 g	Lemon juice	:-(:-(	:-(	:-)	:-):-)
1 oz.	7	1	6	0	33 mg	0	Lime	:-(:-(	:-(	:-)	:-):-)
1 med.	135	4	126	5	323 mg	16 g	Mango	:-(	:-(	:-)	:-)
1 med.	63	5	54	4	286 mg	5 g	Nectarine	:-|	:-|	:-)	:-|
1 med.	69	4	63	2	232 mg	6 g	Orange, navel	:-(:-(	:-(	:-)	:-):-)
1 med.	119	6	109	4	781 mg	11 g	Papaya	:-(	:-(	:-)	:-)
1 med.	59	5	51	3	285 mg	6 g	Peach	:-|	:-|	:-)	:-)
1 med.	103	2	99	2	212 mg	12 g	Pear	:-)	:-)	:-|	:-(
1 cup	83	3	78	2	180 mg	9 g	Pineapple	:-(	:-(	:-)	:-):-)
1 med.	30	2	27	1	104 mg	3 g	Plum	:-|	:-|	:-)	:-)
1 med.	234	16	191	27	666 mg	19 g	Pomegranate	:-(	:-(	:-)	:-)
1 med.	23	1	22	0	70 mg	1 g	Prune, dried	:-(	:-(	:-|	:-|
1 oz.	83	2	80	1	231 mg	10 g	Raisin	:-(	:-(	:-|	:-|
1 cup	64	5	52	7	186 mg	3 g	Raspberry	:-|	:-|	:-)	:-)
1 stalk	11	2	8	1	147 mg	1 g	Rhubarb	:-|	:-|	:-)	:-)
1 cup	46	3	39	4	220 mg	4 g	Strawberries, whole	:-|	:-|	:-)	:-)
1 med.	47	2	43	2	146 mg	5 g	Tangerine	:-(	:-(	:-)	:-)
1 cup	46	3	41	2	170 mg	6 g	Watermelon, diced	:-(	:-(	:-)	:-)

*Limit due to high fructose content. Do a two-week fructose fast twice a year.

Winters and Fruit

Because of fruit's high potassium content, along with fast-acting sugars such as glucose, it can really cause serious blood-sugar issues for your season-type. Your best fruits are bananas and pears, and every other fruit is either a "neutral" or an "avoid." Consuming excess "avoid" fruits can be especially detrimental for you when it's cold outside; however, when the weather gets hot, you may find that you are able to tolerate consuming a little fruit listed as "avoid." You usually do better with lower-glycemic fruits, such as cherries and peaches, while high-glycemic fruits such as watermelon can quickly throw you out of balance unless you have consumed enough purine-rich foods for your main course.

Autumns and Fruit

If you are an Autumn, first read about how fruits affect Winters. Much of this applies to you as well. The main difference is that you can handle the potassium and the quick-acting sugars in fruit a little better than Winters can, especially when it's colder outside. You should still stick to bananas, pears, and low-glycemic fruits such as cherries whenever possible.

Summers and Fruit

Fruit is a mixed blessing for Summers. Due to the high level of potassium and simple sugars contained in most fruit, a piece of fruit is like rocket fuel for you. Nothing will give you a burst of energy, a sense of well-being, and mental clarity the way a piece of fruit does. The problem is that because fruit makes most Summers feel so good, they tend to eat way too much of it. I rarely meet a Summer who isn't a fruit and sugar addict. The problem, as explained in the fructose section, is that all of this fruit will cause you to become insulin resistant, and once this happens, you can no longer store or use sugar for energy properly. Because you rely on sugar for energy, this will cause your energy to plummet to extremely low levels. Many Summers are actually stuck in this state for most of their lives, never really knowing what's wrong with them. The insulin resistance will also cause you to suffer from chronically high insulin levels, which will make your cholesterol levels sky-rocket and make your cells too non-porous. When this happens, even oxygen has a hard time getting into your cells, and you produce much of your energy without oxygen, which creates a lot of metabolic acids. These have a difficult time exiting the cells, and you now have the low-oxygen, high-acid environment that is perfect for cancer to thrive in. I mention all of this because I rarely see a Summer who does not have these problems, to some degree. Do yourself a favor and undertake at least a two-week fructose fast. This will most likely be a very difficult two weeks for you, especially if you do not make sure you consume plenty of potassium from other potassium-rich foods. At the end, however, you should regain some of your insulin sensitivity and have a new lease on life.

Yet be warned that your season-type has a very easy time getting re-addicted to fruit. After a two-week fructose fast, you will feel so much better, especially when you eat fruit, that you can quickly fall into the trap of consuming too much fruit again. The best strategy for you is to strictly limit yourself to 15 grams of fructose per day and to eat no foods that contain added sugar. Often, the best way for your season-type to consume fruit is to have your first piece in the morning on an empty stomach. Nothing will jump-start your metabolism first thing in the morning like a piece of fruit, especially something like an orange. You will find that 15 to 30 minutes after eating your morning fruit, your system will be primed to handle a nice grain-based breakfast much better. Your other fruit is best eaten either as a dessert to satisfy your sweet tooth, as a mid-afternoon snack, or at the very beginning of your work-out to give you the potassium and sugar necessary to fuel your muscles. Most fruits will cause your blood to make a shift to the acidic direction. Because most Summers have blood that is too alkaline, especially when it's hot outside, this is one of the many benefits of consuming fruit for Summers.

Citrus fruits cause your blood to make the biggest shift in the acidic direction, so citrus fruits are especially recommended when it's hot outside to help balance you out. When it's colder outside, your blood tends not to be as overly alkaline as it is when it's hot, so you can choose whatever fruit most appeals to you. What purines are to Winters, an orange or a grapefruit is to you, with the only difference being that Winters can eat virtually unlimited purines to help balance out their metabolism, while Summers are limited to about three oranges a day if you want to keep your fructose consumption at around 15 grams daily. When it's warm outside, don't waste your limited fruit allowance on fruits such as bananas, which can move your blood pH in the wrong direction. Use fruits such as citrus and, to a lesser degree, melons as a way to bring yourself back into balance.

The other important component of fruit that helps the Summer season-type is potassium, and for this reason, the potassium content of various fruits is listed, along with the fructose content. When choosing fruits, try to pick those that have a high potassium content and a low fructose content. Following is an example of what I am talking about:

Fruit	Fructose	Potassium
1 apple	13 g	195 mg
15 apricots	15 g	1,365 mg
4 cups strawberries	16 g	880 mg
3 oranges	18 g	696 mg

One apple has 13 grams of fructose, which is nearly your entire daily limit of fructose, while 15 apricots have only 15 grams of fructose. That same apple has only 195 mg of potassium, while the 15 apricots have 1,365 mg of potassium. The extra 1,170 mg of potassium that you, as a Summer, get from eating the apricots, as opposed to the apple, can mean the difference between low energy and high energy. The more you choose fruits high in potassium, relative to their fructose content, the more fruit and the more potassium you get in a day.

Eating three oranges gives you 18 grams of fructose and 696 mg of potassium; in addition, citrus fruits are especially good at shifting your usually overly alkaline blood back into the acidic direction. When it's hot outside, you are more prone to having blood that becomes overly alkaline. The point is that fruit, in a way, can be like medicine for you, so don't waste your 15 grams of fructose by eating something like an apple. Choose fruits such as apricots to get the maximum amount of potassium possible or citrus fruits when it's especially hot outside, to help keep your blood pH balanced.

Springs and Fruit
If you are a Spring, first read about how fruit affects Summers. Much of this applies to you as well. The main difference is that your blood does not tend to get as overly alkaline as a Summer's blood does. This means you are a little freer to choose fruits that appeal to you when it's hot outside, rather than having to choose fruits such as citrus that have the greatest ability to balance your blood chemistry. Odds are that you have over-relied on fruit and sugar for energy to some degree for many years, so it's highly recommended that you do at least a two-week fructose fast as well.

Fruit Summary for All Season-Types
Due to their high levels of potassium and simple sugars, fruits can have a very potent effect on our metabolism. With the exception of bananas, fruit will usually cause a Winter to get further out of balance. Most fruits are the most balancing food there is for

Summers and Springs; however, because it gives them such a burst of energy and sense of well-being, these two season-types often eat too much fruit, resulting in excess fructose consumption and all of the negative effects that go along with that. Start to see fruit as the powerful metabolic agent it is, and remember to always limit your daily consumption of fructose to no more than 15 grams a day, which includes any fructose from processed sugar as well. It's also advised that you do a two-week fructose fast twice a year, to help ensure that you do not succumb to any of the negative metabolic effects of consuming too much fructose.

Fats, Oils, Nuts, and Seeds

On the opposite page is the chart of fats, oil, nuts, and seeds. I have already talked at length about fats and oils. On the Four Seasons Diet, it's highly recommended that you limit your intake of fats and oil to the ones marked with an asterisk. Most processed foods contain oils and fats that are not recommended for consumption. Although oils may seem like benign substances, remember from the section on vegetable oils that omega-6 fats can have a dramatic negative effect on our metabolism and in excess can hinder the ability of our cells to produce energy. Now, almost every processed food that exists contains omega-6 fats, so it will take a little work on your part to eliminate them from your diet. Remember that all of the new evidence shows that saturated fats such as butter, which have been blamed for years as the cause of heart disease, are not the real culprit. For Winters and Autumns, saturated fat consumption is one of the keys to good health.

Winters and Fats, Oils, Nuts, and Seeds

As a Winter, you need a high-protein and high-fat diet. Remember that your metabolism tends to cause your cells to become too porous, which is part of the cause of your erratic blood-sugar issues. Fats and oils that are high in saturated fat, such as butter, cream, sour cream, and cream cheese, are crucial for your well-being, especially when it's cold outside. These foods will help keep your cells from becoming too porous. When it's warmer outside, your need for saturated fat goes down, but this type of fat should still be the principal fat you consume. Olive oil and coconut oil are also good choices for you; however, they will not have the same positive metabolic effect that the longer-chain saturated fats will. You can increase your consumption of olive oil and coconut oil as it gets warmer, but when it's cold, try to get at least half of your fat from longer-chain saturated fats.

Nuts that are heavily salted are your ideal snack food. Although I do not recommend snacks, until you balance out your metabolism, you may find that you are hungry between meals. Nuts are a perfect combination of protein and fat that you require in a snack food, as long as there is enough salt added. If you need a snack, dry roasted and salted nuts, peanut butter on a few saltine crackers, or a handful of salted macadamia nuts, brazil nuts, or pecans are perfect options for you.

Calories per Serving							Recommended % of Calories			
							Winter	Autumn	Spring	Summer
		Protein				Protein:	35-45%	30-35%	25-30%	20-25%
			Carbohydrates			Carbohydrates:	25-35%	35-50%	50-60%	60-70%
				Fat		Fat:	25-35%	20-30%	15-20%	10-15%
Serving Size	Total Cal	P Cal	C Cal	F Cal	Pur=Purines* Pur	Purines*:	High Winter	Medium Autumn	Low Spring	Very Low Summer
						FATS & OILS				
1 tbsp.	119	0	0	119		Almond oil	:-|	:-|	:-|	:-|
1 tbsp.	100	0	0	100		Butter**	:-)	:-)	:-(	:-(
1 tbsp.	124	0	0	124		Canola oil	:-(	:-(	:-(	:-(
1 tbsp.	116	0	0	116		Coconut oil**	:-)	:-)	:-)	:-)
1 tbsp.	124	0	0	124		Corn oil	:-(	:-(	:-(	:-(
1 tbsp.	119	0	0	124		Cottonseed oil	:-(	:-(	:-(	:-(
1 tbsp.	52	0	0	52		Cream, heavy**	:-)	:-)	:-(	:-(
1 tbsp.	122	0	0	122		Fish oil**	:-|	:-|	:-)	:-)
1 tbsp.	120	0	0	120		Flaxseed oil**	:-(	:-(	:-)	:-)
1 tbsp.	112	0	0	112		Ghee**	:-)	:-)	:-(	:-(
1 tbsp.	119	0	0	119		Lard**	:-)	:-)	:-(	:-(
1 tbsp.	124	0	0	124		Olive oil**	:-)	:-)	:-)	:-)
1 tbsp.	116	0	0	116		Palm oil**	:-)	:-)	:-(	:-(
1 tbsp.	116	0	0	116		Palm kernel oil**	:-)	:-)	:-)	:-)
1 tbsp.	119	0	0	119		Peanut oil	:-|	:-|	:-|	:-|
1 tbsp.	119	0	0	119		Safflower oil	see *** below			
1 tbsp.	119	0	0	119		Sesame oil	:-|	:-|	:-|	:-|
1 tbsp.	119	0	0	119		Sunflower oil	see *** below			
						NUTS & SEEDS				
1 oz.	162	21	25	117		Almonds	:-|	:-|	:-)	:-)
1 oz.	185	14	14	157		Brazil nuts	:-)	:-)	:-|	:-|
1 oz.	155	18	35	103		Cashews	:-(	:-(	:-)	:-)
1 oz.	55	2	50	3		Chestnuts	:-(	:-(	:-)	:-)
1 oz.	185	7	27	151		Coconut, meat, dried	:-)	:-)	:-|	:-|
1 oz.	177	15	19	144		Filberts	:-)	:-)	:-|	:-|
1 oz.	184	12	21	151		Hickory nuts	:-)	:-)	:-|	:-|
1 oz.	203	8	16	179		Macadamia nuts	:-)	:-)	:-|	:-|
1 oz.	164	23	25	116		Peanuts, dry roasted	:-)	:-)	:-|	:-(
1 oz.	199	9	16	174		Pecans	:-)	:-)	:-|	:-|
1 oz.	190	13	15	162		Pine nuts	:-(	:-(	:-)	:-)
1 oz.	157	20	32	105		Pistachios	:-|	:-|	:-)	:-)
1 oz.	151	24	20	107		Pumpkin seeds	:-)	:-)	:-|	:-|
1 oz.	86	10	16	60		Sesame butter, tahini	:-|	:-|	:-)	:-)
1 oz.	164	20	23	121		Sunflower seeds	:-(	:-(	:-)	:-)
1 oz.	185	15	16	154		Walnuts	:-)	:-)	:-|	:-|

* + = medium, ++ = high, +++ = very high
**These are the healthiest oils and should be the primary ones consumed.
***Cold-pressed high oleic is :-|. Commercially processed or high linoleic is :-(.

Autumns and Fats, Oils, Nuts, and Seeds

If you are an Autumn, first read about how fats, oils, nuts, and seeds affect Winters. Much of this applies to you as well. The main difference is that your cells do not tend to become overly porous to the same extent that a Winter's cells do. This means that you do not have to rely on eating large amounts of long-chain saturated fats as a way of keeping your cells from getting too porous. Although you may still benefit from adding more of these fats to your diet when the weather is cold and from lowering your consumption a little when it's warm, you do not have the same biological imperative that a Winter has to consume these fats to stay healthy. You are much freer to eat the recommended fats and oils that appeal most to you.

When it comes to snacking, nuts are also an excellent choice, but you are free to add a few more carbohydrates to your snacks. Rather than a handful of roasted salted peanuts, you may choose half of a peanut butter sandwich or some nuts and raisins.

Summers and Fats, Oils, Nuts, and Seeds

As a Summer, your ideal diet is low in protein and fat and especially low in long-chain saturated fats. Just as Winters tend to have cells that become too porous, you have cells that are often too nonporous. If you have eaten large quantities of fruit and sugar your entire life, odds are that you are insulin resistant, and the high levels of insulin, along with excess saturated fat consumption, are causing your cells to become nonporous. After your two-week fructose fast, it's recommended that you also eliminate foods that contain long-chain saturated fats for a month. This includes cheese, low-fat or full-fat milk, and butter. The Four Seasons Diet will help keep your insulin at healthier levels, and after a month of not eating any long-chain saturated fats, you should begin to feel as if you have more oxygen and air when you do simple things such as walking up the stairs. During this time, focus on oils such as extra-virgin olive oil, coconut oil, and one to three teaspoons per day of cold-pressed flaxseed oil mixed into nonfat milk, nonfat yogurt, or protein powder smoothies. Once you feel higher energy and oxygen levels, it's alright to add back a little long-chain saturated fats, especially when it's cold outside. These fats, however, should be secondary to fats such as olive oil, coconut oil, and flaxseed oil. Use your long-chain saturated fats and oils as side dishes, as opposed to staples the way a Winter does. A little butter or cream now and then won't kill you. You may also choose to consume low-fat milk and yogurt when it's cold outside and switch to nonfat when it gets warmer. You may find that you do best eliminating all long-chain saturated fats when the weather is hot, unless you are burning a lot of fat exercising.

It's very easy for you to overdo nuts, because they are high in protein and fat, and your diet is low in protein and fat. Peanuts and peanut butter are especially bad for you and will quickly throw you out of balance if you eat them regularly. Limit nuts to occasional and light use, such as sprinkling some sunflower seeds on top of your salad or having a few almonds with some fruit for a snack.

Springs and Fats, Oils, Nuts, and Seeds
If you are a Spring, first read about how fats, oils, nuts, and seeds affect Summers. Much of this applies to you as well. The main difference is that your cells do not tend to become as nonporous as a Summer's cells. This means you are much freer to consume fats such as butter and cream. You still tend to do best using olive oil, coconut oil, and a little flaxseed oil, but you do not have to be as strict about eliminating butter, cream, and cheese when it's hot outside. You still need to keep your fat consumption low, but you can choose more of the fats that appeal to you, rather than having to choose fats as a way to keep yourself balanced.

Fats, Oils, Nuts, and Seeds Summary for All Season-Types
Long-chain saturated fats will tend to make the cells less permeable, and oils such as flaxseed oil and olive oil tend to make the cells more permeable. For this reason, Winters should consume the most long-chain saturated fats, followed by Autumns, Springs, and finally Summers. All season-types can handle greater amounts of long-chain saturated fats, such as butter and cream, when it's cold outside, and fewer of these fats when it's hot outside. Nuts that are heavily salted are a great snack food for Winters and Autumns but a poor choice for Summers and Springs.

Sample Meals

Now that you have a good understanding of the effects that various foods have on your season-type, you're probably wondering what foods you should prepare for healthy meals. I have come up with a few easy sample meals with good food choices for all of the season-types. Whenever possible, I have attempted to make the meals as similar as possible for the four season-types, for a number of reasons. First, I want you to understand how a few minor changes to a meal can make it more suitable or less suitable for your season-type. Second, most people have family considerations to think about when preparing food. In a household where everyone is the same season-type or two close season-types, such as Winters and Autumns, it's fairly easy to make the same meal for everyone. It's more challenging when you have a household with opposite season-types, such as Winters and Summers. You should also consider the season-types of your children when you prepare meals. Usually, children will take after the season-type of one of the two parents, and sometimes they will be more like one of their grandparents than like one of their parents.

Helping your children understand how food choices affect them can really benefit them in school, not to mention in life in general. Remember that eating contrary to your-season type will cause lower energy levels, along with problems with mood, concentration, and general overall well-being. A Winter mother feeding her Summer child Winter foods is likely to have a child with low energy levels and lack of concentration. Similarly, a Summer father feeding his Winter child Summer foods will probably have a child with erratic blood sugar and weight-gain issues.

After the sample meals, you will find explanations to help you understand why some often very subtle changes were made for the various season-types. Do not feel as though you need to stick to these meals or even try them, for that matter. The purpose is to let you see enough sample meals, with explanations, so that you can easily learn to modify your favorite meals for your season-type. Even if you have a family with one of each season-type, after reading about the sample meals you should be able to continue to make your family's favorite meals, by using simple solutions to help each season-type eat in a way that's best for him or her.

Breakfast

All of these meals are very basic, without seasonings or

extra ingredients that might add more flavor. The purpose of each meal is to provide a few good, simple examples of meals and snacks for you and your family.

Winter Breakfast #1			
Breakfast Sandwich	P	C	F
9 oz. Canadian bacon	204	12	162
1 egg sunny side up	25	1	45
1 English muffin	24	124	9
1 banana	4	98	3
Calories:	257	235	219
711	36%	33%	31%

Autumn Breakfast #1			
Breakfast Sandwich	P	C	F
6 oz. Canadian bacon	136	8	108
1 egg sunny side up	25	1	45
1 English muffin	24	124	9
1 banana	4	98	3
Calories:	189	231	165
585	32%	39%	28%

Spring Breakfast #1			
Breakfast Sandwich	P	C	F
4 egg whites	64	0	0
2 oz. part skim mozzarella	48	6	78
2 English muffins	48	248	18
1/4 of a large cantaloupe	8	60	3
Calories	168	314	99
581	29%	54%	17%

Summer Breakfast #1			
Breakfast Sandwich	P	C	F
2 egg whites	32	0	0
1.5 oz. part skim mozzarella	36	5	58
2 English muffins	48	248	18
1/2 of a large cantaloupe	16	121	6
Calories	132	374	82
588	22%	64%	14%

After each food item, the calories from protein (P), carbohydrates (C), and fat (F) are listed. At the bottom, the total calories for a meal are listed under the word *calories*, and to the right of the word *calories* are the total calories for protein, carbohydrates, and fat. Under that is the percentage of calories from protein, carbohydrates, and fat: most of the meals fall within the recommended range for each season-type. Don't worry about counting calories right now. Just read over all of these meals to start, until you become comfortable with how to adjust meals for the season-types.

The first breakfast is a simple breakfast sandwich. Winters need the most protein that contains purines, so the centerpiece of their sandwich is a large piece of Canadian bacon. Canadian bacon is a great meat option for Winters and Autumns because it has a good mix of protein and fat. Lower-fat ham is also a good choice for many meals. The problem with sausage and regular bacon is that they often contain twice as many calories from fat as from protein. Ideally, Winters and Autumns need more protein than fat. While it's all right for Winters to consume more calories from fat for one meal, they should try to stick within their diet plan during the course of a day. For Winters, breakfast is often the most important meal, and if they are going to go heavier on the fat and higher in the calories, breakfast is the meal for Winters to splurge. The main protein difference for Autumns is that their serving size of Canadian bacon is smaller than the size of the serving for Winters.

If you look at the Summer and the Spring sandwiches, you'll notice that they do not contain Canadian bacon. Remember, the Summer's and the Spring's diets are lower in protein, lower in purines, and lower in fat. Their protein consists of egg whites mixed with part-skim mozzarella cheese. Egg whites are often Summers' and Springs' best friend for breakfast because they contain no purines and no fat and are a complete source of high-quality protein. In fact, the protein from egg whites is superior in many ways to the protein from meats such as beef. Egg whites can be fried in a low-fat cooking spray to keep the fat to a minimum.Some people feel guilty about throwing the yolks away; however, gettingprotein from egg whitesis far more economical and environmentally friendly than from meat or poultry. For example, if you purchase egg whites from the store that have already been pre-separated, they cost about half the price per gram of protein when compared to buying chicken. Raising animals for meat is also a lot harder on the environment than raising chickens for eggs is, so you can feel good about consuming egg whites for your protein for several reasons.

Next in the Winter's sandwich is one egg, sunny-side up. If you are going to eat whole eggs, the yolk should always be left runny. When you keep the yolk runny, the fat contained in it is extremely beneficial. Once you cook an egg yolk and it turns solid, the cholesterol in the yolk oxidizes, and it becomes unhealthy for you when you eat it. The Winter and the Autumn get only one sandwich, so this egg can be added to the single sandwich or eaten on the side, if that's preferred.

The Summers and the Springs each get two sandwiches, and the eggs can be added to the middle of each sandwich, or you can make four open-faced half sandwiches, if you prefer that. All season-types can add seasonings and veggies to their sandwiches, per their preference. Winters are fine adding generous amounts of salt to their eggs, while Summers and Springs are probably getting enough salt from the English muffins for their entire meal. Feel free to add salsa, tomatoes, hot sauce, ketchup, or any other lower-calorie options that do not radically affect the calorie percentages of each meal. Just make sure if you use foods such as ketchup that they do not contain fructose or, if they do, that you count the fructose toward your 15 grams a day.

Finally, the four breakfasts include fruit.The Winter and the Autumn get one banana, as this is by far the best fruit for Winters and Autumns to consume, especially when it's cold outside. The Spring gets ¼ of a cantaloupe, and the Summer gets ½ of a cantaloupe. You can substitute other fruits with a similar calorie count, if you choose. Melon is an excellent choice, however, because the sodium in the English muffins and the cheese needs to be counterbalanced with potassium for this meal to work for Springs and Summers. Melons are especially high in potassium and also help balance a Spring's and a Summer's blood chemistry better than almost any other fruit, with the exception of citrus fruits.

The next breakfast is the Mexican dish huevos rancheros. Starting with the protein and fat content of the four different versions of this breakfast, you will notice that the Winter's and the Autumn's protein and fat come from eggs and lean ham, while the Spring and the Summer versions have egg whites and cheddar cheese. All four versions have beans, with the Winter getting the smallest amount and the Summer getting the largest. The other difference in the beans is that the Winter and Autumn versions use higher-purine pinto beans, while the Spring and Summer versions use moderate-purine black beans. All four versions include two corn tortillas. All four versions have salsa, or else you can use enchilada sauce, if you prefer. The Spring and Summer versions also have added tomatoes and fresh onions. These are two vegetables that really help balance the blood chemistry of these two season-types, and it's usually alright for Summers and Springs to add fresh tomatoes and onions to any meal of their choosing. Finally, the Spring and Summer versions have brown rice, but because the beans are high in fiber, you can probably get away with adding white Spanish-style rice, if you prefer. Just watch the sodium content, because many Spanish rice mixes are very high in sodium. Once again, you can feel free to add spices and extra minor ingredients, per your preference.

Beans are very high in potassium, so the Winter and the Autumn will do best to add salt to their beans to help counter the negative effect that excess potassium can have on them. A cup of beans has almost as much potassium as two bananas, so it's especially important for a Winter to be generous with the salt shaker when eating beans. Fruit and beans are consistently the two foods highest in potassium, so Winters and Autumns should always make sure they consume enough salt when they eat these foods.

If you are making this type of dish for a large family, it's best to buy beans without salt and not to add any fat, salt, or oil to foods you cook, such as beans or rice, especially if you have any Summers in the family. Try to get in the habit of keeping foods such as olive oil, butter, and table salt on the table where they belong. This way, all family members can add these to their meals in levels that are most beneficial to them. It can oftentimes be very difficult for a Winter or an Autumn to fully understand why a Spring or a Summer needs foods that are prepared without added salt or fat. Just try to remember that in the same way that Winters may need meat or other high-purine foods to feel their best, Summers and Springs need low-fat and low-salt foods to feel their best.

Winter Breakfast #2			
Huevos Rancheros	P	C	F
2 eggs sunny side up	50	4	90
8 oz. lean ham	176	0	96
1/2 cup pinto beans	27	91	4
2 corn tortillas	16	112	18
Salsa	2	8	0
Calories	271	215	208
694	39%	31%	30%

Autumn Breakfast #2			
Huevos Rancheros	P	C	F
2 eggs sunny side up	50	4	90
4 oz. lean ham	88	0	48
3/4 cup pinto beans	41	137	6
2 corn tortillas	16	112	18
Salsa	2	8	0
Calories	197	261	162
620	32%	42%	26%

Spring Breakfast #2			
Huevos Rancheros	P	C	F
4 egg whites	64	0	0
1 oz. cheddar cheese	30	2	81
3/4 cup black beans	40	125	6
2 corn tortillas	16	112	18
Salsa	2	8	0
1/2 a medium tomato	3	17	2
fresh diced onions	1	5	0
1/2 cup brown rice	7	95	7
Calories	163	364	114
641	25%	57%	18%

Summer Breakfast #2			
Huevos Rancheros	P	C	F
4 egg whites	64	0	0
1 oz. cheddar cheese	30	2	81
1 cup black beans	53	166	8
2 corn tortillas	16	112	18
Salsa	2	8	0
1/2 a medium tomato	3	17	2
Fresh diced onions	1	5	0
1 cup brown rice	15	189	14
Calories	184	499	123
806	23%	62%	15%

This next breakfast is about as basic as it gets for Winters and Autumns. It consists of a piece of pork tenderloin with eggs and a bowl of oatmeal. Protein and fat are the two most important elements of the Winter and Autumn breakfasts, especially for the Winters. If you eat meat, it's usually best to start with that choice first when planning your breakfast. For example, pork tenderloin is relatively low in fat, compared to many other meats you might have for breakfast. You might also choose a steak for breakfast or a piece of salmon. Remember that protein and purines are crucial, and they are often hardest to get for breakfast. Meats such as sausage and bacon are often too low in protein and too high in fat, while other meats high in purines might not appeal to you for breakfast. When it's cold, your need for purines in the morning rises considerably. When starting the Four Seasons Diet, Winters and Autumns should try to get purines for breakfast in their first week. Then they should try skipping purines for one breakfast to see what the effect is. Try having just an egg and cheese omelet without any purines. You may find that if you skip your morning purines, you don't feel as good as you have been after breakfast. You may notice that your old blood-sugar problems have returned, and that you are hungry again a few hours after eating. In the section on being a vegetarian for your season-type, I'll give you a few tips on supplements you can take that will make up for the lack of meat.

The rest of this meal is a simple serving of oatmeal, which is probably the best breakfast cereal there is for Winters and Autumns. Tailor your serving size so that you fall within your recommended percentage of carbohydrates. Remember to avoid quick-cook instant oatmeal, because it has a much higher glycemic index. Either pre-make your steel-cut oatmeal, pour it into a pan, cool it in the fridge, and cut it into squares to eat during the course of a few meals, or keep reading to learn about another easy option that I recommend for Summers and Springs.

As I mentioned earlier, quick-cook oats should be avoided, due to their higher glycemic value. In the muesli for Summers and Springs, I recommend "old-fashioned" rolled oat flakes, which are not the quick-cooking type. The Summer and Spring diets are both very high in grains, and oftentimes a large serving of grains for a meal can be a little overwhelming. This is especially true of a grain such as oats, which tends to swell up a lot when cooked. Eating old-fashioned oats uncooked with milk is often much more enjoyable than forcing down a bowl of cooked oatmeal three times

Winter Breakfast #3			
Pork & Oatmeal	P	C	F
8 oz. pork tenderloin	154	16	76
2 eggs sunny side up	50	2	90
Small bowl of oatmeal	28	169	33
Calories	232	187	199
618	38%	30%	32%

Autumn Breakfast #3			
Pork & Oatmeal	P	C	F
8 oz. pork tenderloin	154	16	76
1 egg sunny side up	25	1	45
Large bowl of oatmeal	37	226	44
Calories	216	243	165
624	35%	39%	26%

Spring Breakfast #3			
Homemade Muesli	P	C	F
1 cup rolled oat flakes	37	226	44
1 oz. raisins	2	80	1
1 cup lowfat milk	41	51	26
2 tbsp. sunflower seeds	10	22	60
Protein powder	80	0	0
1/2 tsp. cinnamon			
Calories	170	379	131
680	25%	56%	19%

Summer Breakfast #3			
Homemade Muesli	P	C	F
1 cup rolled oat flakes	37	226	44
1 oz. raisins	2	80	1
1 cup nonfat milk	42	54	5
1 tbsp. sunflower seeds	5	11	30
1 tsp. brown rice syrup	0	20	0
Protein powder	30	0	0
1/2 tsp. cinnamon			
Calories	116	391	80
587	20%	67%	14%

as large. You can get creative when making your muesli. I kept this recipe simple, with old-fashioned rolled oat flakes, raisins, sunflower seeds, and cinnamon. Summers should use nonfat milk, while Springs can get away with low-fat milk. I recommend a little high-quality protein powder, about enough to add about 30 calories' worth of protein for a Summer and almost triple this amount for Springs. This equates to about 7 or 8 grams of protein for a Summer and 20 grams for a Spring. You could also use some nonfat Greek-style yogurt instead, which is higher in protein, lower in sugars, and lower in calcium than regular yogurt. An excellent protein powder for this muesli recipe is Sunwarrior raw vegan vanilla-flavored rice protein. Sunwarrior rice protein is processed in a special way that makes it the highest-quality vegetable protein available. This protein is my preferred choice for muesli, because the flavor goes really well with oats, and it mixes easily with just a little milk. You could also use egg white protein powder, whey protein powder, or casein protein powder. Whey and casein are high in calcium, so Summers and Springs need to make sure not to consume too much of these two protein powders. (I offer Sunwarrior rice protein at a discount price on my website: FourSeasonsDietBook.com.

Summers can also add a little fructose-free sweetener such as brown rice syrup or barley malt powder. The barley malt powder goes especially well with the muesli, is fructose free, and is full of vitamins and minerals. Another nice thing about making your own muesli vs. store-bought cereals is that you can control the sodium and fructose levels much easier. Many store-bought cereals are very high in sodium and added sugars. (I also offer barley malt powder on my website.

This is another simple breakfast for Winters and Autumns, consisting of a bowl of oatmeal with a banana and a serving of Canadian bacon. You can flavor the oatmeal with a little cinnamon, a small pat of butter, and a little milk, if you like. If a Winter is going to eat fruit and cereal in the morning, this is the way to do it. Oatmeal has moderate amounts of purines and has an extremely low glycemic index, so it won't cause blood-sugar issues the way processed cereals can. Bananas, although high in potassium, do not have the same acidifying effects on the blood that other fruits have, and they are therefore the best fruit for Winters and Autumns. Feel free to add as much salt to the oatmeal and Canadian bacon as you feel is necessary. The Canadian bacon should satisfy your protein and fat requirements.

This is a pretty basic breakfast for Summers and Springs, consisting of cereal and egg whites. Wheatabix is a relatively good cereal because it's whole grain and is very low in fructose. It's sweetened with barley malt (along with just a little sugar), which is one of the recommended fructose-free sweeteners in the Four Seasons Diet.

Winter Breakfast #4			
Bacon & Oatmeal	P	C	F
12 oz. Canadian bacon	272	16	216
1 cup cooked oatmeal	24	116	27
1 banana in oatmeal	4	98	3
Calories	300	230	246
776	39%	30%	32%

Autumn Breakfast #4			
Bacon & Oatmeal	P	C	F
6 oz. Canadian bacon	136	8	108
1 cup cooked oatmeal	24	116	27
1 banana in oatmeal	4	98	3
Calories	164	222	138
524	31%	42%	26%

Spring Breakfast #4			
Egg Whites & Cereal	P	C	F
1 orange	4	63	2
1 1/4 cup wheatabix cereal	24	176	13
1 cup low-fat milk	41	51	26
1 tsp.flax oil blended in milk	0	0	40
4 egg whites	64	0	0
Calories	133	290	81
504	26%	58%	16%

Summer Breakfast #4			
Egg Whites and Cereal	P	C	F
1 orange before breakfast	4	63	2
1 1/2 cups wheatabix cereal	29	211	16
1 cup low-fat milk	41	51	26
1 tsp.flax oil blended in milk	0	0	40
2 egg whites	32	0	0
Calories	106	325	84
515	21%	63%	16%

The orange should ideally be eaten about a half hour before your main breakfast, because citrus is a great way for Summers to get their systems going first thing in the morning. When you have cereal with milk for breakfast, you can always add a few egg whites on the side, fried in low-fat cooking spray, as a way to get a little extra protein. As another option, you can blend a little protein powder with milk and flaxseed oil and pour this over your cereal in the morning.

The next four breakfasts suggest a few versatile options for potatoes. Rather then frying potatoes in oil, you can boil a pot of them or bake a bunch of them and stick them in the refrigerator overnight. In the process of cooling the potatoes, some of the regular carbohydrates get converted to resistant-carbohydrates, and they will have a lower glycemic index and will make you feel fuller faster, as long as they are not reheated. They will also help keep you full between meals. Another nice thing about cooking potatoes in this manner is that you can add fat, if you still need fat in a particular meal, or you can eat them without fat. In this breakfast, I recommend serving the potatoes without any added fat, and I have added nonfat sour cream to this meal, although if you prefer ketchup, you can add that instead. Winters and Autumns need to be sure to add plenty of salt to this meal to help counterbalance the potassium in the potato. The salmon is high in fat and purines and is an excellent protein choice for Winters and Autumns.

For Summers and Springs, potatoes can be very versatile for breakfast because they are low in fat, which gives you a lot of options for adding other sources of fat. They are also high in potassium, which is great for Summers and Springs. In these two breakfasts, I include a mix of egg whites as a way to get protein without fat, which allows you to add cheese to this meal. The potato and the eggs can be topped with nonfat sour cream, salsa, fresh tomatoes, and fresh onions. Summers should start this breakfast off with an orange or another type of fruit, ideally eaten about half an hour before the main breakfast, as a way to get enough carbohydrates in their meal. They can also eat the orange or another piece of fruit with breakfast, if they prefer.

Winter Breakfast #5			
Salmon	P	C	F
9 oz. salmon	214	0	238
3/4 potato, cooked & cooled	16	191	2
2 tbsp. nonfat sour cream	8	16	0
Calories	238	207	240
685	35%	30%	35%

Autumn Breakfast #5			
Salmon	P	C	F
7 oz. salmon	166	0	185
1 potato, cooked & cooled	21	254	3
2 tbsp. nonfat sour cream	8	16	0
Calories	195	270	188
653	30%	41%	29%

Spring Breakfast #5			
Eggs & Potato	P	C	F
1 potato, cooked & cooled	21	254	3
4 egg whites	64	0	0
1/2 a medium tomato	3	17	2
Salsa	2	8	0
1 oz. cheddar cheese	30	2	81
2 tbsp. nonfat sour cream	8	16	0
Calories	128	297	86
511	25%	58%	17%

Summer Breakfast #5			
Eggs & Potato	P	C	F
1 orange	4	63	2
1 potato, cooked & cooled	21	254	3
4 egg whites	64	0	0
1/2 a medium tomato	3	17	2
Salsa	2	8	0
1 oz. cheddar cheese	30	2	81
2 tbsp. nonfat sour cream	8	16	0
Calories	132	360	88
580	23%	62%	15%

Lunch

The first lunch is a basic chicken and rice dish. Light-meat chicken is being used because it can be eaten by all four season-types. Even though it contains purines, the amount of chicken in the Summer and Spring lunches is relatively small. Going with a lean meat for the Winters and the Autumns also allows them to add some extra fat, in the form of butter for the rice and vegetables and olive oil for the salad. This is something Winters and Autumns should always be mindful of when choosing a meat. If they choose a fattier meat, they will have to watch their consumption of other fats, such as butter, cheese, and salad dressing. Eating a high-fat meat such as salmon or fatty beef will easily provide plenty of fat calories for your meal. If you add too many other fats when you consume these proteins, you can boost your percentage of fat calories from a given meal to 60 percent or higher.

The steamed corn and the spinach salad are both excellent vegetables for Winters and Autumns. By adding butter to the corn and the rice, you will help slow down the rate at which the carbohydrates enter your system, giving you a lower overall glycemic effect. As usual, Winters and Autumns should feel free to salt their corn and rice. The olive oil is intended for your salad dressing, and, as with other meals, you may want to add spices or other minor ingredients that do not radically alter the nutritional profile of a meal.

The Summer and Spring lunches have small servings of chicken. You could just as easily consume a piece of white fish, egg whites, or a protein smoothie. Chicken was used primarily to show how you can make one meal to serve all of your family's season-types. The Summer and Spring lunches get much smaller portions of chicken but much larger portions of rice. A lettuce, tomato, and onion salad has also been substituted for the Winter's and the Autumn's spinach salad, although you could use spinach for convenience. Ideally, if you have a household with several different season-types, it's good to buy a variety of several common foods, and greens are one of those potential items. Spinach is the best salad for Winters and Autumns, and a darker lettuce other than spinach, such as romaine, is best for Summers and Springs. Feel free to add other vegetables per individual preference. As you can see, most of the fat in the Summer and Spring lunches comes from the olive oil for the salad. It's good to measure out your food quantities for at least a few weeks so that you can get used to portion sizes. For example, 3 ounces of chicken and a quarter tablespoon of olive oil may seem extremely paltry for the Summerswho are consuming these portions for the first few weeks.

Winter Lunch #1			
Chicken & Rice	P	C	F
8 oz. chicken, light meat	222	0	24
1/2 cup steamed corn	6	73	9
1/2 cup brown rice	7	94	7
1 tbsp. butter (corn & rice)	0	0	100
Spinach salad	6	12	2
1/2 tbsp. olive oil (salad)	0	0	62
Calories	241	179	204
624	39%	29%	33%

Autumn Lunch #1			
Chicken & Rice	P	C	F
6 oz. chicken, light meat	166	0	18
1/2 cup steamed corn	6	73	9
1 cup brown rice	15	189	14
1/2 tbsp. butter (corn & rice)	0	0	50
Spinach salad	6	12	2
1/2 tbsp. olive oil (salad)	0	0	62
Calories	193	274	155
622	31%	44%	25%

Spring Lunch #1			
Chicken & Rice	P	C	F
5 oz. chicken, light meat	139	0	15
1/2 cup steamed corn	6	73	9
1 1/2 cups brown rice	22	283	21
Lettuce, tomato, onion salad	3	20	3
1/2 tbsp. olive oil	0	0	62
Calories	170	376	110
656	26%	57%	17%

Summer Lunch #1			
Chicken & Rice	P	C	F
3 oz. chicken, light meat	83	0	9
1/2 cup steamed corn	6	73	9
1 1/2 cups brown rice	22	283	21
Lettuce, tomato, onion salad	3	20	3
1/4 tbsp. olive oil	0	0	31
Calories	114	376	73
563	20%	67%	13%

This is the ideal amount for their metabolism, however, and they have probably spent many years eating too much fat and protein, which is one of the main reasons they have probably suffered from low energy levels most of their lives. Once Summers get used to smaller portions of meat and fewer fats and oils, it will become second-nature to them.

Summers can add a little salt, if they feel the need, but a light amount is key with this meal. This meal is not overly high in potassium, and anything more than minimal amounts of salt will upset a Summer's potassium balance.

The next lunch is an easy Mexican-style meal. For protein, the Winter and the Autumn get beef, and the Spring and the Summer get white fish, along with the protein in the beans and the cheese. The Winter and Autumn lunches get a small serving of pinto beans, and the Summer and Spring lunches get a serving of black beans. If you are making one meal for a large family, you need to decide which beans to use. The pinto beans are higher in purines than the black beans and are better for the Winters and the Autumns. The black beans are better for the Summers and the Springs. When making decisions such as this, it's best to factor in several other important variables. For example, the Winter and Autumn lunches are already getting a higher-purine meat for their main course, so it's not crucial that they get higher-purine beans. Conversely, the Summers and the Springs are not consuming any other purines with this meal, so the pinto beans may not be that bad for them. Given that there are some pros and cons for all four season-types, probably the most important factor in this decision becomes the weather outside. If it's colder, and you want to serve only one type of bean, go with the higher-purine pinto beans, and if it's warmer, go with the lower-purine black beans. Remember, the colder it gets, the more Winters and Autumns need higher amounts of purines, and in colder weather, the more Summers and Springs can handle some purines. Conversely, the hotter it gets, the more imperative it is that Summers and Springs follow a lower-purine diet, and in hotter weather, the less crucial purines become for Winters and Autumns. If you start the Four Seasons Diet during the winter months or the summer months, remember that as the seasons change, you may have to slightly modify your meals. Purines and fats, more specifically saturated fats, are two items that can be consumed in larger amounts the colder the weather gets.

All four lunches include Mexican "queso" white cheese;

however, if you prefer, you can use cheddar, jack, or some other cheese more to your liking. Most cheeses have pretty similar calorie counts, so it's usually safe to substitute an ounce of one cheese for another.

Winter Lunch #2			
Mexican	P	C	F
12 oz. beef sirloin	153	0	86
1/2 cup pinto beans	27	91	4
1 corn tortilla	8	56	9
Fresh salsa	2	8	0
1 oz. Mexican queso cheese	24	4	72
Spinach salad	6	12	2
Calories	220	171	173
564	39%	30%	31%

Autumn Lunch #2			
Mexican	P	C	F
8 oz. beef sirloin	102	0	57
3/4 cup pinto beans	41	137	6
2 corn tortillas	16	112	18
Salsa	2	8	0
1/2 oz. queso cheese	12	2	36
Spinach salad	6	12	2
Calories	179	271	119
569	31%	48%	21%

Spring Lunch #2			
Mexican	P	C	F
4 oz. fish, roughy	78	0	7
1 oz. Mexican queso cheese	24	4	72
3/4 cup black beans	40	125	6
2 corn tortillas	16	112	18
Salsa	2	8	0
1/2 a medium tomato	3	17	2
Fresh diced onions	1	5	0
3/4 cup brown rice	5	126	9
Calories	169	397	114
680	25%	58%	17%

Summer Lunch #2			
Mexican	P	C	F
4 oz. fish, roughy	58	0	5
3/4 oz. Mexican queso cheese	18	3	54
3/4 cup black beans	40	125	6
2 corn tortillas	16	112	18
Salsa	2	8	0
1/2 a medium tomato	3	17	2
Fresh diced onions	1	5	0
1 cup brown rice	15	189	14
Calories	153	459	99
711	22%	65%	14%

The main exception is part-skim mozzarella cheese, which is lower in fat. Usually, when this cheese is listed in a meal, it's to keep the fat calories within the recommended range for a particular season-type, so take note if you are substituting this cheese for another one, and try to keep the total fat calories the same.

The beans are high in potassium, so Winters and Autumns will want to be generous with the salt shakers, while Summers and Springs can add a small amount, if they wish.

The Summer and Spring lunches include brown rice; however, there is enough fiber in the beans that if you prefer, you can use white rice, although brown is still the better option. Feel free to add extra items, such as cilantro and fresh lemon juice, per taste. The Summer and Spring lunches are best eaten by rolling up the beans, salsa, onions, and cheese into the tortillas and eating them like mini-burritos. If you prefer, you could substitute one or two fat-free larger flour tortillas with the same total carbohydrate count for the three corn tortillas and make one or two large burritos out of all of your ingredients. Most corn tortillas are fat-free, while most flour tortillas have added fat, and it's almost always added vegetable oil that is high in omega-6 fats. If you can't find fat-free flour tortillas, stick to corn, and warm them up on a hot frying pan without using any oil or in the toaster for about 20 seconds to help soften them and make them more flavorful.

The next lunch is an example of what you can order when eating out. The menu was inspired by what is available at a national sandwich chain. Most large chain restaurants now make nutritional information available, and by doing a little research online, you can easily prepare in advance if you ever need to eat out. I urge caution when eating out, however, because most restaurants and fast-food places use vegetable oil and high-fructose corn syrup in their breads and other food items. For this reason, when eating out at a fast-food sandwich chain, always go for the bread that's lowest in fat, because this is usually your best choice, even if it's the white bread.

For Winters, the key is finding a high-protein sandwich with fewer fat calories than protein calories and one that is lower in carbohydrates. The best way to accomplish this is to order a 6-inch sandwich, to limit your bread intake. You can then add double meat to up your protein intake. The chain I used for this example did not provide the calorie information of adding the double meat, so I had to get a little creative to figure out the calories. First, I added the calories from two 6-inch Philly cheese steak sandwiches.

This chain does provide the calorie count for bread and cheese, so I simply subtracted the calories from the 6 inches of bread from the extra sandwich, along with the cheese in the extra sandwich. This left me with basically the calories from only the extra meat in the second sandwich or essentially the calories from adding the double meat to a 6-inch sandwich. As you can see, the percentages of calories from protein, carbohydrates, and fat worked quite well for Winters, and they would get a good amount of purines from the meat.

Winter Lunch #3			
Sandwich Shop	P	C	F
6 " Philly cheesesteak w/double meat	276	272	271
Calories	276	272	271
819	34%	33%	33%

Autumn Lunch #3			
Sandwich Shop	P	C	F
12" Philly cheesesteak	156	212	160
Calories	156	212	160
528	30%	40%	30%

Spring Lunch #3			
Sandwich Shop	P	C	F
12" oven roasted chicken	184	368	90
With cheese	16	0	60
Calories	200	368	150
718	28%	51%	21%

Summer Lunch #3			
Sandwich Shop	P	C	F
12" oven roasted chicken	184	368	90
1 orange	4	63	2
Calories	188	431	92
711	26%	61%	13%

The Autumn sandwich choice was much easier; Autumns can simply order a 12-inch Philly cheese steak sandwich to get the proper caloric ratios for their season-type. All season-types need to try to limit their use of added fats, such as mayonnaise and other dressings, which usually contain large amounts of omega-6 vegetable oil and high-fructose corn syrup.

The best choice for the Spring was a 12-inch oven-roasted chicken sandwich with cheese. Even though the cheese is included in this sandwich when you order it, when listing the calorie content on its website, this national chain omits the cheese from the calorie count, in order to make it a lower-fat menu item. Add the cheese back in to get your fat calories, and don't use any mayonnaise or other condiments; the fat from the cheese is probably your healthiest option. The best Summer sandwich choice is a 12-inch oven-roasted chicken sandwich without the cheese. Just make sure you do not add any dressings or mayonnaise. The Summer lunch also includes a piece of fruit, such as an orange or four to five dried apricots for dessert.

Also, do not order any drinks or chips. All of these lunches have adequate calories. Summers should avoid the temptation of eating the baked chips, because these will add more sodium to the meal and potentially upset their potassium balance. The 12-inch oven-roasted chicken sandwich has around 1,200 mg of sodium, which is above the upper limit recommended for a Summer meal, unless Summers are eating large amounts of potassium. The sandwich has some potassium, especially if you add enough veggies, such as tomatoes and lettuce. This is why having fruit for dessert, such as four or five dried apricots, which are extremely high in potassium, or a can of coconut water is your best option for dessert. Coconut water is extremely high in potassium; however, half of the sugar calories are fructose, so be sure to add that to your daily fructose count. Adding drinks or chips will usually add fructose and vegetable oil to your meal, and any time you have the urge to eat these items, re-read the sections on both.

This is a simple lunch of fish, potatoes, and vegetables. The Winter and Autumn lunches consist of perch, which has a little more fat than the Spring and Summer fish, which is roughy. The Winter and Autumn vegetables are cauliflower and carrots with butter, while the Spring and Summer lunches have a fresh salad of lettuce, tomato, onion, and cucumber.

All four lunches include some potato, with the Winter getting the least, and the Spring and the Summer the most. The Winter and the Autumn get a tablespoon of butter, which they can use on their vegetables and potato, while the Spring and the Summer get olive oil to use on their salad and potato.

Winter Lunch #4			
Fish & Veggies	P	C	F
8 oz. perch	182	0	34
Cauliflower & carrots	4	20	30
1/2 potato	10	127	1
1 tbsp. butter	0	0	100
Calories	196	147	165
508	39%	29%	32%

Autumn Lunch #4			
Fish & veggies	P	C	F
8 oz. perch	182	0	34
Cauliflower & carrots	4	20	30
1 potato	21	254	3
1 tbsp. butter	0	0	100
Calories	207	274	167
648	32%	42%	26%

Spring Lunch #4			
Fish & Veggies	P	C	F
8 oz. fish, roughy	158	0	14
Lettuce, tomato, onion, cucumber salad	2	15	1
1 1/2 potato	32	381	4
1 tbsp. olive oil	0	0	124
Calories	192	396	143
731	26%	54%	20%

Summer Lunch #4			
Fish & veggies	P	C	F
6 oz. fish, roughy	118	0	11
Lettuce, tomato, onion, cucumber salad	2	15	1
1 1/2 potato	32	381	4
1/2 tbsp. olive oil	0	0	62
Calories	152	396	78
626	24%	63%	12%

This lunch is designed to illustrate the difference between white sauces and red sauces. All four season-types are using white chicken meat for their protein source, which will allow the Winters and the Autumns to use Alfredo sauce, instead of red sauce, on their pasta and to add butter to their vegetables. If they used dark chicken meat instead of white, the Winters and the Autumns would have to use a red sauce on their pasta and not use butter on their vegetables.

The pasta weights given are their dry weights before cooking. Once the pasta is cooked, simply mix part of it with the white sauce for the Winters and the Autumns and part of it with the red sauce for the Summers and the Springs. It's advised to get nonfat or low-fat red sauce to allow the Summers and the Springs to add their own extra fat. Also, most pasta sauces use vegetable oils that are high in omega-6 fats, instead of extra-virgin olive oil, so steer clear of those brands. Some sauces use olive oil but not extra-virgin olive oil. Olive oil that is not labeled "extra virgin" should be avoided, because this type of oil is often heavily processed and is not as healthy as extra-virgin olive oil.

If you wanted to serve all four season-types both white-meat chicken and red sauce, you would simply add more butter and olive oil to the Winters' and Autumns' meals. In my experience, Winters and Autumns usually have a natural preference for white sauces, while Summers and Springs often gravitate toward the red sauces. People normally develop a preference when they are younger, without ever realizing that it's tied to the fat content of the sauce and their season-type.

The Winter and Autumn lunches add green beans as the vegetable dish, which are one of the better vegetables for these two season-types and which contain a moderate amount of purines.

The Summer and Spring lunches have a fresh salad for their vegetable dish. The olive oil included for Summers and Springs can be used on the salad, added to the red sauce, or a combination of the two.

This lunch is a classic example of how all four season-types can theoretically eat from the same table of food, even if everyone uses a red sauce. The Winter lunch has the highest serving of chicken, followed by Autumns, Springs, and finally Summers. Similarly, the Summer lunch has the largest serving of pasta, followed by Springs, Autumns, and Winters. If everyone eats the same low-fat red sauce, the Winters will add a generous amount of butter and olive oil to their meal, while the Autumns will add less. The Summers and the Springs would not add any butter but simply a little olive oil.

Winter Lunch #5			
Chicken, Pasta & Veggies	P	C	F
8 oz. chicken, light meat	222	0	24
2 oz. pasta (pre-cooked weight)	24	168	9
1/4 cup Alfredo sauce	16	20	99
1 cup green beans	6	35	3
1 tbsp. butter	0	0	100
Calories	268	223	235
726	37%	31%	32%

Autumn Lunch #5			
Chicken, Pasta & Veggies	P	C	F
6 oz. chicken, light meat	166	0	18
3 oz. pasta (pre-cooked weight)	36	252	14
1/4 cup Alfredo sauce	16	20	99
1 cup green beans	6	35	3
Calories	224	307	134
665	34%	46%	20%

Spring Lunch #5			
Chicken, Pasta & Veggies	P	C	F
5 oz. chicken, light meat	139	0	15
4 oz. pasta (pre-cooked weight)	48	336	18
1/2 cup fat-free marina sauce	8	24	0
Lettuce, tomato, onion, cucumber salad	2	15	1
3/4 tbsp. olive oil	0	0	93
Calories	197	375	127
699	28%	54%	18%

Summer Lunch #5			
Chicken, pasta & veggies	P	C	F
3 oz. light chicken	83	0	9
5 oz. pasta (pre-cooked wgt.)	60	420	22
1/2 cup fat-free marina sauce	8	24	0
Lettuce, tomato, onion, cucumber salad	2	15	1
1/2 tbsp. olive oil	0	0	62
Calories	153	459	94
706	22%	65%	13%

Hopefully, you're getting a good picture of how to feed not only yourself, but your entire family. When serving a family, choose low-fat or nonfat items. This will allow everyone to add his or her own proper amount of healthy fat, while eliminating sources of processed vegetable oil. Remember that most fats that are pre-added to foods these days consist of vegetable oil, which is high in omega-6 fats. Cook the chicken, the pasta, and the vegetables without any added salt, and use as little oil as possible. Then let everyone add the amount of salt and healthy oil that is best for him or her. Ideally, every meal will have butter and olive oil on the table for your family members to add. Summers are especially prone to suffering the ill effects of eating too much fat, so leave a measuring spoon on the table to allow people to measure their own oils, or add the proper amount of oil to each plate of food before you put it on the table.

Winters are especially prone to feeling the ill effects of consuming too much potassium, so any time a high-potassium dish is served, such as beans, potatoes, vegetables, or fruit for dessert, be sure to add enough salt to the meal in order to counter the effects of excess potassium if you are a Winter or an Autumn.

The last lunch is a Mediterranean-style plate. Lamb is being used as the concentrated source of protein, although you could use beef or chicken and adjust the level of other foods, as needed. For example, if you were to use white-meat chicken, which is much lower in fat than lamb, you would have to make up the loss of fat from the lamb from other sources. Winters and Autumns might switch from fat-free yogurt to whole-milk yogurt, might add more olive oil to their salad, could fry their chicken in butter, or could do a combination of several of these. It helps to think of your concentrated protein sources in terms of how much fat they contain and then base your meal around that. If you are going to eat a high-fat meat, you know the rest of your meal will have to be lower in fat. Likewise, if you want to consume fat from other sources such as butter or full-fat yogurt, you will have to pick a leaner meat, such as chicken.

In this example, because a high-fat meat is used, the rest of the meal is leaner. The next items on the menu are garbanzo beans and fat-free pita bread, as the source for carbohydrates. The lunch also includes a salad and fat-free yogurt for all four season-types.

Winter Lunch #6			
Mediterranean Plate	P	C	F
6 oz. lamb	174	0	255
1/2 cup garbanzo beans	25	91	18
Lettuce, tomato, onion, cucumber salad	2	15	1
1 cup fat-free yogurt	60	73	4
1 piece fat-free pita bread	16	96	0
Calories	277	275	278
830	33%	33%	33%

Autumn Lunch #6			
Mediterranean plate	P	C	F
4 oz. lamb	116	0	170
1/2 cup garbanzo beans	25	91	18
Lettuce, tomato, onion, cucumber salad	2	15	1
1 cup fat-free yogurt	60	73	4
1 piece fat-free pita bread	16	96	0
Calories	219	275	193
687	32%	40%	28%

Spring Lunch #6			
Mediterranean Plate	P	C	F
2 oz. lamb	58	0	85
1/2 cup garbanzo beans	25	91	18
Lettuce, tomato, onion, cucumber salad	2	15	1
1 cup fat-free yogurt	60	73	4
1 1/2 pieces fat-free pita bread	24	144	0
Calories	169	323	108
600	28%	54%	18%

Summer Lunch #6			
Mediterranean Plate	P	C	F
1 cup garbanzo beans	50	182	36
Lettuce, tomato, onion, cucumber salad	2	15	1
2 pieces fat-free pita bread	32	192	0
1/2 tbsp. olive oil	0	0	62
1 cup fat-free yogurt	60	73	4
Calories	144	462	103
709	20%	65%	15%

If you look at the Summer and Spring lunches, you'll notice that the Summer lunch has no lamb, and the Spring lunch has only 2 ounces of lamb. This is because both the yogurt and the garbanzo beans contain fair amounts of protein, which are adequate for the Summer and almost adequate for the Spring. The Summer lunch contains a little olive oil for the salad, because the rest of the lunch is lower in fat.

Hopefully, you're starting to see the ideal way to eat for your season-type at every meal. Winters need to focus on getting enough high-quality protein, without overloading on the fat. It's very easy for Winters to consume a fatty protein source and then overload on fat in the rest of the meal. Although this will not be as detrimental to them as it would be for other season-types, the goal for Winters is to consume roughly 40 percent of their calories from protein and roughly 30 percent from fat. This ratio will keep them in fat-burning mode and will prevent them from gaining more body fat. If Winters need to gain weight or are highly active, then they might benefit from adding more fat to their diet. The higher the percentage of fat any season-type eats over his or her recommended ratio, the more likely that season-type is to store that excess fat as body fat. Remember from an earlier chapter that a Winter's muscles burn the most fat and therefore store the most fat for energy. This type of stored fat, along with a little body fat, is healthy. Where all of the season-types get into trouble is when they consume so much dietary fat that their muscles cannot store any more, so they begin to store it in places such as their bellies, butts, or thighs.

Snacks

Snacks are not encouraged on the Four Seasons Diet. If you are eating properly for your season-type, you generally should not be hungry between meals. Athletes who burn a lot of calories are the exception. When starting out on the diet, you may find yourself hungry between breakfast and lunch or between lunch and dinner. The first thing to do is analyze what you ate for the previous meal. The usual reasons for being hungry between meals include:

1. Not eating enough purines if you are a Winter or an Autumn.
2. Eating too many carbs if you are a Winter or an Autumn.
3. Eating too much fat if you are a Summer or a Spring.

4. Eating too few carbohydrates if you are a Summer or a Spring.
5. Eating too many high-glycemic-index carbohydrates if you are a Winter or an Autumn.
6. Eating more than 15 grams of fructose per day, especially if you did not do the recommended two-week fructose fast before starting the diet.
7. Consuming too much vegetable oil that is high in omega-6 fats.

There are many other reasons you might be hungry between meals, but these are the most common. It's very easy for Winters to go a few meals in a row without eating enough high-purine foods, and it's also extremely easy for a Summer to consume too much fat, especially when eating out. If you find yourself hungry between meals, think about what you ate for your last meal, and take note. You may need to do some fine-tuning to see what ratios work best for you. Even though each season-type has a recommended ideal ratio of calories from protein, carbohydrates, and fat, some season-types may find that they do better going beyond these extremes. For example, a Winter may find he does best eating 50 percent fat, or a Summer may find she does best eating 15 percent protein. This may be especially true of Winters when it's cold outside and of Summers when it's hot outside. If you find that you need a snack between meals, I'll provide a few recommendations for each season-type.

The best snacks for Winters are usually fatty and salty foods, such as nuts, with lower levels of carbohydrates. The first Winter snack consists of a little peanut butter on a stalk of celery. Snacks do not have to follow the same caloric ratios as the main meals. Rather, they are designed to help get each season-type to the next meal and back on track.

Autumns do best with fatty, salty snacks that have a few carbohydrates in them as well. The first Autumn snack consists of some peanut butter on low-fat crackers. The number of crackers you eat depends on the brand and type of crackers you purchase, so I have not indicated an amount. Whatever type of cracker you purchase will have the nutritional information on the box, so just eat enough crackers to get 12 grams (48 calories) worth of carbohydrates.

Summers do best on higher-carbohydrate snacks and ideally with lower-fat snacks. The first Summer snack is a cup of nonfat yogurt with four apricots. Apricots are a great fruit for a Summer's snack because they are low in fructose for a fruit and are high in minerals such as potassium and iron, which help a Summer produce energy. If you use dried apricots or any dried fruit, make sure they do not contain any added sulfites or sulfur dioxide as preservatives. Ideally, you should soak your dried fruit in water for six to twelve hours before eating it, because it will swell up with water and become more digestible; however, this is not necessary.

Winter Snack #1			
Peanut Butter & Celery	P	C	F
2 tbsp. peanut butter	28	25	135
1 stalk celery	1	5	0
Calories	29	30	135
194	15%	15%	70%

Autumn Snack #1			
Peanut Butter & Crackers	P	C	F
2 tbsp. peanut butter	28	25	135
crackers	6	48	2
Calories	34	73	137
244	14%	30%	56%

Spring Snack #1			
Yogurt & Fruit	P	C	F
1 cup plain low-fat yogurt	41	51	26
4 apricots	8	56	4
Calories	49	107	30
186	26%	58%	16%

Summer Snack #1			
Yogurt & Fruit	P	C	F
1 cup plain nonfat yogurt	42	54	5
4 apricots	8	56	4
Calories	50	110	9
169	30%	65%	5%

The next Winter snack consists of cheese and half a pear. Cheese is a great source of fat and salt for a Winter, and pears are one of the few fruits that are advisable for a Winter to eat.

The Autumn snack is similar to the Winter snack but has a little less cheese and consists of a whole pear, instead of half a pear.The second Summer snack is a smoothie made with strawberries and nonfat milk or yogurt. Strawberries are another excellent fruit for Summers, because they are low in fructose and high in fiber. Remember that consuming too much calcium can slow down Summers and Springs. In the supplement section, I'll explain how you can use magnesium supplementation to help counter the effects of eating a high-calcium, low-magnesium meal.

The Spring smoothie is similar to the Summer smoothie, except that it uses low-fat milk, rather than the nonfat milk of the Summer smoothie.

Instead of the smoothie, both season-types could snack on Greek-style yogurt and add their own fresh fruit. The Spring would use low-fat Greek yogurt, while the Summer would use nonfat. As explained earlier, this type of yogurt is much higher in protein and has only one-third to one-half the amount of calcium of regular yogurt, making it a great lower-calcium yogurt choice compared to regular yogurt for Summers and Springs.

Winter Snack #2			
Cheese & Pear	P	C	F
1.5 oz. of cheese	45	3	121
1/2 a pear	1	49	1
Calories	46	52	122
220	21%	24%	55%

Autumn Snack #2			
Cheese & Pear	P	C	F
1 oz. of cheese	30	2	81
1 pear	2	99	2
Calories	32	101	83
216	15%	47%	38%

Spring Snack #2			
Fruit Smoothie	**P**	**C**	**F**
1/2 cup low-fat yogurt	27	33	16
1/2 cup low-fat milk	20	25	13
1 cup strawberries	3	39	4
Calories	**50**	**97**	**33**
180	28%	54%	18%

Summer Snack #2			
Fruit Smoothie	**P**	**C**	**F**
1/2 cup nonfat yogurt	30	36	2
1/2 cup nonfat milk	21	27	2
1 cup strawberries	3	39	4
Calories	**54**	**102**	**8**
164	33%	62%	5%

The final Winter snack consists of a handful of salted peanuts, which are a great snack to help a Winter make it through to the next meal. The Autumn snack consists of a little fewer peanuts, with a small amount of added raisins.

The final Summer snack consists of two almonds and 1½ ounces of raisins. Almonds tend to be the best nuts for Summers and Springs, and two almonds contain just a small amount of fat and protein. Nuts are one of those foods that should be used cautiously by Summers and Springs. They are very high in fat, and eating too many of them will often cause Summers' and Springs' energy levels to plummet and will increase their hunger. This is why the Summer snack includes only two almonds. One of the best Summer snacks is a half or a whole potato that has been cooked and then cooled in the refrigerator, then eaten cold. This snack is high in carbohydrates, high in resistant-carbohydrates, high in potassium, low in protein, and low in fat, and a half of a potato is often enough of a snack to fill up Summers and fuel them for two to three hours if they feel the need for a snack.

The Spring snack is the same as the Summer snack, except it consists of four almonds, instead of two. Even though the amount of almonds seems very paltry, I included them in this snack to illustrate a way that a Summer or a Spring could consume nuts without any ill effects; in other words, in small quantities. In reality, the Summer and the Spring snacks could just as easily be the raisins without the added nuts, because it's really the sugar that will help get them to the next meal.

Winter Snack #3			
Salted Nuts	P	C	F
25 g salted peanuts	26	20	113
Calories	26	20	113
159	16%	13%	71%

Autumn Snack #3			
Nuts & Raisins	P	c	F
15 g salted peanuts	16	12	68
1/2 oz. raisins	1	40	1
Calories	17	52	69
138	12%	38%	50%

Spring Snack #3			
Nuts & Raisins	P	C	F
4 almonds	4	3	25
1 1/2 oz. raisins	3	120	3
Calories	7	123	28
158	4%	78%	18%

Summer Snack #3			
Nuts & raisins	P	C	F
2 almonds	2	1	12
1 1/2 oz. raisins	3	120	3
Calories	5	121	15
141	4%	86%	11%

Dinner

By now, you should be getting a fairly good idea of how to prepare meals for a family composed of different season-types. For this dinner, I chose a variation of a standard American dinner, consisting of pork chops, mashed potatoes, and applesauce. I chose this dinner because it's a good illustration of some of the changes you may need to make to a meal in order to serve all four season-types. For example, in this example pork tenderloin is used, instead of pork chops. If your entire family consisted of Winters and Autumns, you could get away with pork chops; however, chops are too high in fat to work for Summers and Springs. You could use pork tenderloin or lean ham as a way to feed the same meat to all four season-types. You could also serve pork chops to the Winters and the Autumns and another meat to the Summers and the Springs. The point of this meal is to get you to understand how food choices might really work great for one or two family members, while undermining other family members.

In this case, if you choose pork tenderloin for everyone, the Winter gets the biggest portion, followed by the Autumn, the Spring, and finally the Summer. The next item on the menu is mashed potatoes. This is another dish that often has to be specially prepared for Springs and Summers. For example, adding whole milk, butter, and salt to the entire batch will simply overload Summers and Springs with both fat and salt. In this example, the potatoes are simply potatoes mixed with nonfat milk and no added salt or butter. This allows every family member to add the amount of butter and salt that's best for him or her. The serving sizes equates to about half a potato's worth of mashed potatoes for the Winter, three-fourths of a potato for the Autumn, and a full potato for the Spring and the Summer. The proportions given are in keeping with the ideal nutrient ratios for each season-type, so if you add more of one food, try to add a little of the others as well. For example, if the Summer was still hungry and ate another serving of potatoes, try to add a corresponding amount of tenderloin to the Summer's meal as well.

Each season-type gets a cup of unsweetened applesauce with his or her dinner. Always try to buy products such as applesauce without any added sugar. As you adopt a low-fructose diet, your taste buds will gradually get used to food without added sweeteners. Remember that it's the fructose in large part that is causing your food cravings. Adding a little sugar here and there will quickly put you over your daily 15 grams of fructose, which may stoke your hunger hormones and suppress your feel-full hormones. Do your entire family a favor, and strictly limit the amount of sugar you bring into the house.

The last item on the menu is the butter, which each individual can add to his or her mashed potatoes. A healthier choice for the Summers and the Springs would be to add olive oil to the potatoes, but a little butter every now and then should be alright. There is nothing wrong with adding olive oil to mashed potatoes, however. Part of changing your diet involves changing your thinking.

Winter Dinner #1			
Pork & Mashed Potatoes	P	C	F
12 oz. pork tenderloin	231	24	114
Mashed potatoes	20	139.5	2
1 tbsp. butter for potatoes	0	0	100
1 cup applesauce	0	27	0
Calories	251	190.5	216
658	38%	29%	33%

Autumn Dinner #1			
Pork & Mashed Potatoes	P	C	F
8 oz. pork tenderloin	154	16	76
Mashed potatoes	31	209	4
1/2 tbsp. butter for potatoes	0	0	50
1 cup applesauce	0	27	0
Calories	185	252	130
567	33%	44%	23%

Spring Dinner #1			
Pork & Mashed Potatoes	P	C	F
6 oz. pork tenderloin	116	12	57
Mashed potatoes	41	279	5
1 cup applesauce	0	27	0
1/2 tbsp. butter for potatoes	0	0	50
Calories	157	318	112
587	27%	54%	19%

Summer Dinner #1			
Pork & Mashed Potatoes	P	C	F
4 oz. pork tenderloin	77	8	38
Mashed potatoes	41	279	5
1 cup applesauce	0	27	0
1/4 tbsp. butter for potatoes	0	0	25
Calories	118	314	68
500	24%	63%	14%

A hundred years ago, potatoes and butter were staples in most households, while olive oil was relatively rare. We developed many of our traditional ways of serving foods based on what was available at the time. When eating for your season-type, don't be afraid to throw away convention and do what's best for you. The point of many of the sample meals is not to get you to make them the way I have described, but rather to prompt you to think about how to make meals that you and your family enjoy and that are also healthy for all of the season-types in your household.

This is another meal where part of the goal is to eliminate the conventional way you may have been doing things. In Mexico, tacos are usually made with soft corn tortillas, not the hard crunchy shells we normally eat here in America. The problem with these hard shells is that they are usually made with hydrogenated vegetable oil or vegetable oil that is high in omega-6 fats, neither of which is recommended on the Four Seasons Diet. Also, the amount of fat added to many of these products would be almost half of the fat calories a Summer would obtain from an entire meal, so adding in these types of products would mean the Summer would have to eliminate other foods that add flavor and nutrition, such as cheese. It's best to get in the habit of eliminating processed foods that contain added vegetable oil, whenever possible, and to replace them with fat-free versions that allow you to add your own fat. The beans are another example. Instead of buying refried beans with added vegetable oil, simply buy whole beans and add your own spices and a dash of olive oil or another healthy fat for flavor. You can also purchase fat-free refried beans, if you prefer.

This dinner uses lean ground beef, because it's the most versatile for all of the season-types. Cheddar cheese is added for extra flavor and fat; however, you could use Mexican Queso cheese or part-skim mozzarella, which is lower in fat and allows you to use more cheese and still keep your fat at the optimum level for your season-type. The Winter dinner relies mainly on black beans for carbohydrates, with one added tortilla. As with the other meals, the Summer dinner has the smallest serving of meat and the largest amount of tortillas and rice.

For flavor, add spices to the meat, beans, and rice. In addition, you can add fresh lettuce, tomatoes, and onions. Another good thing to have for all of the season-types is fat-free sour cream. This is a tasty condiment that can be used by all of the season types in a household, and because only small servings are normally used, it adds negligible amounts of protein and carbohydrates. This is in contrast to regular sour cream, which can add more than 20 calories of fat per tablespoon and can quickly overload a Summer and a Spring with fat calories.

Winter Dinner #2			
Mexican Style Tacos	P	C	F
8 oz. 95% lean ground beef	246	0	120
1 oz. cheddar cheese	30	2	81
1 corn tortilla	8	56	9
3/4 cup black beans	40	125	6
Fresh salsa	2	8	0
Calories	326	191	216
733	44%	26%	29%

Autumn Dinner #2			
Mexican Style Tacos	P	C	F
4 oz. 95% lean ground beef	123	0	60
1 oz. cheddar cheese	30	2	81
2 corn tortillas	16	112	18
3/4 cup black beans	40	125	6
Fresh salsa	2	8	0
Calories	211	247	165
623	34%	40%	26%

Spring Dinner #2			
Mexican Style Tacos	P	C	F
4 oz. 95% lean ground beef	123	0	60
1/2 oz. cheddar cheese	15	1	41
2 corn tortillas	16	112	18
3/4 cup black beans	40	125	6
Fresh salsa	2	8	0
1 cup brown rice	15	189	14
Calories	211	435	139
785	27%	55%	18%

Summer Dinner #2			
Mexican Style Tacos	P	C	F
2 oz. 95% lean ground beef	61.5	0	30
1/2 oz. cheddar cheese	15	1	41
3 corn tortillas	24	168	27
3/4 cup black beans	40	125	6
Fresh salsa	2	8	0
1 cup brown rice	15	189	14
Calories	158	491	118
767	21%	64%	15%

The next dinner is a basic Chinese-style stir-fry. The meat used is white-meat chicken, because it's the most versatile for all four season-types. For the vegetables, it's recommended that you get a mixture of vegetables beneficial for all of the season-types in your house, and allow everyone to pick more of the vegetables that are best for him or her. For the Winters and Autumns, this would include green beans, snow peas, or cauliflower. For Summers and Springs it would be broccoli, onions, or bell peppers. Fry all of the vegetables in a tablespoon of sesame oil for a family of four. This is an oil that is alright to use on occasion, and the amount used will provide about 27 calories of fat per person. It's recommended that you do not fry the vegetables in any sauce, but rather have the sauce on the side for everyone to add according to his or her season-type. Most Asian-style sauces are very high in sodium, which is fine for Winters and Autumns but can cause problems for Summers and Springs. Except for the vegetables, this meal is not very high in potassium, so it would be easy for Summers and Springs to overload on sodium. For example, a cup of broccoli has only around 250 mg of potassium, while a tablespoon of soy sauce can have roughly 1,000 mg of sodium. For this reason, it's best to put the teriyaki or soy sauce on the table and let people choose an amount that is best for their season-type.

After a high-sodium, lower-potassium meal such as this, it's often beneficial for Summers and Springs to have a piece of higher-potassium fruit, such as cantaloupe, apricots, or Kiwi fruit. Half a cantaloupe, for example, has nearly 800 mg of potassium, which will help rebalance Summers and Springs if they consume too much sodium. Another great source of potassium is coconut water, which contains approximately 600 mg of potassium per cup. The same one-cup serving contains approximately 10 grams of sugar, half of which consists of fructose. If you drink coconut water, be sure to add the fructose to your daily count.

All four dinners have added butter for the rice. It would be more beneficial for the Summers and the Springs to add coconut oil or olive oil to their rice, instead of butter. Coconut oil has a little flavor and can take some getting used to; however, most people find that as they begin to use coconut oil regularly, it actually enhances the flavor of their food.

The best rice to use is longer-grain rice and preferably long-grain brown rice. Long-grain rice is higher in resistant-carbohydrates than shorter-grain rice is. As with all meals containing carbohydrates such as rice, you can add some resistant-carbohydrate powder to obtain additional carbohydrates. This will be especially beneficial for Winters and Autumns.

Winter Dinner #3			
Chinese Stir-Fry	P	C	F
8 oz. chicken, light meat	222	0	24
Mixed vegetables	8	40	27
1 cup brown rice	15	189	14
1 1/2 tbsp. butter for rice	0	0	150
Calories	245	229	215
689	36%	33%	31%

Autumn Dinner #3			
Chinese Stir-Fry	P	C	F
6 oz. chicken, light meat	166	0	18
Mixed vegetables	8	40	27
1 cup brown rice	15	189	14
1 tbsp. butter for rice	0	0	100
Calories	189	229	159
577	33%	40%	28%

Spring Dinner #3			
Chinese Stir-Fry	P	C	F
5 oz. chicken, light meat	139	0	15
Mixed vegetables	8	40	27
1 1/2 cups brown rice	22	284	21
1/2 tbsp. butter for rice	0	0	50
Calories	169	324	113
606	28%	53%	19%

Summer Dinner #3			
Chinese Stir-Fry	P	C	F
3 oz. chicken, light meat	83	0	9
Mixed vegetables	8	40	27
1 1/2 cups brown rice	22	284	21
1 tsp. butter for rice	0	0	33
Calories	113	324	90
527	21%	61%	17%

You can mix a tablespoon of resistant-carbohydrate powder into your rice with some teriyaki sauce, soy sauce, or another sauce, which adds moisture and a way to get all of the benefits from consuming resistant-carbohydrates.

This next dinner is an extreme example of how challenging it can be for many common dinners to still satisfy every season-type. For this dinner, I reviewed the nutritional menu of a national pizza chain to see whether it would be possible to come close to meeting the requirements of all four season-types. While I do not advocate eating this pizza as a meal, I am using it to illustrate how you can almost always find ways to make choices for every season-type.

Pizza can be a very challenging way to feed every season-type. First, most pizza is very high in fat in relation to protein and high in fat in general. This makes it tough to feed almost every season-type. Most of the pizzas were simply too high in fat, relative to protein, to allow them to meet the ideal ratios. Often, pizzas with toppings such as Canadian bacon and pineapple can be higher-protein options; however, this would not work for Summers and Springs.

To make this meal work, I looked for two things from the nutritional menu. First, I looked for the menu item that was highest in protein, relative to fat and carbohydrates. In this case, that food item happened to be baked chicken wings. The next thing I looked for was the food item on the menu that had the lowest percentage of fat. In this case, the pizza chain has a lower-fat pizza option, and I chose the chicken, onion, and pepper pizza. This pizza has about 23 percent of its calories as fat, which is actually lower than the percentage of fat for non-pizza items, such as breadsticks and pasta. The breadsticks were 32 percent fat, and the best pasta option was 40 percent fat.

By ordering these two items, it's possible to feed a family of all four season-types and get very close to meeting the ideal percentage of macronutrients. First, Winters get two slices of pizza and three baked wings to keep their protein high and carbohydrates low. Next, Autumns get three slices of pizza and one and a half baked wings.

The Summer and the Spring each get three slices of pizza, which puts them close to the right ratios of nutrients. The problem for these two season-types is that three slices of pizza contain more than 1,500 mg of sodium, which will cause both season-types problems unless they add some potassium to their meal. One trick these season-types can use when they know they are going out to a restaurant such as this is to bring a can of coconut water or some dried apricots with them. It will add extra carbohydrates to the meal, along with a lot of potassium. Ideally, Summers and Springs want at least four times as much potassium as sodium in a meal.

Winter Dinner #4			
Pizza	P	C	F
2 slices chicken, onion, pepper	88	182	79
3 baked wings	120	12	180
Calories	208	194	259
661	31%	29%	39%

Autumn Dinner #4			
Pizza	P	C	F
3 slices chicken, onion, pepper	132	276	120
1 1/2 baked wings	60	6	90
Calories	192	282	210
684	28%	41%	31%

Spring Dinner #4			
Pizza	P	C	F
3 slices chicken, onion, pepper	132	276	120
Calories	132	276	120
528	25%	52%	23%

Summer Dinner #4			
Pizza	P	C	F
3 slices chicken, onion, pepper	132	276	120
17.5 oz. coconut water	0	76	0
Calories	132	352	120
604	22%	58%	20%

By adding the coconut water, they get less than half as much potassium as they get sodium; however, this is far better than the alternative of getting almost no potassium. If you feel uncomfortable bringing coconut water into the restaurant with you, drink it either before you go in or after you leave. Similarly, Summers and Springs could eat a piece of high-potassium fruit, either before or after dinner, to help balance them out.

Although this meal is less than ideal for many reasons, I am giving you the best-case scenario from a metabolic standpoint, if you choose to eat pizza out. Eating the same meal at home gives you more options. You could order a different pizza with more fat, and then the Summers and the Springs could eat one piece of pizza and either some pasta or bread or something else lower in fat and higher in carbohydrates. If that pizza was still low in protein compared to fat, the Winters and the Autumns could eat some extra lean protein. The two most important considerations in a meal like this is for Winters to make sure they do not overload on carbohydrates, and for Summers to make sure they do not overload on fat. Those two season-types will have the hardest time, metabolically speaking, if they do not make an extra effort in planning a meal like this.

Of course, the other option is for everyone to eat the pizza and not worry about it. One of the many great things about the Four Seasons Diet is that if you are strict for most meals, you will be able to cheat occasionally, without feeling as bad as you would if you were not on the diet. Remember that most Summers have high levels of blood fat from following a traditional Western diet, especially if they have belly fat and insulin resistance. If you recall from an earlier chapter, belly fat is continually releasing fat into the bloodstream and overloading the Summer's metabolism. Once Summers have been on the Four Seasons Diet for a while, they will usually lose the excess belly fat, will no longer be insulin resistant, and will have a blood pH that is much more closer to ideal. The effect from eating one high-fat meal in this state is far different from what the effect would have been before they started the diet. They may feel a little tired or hungry but nothing like before. The danger at this point would be to go back to eating a high-fat meal for the next several meals, because the salty pizza probably tasted pretty darn good to someone on a lower-fat, lower-salt diet. If Summers were to eat like this for a few days, they would likely find their old problems starting to return.

Winters may have a similar experience. The high level of carbohydrates in the pizza may not affect them as these carbs would have before. Winters may actually feel pretty darn good and energized after splurging on a high-carbohydrate meal such as this. I wish I had the answer to how often you can deviate from your diet and splurge, but, ultimately, the real problems are the hormones and the addictions that your body has to deal with that will undermine you. People who are reading this and are over forty can probably attest to times in their lives when they suddenly realized they had put on an extra ten or twenty pounds during the course of a few months. When this happened, it usually meant they had fallen back into a state of imbalance that would take weeks or months to fix.

As a general rule, it's almost universally acceptable for everyone to splurge on one meal a week and eat whatever he or she wants. The biggest hurdle will be fighting the cravings the next day for more of what you had the night before. If you splurge for one meal, acknowledge it, take ownership of it, and take control of it. Pledge to be strict for the next few days, and you can be almost certain you will not feel any ill effects from one weekly splurge. Also, make a mental note of how hard it is to be strict during the next few days after a splurge. If you find that it's easy, enjoy your weekly splurge as a reward for sticking to your diet the rest of the week. If you find it hard or, worse, you splurge in the next day or two, maybe it's time to reconsider whether you're someone who can handle a weekly splurge.

If you do splurge, it helps to be extra diligent about whatever you splurged on, in relation to your season-type. For example, Winters usually find that carbohydrates are their downfall, so if you splurge on pasta or bread for a meal, try to keep your carbohydrates as close as possible to your recommended 25 to 35 percent the next day. For Summers, if you splurge on a high-fat meal such as pizza, try to keep your fat intake as close as possible to the recommended 10 to 15 percent the next day. For all season-types, if you splurge on sugar, fruit, or other high-fructose foods, it's advised to either eliminate all sugar and fruit the next day or cut back to 7 to 8 grams of fructose, rather than the regular 15 grams. Fructose is one of the easiest things to find yourself addicted to. Remember that it doesn't take long for excess fructose consumption to increase your hunger hormones, suppress your feel-full hormones, and increase your brain's pleasure from eating food. If you want to control your food cravings, the easiest single thing you can do is to control your fructose consumption. Restrict yourself to no more than 15 grams a day, and if you splurge on fructose, either eliminate fructose the next day or reduce your consumption to 7 to 8 grams.

The final dinner is a simple roast beef sandwich. Lean roast beef is a very versatile meat because it's fairly low in fat and can usually be eaten by all four season-types in a meal. It's also a great deli meat to keep on hand for the Winters and the Autumns in the house as a snack or an extra way to add a little fairly lean protein to any meal that might otherwise be too low in protein for them. If you are going to make deli meat a regular part of your diet, keep in mind that many of them contain ingredients you should avoid, such as nitrites and MSG. It's well worth the extra money to purchase deli meats that contain no added artificial ingredients, nitrates or nitrites, MSG, or preservatives and are from animals raised without the use of antibiotics or hormones.

The Winter gets one sandwich with a large serving of roast beef and cheese. All of the season-types can feel free to add whatever vegetables they want to their sandwiches, such as lettuce, tomato, and onions. Mayonnaise is generally not recommended, because it usually contains large amounts of vegetable oils high in omega-6 fats. Some brands advertise that they use olive oil, but most of them use a blend of olive oil and other vegetable oils that are high in omega-6 fats, which are not recommended. Your best option is to buy a reduced-fat mayonnaise, if you feel you need the added flavor.

The Autumn gets one and a half sandwiches with less overall meat and cheese than the Winter's one sandwich. The Summer and the Spring get one and a half sandwiches with even less meat than the Autumn's. They also get a cup of fat-free minestrone soup, and the Summer gets a piece of fruit for dessert. The Summer and the Spring sandwiches should contain lots of veggies, especially tomatoes and onions, which are especially good for these two season-types.

This meal illustrates the stark differences between the four season-types. Winters get a big serving of meat and cheese with their sandwich, while Summers get three pieces of bread with lots of veggies and a little meat in between, and the Autumn and the Spring fall somewhere between the two.

Winter Dinner #5			
Roast Beef Sandwich	P	C	F
6 oz. roast beef	168	0	54
2 oz. part-skim mozzarella	58	6	78
2 pieces of bread	48	176	24
Calories	274	182	156
612	45%	30%	25%

Autumn Dinner #5			
Roast Beef Sandwich	P	C	F
3 oz. roast beef	84	0	27
2 oz. part-skim mozzarella	58	6	78
3 pieces of bread	72	264	38
Calories	214	270	143
627	34%	43%	23%

Spring Dinner #5			
Roast Beef Sandwich	P	C	F
2 oz. roast beef	56	0	18
1 oz. part-skim mozzarella	29	3	39
3 pieces of bread	72	264	38
1 cup low-fat minestrone soup	12	68	13
Calories	169	335	108
612	28%	55%	18%

Summer Dinner #5			
Roast Beef Sandwich	P	C	F
2 oz. roast beef	56	0	18
3 pieces of bread	72	264	38
1 cup low-fat minestrone soup	12	68	13
Fruit for dessert	4	98	3
Calories	144	430	72
646	22%	67%	11%

Putting It All Together

Hopefully, these sample meals have given you a good understanding of how to prepare meals for your season-type, as well as for the season-types of all members of your household. Oftentimes, it helps to keep a few "power" foods on hand for your two extreme season-types, the Winters and the Summers. This is because they are the ones who may have the hardest time creating meals that fall within their dietary ratios. For Winters, power foods would be higher in protein and purines, with only a moderate amount of fat, such as lean roast beef or lean ham from the deli. For Summers, power foods would be high in carbohydrates and lower in fat, such as cooked and refrigerated potatoes, fruit, coconut water, apricots, or low-fat pita bread.

If a meal is a little low in protein, it's relatively easy for Winters to grab a few slices of roast beef or ham out of the refrigerator to help balance their meals. Likewise, if a meal is lower in carbohydrates and higher in fat, a Summer can always grab a piece of pita bread or a cold potato. Cold potatoes can be especially versatile for Summers because they go with just about any dish, are low in fat, have a fairly low glycemic index when eaten cold, are low in sodium, and have around 1,600 mg of potassium per potato. This amount of potassium is good at countering the effects of a high-sodium meal for Summers. For example, if you are eating an Asian stir-fry that is high in sodium, in addition to your rice add a pre-cooked potato from the refrigerator or half of a potato cut into cubes or slices. You can add it cold on top of your stir-fry or eat it as a side dish.

Dried apricots are also a great way to add potassium to meal that is too high in sodium for a Summer. Apricots are relatively low in fructose and high in potassium for a fruit. A dessert of four to five apricots after a meal that's high in sodium is a great way for Summers to get their sweet tooth fix, along with enough potassium to balance out their season-type.

First, Count Calories and Do the Math—Then Improvise

Although it's a good idea to count your calories and figure out your ratios for the first few weeks, try not to become too obsessed with it in the long term. The whole point of tracking your ratio of protein, carbohydrates, and fat is to get you accustomed to what a proper meal looks like and, more important, feels like. If you count your calories for a few weeks and keep a mental note of the reaction you have to each meal, it will eventually become second-nature to create meals that work for you, without having to count calories.

Let's take the last sandwich dinner as an example. Winters have probably eaten way too many carbohydrates for most of their lives, while Summers have probably consumed way too much fat during their entire lives. By counting out your meat, bread, and cheese, you'll quickly learn what works for you, and soon you'll be able to make a sandwich without having to think about it. Winters may be surprised at first to see how much meat and cheese their sandwich contains and how little bread they get. Similarly, Summers may be shocked to learn that their sandwich is basically bread and vegetables, with just the tiniest amount of meat and cheese. Once all of the season-types learn approximately how much meat, cheese, and bread to use when making a sandwich, they can stop using the scale to measure ounces of food and can quit keeping precise track of calories. Following are a few simple guidelines that each season-type will generally find work best for him or her.

Winters need to focus on getting a high-quality source of protein, along with purines, for most meals. Later in this chapter, you'll learn how to eliminate meat if you choose, but for now I'll talk as if you are a meat eater, because more than 90 percent of Winters whom I meet are very meat-centric people. Winters can handle the largest amount of protein and fat, but their problem is that they usually eat too much fat and not enough protein. As a Winter, when you begin to make your meals, remember that 40 percent of your calories should come from protein and 30 percent from fat, with an emphasis on higher-purine proteins and long-chain saturated fats. When making your meals, start with the meat. Choose either a lean meat or a fattier meat. If you pick a lean meat, you'll be able to include other fatty foods, such as cheese, butter, olive oil, and similar items. If you pick a fatty meat, you will often end up getting more fat calories than protein calories and may have to restrict any further fat consumption. In this case, the rest of your meal should be mainly carbohydrates and protein. Vegetables should always make up a good portion of your carbohydrates, because they have a low glycemic index and are usually high in fiber, which is often lacking in the Winter's diet. Resistant-carbohydrate powder can be your best friend at every meal, because it will help you control your carbohydrate cravings, both during and between meals.

Meal Tips for Winters

As a Winter, any time you want to lose weight, simply lower your carbohydrate consumption a little bit, and limit your fructose and omega-6 fats. You'll most likely find that your appetite goes away, and dieting is relatively easy. If you find that you need to gain a little weight, simply increase your carbohydrate consumption, but do not eat more fructose or omega-6 fats, because this could cause your appetite and your weight to get out of control. When preparing your meal, always think first in terms of your protein source and how much fat is in that protein source. Then figure out how much extra fat you can consume, if any, and finally add in your carbohydrates. Going back to our sandwich example, a leaner meat, such as white-meat turkey or lean roast beef, allows you to add in some cheese or another fat. A fatty meat such as bologna can calorically be more than 75 percent fat and only 25 percent protein. If you have a bologna sandwich, you know that your meal will be too heavy in fat and too light in protein, so limit your consumption of any other fats. If you can find a way get some extra lean protein, great. If not, simply take note of your well-being during the next four hours. You may experience a little hunger or a drop in energy and feel the need for a snack. In this case, grab a little lean protein, such as a few pieces of turkey breast out of the refrigerator, and this should help get you through the next meal. This is one of the many advantages of keeping lean protein on hand at all times for your season-type. If you have a sandwich made up of a moderately fat protein, such as pastrami, which is about 30 percent fat and 70 percent protein, you can add just a little more fat, along with some carbohydrates.

The deli counter at the supermarket may be the Winter's best friend when he or she begins the Four Seasons Diet, because most of them have nutritional information on their meats. Try to stock up on the lowest-fat meats you can find, such as low-fat ham, low-fat turkey, and low-fat roast beef. As mentioned earlier, it's well worth the extra money to purchase deli meats that contain no added artificial ingredients, nitrates or nitrites, MSG, or preservatives and are from animals raised without the use of antibiotics or hormones. You can use these low-fat deli meats to add extra lean protein to a meal, because this will be your biggest challenge when creating your meals. Any time you find that your meal is a little low on protein, simply take out some of the lean deli meat to get your meal into balance. These meats can be especially helpful for breakfast, which can be your most challenging meal. Being able to eat a few eggs sunny-side up, with some lean deli ham and a few pieces of toast, will make your world far more simple and enjoyable. Another easy breakfast is half of a potato fried in butter with lean ham. Also, purchase a digital scale to measure your food during your first few weeks on the Four Seasons Diet. When you begin to feel comfortable with the proper portions to use for your meals, you can usually eliminate the scale. At this point, you should begin to focus on how you feel during the four hours after you eat a meal. If you learn to know instinctively how much meat, butter, or bread to use in your meals, life will become easier and more enjoyable for you.

During their meals, Winters also need to watch their intake of sodium vs. potassium and calcium vs. magnesium. Make sure to get plenty of calcium, and any time you eat high-potassium foods, such as potatoes, beans, and fruit, be sure that you consume adequate amounts of salt. Half of a potato has roughly 800 mg of potassium and a cup of black beans has around 600 mg of potassium. When eating these foods in your carbohydrate dish, be extra certain you get enough salt with your meal.

As mentioned earlier, Winters who engage in extremely intense endurance events, such as marathon training, will often need to increase their carbohydrate consumption. The determining factor is your intensity level, which is measured by your pace. Any Winter running five- or six-minute miles will have to increase his or her carbohydrate consumption, while those doing ten- or twelve-minute miles are probably fine on the standard Winter diet. In between those two paces, you'll have to do some experimenting to see what works best for you. You may find that you need to increase your carbohydrates on training days and go back to your standard Winter diet on nontraining days. Remember that fat-burning muscles can burn either fat or sugar for energy. Although they normally prefer to burn fat, if the intensity level gets high, they will begin to burn sugar. Conversely, if you want to lose weight, don't do intense cardiovascular exercise; all that you'll do is burn your stored sugar. Keep the pace moderate and steady, and you'll be sure to burn stored fat for energy.

Meal Tips for Autumns

Autumns are in many ways the most fortunate of all of the season-types. They can eat most of the high-fat and high-protein foods so typically found in the Western diet; however, their well-being is not as dependent on consuming adequate amounts of protein as a Winter's is. Furthermore, they can eat a fair amount of carbohydrates without suffering too many ill effects. Much of what I explained regarding Winters also applies, to some extent, to Autumns. The main issue that Autumns usually have is eating too much fat. Even though it's recommended that they try to keep their fat consumption between 20 and 30 percent of their daily calories, it's very easy to go over this limit, if they're not careful. This is especially true, given that the Autumn diet is higher in protein, and many high-protein foods are often higher in fat. One great piece of advice I gave to Winters also holds true for Autumns. Keeping a ready supply of low-fat deli meat on hand in the refrigerator can really help when you start the Four Seasons Diet. Once you have a reliable source of lean protein, should your meal require a little extra, you can focus your attention on where your fat and carbohydrates will come from. I do not advocate eating deli meats for every meal. Rather, I am saying that if you have already reached your fat limit for any meal but not your protein limit, go ahead and grab a few pieces of lean meat to help keep yourself in balance. Carbohydrate levels are usually much easier to control, because many foods that are high in carbohydrates also tend to be low in fat.

The main thing Autumns need to be aware of is that because they are so close to being balanced much of the time, they might have to change their diet the most as the temperature outside changes. Winters usually have blood that is slightly too acidic, while Summers usually have blood that is slightly too alkaline. Winters usually eat foods that alkalize the blood, such as proteins with purines; they will simply eat less of them when it's hot outside. Autumns usually have blood that maintains the proper pH pretty well, so weather can really affect them almost as much as their diet does. Autumns need to eat more carbohydrates and less protein and fat when it's hot outside. They will also need to eat more protein and fat and fewer carbohydrates when the weather is cold.

Meal Tips for Summers

Of all of the season-types, Summers may initially have the most difficult time creating balanced meals; however, they are often the ones who benefit the most rapidly by adopting the Four Seasons Diet. Most Summers have suffered their entire lives because of eating food that was too high in protein and way too high in fat, which has caused them to have extremely low energy levels. As they get older, most Summers begin to suffer from insulin resistance, which further depletes their energy. When planning a meal, the key for Summers is to find creative ways to make low-fat and low-sodium food somewhat appetizing. The bigger challenge is often eating out in a restaurant, because most restaurant food is high in fat and sodium. When you plan a meal, think of what many people traditionally call "peasant food," because this is often the ideal type of meal for you. For example, in Italy, Sicilian food is considered "peasant food": generous portions of pasta, tomato sauce, and fresh vegetables, and the meals are lower in fat. In contrast, it's the "rich" foods of Northern Italy, high in butter and cream, that often undermine you. Similarly, the "peasant foods" of Latin American countries, such as Mexico, are often ideal choices for Summers. Americanized Mexican food has a lot of cheese, fat, and grease. Real Mexican food, however, features rice, beans, fresh salsas, and fresh vegetables and is lighter on the meat and the cheese. Typically, if cheese is used, it's small amounts of white "queso" cheese for flavor, not mountains of cheese as you would find in American-style Mexican food. Also, most traditional Mexican dishes use lean white fish caught fresh from the ocean. The same can be said of the traditional peasant foods from many other countries.

As a Summer, you can find loads of inspiration from the simple dishes of many nationalities. For example, a Mediterranean-style meal of hummus and pita bread, a Thai-style vegetable dish, Mexican rice with beans and salsa, Indian-style garbanzo beans and potatoes in a spicy sauce, Ethiopian-style bean and vegetable dishes served with their famous injera bread, and many other ethnic dishes are all good choices for Summers. What makes most of these "peasant foods" so ideal for you is that, traditionally, most of these cultures were farmers who did not raise livestock or eat a lot of meat. In countries such as the United States, where grazing land was plentiful, farmers often consumed large amounts of meat and dairy foods. In many countries, however, such as Mexico, the climate and the soil are often more suited to farming, and raising huge herds of cattle is not that easy. These farmers developed a cuisine that focuses on spices and other creative lower-fat ways to create flavorful food. Ethnic restaurants are often your best choices when eating out, as long as you make sure you do not get too much vegetable oil in your meal. Sadly, most American ethnic restaurants have switched from traditional oils, such as olive oil and coconut oil, to cheaper vegetable oils that are high in omega-6 fats. If you live anywhere close to a major college university,

"university districts" are often full of mom-and-pop ethnic-style restaurants, and because they have to cater to college students on a limited budget, they often serve more traditional-style dishes that are lower in meat and cheese. A Mongolian grill is also a great choice for Summers because you get to choose the vegetables you want, with lots of rice, while going lighter on the meat and the fat.

When you make meals at home, the fat in your meal is by far the most important consideration. Summers need so little fat that they have to find ways to use fat to add flavor to their food without going overboard. Luckily, many low-fat cookbooks are out there, so if you need help with menu ideas, purchase one with recipes that appeal to you, or go online to look for creative ideas. For a Summer, it's often easiest to start with your carbohydrate dish, because that's where most of your calories will come from. When choosing proteins, try to go as lean as possible; otherwise, you'll find that all of your fat calories are in your protein dish, leaving you no fat for the rest of your meal. For your meat dish, white fish is often your best choice, because this is lowest in purines and fat. Other good choices are light turkey and chicken, although these are higher in purines and fat. I do not recommended soy protein, and I'll explain the reasons in Chapter 8; however, one great way for Summers to get protein is by using egg whites. Egg whites can be cooked and seasoned in a way that goes with just about every dish you can come up with. Either fry them in low-fat cooking spray, or hard-boil a dozen and keep them in the refrigerator for when you need them. Simply throw away the yolks, or, if you fry them, rather than throwing out the runny yolks, you can add a few to your dog's food. Do not feed cooked yolks to your pets, however, because once the yolk is cooked, it is not recommended for people or animals. You can fry up the egg whites with some Mexican seasonings and use them in traditional-style tacos with soft corn tortillas, rice, beans, and salsa. You can add them to Asian stir-fry dishes. You can add the hard-boiled whites to potatoes with a little fat-free dressing and some healthy extra-virgin olive oil to make an easy potato salad. In virtually any dish that traditionally contains meat, you can substitute egg whites. They are an extremely high-quality, fat-free protein that has higher biological value than even meat. Do not feel guilty if you end up throwing away the yolks, because getting your protein from egg whites is cheaper than getting it from meat, and getting eggs from chickens is more sustainable and environmentally friendly than raising animals for meat.

Once you have your protein and carbohydrate sources

figured out, it's best to see how much fat you have left after subtracting the fat from the protein and carbohydrate dishes. Many carbohydrates, such as grains, contain a fair amount of fat, so be sure to factor this in. For example, let's say you are making Mexican-style tacos using egg whites for your protein. Factor in the fat from any corn tortillas or rice. Then figure out how much fat you have left to use and decide how you are going to add flavor to your meal. For many Summer dishes, this one included, adding fresh tomatoes and onions with a little salt and olive oil is a great way to create flavor and texture. Also, lower-fat cheeses, such as part-skim mozzarella or Mexican-style white cheeses that are served in small crumbles, are great ways to add flavor with only a little fat.

If you are looking to lose weight, completely eliminate all sources of long-chain saturated fats, such as those found in most fatty meats and fatty dairy products. Saturated fats tend to get stored by Summers and are not burned for energy the same way they are for other season-types. You'll be amazed at how quickly you lose weight once you limit your fat to 15 percent of your daily calories, and restrict your consumption of fats and oils to healthy ones, such as olive oil and coconut oil. Any time you want to gain weight, simply add in more long-chain saturated fats, such as cheese and fatty meats. If you are happy with your weight, you can eat some of these fats as long as you don't go overboard. They will have a tendency to increase the hunger of Summers if too much is consumed. As a general rule, if Summers have excess belly fat, they need to keep their consumption of these fats down to a minimum in order to lose that fat. Summers who want to lose their belly fat could cut their fat intake down to 10 percent or even lower for a short while, as a way to quickly eliminate the harmful belly fat.

In addition, Summers should also watch their sodium vs. potassium and calcium vs. magnesium consumption. Try to keep sodium and calcium consumption at moderate levels, and make sure to get plenty of potassium and magnesium. Nonfat dairy is a great way for Summers to get fat-free, purine-free protein; however, too much can often cause a Summer to get out of balance, due to the high levels of calcium. One trick for Summers is to eat Greek-style yogurt, rather than regular yogurt and milk. Greek yogurt has nearly twice the protein of regular yogurt and dairy products and only one-half to one-third the level of calcium. This type of yogurt is a great way to get high-quality, nonfat concentrated protein without overloading on too much calcium. For every meal, Summers should also make sure they get plenty of potassium relative to sodium. Foods such as potatoes, beans, fruit, and many vegetables are high in potassium. Concentrated sources of sodium, such as soy sauce, teriyaki sauce, soups, cured meats, cheese, snack foods, and pickled foods, can cause a lot of problems for Summers. Whenever you eat any of these high-sodium foods, make sure you offset them with enough foods that are high in potassium. Also, do your best to find low-sodium alternatives, or cut down on your consumption of regular items high in sodium. For example, one tablespoon of soy sauce can have nearly 1,000 mg of sodium. Look for lower-sodium ways to add flavor to your Asian dishes, or get accustomed to adding less soy sauce to your rice and stir-fry dishes.

Meal Tips for Springs

Springs are similar to Summers in their requirements but have a much easier time keeping themselves in balance. Much of what applies to Summers also applies to Springs. Springs can have a little more fat and protein than Summers, however, and are not as prone to suffering the ill effects caused by consuming an excess of either. The main thing Springs need to focus on is not getting too much fat in their diet. They are not quite as sensitive as Summers, however, when it comes to eating too much fat. Summers may quickly find themselves out of balance from one or two high-fat meals, whereas it might take several meals containing excess fat for a Spring to begin to feel the adverse effects.

Advice for All Season-Types

Some advice applies to all season-types. All season-types should consume more long-chain saturated fats and purines when it's cold outside than they do when the weather is hot. Chart 7.98 will help you get a better idea of how to put this into practice for your season-type.

CHART 6.98 PURINE AND LONG-CHAIN SATURATED FAT CONSUMPTION

	Cold Outside	Moderate Outside	Hot Outside
Winter	Very High	High	Moderate
Autumn	High-Moderate	Moderate	Moderate-Low
Spring	Moderate	Moderate-Low	Low
Summer	Moderate	Low	Very Low

All season-types should limit their consumption of fructose

to no more than 15 grams a day. I know I have been repeating this over and over; however, that is because I know this will be the hardest rule for many people to follow. If you want to lessen your hunger hormones and increase your feel-full hormones, you have to control your fructose consumption. Once your body actually knows it's full and not hungry, weight loss becomes nearly effortless. Many people are surprised by how much their appetite disappears by following this one simple rule. It's as though your body has been trying to send you the signal for years that it wasn't hungry, only the fructose was interfering with your hormonal messages. Don't be surprised if you suddenly find that you're eating only half of your normal amount of food for a while after your first fructose fast. When our bodies are getting the proper hormonal messages, they know exactly what our ideal weight is and will send the message to us very clearly. You may find that you go through a long period of not being hungry, while you effortlessly lose weight. When you are in this state, you are burning a lot of fat for energy. Summers and Springs usually experience decreased energy levels as they approach their ideal weight. Once they reach their ideal weight, insulin sensitivity is usually restored, along with their appetite. If they focus on eating the right amount of carbohydrates and limiting their fructose, they will often experience more energy than they have in years, as long as they remember to limit their fructose consumption to no more than 15 grams a day.

All season-types also need to limit their consumption of processed vegetable oils that are high in omega-6 fats. This will eliminate a lot of the processed foods you may currently be eating. If you purchase processed or canned foods, look for the fat-free versions and add your own healthy fats, according to what's best for your season-type. For example, if purchasing pasta sauce, buy a fat-free kind and let every family member add his or her own extra-virgin olive oil, based on each person's season-type. Limit your fat consumption to the ones listed on the diet charts with two asterisks next to them, as much as possible. Any time you have the urge to eat foods that are high in processed vegetable oils, remember the cows that got fat when fed vegetable oil and the ones that got lean when fed coconut oil. Or think about all of the studies linking omega-6 fats to breast cancer, as well as other cancers. Our need for omega-6 fats is very low, and most people will get plenty by eating the fats and oils recommended in the Four Seasons Diet. It's the omega-3 fats that are usually a little lacking in our diet, so be sure to add flaxseed oil or cod liver oil to your daily diet.

After Every Meal, Assess How You Feel

All season-types need to pay attention to how their food is making them feel. Once you limit your consumption of foods that contain fructose and get your body's hormonal messages working properly, you will become much more in tune with your body. I have explained how Winters and Autumns need more calcium and sodium, while Summers and Springs need more magnesium and potassium. Yet it's important not to take this to an extreme. Balance is the key when it comes to calcium/magnesium and sodium/potassium, and each season-type has a slightly different balance that makes him or her function optimally. Summers who eliminate all sodium from their diet, for example, may feel better for a week or two as they get back into balance, but then they can quickly get out of balance the other way and have too little sodium. This type of trap can be easy to fall into. For example, Winters might cut back on potassium and feel great for a few weeks or a month and think they have it all figured out. If they have cut back too far, however, they will get out of balance the other way.

Remember, after every meal, to make a mental note of what you ate and how you feel until the next meal. You should have steady energy, mental clarity, and a positive mood (assuming nothing negative is going on in your life) and should not experience hunger to any great degree.

If you feel bad after a meal, it can usually be traced back to something that is affecting your season-type. Go though the following checklist of seven items, which account for most problems you may experience:

1. Have you been following the 15 grams of fructose rule? If the answer is no, go back on a mini-fast for a few days or do a full two-week fast, if necessary. There is no reason to try to analyze anything else if you are not following this rule, because overconsumption of fructose will throw every season-type out of balance. This is the most important rule of the Four Seasons Diet. Remember that fructose changes your brain chemistry, so that it becomes like the brain of a drug addict. If you find it hard to quit consuming fructose, keep in mind that your brain is similar to the brain of a cocaine or heroin addict, and acknowledge the difficulty with quitting fructose as the serious addiction it is.
2. Have you been limiting your consumption of processed

vegetable oils, such as corn oil, canola oil, safflower oil, and soybean oil?

3. Are you getting the proper amount of purines for your season-type—that is, a Winter might not be getting enough or a Summer might be getting too many?
4. Are you getting the right level of protein, carbohydrates, and fat for your season-type in relation to the temperature outside? Also, are you getting the proper amount of long-chain saturated fats for your season-type?
5. Are you maintaining the proper ratio of calcium and magnesium for your season-type?
6. Are you maintaining the proper level of sodium and potassium for your season type?
7. Are you sticking to three meals a day or snacking only when it's absolutely necessary?

Don't Backslide into Old Habits

The other trap that is easy to fall into is going back to your old way of doing things. Once you balance your hormones, weight, and energy levels, it's easy to forget how bad you used to feel. Any season-type can fall off the Four Seasons Diet when this happens. Winters may feel so good after following the diet for a while that excess carbohydrates do not affect them at first, the way they used to. Rest assured, however, a few days of bingeing on carbs may be all it takes to throw a Winter out of balance again. A similar thing can happen to Summers with regard to eating too much fat, especially cheese. Summers who are in balance may be able to handle their first cheese pizza dinner, and because it does not make them feel bad, they soon start to work more fat into their diet. In both cases, once these season-types are in balance, it's the longer-term metabolic effects of eating the wrong foods that does the most damage. For example, unrestrained cheese consumption can quickly result in excess belly fat and insulin resistance for many Summers. Once this happens, you won't be able to go back to your Summer diet and instantly feel good again. You may find that you have to go through the same long process of getting back into balance that you did when you first started the diet.

Once you know the basic rules for your season-type, stick to them with only minor adjustments. If you're a Summer, and you binge on cheese pizza, go back to the strict Summer diet for at least a few days, or, better yet, consume less fat than normal the next day, to help your body burn off the excess fat from the pizza meal.

Once you know your season-type, unless you are changing your workout routine and burning different fuels for energy, the diet for your season-type will likely be the diet you will follow for the rest of your life, if you want to maintain your health. It can be frustrating for a Winter to give up all of those carbs and for a Summer to give up all of that cheese, but at least you now have the knowledge to choose your path in life. It's likely that many of you will have great success eating for your season-type and then will find that you gradually stop adhering to your diet plan. If this happens, and you wake up one day overweight or feeling horrible again, just start over, go on another two-week fructose fast, and be assured that within a month, you can get yourself back into balance. You may find that this happens several times; however, eventually you will get accustomed to your diet and hopefully will grow tired of feeling bad and gaining weight, over and over again.

Being a Vegetarian for Your Season-Type

Summers often thrive on a vegetarian diet, and Springs have a relatively easy time adopting a vegetarian lifestyle. It is a little more challenging for Autumns and especially for Winters to become vegetarians; however, I believe it is possible for Winters to do well on a vegetarian diet. It simply takes a little more work for Winters than for the other season-types. In a later section, you'll learn about the many benefits of an all-natural vegetarian diet, and you'll read about studies that show it adds about ten years to your life.

If you are a Winter or an Autumn and are not yet a vegetarian, I recommend that you get the Four Seasons Diet working for you first by following a traditional diet, before you attempt to become a vegetarian, so that you can see how you are supposed to feel when you get your correct ratio of protein, carbohydrates, and fat. Once you have the diet working for you, you can begin to make some of the changes I will recommend.

If you are a Winter or an Autumn who is already a vegetarian, there is a good chance you have struggled a bit with getting the vegetarian diet to work for you. Following is some advice for these two season-types in regard to adopting a vegetarian lifestyle.

First, limit your consumption of medium- and high-glycemic starches and grains, especially those that have been processed, such as white flour and white rice. Your best sources for carbohydrates include lower-glycemic ones, such as beans, lentils, nonstarchy vegetables, and resistant-carbohydrates. By limiting your carbohydrates to those that have a low glycemic index, you will be able to consume a higher percentage of carbohydrates and a lower percentage of protein than if you ate medium- or high-glycemic carbohydrates. Beans and lentils are very high in purines and are a great way for Winters and Autumns to get purines when they do not eat meat. The best vegetarian source of purines is brewer's yeast, which can be purchased at most health food stores. It is high in purines, and just one teaspoon of brewer's yeast has as many purines as a pound of beef or half a pound of salmon. It is not the best-tasting supplement in the world and is usually mixed with a little water and swallowed, or else purchased in tablet form, if you want to avoid the terrible taste. If you purchase it in tablet form, 1,000 mg of brewer's yeast is all you need to get the purine equivalent of eating a pound of beef.

For any Winter or Autumn who wants to be a vegetarian, brewer's yeast tablets should be an essential part of your diet, unless you are eating plenty of beans and other high-purine foods. For any meal that does not include a high-purine food such as beans, simply consume 500 to 1,000 mg of brewer's yeast, depending on the weather outside. Remember, you need more purines when it's cold outside and fewer when it's hot.

By making sure to add plenty of high-purine vegetarian foods to their meals, or brewer's yeast tablets, if necessary, Winters and Autumns can easily meet their purine needs without having to eat meat. The next challenge for them is finding a way to get enough vegetarian protein. Winters and Autumns will probably find that they need less protein if they follow a vegetarian diet than if they are eating meat. This is because research shows that when meat is cooked, the proteins coagulate, and up to 50 percent of the proteins may be hard to digest or even indigestible. Simply heating meat to 110 degrees Fahrenheit has been shown to destroy the amino acids tryptophan and lysine, while cooking meat above 117 degrees for longer than three minutes causes more serious changes to occur. This includes the coagulation of proteins, the denaturing of some proteins, and the creation of cancer-causing compounds, such as heterocyclic amines, polycyclic aromatic hydrocarbons, and n-nitroso compounds.

Dairy foods can be an excellent source of high-quality protein for Winters and Autumns, and earlier I mentioned Greek-style yogurt, which has twice as much protein as regular yogurt and is relatively low in carbohydrates, if you stick to the unsweetened versions. Another excellent way to get extra protein is with a whey or casein power protein supplement. Whey and casein are excellent sources of protein for Winters and Autumns because they are high in calcium, and these two season-types need to keep their calcium levels higher than the other two season-types do. Whey and casein are low in purines, however, so if you consume whey or casein for your protein, just make sure to eat another high-purine food or take a brewer's yeast tablet. When you purchase whey or casein protein, make sure it doesn't contain any added sugar or sucralose. Sucralose is an artificial sweetener that is often contained in protein powders, and later on you'll learn why it's best to avoid this additive.

Other vegetarian sources of protein that are high in purines include spirulina (also known as blue-green algae) and bee pollen. In fact, spirulina is a superior source of protein that contains all of the essential protein building blocks and is up to 70 percent protein. Beef, by contrast, is only about 22 percent protein and, as you will learn later, is often loaded with toxic chemicals, creates potentially cancer-causing compounds when cooked, and is not environmentally sustainable.

If you think of traditional Indian food, these are the types of dishes that are often ideal for vegetarian Winters and Autumns. Indian recipes may feature beans and lentils for a main course, often served with a type of cheese called paneer. Paneer is most similar to our mozzarella cheese and is a bit lower in fat than other cheeses; however, it is still a high-fat food. In the following charts, I'll go over some of the sample meals I created earlier for Winters and Autumns and give you a vegetarian version that should work for your season-type.

Vegetarian Breakfast
If you recall, the first sample breakfast was a sandwich with Canadian bacon and eggs. In this example, the Canadian bacon has been replaced by a whey protein shake, which is consumed separately, and more cheese has been added to both sandwiches to increase the fat content. In addition, both season-types would want to take a 500 mg brewer's yeast tablet, because this meal has no purines in it. Switching out meat for either a whey protein shake or a casein protein shake, plus adding a brewer's yeast tablet, is something Autumns and Winters can do when looking to replace meat in any meal. Also, remember that much of the protein contained in cooked meat is not usable by the human body, so you

may find that you actually need a lower percentage of calories from protein when you consume whey or casein protein powder. You may need to experiment a little and see what works best for you.

Winter Vegetarian Breakfast #1			
Breakfast Sandwich	P	C	F
Whey protein shake	104	4	0
1 egg sunny side up	25	1	45
2 oz. cheddar cheese	60	4	162
1 English muffin	24	124	9
1 banana	4	98	3
Calories	217	231	219
667	33%	35%	33%

Autumn Vegetarian Breakfast #1			
Breakfast Sandwich	P	C	F
Whey protein shake	104	4	0
1 egg sunny side up	25	1	45
1 English muffin	24	124	9
1 oz. cheddar cheese	30	2	81
1 banana	4	98	3
Calories	187	229	138
554	34%	41%	25%

Vegetarian Lunch
Lunch #2 was originally a Mexican dish with beef sirloin, and here I simply removed the sirloin and added some fried egg whites and extra cheese. Frying egg whites in low-fat cooking spray is a great way to get high-quality vegetarian protein that is low in fat. Egg whites have a very neutral flavor, so you can use your allowed fat calories on items such as butter and cheese, which can add flavor to these dishes. Because both of these dishes already contain purines in the beans, there is no need to add any brewer's yeast to this meal.

Winter Vegetarian Lunch #1			
Mexican	P	C	F
Seven fried egg whites	112	4	0
1/2 cup pinto beans	27	91	4
1 corn tortilla	8	56	9
Fresh salsa	2	8	0
2 oz. Mexican queso cheese	48	8	144
Spinach salad	6	12	2
Calories	203	179	159
541	38%	33%	29%

Autumn Vegetarian Lunch #1			
Mexican	P	C	F
Six fried egg whites	96	4	0
3/4 cup pinto beans	41	137	6
2 corn tortillas	16	112	18
Salsa	2	8	0
2 oz. Mexican queso cheese	48	8	144
Spinach salad	6	12	2
Calories	209	281	170
660	32%	43%	26%

Vegetarian Dinner

The last dish is the Chinese stir-fry dish used in Dinner #3, with the chicken replaced by a whey protein shake. Similar to the way that meat-eating Winters and Autumns should always keep some lean deli meat in the fridge in order to get extra protein when needed, vegetarian Winter and Autumns should always have some sugar-free (and without artificial sweeteners, such as aspartame or sucralose) whey, casein, or egg white protein powder handy for the same reason. I chose this meal for the last example because rice and veggies are high in carbs and low in protein, so in these two cases I had to use more whey protein in the shakes. The nice thing about powdered protein is that you can use as little or as much as you need to get the extra protein that might be missing in the rest of your meal. You could just as easily fry up some egg whites and throw them in with the stir-fry. Because they are bland, they will simply absorb the taste of the stir-fry sauce. Egg whites that have already been separated from the yolks can be purchased in most grocery stores these days, but cracking and separating them yourself takes less than a minute. Each egg white has about 16 calories, so for Winters to get enough protein in this dish, they would need about a dozen egg whites.

Winter Vegetarian Dinner #1			
Chinese Stir-Fry	P	C	F
Whey protein shake	208	8	0
Mixed vegetables	8	40	27
1 cup brown rice	15	189	14
1 1/2 tbsp. butter for rice	0	0	150
Calories	231	237	191
659	35%	36%	29%

Autumn Vegetarian Dinner #1			
Chinese Stir-Fry	P	C	F
Whey protein shake	156	6	0
Mixed vegetables	8	40	27
1 cup brown rice	15	189	14
1 tbsp. butter for rice	0	0	100
Calories	179	235	141
555	32%	42%	25%

7
Fine-Tuning

Adjusting the Four Seasons Diet for lifestyle and climate.

Ideally, your intake of protein, carbohydrates, and fat should match as closely as possible the amount of each of these macronutrients that your body prefers to burn for energy. When you eat the same mix of fuels that you are burning for energy, your body will communicate with you in many subtle ways. By noticing how each meal affects your appetite, energy levels, and emotional well-being, you will learn how to fine-tune your diet in a way that works best for you.

During each meal, you should pay attention to how that meal affects your appetite and feelings of satisfaction while you are eating the meal and afterward. If you are consuming your ideal mix of fuels, your appetite will slowly diminish by the end of each meal, and your feelings of satisfaction will go up. You will also feel satisfied until the next meal or snack, if you choose to snack. When you consume the wrong mix of fuels, you may feel hungrier afterward than when you started eating, even though your stomach is full, or you might develop a craving for sweet foods or carbohydrates. You may also find that your energy plummets or that you become hyper or jittery. These are signs that you consumed the wrong mix of fuels at that meal.

The most common problem for Summers is eating too much fat, especially if they have an excess of belly fat. Belly fat continually releases blood fat into the body, which will keep the Summer in a constant state of low and erratic energy. The first thing that Summers, as well as every other season-type, need to do is a two-week fructose fast and limit their fructose consumption after that. This will allow their bodies' hormonal messengers to begin to work properly again and actually tell them when they are hungry or full. Once Summers have finished their fructose fast and are limiting their fructose consumption, the next step is to get rid of their belly fat, if they have it. This is easy for Summers to accomplish by simply cutting down on the amount of fat they eat during this phase of their dieting. Because belly fat is continually releasing fat into the bloodstream, Summers can reduce the amount of fat they eat to 10 percent of their daily calories or even

250

less for a very short time, while their bodies burn off this fat. This will happen very quickly if Summers limit their fat consumption.

Belly fat is one of the main reasons that Summers often have low appetites or can easily skip a meal or two and feel alright. When Summers with belly fat skip a meal, they continue to release belly fat as blood fat to supply them with a modest amount of energy and in the process help balance out their bodies by lowering the amount of belly fat they have stored. Remember that your diet should match what you burn for energy; however, for a Summer with belly fat, the body's release of belly fat has the same effect as eating fat, which is to increase blood fat. This causes the Summer's body to burn more fat for energy, which decreases sugar-energy production and makes a Summer's energy levels plummet. When Summers with belly fat eat a standard American high-fat meal, they are overloaded with the fat from the meal, combined with the fat being released by their belly fat, and in the process they often feel much worse after eating. Summers often skip breakfast or even eat only one meal a day because they claim it makes them feel better. It's common for many Summers to have excess belly fat, along with being insulin resistant. The result is that they have low energy levels and usually feel tired after eating a meal. Many Summers in this state find that it's best to skip eating meals and to limit themselves to one daily meal, as a way to maintain moderate energy levels.

This is an example of what happens when you eat the wrong mix of fuels for your season-type. Let's say that certain Summers eat one meal a day, with more fat than they prefer to burn for energy. The result is that they store most of the excess fat, oftentimes as belly fat. As long as they skip a meal or two a day, they can keep this up, while having a moderate energy level, using the 23 hours of not eating every day as a way to burn off the excess fat they eat. The reality is that their energy levels will be only a fraction of what they could be if they learned to eat right for their season-type.

Once Summers burn off their belly fat, they should be able to eat three meals a day and actually feel energized after eating, rather than tired or sleepy afterward, as they usually do. After Summers have gotten rid of their belly fat and begun to limit their fructose consumption, they can begin the maintenance part of the Four Seasons Diet, which simply consists of learning to limit their fat intake at each meal, as way to control their appetite and keep their energy levels high. When Summers eat a meal with too much fat, their appetites can often get out of control. Remember, Summers' bodies are looking to keep their stored-sugar levels high, and until this happens, they will continue to feel hungry. When they eat a meal that is high in fat, they simply overeat in order to get enough carbohydrates, and then they store the excess fat. Even lean Summers who overeat fat for just a few days will quickly throw their bodies out of balance until they burn off the excess fat again. If you binge for a weekend on too much fat, the easiest solution is to drastically cut back on your fat calories for a few days until you burn off the fat again.

A Summer with an appetite problem is almost always a Summer who eats too much fat or fructose. This is another reason Summers need to limit their fructose consumption, because 30 percent of fructose gets converted into fat. While you learn to fine-tune your diet, always start by eating a lower amount of fat, and keep in mind that you will tend to store almost all of your excess dietary fat as body fat or belly fat. If you are undereating fat, your body will soon begin to look emaciated or too skinny, and this will be one of the signs to increase the amount of fat you eat.

A Winter's appetite problems are caused by the exact opposite situation: overeating too many carbohydrates, especially higher-glycemic carbohydrates. Summers who eat too much fat often begin to feel a ravenous appetite while they are eating. Winters who eat too many carbohydrates, however, often experience their hunger after a meal. They may actually feel good or notice a nice burst of energy when they eat too many carbohydrates. Their appetite problem usually occurs after their meal is finished, when their blood sugar crashes to well below their baseline level. Remember that your baseline level of blood sugar is the level you had before you started eating a meal. Although a person with a normal blood-sugar response usually experiences an increase in blood sugar after a meal, followed by a gradual return to baseline, Winters often experience a quick increase in blood sugar, followed by a rapid plunge that takes them below their baseline. Winters need to pay close attention to the amount of carbohydrates they eat at each meal, along with the glycemic index of those carbohydrates. If Winters are looking to lose weight, they will find it easier if they restrict their carbohydrates to those with lower glycemic indexes and limit their carbohydrates to no more than 35 percent of their total daily calories. This will help keep their blood sugar stable and prevent them from snacking between meals. This, combined with slightly cutting back on total calories, will allow Winters to stay in fat-burning mode for most of the day, enabling them to gradually and easily lose the weight they want, while maintaining their energy levels without any significant hunger.

It's also imperative that Winters do the two-week fructose fast and limit their fructose consumption after that, so that their feel-full hormones can begin to work properly. When Winters who need to lose weight do the fructose fast, they will begin to hear the message their bodies have been trying to send them for a very long time, which is that they are not really hungry after all. When they combine this with eating only low- to medium-glycemic index carbohydrates, they will find it relatively easy to lose weight and get down to the weight their bodies prefer.

Summer Weight Loss Secret

Summers often have hard time losing those last few stubborn pounds of fat if they eat three meals a day. This is because the Summer diet is high in carbohydrates, which keeps a person's level of stored sugar high. Although this is good at helping Summers produce energy, they will tend not to burn as much fat when their stored sugar levels are high, compared to when they are low.

The best strategy for a Summer and, to a lesser extent, a Spring is simply to eat two meals a day. This can mean you skip breakfast and eat only lunch and dinner. If you work out after breakfast, it can also mean you eat breakfast but then skip lunch and don't eat again until dinner. Once you work out, you will deplete your level of stored sugar, and if you skip lunch, your body will begin to burn off those last few stubborn pounds.

This is because Summers eating three meals a day will tend to keep their stored sugar levels between 70 and 100 percent of their maximum, and it's tough to burn off those last few pounds of fat when your stored sugar reserves are this high. By skipping one meal and allowing your stored sugar reserves to get down to 40 to 60 percent of their maximum, you will begin to burn off more fat during the five or so hours after you skip a meal.

Eating this way will also help Summers maintain a higher level of insulin sensitivity and will keep their cells more permeable. Remember that most Summers are insulin resistant and have cells that are too impermeable. So any time you feel out of balance as a Summer, as if your body is not storing and using sugar properly, you can try to switch to two meals a day as a way to restore insulin sensitivity and to lose those last few stubborn pounds in the process.

Changing the Mix

The main principle behind the Four Seasons Diet is that you eat foods in the same ratio that your body prefers to burn for energy. The ratios given are what your recommended ratios should be for a 24-hour period. Although many people may find that this ratio works great for every meal, others learn that they do better if they change the ratios up a little bit at each meal, but keep the overall ratios the same during a 24-hour period.

The most common change people make concerns their intake of protein. Some people find that they need more of their daily protein in the morning, while other people require more at night. You may have to experiment a little to see what your body prefers. If, after a particular meal, you find that your appetite has not been satisfied, you have less energy, or your emotional well-being is not good, these are signs that you did not eat in a way that worked for your body. Do your best to keep track of which meals make you feel better and which ones make you feel worse. You may begin to discover patterns, such as the lowest-fat meals make you feel best or the lowest-carbohydrate meals make you feel great. Although the ratios are very good guidelines, some people may need to be very strict when it comes to consuming enough of one variable, such as protein, while they do not need to be as strict about eating too much of another variable, such as carbohydrates.

Adjust Your Diet in Hot or Cold Weather

As the weather changes, most people will need to modify their ratios slightly. Usually, the colder it gets, the greater the need for fat, especially saturated fat. For Summers, this may mean they eat no saturated when it's hot outside and a little bit when it's cold. Conversely, Winters, might eat modest amounts when it's hot outside and large amounts when it's colder. Remember that the colder it gets, the more permeable the cells will become, and the hotter it gets outside, the less permeable they will become. Dietary saturated fat and cholesterol make the cells less permeable, so both can be consumed in greater amounts in colder weather. Studies show that we burn more fat when we are cold, and that the amount of extra fat we burn is largely controlled by the availability of our stored sugar.

To understand how that process works, you need to

first grasp how the cold affects the way we burn calories to stay warm. Water conducts heat and cold nearly 25 times as much as air does. This is one reason a swimmer who swims across the English Channel can burn off nearly 14 pounds of body fat, while a marathon runner would be lucky to burn off half a pound of fat by running a marathon. Swimmers probably burn more calories keeping their bodies warm than they actually burn swimming. This is also the reason swimmers such as Michael Phelps can consume 12,000 calories a day. Spending hours a day in a pool, even if the water is 80 degrees, will burn far more calories than being outside in a bathing suit when it's 80 degrees.

Although most of us do not swim when it's cold, the humidity outside can also have a dramatic effect on how much the cold actually makes our bodies colder. When it's cold and humid, our bodies have to work harder to stay warm than when we are in the cold and it's dry. Thirty degrees in rainy, humid Seattle will feel far colder than 30 degrees in Denver, where it tends to be much drier. Likewise, 80 degrees might feel oppressive in Florida, due to the humidity, and very comfortable in Arizona, where it's dry.

Why the Season-Types Burn Different Fuels to Stay Warm

The other thing to keep in mind is that each season-type following his or her proper diet will tend to burn different amounts of fat and carbohydrates to stay warm. One study looked at the fuels the body uses to stay warm when fed a high-carbohydrate diet, similar to what a Summer should consume, vs. a low-carbohydrate diet, which is the diet recommended for a Winter. To mimic the cold, subjects were placed in a liquid-conditioned wet suit at 50 degrees, which would be similar to being in the water or in a very humid environment. Researchers found that when it's above 70 degrees, people on a high-carb diet, similar to the Summer diet, burn no fat to stay warm. When the same people are exposed to the cold, they burn about twice as many calories to stay warm (not total calories, but calories spent to maintain body heat) and use more than 80 percent carbohydrates to generate body heat and about 20 percent fat. This is the reason Summers need to eat a little more fat when they are cold. The cold will also tend to make the cells more permeable, which is the reason Summers can usually get away with eating more saturated fat when it's colder outside. Those with a diet similar to the Winter diet burned an equal mix of fat and carbohydrates to stay warm when it was 70 degrees, and when they were exposed to the cold, they also burned about twice the calories to stay warm; however, they still used a fairly even mix of fat and carbohydrates in the process. The cold temperatures will make the cells more permeable and also lower the blood pH, and this is the reason a Winter needs more saturated fat and purines when it's colder outside.

Weight Loss Tips

If you are trying to lose weight, evidence suggests that by keeping yourself slightly cold, you can burn double to triple the amount of fat as when you are warm. Similarly, when you drink ice water, you will burn more calories than when you drink water at room temperature, because your body has to burn more calories in the process of getting the ice water up to body temperature. The amount of extra calories burned is a little less than 20, so if you switch to drinking ice water, you can hope to burn only about an extra 100 calories a day, but that equates to nearly a pound of body fat in one month. Taking a cold shower vs. a hot shower will also cause you to burn more fat calories. Taking a hot shower in the summer months can be disastrous for Summers, however, because when it's hot outside, their bodies' cells are usually too nonpermeable and their blood pH is often too alkaline. When it gets hot outside, Summers are advised to take cooler showers than normal and to finish the shower with slightly cold water, so that they feel slightly cold when they are done showering.

Exercise

Exercise has perhaps the greatest potential to make you modify the diet for your season-type. To understand how exercise affects your need to modify your diet, remember these key principals:

1. Your daily intake of protein, carbohydrates, and fat should be similar to what your body prefers to burn for energy.
2. Sugar-burning muscles burn sugar for energy, while fat-burning muscles can burn either fat or sugar for energy.
3. Fat-burning muscles will burn fat for energy at lower intensities and then switch over to burning sugar for energy at higher intensities.

Keeping these principles in mind with regard to your particular season-type will help you modify your diet according to the way you prefer to exercise.

How Summers Can Modify Their Diet When Exercising

Summers are probably the easiest season-type to understand, because they have the highest proportion of sugar-burning muscles and the lowest proportion of fat-burning muscles. This means that even at rest, Summers are burning mainly sugar for energy. Summers do have some fat-burning muscles and will use these when they engage in lower-intensity exercise. For example, Summers who go on a long walk or hike will often use their fat-burning muscles in conjunction with their sugar-burning muscles. If Summers engage in a lot of lower-intensity exercise such as this, they will need to slightly increase their fat intake to match what they burn for energy. When Summers reach their ideal weight and understand these principles, it becomes pretty easy for them to gauge their need for fat. If they eat too much fat, they will begin to store more fat and will soon notice it. If they are not eating enough fat, they often start to look too gaunt and emaciated and will realize that it's time to eat more fat. Summers usually have more defined muscles, and their tendons are more visible when they are lean, compared to the other season types. This is because fat-burning muscles store more fat for energy, and since Summers have very few fat-burning muscles, when they are lean you can often see every muscle clearly defined. Summers are also the season-type most prone to obesity the older they get. This is primarily because they do not burn very much fat for energy and will store the fat they do not burn.

For these reasons, Summers have the easiest time modifying their diet in relation to their exercise. The main factor Summers need to consider is whether they want to lose fat, maintain their fat level, or gain fat. Because Summers mainly always burn sugar for energy, they should increase their fat consumption only if they begin to look a little thin or gaunt, or if they engage in long-duration, low-impact exercise and are beginning to feel their energy levels drop.

How Winters Can Modify Their Diet When Exercising

Winters have the hardest time of all of the season-types when it comes to modifying their diet in relation to exercise. The general rule for Winters is that the higher their level of intensity, the more carbohydrates they will need to add to their diet. For example, Winters at rest are burning only around 20 percent carbohydrates for energy. When they increase their level of activity, as measured by their VO_2 max, they burn more carbohydrates. A person's VO_2 max represents the maximum amount of oxygen he or she can use to produce energy. For example, at 100 percent VO_2 max, people are using 100 percent of the oxygen their bodies take in during intense maximal exercise. A 50 percent VO_2 max means people are using only about half of their maximal oxygen uptake. As Winters boost their percentage of VO_2 max, they increase the amount of carbohydrates they use for energy. When they get somewhere between 55 and 70 percent of their VO_2 max, they begin to burn about 50 percent carbohydrates and 50 percent fat for energy. When they get to around 80 to 90 percent of their VO_2 max, they are burning around 80 percent carbohydrates for energy, and over 90 percent VO_2 max, they are burning mainly carbohydrates for energy.

Winters can use this to either modify their workout to achieve a desired result, such as burning fat, or modify their diet, if they want to push themselves to a more elite level of fitness. For most people reading this book, your desire is probably to lose a little weight and be in overall good shape. The biggest mistake people make when they are mainly looking to lose body fat is that they work out too intensely. If Winters go to the gym and exercise on the treadmill at an intense 80 percent VO_2 max, they will be burning mainly carbohydrates for energy, whereas if they take the intensity way down to under 50 percent VO_2 max, they will burn primarily fat for energy.

If your goal is simply to burn off body fat, then lower-intensity, longer-duration exercise should be your primary focus. Think of going on a brisk walk for an hour, a 5- to 10-mile jog at a moderate pace, or a long bike ride at a moderate pace. These will all help you burn mainly fat for energy. The faster your pace, the higher your intensity, the less fat and the more carbohydrates you will burn. Some people advocate training at higher intensities, because they claim the body will convert fat into glucose in a process called *gluconeogenesis*. The truth is, only glycerol can be converted to glucose—not fatty acids. Remember that fats are stored as triglycerides, which consist of three fatty acids bound together to one glycerol molecule. When the body burns fat for energy, it releases the fatty acids from the glycerol, and the fatty acids get burned in a process called *beta-oxidation*. If you run at an intense pace, hoping to turn fat into sugar for energy, the best you can hope for is that you will turn some glycerol into energy, leaving you with three fatty acids to deal with. In reality, your body will almost completely exhaust your stored-sugar reserves before it begins to convert glycerol into glucose, and when you totally run out of stored sugar, you will most likely find yourself craving carbohydrates. This is the reason you are better off burning body fat by adopting a slow-enough pace to simply let your fat-burning muscles burn the fat for energy.

At the opposite end of the spectrum is the Winter who is looking to be an elite distance runner or a cyclist. At the elite levels of training, a higher VO_2 max is often used for conditioning purposes. When Winters train in this manner, they burn a greater percentage of carbohydrates the higher their level of intensity. As a result, they will need to increase the amount of carbohydrates they consume, in order to replenish their stored-sugar reserves. Oftentimes, Winters who are elite endurance athletes will need to eat exactly the same way a Summer or a Spring eats, especially on training days. On nontraining days, they may still find that they need to eat larger quantities of carbohydrates, in order to help keep themselves in sugar-burning mode on training days. Other athletes may find that they do better eating more fat and fewer carbohydrates on nontraining days. If you are a Winter endurance athlete who is training at an elite level of fitness, you will have to do some trial-and-error testing to see what works best for you, but at least now you have an understanding of how you need to modify your diet in relation to your training. All of the other Winters who are simply looking to lose a little weight or stay lean, if they are already at their ideal weight, should simply keep their intensity at a more moderate pace and increase the amount of time they spend training.

How Springs and Autumns Can Modify Their Diet When Exercising

Springs are most like Summers but burn a little more fat and fewer carbohydrates for energy. While a Summer will burn almost exclusively carbohydrates at even a modest VO_2 max, Springs will burn a little more fat at a modest VO_2 max, but at anything above about a 50 percent VO_2 max, Springs burn mainly carbohydrates for energy. Autumns are most like Winters but burn a few more carbohydrates and less fat for energy. Usually, Autumns will burn a fairly even mix of fat and carbohydrates at a moderate pace, but as they increase their intensity, they begin to burn mainly carbohydrates. Once again, Springs and Autumns will need to do some experimenting with their diets to see what works best for them at different levels of intensity.

High-Intensity Interval Training (HIIT) for Summers and Springs
Although traditional cardio training works well for Winters and Autumns, there is another type of cardio training called HIIT, which stands for *high-intensity interval training*, that is ideally suited for Summers and Springs.

HIIT is a form of cardio training that consists of a warm-up period, followed by performing an all-out sprint-type exercise for anywhere from 10 seconds to a minute, followed by 1 to 4 minutes of lower-intensity cardio exercise. This sprint/low-intensity cycle is performed anywhere from 4 to 10 times, with the usual goal of finishing the entire cardio session in 12 to 20 minutes. The all-out sprint exercise can consist of anything that allows you to work at maximum intensity, such as sprinting, running up a long flight of stairs as fast as you can, running on a treadmill set to maximum incline, or cycling on a stationary bicycle set to a higher level of resistance. If you do the sprint portion correctly, you should be working at a minimum of 105 percent of your maximum VO_2 threshold, preferably higher. After each sprint session, you should find that you are breathing quite heavily while you do the lower-intensity portion of the routine. The lower-intensity portion of the routine can consist of lightly jogging, walking on a treadmill set at the maximum incline, or lightly pedaling on the stationary bicycle. Ideally, your breathing and heart rate will go down just a little bit before it's time for your next all-out sprint.

HIIT training is a very intense form of exercise, and if you engage in it, it's important to take at least one day of rest in between training sessions in order to recover properly. Most people who do HIIT, for example, either do a Monday / Wednesday / Friday session or a Tuesday / Thursday / Saturday session, giving them three days of HIIT training with four days of rest per week. Doing HIIT training more than three days a week is actually counterproductive, so if you are a driven person who wants to maximize your results, work out intensely for three days a week doing HIIT and give yourself the necessary four days of rest.

HIIT training is an extremely demanding form of cardio exercise that is not suited for everyone. Prior to beginning HIIT training, you should get an okay from your physician that it's safe for you to do this type of training. It's best to start off with a shorter sprint time of around 10 seconds and then slowly work your way up to longer sprint times. If you have not done cardio training for a long time, and you do HIIT correctly, you will find that 10 seconds of all-out effort will be extremely demanding, both mentally and physically; however, HIIT has great benefits, especially when you factor in the amount of time it takes when compared to traditional cardio regimes. In fact, multiple studies show that 10 to 20 minutes of HIIT training three times a week has cardio benefits that are comparable to five hours a week of traditional cardio training.

There are many reasons that this type of exercise is ideal for Summers and Springs. First, studies show that HIIT training is more effective at increasing the oxidative capacity of sugar-burning muscles, while traditional cardio training with a lower VO_2 max is best at increasing the oxidative capacity of fat-burning muscles. This is in large part due to the effects that different types of cardio training have on the enzymes and proteins responsible for energy production. HIIT training increases the enzymes most responsible for producing energy using sugar, such as *phosphofructokinase* and *hexokinase*, so training using HIIT will enable Summers and Springs to have more overall energy during the week. At the same time, HIIT increases the amount of sugar that muscles will store for energy, further helping Summers and Springs maintain a high energy level. One study showed that HIIT training can boost the amount of sugar that muscles will store by 26 percent.

Another key enzyme involved in energy production is called *succinate dehydrogenase*, often referred to as SDH. One study examined how different types of cardio training affected levels of this key energy enzyme in both fat-burning muscles and sugar-burning muscles. The study found that traditional lower-intensity, longer-duration cardio exercise increased SDH enzymes only in fat-burning muscles, and that the amount of SDH increase was 32 percent. The study also found that HIIT type cardio training increased SDH enzymes only in sugar-burning muscles, and that the amount of increase was 49 percent. So, although both types of cardio training have comparable cardio benefits, traditional cardio appears to have more benefits for people with a higher proportion of fat-burning muscles, while HIIT cardio appears to have more benefits for those with a greater proportion of sugar-burning muscles.

Besides helping to boost key energy proteins and enzymes in sugar-burning muscles, HIIT training has numerous other benefits for Summers and Springs. As explained earlier, Summers and Springs often suffer from poor insulin sensitivity and from insulin resistance. Studies show that a mere two weeks of HIIT training can lower insulin levels by 37 percent (measured as the area under the insulin curve), while improving insulin sensitivity by 23 percent. It does this in part by helping to increase the amount of a protein called GLUT 4 by 20 percent after just one week of HIIT training. GLUT 4 is an important regulator of insulin sensitivity.

In addition, two weeks of HIIT training have been shown to lower levels of blood fats by 26 percent. Lowering blood fats helps improve both insulin sensitivity and the overall energy level of Summers and Springs, because excess blood fats are a common problem for these two season-types that often contributes to their lack of energy.

Another benefit of HIIT training for Summers and Springs is that it will tend to put them into fat-burning mode for several hours after their HIIT sessions. Summers and Springs do not burn very much fat for energy, and as a result, they can easily accumulate excess body fat when they eat too much dietary fat. It can be difficult for Summers, especially, to burn this fat off because they burn mainly carbohydrates for energy. HIIT training helps deplete levels of stored sugar, and after a good HIIT session, the body will switch to fat-burning mode, as it attempts to replenish stored-sugar levels. In addition, after a HIIT training session, fat is released into the bloodstream, which contributes to the one to three hours of fat burning that occurs after a good HIIT session. During this time, the body is burning fat while it works to significantly increase its levels of stored sugar, both of which have an overall positive benefit for Summers and Springs.

HIIT training has also been found to decrease unhealthy LDL cholesterol, and this is probably due in large part to the fact that HIIT lowers overall insulin levels. One of the main reasons Summers and Springs often suffer from low energy is that their cells are no longer responsive to insulin, so they don't store enough sugar for energy to fuel the high sugar needs of their season-types. When this happens, the body responds by producing excessive amounts of insulin, which, as you have learned, is the root cause of many of the other health issues that Summers and Springs tend to suffer from.

In effect, when you cardio train using HIIT, your body begins to adapt to the training by boosting the amount of sugar it stores in the muscles, because HIIT training requires large amounts of stored sugar as fuel. In addition, the muscles respond by increasing the number of enzymes responsible for sugar-energy production in sugar-burning muscles. The net result is that the body quickly becomes more insulin sensitive, and insulin levels begin to decrease. Levels of blood fats also drop, except for the one to three hours following HIIT training, during which time they rise while the body is storing more sugar for energy and burning off excess fat. If you wanted to come up with a magic pill to help cure Summers and Springs of many of their health problems, it would do all of the things I just mentioned. HIIT training is that magic pill for these two season-types.

Weight Lifting
Weight lifting is quite different from cardio training. Usually, with weight lifting, the goal of men is gain muscle mass and size, and the goal of women is increase strength without getting bigger, while they firm, slim, tone, and shape their bodies. Weight lifting tends to burn more carbohydrates for energy, often at a VO_2 max of 100 percent or even more than 100 percent if you're working to gain size and strength. When your VO_2 max is beyond 100 percent, you are forced to produce sugar energy without oxygen, and in the process you produce excess acid, which ultimately needs to be eliminated with the help of oxygen. When you are over 100 percent VO_2 max, however, you are already using all of your oxygen for energy production and are therefore accumulating what is called an *oxygen deficit*. Essentially, you are accumulating acidic waste products that need oxygen to be eliminated. This is the reason that when you lift weights, you are often left breathing heavily afterward. Your body is still trying to use oxygen, not for energy, but to get rid of the metabolic acids you produced.

Most season-types who lift weights will burn carbohydrates for a large percentage of their energy. One of the benefits of building muscle is that muscles burn calories even when you are not working out, 24 hours a day. Muscles at rest are similar to a car engine that is parked and idling, burning fuel 24 hours a day. Studies show that muscles burn about an extra 6 calories a day per pound, even at rest. Although this may not sound like a lot, those muscles will burn extra calories when you are moving around as well. For example, let's say you put on an extra 5 pounds of muscles in your legs. Those 5 pounds of leg muscles will burn an extra 30 calories a day while you're sitting, resting, and sleeping. Those extra muscles will also burn more calories as you walk around during the day. Let's say, they burn an extra 30 calories from your regular daily activity. Now you're burning an extra 60 calories a day, which means during the course of a year, they'll burn enough calories to knock off more than 6 pounds of body fat. In addition, even working out with weights lightly only three times a week will burn an extra 600 calories a week. Combine that with the extra calories your muscles burn at rest and moving around, and, suddenly, you're burning an extra 1,000 calories a week, all from simply working out very lightly with weights for three hours a week and gaining 5 pounds of lean muscle. For people who work out at a higher intensity five days a week and gain large amounts of muscle mass, the extra calories burned per week can easily exceed 6,000 calories.

Adjusting your diet for weight lifting is similar in many ways to doing it for cardiovascular training. First, you need to decide what your goals are. If you want to gain maximum muscle mass and size, you need to lift more heavily and intensely, which means you'll burn mainly carbohydrates for energy. If your goal is to trim, tone, and shape your body, you'll work out lighter and less intensely and will use fewer carbohydrates than you would if you were looking to put on size and strength.

Weight Lifting for Summers and Springs

Summers will burn mainly carbohydrates for energy, no matter which way they work out, so they have the easiest time modifying their diet. They will need to increase their calories if they want to gain size and strength and keep their calories the same if they want to trim, tone, and shape. Either way, their diet remains pretty much the same high-carb, low-fat diet they would be following if they did not work out. The same applies to Springs, because they usually burn mainly carbohydrates when weight training.

Weight Lifting for Winters and Autumns

At the opposite end of the spectrum are Winters. Winters who want to gain size and strength will have to work out in a way that increases the amount of carbohydrates they burn for energy, which means they will have to consume more carbohydrates. Winters who want to trim, tone, and shape their bodies will work out at a lower intensity level. They will still burn more carbohydrates than when resting, but will also burn fat during their workout. Autumns are very similar, in that they will continue to burn a mix of carbohydrates and fat, depending on their level of intensity.

For All Season-Types: Should You Eat Before, During, or After Weight Lifting?

For all season-types who lift weights, what you eat before and during your workout will have a huge effect on what you burn for energy during your workout. Many people drink a protein shake prior to working out, in the belief that it will help them burn fat during the workout. Protein shakes before a workout will cause an insulin response that will actually lower the amount of fat you burn for energy. This is especially true if you use a faster-acting protein, such as whey protein. If you want to maximize your fat burning during weight lifting, you're best not eating anything for at least two hours before working out. This will give your insulin a chance to get back to normal levels from your last meal and will put you back into the maximum fat-burning mode for your season-type. As stated earlier, Summers and Springs are never going to burn much fat when they lift weights, while Winters and, to a lesser extent, Autumns can burn a combination of fat and carbohydrates, depending on their level of intensity. If you're a Winter or an Autumn and your goal is to burn fat and tone, trim, and shape your body but not gain huge amounts of muscle, then your best strategy is not to eat at least two hours, preferably longer, before you work out. This will put you into your maximum fat-burning mode while you work out, helping you burn more fat and fewer carbohydrates than you would if you ate right before you worked out.

For anyone who wants to gain maximum size and strength, the best approach is to consume a high-glycemic carbohydrate drink, such as dextrose or maltodextrin, while you work out (avoid most commercial drinks because they contain fructose, either as HFCS or as sucrose). The best strategy is to consume about 50 grams of carbohydrates for every hour you work out. Start drinking the high-glycemic carbohydrate shake a few minutes before you start your workout, and space out the drink so that you consume an even amount during the first three-quarters of your workout. For example, if you work out for an hour, you would drink your 50 grams of high-glycemic carbohydrates during the first 45 minutes of your workout, taking a sip right before you start working out, followed by equal sips every 5 to 10 minutes during your workout. This will help keep your insulin and blood-sugar levels slightly elevated during your workout, which will keep you in sugar-burning mode and allow you to work out more intensely than if you did not consume a drink during your workout. If you want to lose weight or maintain your existing weight, and do not want to gain a lot of size or strength, it's best to skip the workout drink and rely on your stored sugar and stored fat to energize you.

Your post-workout meal also depends on your ultimate goal. If you are a Summer or a Spring who is trying to lose those last few stubborn pounds, you can skip your post-workout meal. Exercising should help reduce your levels of stored sugar, and this will help you burn more fat than you normally would. If you skip your post-workout meal and do not eat for about four to five hours after your workout, you will burn off the remaining pounds that are often the most difficult to lose.

People who are looking to tone, trim, and shape their bodies can wait until they feel hungry for their next meal. When you work out with weights, you will continue to burn extra calories after you work out, and your appetite will be naturally suppressed from the weight lifting for an hour or two. Once you get hungry, you can eat your normal meal, with perhaps a few more carbohydrates than normal if you are a Winter or an Autumn.

If you want to gain maximum muscle mass and strength, you will have to take a very different approach. In addition to consuming 50 grams of carbohydrates during your workout, you may also want to consume another 50 grams of a carbohydrate drink with about 10 grams of protein immediately after your workout to help replenish the stored muscle sugar you burned during your workout. When you maintain higher insulin levels, you will be able to gain strength and size a lot easier. The problem is that excess insulin over a prolonged period of time can also have negative metabolic consequences. If you are young, you may be more immune to many of these consequences; however, once you get into your early thirties, keeping your insulin levels high all of the time can be counterproductive to your workouts.

As you begin to age, if you are trying to gain size and strength, you can cycle between a week or two of keeping your insulin levels high by eating a lot of carbs to gain size and strength (gaining periods), followed by a week of two of keeping your insulin levels lower by not eating after you work out, as a way to lose any excess fat you gained during the "gaining periods." As you age, if you do not adopt a strategy such as this and instead keep your insulin levels and food intake high all the time, it will eventually become very counterproductive to your workouts. This is because the high insulin levels will make your cells too impermeable, and your muscles won't get the oxygen they need to fuel intense workouts.

Most of human history consisted of times of "food excess," followed by times of "food shortages," and humans have adapted over thousands of years to these periods of excess and shortages. You can use this to your advantage if you learn to listen to your body and eat a little "excess" food for a week or two in a forced "growth period," followed by a week of two of a "shortage" period, when you eat less food as a way to keep your cells from getting too impermeable due to too much insulin produced during the "excess" period. When you are in the "excess" food consumption mode, you will know it's time to quit when you become a bit more winded during your workouts. When you are in the food "shortage" mode, you will know it's time to quit if you experience a sudden drop in strength.

If you are in "excess mode" and consume a high-carb post-workout drink, you should also be sure to eat your next meal within an hour or two after your drink, to help your muscles recover and store even more sugar. Summers and Springs can eat their regular higher-carbohydrate diet, while Winters and Autumns will need to experiment a little. They may find that the extra carbohydrates from the workout drink and the post-workout drink are all their muscles need to help maximize their growth. They may also need to eat a few more carbohydrates in their next meal or maybe even for the next several meals. It's recommended that Winters and Autumns who want to gain size and strength start off by not consuming any workout drink or post-workout drink. They can then add the workout drink to see how that affects them, and if they are alright with that for a week or two, they can try adding the post-workout drink. If that works for them as well, they can slowly add in more carbohydrates for the next meal. It's imperative that Winters and Autumns slowly add in more carbohydrates and gauge how their bodies react, because nothing will imbalance them as much as consuming too many carbohydrates.

Summers and Springs who want to gain size and strength may find it necessary to add extra protein to their diet. Oftentimes, this can be done for the last meal of the day, after they have already replenished their stored-sugar levels. Remember that if you consume too much protein with your carbohydrates, you will tend not to store as much sugar for energy. The first goal of Summers and Springs should be to restore their levels of stored sugar, because these are usually replenished more quickly the first 1 to 4 hours after a workout. Extra protein can then be added when stored-sugar levels have been replenished, to help build and repair muscle. Summers and Springs can also consume their extra protein as a single protein shake before going to bed, because this will help them build muscle while they sleep.

Various types of protein have different speeds with which they release their proteins into the body. Whey protein, for example, is an extremely fast-acting protein and will quickly release protein into the system after it's consumed. At the opposite end of the spectrum is casein protein, which releases its proteins very slowly. Usually, whey protein is recommended after a workout, while casein protein is recommended right before going to bed. This is because the whey protein after a workout is more effective in acting as a signal that elevates protein synthesis, assisting in the growth and repair of muscles. Although fast-acting whey helps in protein synthesis, slower-acting casein is superior at helping to suppress protein breakdown. This makes it especially useful when taken right before bedtime, as it will help minimize protein loss at night.

The only downside to whey protein and casein protein for Summers and Springs is that they are both high in calcium, which can decrease sugar-energy production, especially if not enough magnesium is taken, either with supplements or in the diet. For this reason, Summers and Springs may want to limit their consumption of whey and casein protein to once a day and consider using egg whites as a protein source. Egg whites are digested more slowly than whey protein is but more quickly than casein. They can be used as a great protein source with any meal and supply all of the essential amino acids necessary for muscle growth and repair. In addition, egg whites do not contain any calcium, which can slow down energy production for Summers and Springs in excessive amounts. Yet egg whites do contain more than 50 mg of potassium per egg white, which can help speed up energy production for these two season-types. Each large egg white contains about 4 grams of protein, so six egg whites supply 24 grams of protein and more than 300 mg of potassium.

Supplements for Your Season-Type

An entire book could be devoted to how to properly fine-tune the supplements you take for your season-type. Each vitamin and mineral can affect the season-types differently, and even among the same season-types, there are often some differences. For example, while most Summers tend to have blood that is slightly too alkaline, sometimes Summers have blood that is a little too acidic, in which case their nervous systems may be stuck in fight-or-flight mode. Each synthetic vitamin and mineral often comes in different forms, and those forms will affect a person differently, depending on various factors. Calcium can be purchased as calcium lactate, calcium orotate, calcium citrate, and calcium gluconate, along with many other forms. One form of calcium will affect a person differently from another form, and there is a science to knowing which one to take. Rather than begin to try to explain the countless rules with regard to supplementation and the season-types, I have decided to simply give you a brief overview of some of the most common supplementation guidelines and how they apply to the various season-types.

Variable Supplement Requirements
Some vitamins and minerals play a prominent role in producing energy using sugar, while others mainly produce energy using fat. Oftentimes, a season-type who produces energy using predominately fat or sugar will deplete the vitamins and minerals that help produce energy the way he or she prefers. Other times, a particular season-type may not have a deficiency in a particular vitamin or mineral; however, some vitamins and minerals work in pairs with other vitamins and minerals, and the ratio between the two pairs may have a tremendous effect on how a person produces energy.

<u>Calcium/Magnesium and Sodium/Potassium</u>
Calcium/magnesium and sodium/potassium are two examples of minerals that work in pairs. Higher levels of calcium and sodium relative to magnesium and potassium will tend to slow down the rate at which you produce energy using sugar. The key is often to find the balance that works best for you and your season-type. Winters usually do best with higher calcium and sodium diets, while Summers do best with less calcium and sodium and higher levels of magnesium and potassium. Autumns and Springs often need to do a little more experimentation to see what works best for them; however, because they tend not to be as out of balance as Winters and Summers, they are usually not as sensitive to fluctuations in vitamin and mineral balances.

Even when supplementing with potassium, however, it's important to know the proper form to take. Potassium chloride and potassium phosphate will both increase sugar-energy production, while potassium citrate will slow it down. The good news is that if you get your potassium from the food you eat, you do not need to worry about these differences.

Vitamin C

Various forms of synthetic vitamins and minerals can have a dramatic effect on a person's metabolism. On one hand, vitamin C taken as ascorbic acid tends to make the blood more acidic and is usually the type recommended for Summers and Springs. Vitamin C as calcium ascorbate, on the other hand, tends to make the blood more alkaline and is usually the form recommended for Winters and Autumns. As mentioned previously, Winters usually have blood that is slightly too acidic, while Summers usually have blood that is slightly too alkaline. Sometimes, however, a Winter can have alkaline blood, while a Summer has acidic blood, in which case they tend to suffer from a different set of problems. Normally, a Winter with acidic blood experiences erratic energy production, and a Summer with alkaline blood has low energy production. When a Winter's blood becomes alkaline, however, he or she tends to have a nervous system stuck in rest-and-relax mode, while a Summer with acidic blood has a nervous system stuck in fight-or-flight mode. I mention this because whenever you begin taking a new vitamin or mineral, it's important to keep track of how it makes you feel, and adjust what you are taking accordingly.

Foodlike Vitamins

It would be wonderful if we could get all of our vitamins and minerals from the food we eat, but, sadly, our soil has become depleted of many minerals, and as a result our food is often lacking in the nutrients it once had. Some foods contain less than 1 percent of the minerals they contained 100 years ago, so unless you know your food is coming from a farm with mineral-rich soil, you are probably best to use vitamin supplements.

Several companies are making vitamin supplements that are more like food and less like synthetic vitamins. These foodlike vitamins are usually more expensive than synthetic vitamins; however, they do not create the same potential problems because you do not have to worry about which form of a vitamin or a mineral you are taking. These foodlike vitamins do not have the same potential to drastically change the blood pH, as synthetic ones can, so if you can afford to take them, you will have a much easier time keeping yourself balanced.

Vitamin and Mineral Protocols

The two most common imbalances among the season-types are people who burn predominately fat for energy and have slightly acidic blood, and people who burn mainly sugar for energy and have slightly alkaline blood. The following vitamin and mineral protocols can help both of these groups maintain high levels of energy and proper balance in their bodies. If you follow these protocols, it's recommended you take a foodlike natural vitamin supplement containing around 100 percent of the daily recommended value for most vitamins and minerals and then use the protocols to give your body the extra vitamins and minerals it needs for your season-type.

The following additional vitamins and minerals are recommended for people who burn predominately fat for energy, that is, Winters and Autumns:

CHART 7.1 VITAMINS AND MINERALS FOR WINTERS AND AUTUMNS

Vitamin/Mineral	Amount
A	1,000 IU
E	100 IU
B12	100 mcg
C	100 mg
Niacinamide	100 mg
Pantothenic Acid	50 mg
Inositol	100 mg
Choline	100 mg
Calcium	300 mg
Phosphorous	300 mg
Iodine	100 mcg
Zinc	10 mg

The following additional vitamins and minerals are recommended for people who burn predominately sugar for energy, that is, Summers and Springs:

CHART 7.2 VITAMINS AND MINERALS FOR SUMMERS AND SPRINGS

Vitamin/Mineral	Amount
A	1,000 IU
D	1,000 IU
C	500 mg
B1 (thiamine)	5 mg
B2 (riboflavin)	5 mg
B6	5 mg
Niacin (B3)	50 mg
Para Amino Benzoic Acid	50 mg
Folic Acid	100 mcg
Biotin	400 mcg
Potassium	200 mg
Magnesium	300 mg
Iron	50 mcg
Copper	1 mg
Manganese	5 mg
Chromium	100 mcg

As of the writing of this book, I am working on coming up with a good supplement that meets these recommended guidelines. Anyone interested in purchasing supplements that meet these recommendations should check my website at FourSeasonsDietBook.com and click on the "Supplements" tab.

Women, and How They Can Balance Themselves throughout the Month

Women who are premenopausal have an extra concern when it comes to keeping their season-type balanced. This is because as their hormones change during their cycle, their blood pH tends to change as well. Assuming a 28-day cycle, the following changes are the most common that occur. Usually, around days 10 to 16, estrogen levels are higher than normal, and blood pH tends to decline and become more acidic. From days 18 to 24, progesterone levels are higher than normal and blood pH tends to become more alkaline. According to some experts, these changes in blood pH contribute to making both PMS and cramping more severe. The little research that has been conducted on this topic has found that if a women keeps her blood pH more stable during her monthly cycle, she may experience great relief from both PMS and cramping symptoms.

Of course, these hormonal changes affect the various season-types differently. For example, Winters, who tend to have overly acidic blood, may tend to feel much worse on days 10 to 16 as blood pH drops and may actually feel better during days 18 to 24 as blood pH rises. Conversely, Summers may feel better from days 10 to 16 as blood pH falls and feel worse during days 18 to 24 as blood pH rises. Usually, once you figure out what your blood pH is doing on these days, you can easily modify your diet to help your body maintain proper pH, with the potential for minimizing or completely alleviating cramping and PMS.

If you begin to follow the Four Seasons Diet for your season-type and minimize your consumption of fructose and processed vegetable oils, you may find that your cramping and PMS symptoms have already been diminished as your new diet has helped balance out your blood pH. You may still have some PMS and cramping, however, especially when the weather is most adverse for your season-type.

Guidelines for Winters during Their Monthly Cycle
For example, Winters usually have blood that is too acidic. By following the Four Seasons Diet for their season-type, they should begin to balance out their blood pH and find that much of their PMS and cramping disappears. When it's cold outside, they may still suffer from some symptoms, or if they do not tweak their diet at certain times of the month, they might still have symptoms. Following are the most common guidelines a Winter should follow during her monthly cycle.

Winter days 1–9. This is the time of the month when your blood pH is least affected by your hormones. During this time, you should follow the standard diet for your season-type.

Winter days 10–16. On these days, your blood pH may become more acidic as your estrogen levels begin to rise. During this time, you should follow a very strict Winter diet, and you may find you need to add more purine-rich proteins, along with more fat and a little fewer carbohydrates.

Winter days 17–18. Now your blood pH is beginning to get back to normal, and you should transition back to your normal Winter diet for a few days.

Winter days 19–24. On these days, your blood pH may become more alkaline as your progesterone levels begin to rise. You may find that you do better if you are a bit less strict in following a Winter diet and eat a little more as an Autumn does. You may feel better if you eat fewer purines than normal, and even a bit less protein and a little more carbohydrates may work better for you.

Winter days 25–28. Transition back to a normal Winter diet.

Guidelines for Summers during Their Monthly Cycle
Summers usually have blood that is too alkaline. By following the Four Seasons Diet for their season-type, they should begin balance out their blood pH and may find that much of their PMS and cramping disappears. When it's hot outside, they may still suffer from some symptoms, or if they do not tweak their diet at certain times of the month, they might have symptoms. Following are the most common guidelines a Summer should follow during her monthly cycle.

Summer days 1–9. This is the time of the month when your blood pH is least affected by your hormones, so you should follow your normal Summer diet.

Summer 10–16. During this time, your blood pH may become more acidic as your estrogen levels begin to rise. You may actually feel more balanced, as your pH levels begin to fall from their normally high levels. You may feel best sticking to your Summer diet, or you might do better eating a little more like a Spring and adding a bit more purines and protein.

Summer days 17–18. During this time, your blood pH is beginning to get back to normal, and you should transition back to your normal diet for a few days.

Summer days 19–24. On these days, your blood pH may become more alkaline as your progesterone levels begin to rise. This is when you will have to follow a very strict Summer diet, especially when it's hot outside. You may need to completely eliminate purine proteins from your diet and eat less protein and more carbohydrates than you normally do.

Summer days 25–28. Transition back to a normal Summer diet.

Winters usually have overly acidic blood; however, sometimes they can have blood that is too alkaline. Likewise, Summers usually have overly alkaline blood but sometimes can have blood that is too acidic. If this is the case, the previous protocols may not work but might actually make the symptoms worse. If this happens, then at least you are now aware of the powerful effect food can have on your monthly cycle. If the most common protocol listed previously does not work for your season-type but actually makes your symptoms worse, you can try to modify your diet in the opposite direction from that listed on the protocol. Unfortunately, there are too many possible combinations to go over at that point, and it becomes far more individualistic, so the best thing to do is experiment each month until you find what works best for you.

Keep in mind that during days 10 to 16, your blood will tend to become more acidic than normal, and from days 18 to 24, your blood will become more alkaline than normal. You may also notice that your symptoms are greatly affected by the temperature outside, so what may work for you during the summer may have to be modified in the winter, and vice versa.

Guidelines for Autumns and Springs during Their Monthly Cycle
Autumns and Springs are not nearly as predictable as Winters and Summers when it comes to blood pH. For this reason, if either of these two season-types suffers from cramping or PMS, it's recommended that Autumns try to follow a protocol similar to the Winter's, and Springs try to follow a protocol similar to the Summer's. If this makes your symptoms worse, you at least know that food is contributing to your cramping or PMS symptoms and can attempt to modify your diet in the opposite direction to alleviate your symptoms. You may need to change your diet for several monthly cycles to find what works best for you. If you live someplace that has large seasonal fluctuations in temperature, just be prepared to discover that what works in the winter months may not work in the summer months and vice versa.

General Guidelines for All Women

All women who are looking for relief from PMS and cramping will find that the more they limit their consumption of fructose, processed vegetable oils, and processed food in general, the fewer symptoms they will have. In primitive cultures where people eat natural foods, women do not suffer from cramping and PMS the way women who eat processed foods do. Even childbirth in these cultures appears to be far easier and much less painful that what Western women experience. You will learn more about the advantages of eating natural foods a bit later.

In general, all women should make sure to take adequate vitamin D, in the form of D_3, if they are taking it in supplement form, because proper vitamin D levels have been shown to alleviate PMS and cramping. In addition, evidence suggests that 75 percent of breast cancer could be prevented with proper vitamin D levels. The recommended range of serum vitamin D levels is between 40 and 60 ng/ml (100–150 nmol/L) and can be measured by a simple blood test.

Men's Health

Men do not suffer from the metabolic consequences of monthly hormonal fluctuations as women do; however, they do suffer from a gradual decline in testosterone levels as they age. Most men, given the choice between muscle strength, high energy levels, and normal sexual function or muscle weakness, low energy levels, and sexual dysfunction, would obviously choose the former. Having adequate testosterone levels is one key to maintaining the positive male traits most men desire.

Multiple studies show that maintaining insulin sensitivity is essential to keeping your testosterone levels and energy levels high. As men become insulin resistant, their testosterone levels begin to drop in a very linear fashion; the more insulin resistant a man becomes, the lower his testosterone levels get. Insulin resistance also impairs mitochondrial function; mitochondria are the energy producers of the cells in our bodies.

The benefits of higher testosterone go beyond simply increasing muscle mass and libido. Bringing low testosterone levels back up to normal lessens the risk of heart disease in men by approximately 60 percent. Testosterone has also been shown to help prevent mental decline in aging men. Good insulin sensitivity is the key to keeping your testosterone levels high, and this can be accomplished by eating according to your season-type, limiting your fructose consumption to 15 grams a day, and avoiding most processed vegetable oils that are high in omega-6 fats. In addition, men should not eat many soy products, as you will read about in Chapter 8.

Part IV
Eat Right For Your Season

8
Reasons to Avoid Soy

Why this so-called wonder food may not be so wonderful.

Eating right for your season-type means eating protein, carbohydrates, and fat in the same proportion that your body prefers to burn for energy. It also means eating the types of protein, carbohydrates, and fat that are best for your season, while limiting those that are detrimental. There are some foods, however, that are detrimental to all of the season-types, and regular consumption of processed soy foods is not recommended as part of the Four Seasons Diet. There is currently a lot of controversy surrounding the safety of processed soy foods for human health. Many scientific studies have been conducted on soy, and although some research suggests there are positive benefits to consuming soy, other studies demonstrate that eating soy products causes some very serious health problems. Controversy even exists concerning whether it should be legal to add soy protein isolates to food. According to many soy opponents, modern processed soy protein products, such as soy protein isolate, never properly received GRAS status from the U.S. government for use as a food additive. GRAS status means that a food is "generally recognized as safe" for human consumption. It's up to all of us to make our own decisions about whether to include soy as a regular part of our diet, so I'll do my best to provide some history and scientific facts about soy. Then you can make an informed choice.

The Use of Soy in Ancient Times

Sixty years ago, it was nearly impossible to find foods containing soy in the United States, with the exception of hydrogenated soybean oil and soy sauce. Currently, however, soy in some form is contained in many foods, such as bread, nutrition bars, soy milk, tofu, canned tuna, and a host of processed foods. Historically, soy was not grown as a "food crop" but as a "cover crop." Cover crops are plants that are used to increase soil fertility, as opposed to plants that are a source of food. Growing food crops such as wheat or rice depletes the soil of nitrogen, and in order to keep farmland

279

productive, the soil's nitrogen needs to be replenished. Although this is now often done with man-made fertilizers, for most of human history that was not possible.

Ancient farmers relied on manure from cows and other animals, along with cover crops, which were known as "green-manure," due to their ability to replenish nitrogen in the soil, as animal manures do. Cover crops are plants that have a unique ability to pull nitrogen out of the air and bring it down into the soil, where it can be used in the future by plants that need it. Soybean cultivation originated in China thousands of years ago when the Chinese discovered that soy served as an excellent cover crop. The soybeans were not eaten in large quantities, except in times of great famine, because the ancient Chinese had probably figured out that natural soybeans are quite detrimental to human health, even if they are boiled or cooked. Eating unfermented soy products would have caused people serious gastric distress, along with other noticeable physical health consequences. Usually, most of the soybeans were plowed back into the soil, to help increase the fertility of the land.

At some point, the Chinese discovered that if soybeans were fermented for a long period of time, many of the harmful compounds they contained were greatly reduced. These harmful compounds are the opposite of nutrients that help nourish the human body and are referred to as *anti-nutrients*. Gradually, the use of soybeans as a cover crop and an ingredient in fermented foods spread throughout Asia. Contrary to popular belief, however, Asians did not and do not consume large amounts of foods that contain soybeans. In Japan, for example, only a few teaspoons of soy foods are eaten per person each day, usually in the form of fermented foods such as miso, soy sauce, and natto. In Asia, foods derived from soybeans have typically been served as condiments and generally not as a main course. Yet even though fermenting soy into foods for condiments destroys many anti-nutrients, it does not completely eliminate them.

Anti-Nutrients in Soy

Soybeans are now highly processed to reduce the levels of these anti-nutrients, but processing cannot get rid of all of them. In fact, soy is considered one of the foods most likely to cause an allergic response in many people. A number of anti-nutrients contained in soy are worthy of further discussion.

Trypsin Inhibitors: Anti-Nutrients That Inhibit Protein Digestion and Cause Pancreatic Stress

Soybeans are very high in trypsin inhibitors, which hinder the body's ability to properly digest protein. Although many foods contain trypsin inhibitors, they are usually deactivated when foods are cooked. What makes soy unique is its high level of trypsin inhibitors, along with the fact that cooking and processing do not fully get rid of these potentially harmful anti-nutrients, as occurs in other foods. The most effective way to eliminate these harmful compounds may be the old-fashioned fermentation techniques that are used to make products such as soy sauce, miso, natto, and tempeh. Modern processors rely on extra heating, rather than using the more lengthy and expensive ancient fermentation techniques. The problem with the modern processing techniques is that excess heating will damage the proteins contained in soy, which can make it hard for the body to properly digest and assimilate them. The solution that modern processors have come up with is to heat soybeans long enough to destroy many of the trypsin inhibitors but not long enough to severely damage the proteins. As a result, most commercially available products made with soy contain a reduced, yet still high, level of trypsin inhibitors. Although the soy industry says this reduced level is adequate to protect human health, many health experts feel this degree of reduction is not enough. In fact, one of the leading experts on trypsin inhibitors (Professor Irvin Liener) was so worried about the amounts of these harmful anti-nutrients that remained in modern processed soy products that he wrote to the FDA in 1998 expressing his concerns. In the letter, he states,

> I would like to take issue with the information found on page 62979 as it pertains to the risk of human exposure to trypsin inhibitors. The impression one gets from reading this section is that there is little cause for concern as far as the human exposure to soybean trypsin inhibitors is concerned. What is particularly disturbing is the fact that no reference is made to any of the articles which I have published which questions [sic] the safety of soybean trypsin in the human diet.

Professor Liener then lists his four research studies on trypsin inhibitors.

Much of the research done on trypsin inhibitors was conducted on animals, which may be affected differently by these anti-nutrients than humans are. What we really need is more research done on humans, to test the effects that these anti-nutrients have on the human body. In the meantime, the soy industry is claiming that the level of anti-nutrients in soy is low enough that there is no reason to be alarmed, while Professor Liener warns that there is cause for concern and more testing is needed. If you are going to eat soy foods and want to limit your intake of trypsin inhibitors, try to focus on naturally fermented soy products, such as soy sauce, miso, tempeh, and natto, because they come much closer to deactivating trypsin inhibitors than modern processing techniques do.

Trypsin inhibitors can be especially hard on the pancreas, because they make it harder for the pancreas to produce the trypsin and the proteases the body needs. The pancreas often compensates for excess amounts of this anti-nutrient by actually increasing both the number of cells the pancreas contains and its overall size. All of this causes pancreatic stress, which, according to some experts, can lead to pancreatitis, as well as to pancreatic cancer. In fact, many health experts have expressed concern that the rise in deaths from pancreatic cancer in America has mirrored the rise in our consumption of soy. During the 1980s, researchers who studied the damage done to the pancreas by these anti-nutrients and noted the rapid increase in pancreatic deaths began to question whether there was a connection to the trypsin inhibitors contained in modern processed soy foods. Once again, more research is needed to determine whether processed soy foods are safe for human consumption and to ascertain whether there is a connection between pancreatic cancer and the trypsin and protease inhibitors contained in soy.

The soy industry claims that trypsin and protease inhibitors in soy products do not pose a risk to human health. If you do your own research on soy, you are likely to find many sites sponsored by the soy industry that seem at odds with much of what I am saying. For example, the Soyfoods Association of North America consists of members that have an interest in promoting soy, such as Archer Daniels Midland, Boca Foods (a subsidiary of Kraft), Kellogg Company, White Wave (Silk Soymilk), and many other companies that produce soy foods. Part of the association's stated mission is to promote the growth of the soy foods industry by "proactively promoting and upholding the benefits of soy-based foods to consumers, health professionals, researchers, media, government officials, and industry partners." The Soyfoods Association maintains a website at http://www.soyfoods.org/soy-information/faq, which presents information in a question-and-answer format. On May 12, 2012, the website contained the following statements regarding protease inhibitors, as question 11 of the question-and-answer section.

> **11. What are trypsin inhibitors and are there any risks associated with consuming either [sic] trypsin inhibitors? What is lysinoalanine, and are there any risks associated with consuming lysinoalanine?**
>
> **Answer:** Trypsin inhibitors are small proteins that are also present in many other plant products including raw legumes, cereals, potatoes, and tomatoes. Some groups have raised questions about the safety of consuming raw soybeans because they contain trypsin inhibitors, which may reduce the efficiency of protein digestion. However, trypsin inhibitors are mostly destroyed when soybeans are heat processed to make soy foods. Therefore, because humans do not consume uncooked soybeans, there are no risks associated with consuming trypsin inhibitors. In addition, small amounts of trypsin inhibitors that remain in a food may have beneficial health effects in reducing tumor growth and preventing the spread of some cancers.
>
> Lysinoalanine is an amino acid that is found in proteins of cooked foods. Some have questioned the safety of the lysinoalanine in soy, but proper processing of soybeans minimizes any formation of lysinoalanine. (17 – 19) Lysinoalanine may be produced during modern processing; however, no evidence of adverse effects such as kidney lesions have ever been associated with human [sic—humans] consuming lysinoalanine or processed soybeans.

At the end of the statement, the association cites Research Studies 17–19, which stands for three sources it is quoting when making this claim.

    To the average reader, it would appear that there are three sources that back up the Soyfoods Association's claim that there are no risks associated with consuming trypsin inhibitors. I wanted to be fair to both sides of the soy debate, so I decided to track down these sources. I was expecting to find studies that claimed that the level of trypsin inhibitors in processed soy foods was safe for human health. Instead, the studies actually say the following:

Research Study #17: "Compositional Changes in Trypsin Inhibitors, Phytic Acid, Saponins, and Isoflavones Related to Soybean Processing"

This article breaks down the quantity of trypsin inhibitors left in soy after processing. Remember, the Soyfoods Association of America website claims, "However, trypsin inhibitors are mostly destroyed when soybeans are heat processed to make soy foods. Therefore, because humans do not consume uncooked soybeans, there are no risks associated with consuming trypsin inhibitors."

    This research article gives the following numbers on trypsin inhibitors in soybeans and soy products. I have rounded to the nearest whole number.

Sample	Mg/g
Whole soybeans	17–27
Raw soy flour	28–32
Toasted soy flour	8–9
Soy protein concentrate	5–7
Soy protein isolate	1–30

    Note that soy protein concentrate has about 30 percent of the original trypsin inhibitors contained in raw soybeans. The implication of the Soyfoods Association's statement, two paragraphs above, is contradicted by the data in this research study, because there *is* a risk of consuming a high level of trypsin inhibitors in soy protein isolate, so people don't have to eat raw soybeans to consume those anti-nutrients. The Soyfoods Association also states that "some groups have raised questions about the safety of consuming raw soybeans." First, there is almost universal agreement that consuming raw soybeans is not healthy. Second, most of the groups raising concerns about trypsin inhibitors in soybeans are not worried about raw soybeans because these are seldom consumed, but rather they do care about the high levels of trypsin inhibitors that remain in processed soy foods. These health experts feel that the 30 percent of trypsin inhibitors that remain in many processed soy foods are still serious cause for alarm.

Soy contains extremely high levels of trypsin inhibitors that are also very heat stable, which means they are not easy to eliminate by processing. The Soyfoods Association states that trypsin inhibitors are present in many foods, including potatoes. Though this is technically true, what they fail to tell you is that the level of trypsin inhibitors in these foods is much less than in soy, and that in other foods, trypsin inhibitors are largely destroyed by cooking. For example, boiling sweet potatoes for 15 minutes was found to deactivate nearly 100 percent of the trypsin activity. What is most disturbing about many statements made by people in the soy industry is that while their statements may be "technically true," if you fully understand what they are saying, the average person reading many of these statements will be led to believe something that is often very far from the truth.

Research Study #18: "The Bowman-Birk Inhibitor from Soybeans as an Anticarcinogenic Agent"
There are many protease inhibitors in soy. The one that affects protein digestion is the trypsin inhibitor. Another protease inhibitor is the Bowman-Birk inhibitor, which is the one this article is referencing. This article is about the potential of a purified extract of the Bowman-Birk inhibitor (called BBIC or Bowman-Birk inhibitor concentrate) as a potential cancer therapy and is not about consuming soy for anticancer benefits. In fact, this study states that "there are several agents in soybeans, soybean flour, and various commercial preparations of soybeans that can enhance the development of cancer. These compounds are removed from BBIC."

In spite of this statement, the Soyfoods Association states that "in addition, small amounts of trypsin inhibitors that remain in a food may have beneficial health effects in reducing tumor growth and preventing the spread of some cancers." Hopefully, you now see how studies are being cleverly spun in order to promote soy. Although the Soyfoods Association's statement may be "technically correct," most people will be easily confused by it and will likely think that the statement has a different meaning.

Research Study #19: "Lysinoalanine in Food and in Antimicrobial Proteins"

This article has to do with a compound in processed soy called lysinoalanine, which is different from protease inhibitors, so the Soyfoods Association's citing of the article to support its argument for the safety of consuming protease inhibitors in soy foods is inaccurate.

Soy Isoflavones: Beneficial or Harmful?

Most of the positive press that soy has received lately concerns its high concentration of another anti-nutrient called *isoflavones*. The isoflavones contained in soy have received a lot of media coverage regarding their possible beneficial effects on minimizing the risk for developing breast cancer. To understand why many health professionals have concerns about isoflavones, however, you first need to understand what they are and why they are contained in plants in the first place.

Isoflavones, also known as *phytoestrogens*, are compounds found in many plants that are very similar in nature to human estrogen. The best theory currently as to why many plants are high in phytoestrogens is that they act as nature's way of keeping herbivores from overpopulating a specific area by controlling fertility. This theory states that as herbivores begin to overpopulate an area, they are forced to eat plants that have high amounts of phytoestrogens. Herbivores would usually ignore these plants when there is no scarcity of food, in favor of choosing plants that do not contain high levels of these anti-nutrients. The theory is that these phytoestrogens affect herbivores in such as way as to keep them from reproducing, which brings the population back to a more sustainable level. For example, it was found that sheep in Australia that ate large amounts of clover, a plant high in isoflavones, became infertile. There are stories of Buddhist monks who took vows of celibacy and ate large amounts of soy foods because soy was found to decrease their sexual desires. Many health experts believe that the isoflavones in soy helped diminish the monks' sexual urges.

Just as there are two conflicting beliefs about trypsin inhibitors and human health, there are also two opposing arguments about whether isoflavones are helpful or harmful to humans. In the Bibliography, I have listed all of the research articles that I used to support my arguments. When discussing both sides of the soy debate, I also gave the exact titles of many articles in this chapter. I did this because while researching soy, I became disturbed by comments made by many medical professionals, who basically said that not a single study has been conducted that shows soy to be harmful. I wanted to help readers refute those comments. If you choose to research soy on your own, you will come across many websites that promote soy, often paid for by the soy industry, which cite the positive research and often claim there is no negative research. As you will discover in this chapter, however, while many studies do show possible benefits from eating soy foods, many others also demonstrate potentially serious and harmful effects from consuming the anti-nutrients contained in soy.

The isoflavones produced by soybeans are close enough to human estrogen that they can latch onto the receptor sites normally used by human estrogen, effectively blocking human estrogen. Because they are not identical to human estrogen, however, they can have a very different effect on the human body, and this is what the proponents claim produces the benefits and what the opponents say causes all of the harm.

The first round in the isoflavone debate probably goes to the opponents of soy, because the human body was designed to use human estrogen, not plant estrogen, and after I researched both sides of the debate, it became clear that a lot of research is still necessary before the full truth about soy isoflavones is known. In cases such as this, it's better to err on the side of caution.

Isoflavones and Breast Cancer
Many women are currently making an effort to consume products that contain soy isoflavones because they have been told that it will help reduce their risk of developing breast cancer. Perhaps the most famous study concerning isoflavones and breast cancer was the Shanghai Women's Health Study, which was conducted from 1997 to 2002 and consisted of surveys done on approximately 75,000 women. This study asked women what foods they had eaten in the previous year, as well as during their adolescence, and then followed up at later dates to see which women ended up getting cancer. A good summary of this study is in the following research article:

Research Study: "Adolescent and Adult Soy Food Intake and Breast Cancer Risk: Results from the Shanghai Women's Health Study"
This study found a small but statistically significant association between the consumption of soy and a lower risk of breast cancer among premenopausal women. This study also analyzed other

studies that had been done on the association between breast cancer risk and the consumption of soy foods. Of the eleven studies that analyzed "white women" (i.e., Western studies vs. Asian studies), only one study found that soy consumption was associated with a lower risk of breast cancer. The other ten studies found no such association. The Asian studies were more likely to show that soy consumption was associated with a lower risk of breast cancer; however, this study admits that those studies inevitability suffer from what is called *selection and recall biases*. When this study looked at women who had been diagnosed with breast cancer and compared them with cancer-free women, it found significant differences in education, occupation, and diets. For example the cancer-free women ate more soy but also ate more fruits and vegetables. The women with breast cancer who did not eat as much soy also had almost double the positive family history of breast cancer, when compared to the cancer-free women. This, of course, makes you wonder how much of the breast cancer was caused by the higher family history of breast cancer, along with a lower consumption of fruits and vegetables, and how much was due to a lower consumption of soy. The researchers state that "high soy intake could be related to certain lifestyles that may be associated with reduced risks of breast cancer." This study made a good effort to look at other studies and said that a study of 37,643 British women found no association between dietary isoflavones and breast cancer.

As mentioned earlier, many medical experts claim that no studies exist that show isoflavones to be potentially harmful. Here is a brief summary of some of those "nonexistent" studies:

Research Study: "Physiological Concentrations of Dietary Genistein Dose-Dependently Stimulate Growth of Estrogen-Dependent Human Breast Cancer (MCF-7) Tumors Implanted in Athymic Nude Mice"_

This study was an expansion of previous studies that showed that the soy isoflavone genistein actually stimulates the growth of human breast cancer cells, in both isolated cells and living organisms. The study was designed to see what response various doses of genistein would have on mice. The study found that the dietary isoflavone genistein actually increased the tumor size in a dose-dependent manner, meaning the higher the dose of isoflavones, the larger the increase in tumor size.

Other studies have also suggested that soy isoflavones can

increase the rate at which breast cancer grows, as well as hinder the treatment of breast cancer. For example,

Research Study: "Phytoestrogens and Breast Cancer: A Complex Story"
This study examined the effect that the dietary isoflavone genistein has on estrogen-dependent breast cancer growth. It found that this isoflavone enhances human breast cancer tumor growth, and that the tumors regressed when the isoflavones were removed from the diet. It also looked at what effect this isoflavone has on breast cancer therapy, such as tamoxifen, a drug commonly used to treat breast cancer. It found that the isoflavone negated the ability of tamoxifen to inhibit breast cancer growth. Sadly, many women who are diagnosed with breast cancer increase their consumption of soy or actually buy isoflavone supplements, in the belief this will help in their battle with breast cancer—though it appears this is the last thing they should do.

Other studies have found similar results. For example,

Research Study: "Phytoestrogen Concentration Determines Effects on DNA Synthesis in Human Breast Cancer Cells"
The data in this study suggested the possibility that "at typical concentrations in humans, phytoestrogens and related flavonoids and lignans stimulate, rather than inhibit, growth of estrogen-dependant tumors."

Another study done on women with breast cancer found similar results:

Research Study: "Effects of Soy-Protein Supplementation on Epithelial Proliferation in the Histologically Normal Human Breast"
This study consisted of women with either benign or malignant breast epithelial proliferation. The women randomly received either a normal diet or a diet with 60 grams of soy supplements containing 45 mg of isoflavones for 14 days. After only 14 days, the women receiving the soy isoflavones had a significantly increased proliferation of breast lobular epithelium. The study found that "short-term dietary soy stimulates breast epithelial proliferation."

Another study found that soy protein could possibly inhibit the body's own immune system from targeting and killing breast cancer:

Research Study: "Low Concentrations of the Soy Phytoestrogen Genistein Induce Proteinase Inhibitor 9 and Block Killing of Breast Cancer Cells by Immune Cells"
This study found that the isoflavone genistein "inhibits the ability of human natural killer (NK) cells to lyse and target breast cancer cells." The study went on to say that "moderate levels of dietary genistein and soy flour effectively induce PI-9 in human breast cancers grown in ovarectomized athymic mice. A significant population consumes levels of genistein in soy products that may be high enough to induce PI-9, perhaps potentiating the survival of some preexisting breast cancers by enabling them to evade immunosurveillance."

Another study found that the isoflavone genistein can cause breast cancer to grow:

Research Study: "Dietary Genistein Stimulates Growth of Estrogen-Dependent Breast Cancer Tumors Similar to That Observed with Genistein"
This study found that dietary genistein, an isoflavone, stimulates the growth of estrogen-dependent human breast cancer cells. It also found that when the isoflavone is removed from the diet, the breast cancer tumors would regress.

Isoflavones and Breast Cancer Summary
Although some studies suggest that the consumption of soy isoflavones may help prevent breast cancer, most Western studies found no such correlation. In addition, numerous studies show that isoflavones may actually cause breast cancer to grow faster and may interfere with popular breast cancer treatments, as well as impede the body's own immune system from fighting off the cancer.

Isoflavones and Women's Reproductive Health
One thing that most disturbs many health experts about the rapid increase of soy isoflavones in the human food supply is what effect it may have on the sexual development of children, as well as on human reproductive health in general. Several studies examine the effect that these isoflavones may be having on our reproductive health.

Research Study: "Neonatal Genistein Treatment Alters Ovarian Differentiation in the Mouse: Inhibition of Oocyte Nest

Breakdown and Increased Oocyte Survival"
This study found that the isoflavone genistein altered ovarian differentiation during neonatal development, which could lead to alterations in normal ovarian development, possibly hindering normal ovarian function.

While the previous study examined the effect isoflavones have on ovarian function, another study looked at the effect isoflavones have on uterine function:

Research Study: "Dietary Soy Protein and Isoflavones Have No Significant Effect on Bone and a Potentially Negative Effect on the Uterus of Sexually Mature Intact Sprague-Dawley Female Rats"
This study looked at the effect of feeding soy protein and isoflavones to rats. It found that these may have "an adverse effect on the uterus." This is because the 10 percent of the rats fed soy protein and 20 percent of the rats fed isoflavones showed extensive squamous metaplasia in the uterine gland. This means that there were benign changes in the delicate linings of the uterus.

Remember the Buddhist monks who ate soy to help lower their sexual urges and enable them to keep their celibacy vows? An article in the *New Scientist* (vol. 17, no. 45 [November 14, 2003]) states that soy supplements can decrease normal sexual behavior in female rats by as much as 70 percent. According to the article, rats were given doses of isoflavone supplements similar to what many women take. After being fed small doses of soy supplements, the female rats decreased their "encouraging behaviors" to male rats by 70 percent and decreased their "receptive behaviors" by up to 40 percent.

Although many women may get a chuckle out of this last paragraph and change their "Sorry, honey, I have a headache" excuse to "Sorry, honey, I just ate soy," the following studies concerning soy and women's fertility issues are no laughing matter:

Research Study: "Reproductive Effects in Male and Female Rats of Neonatal Exposure to Genistein"
This study administered genistein to rats postnatally for five days after birth, to determine the effects on reproductive function after puberty. The female rats exposed to the higher levels of genistein for only five days showed estrous cycle irregularities. Their fertility was disrupted, and when their ovaries and uterus were examined under a microscope, they showed anatomical changes.

The results indicated that just five days of exposure to genistein caused both abnormal developments of the ovaries in female rats and dysfunction in post-pubertal reproductive performance.

Other studies link early exposure to soy isoflavones to uterine cancer:

Research Study: "Uterine Adenocarcinoma in Mice Treated Neonatally with Genistein"
This study exposed female rats to genistein for the first five days after birth. At eighteen months of age, 35 percent of the rats exposed to genistein had uterine cancer. The study stated that "these data suggest that genistein is carcinogenic if exposure occurs during critical periods of differentiation. Thus the use of soy-based infant formulas in the absence of medical necessity and the marketing of soy products designed to appeal to children should be closely examined."

What is most disturbing about these last two studies is that there were serious consequences to female rats' reproductive systems after they were exposed to genistein for only five days. It begs the question, what is the effect of feeding a baby girl soy-based formula for the first full year of her life? The following study made an attempt to figure out exactly what those effects would be:

Research Study: "Adverse Effects on Female Development and Reproduction in CD-1 Mice Following Neonatal Exposure to the Phytoestrogen Genistein at Environmentally Relevant Doses"
This study treated mice with genistein, the primary isoflavone in soy milk, for the first five days after birth. It had four groups of rats, consisting of a control group that received no genistein, a group that received a low dose of genistein, one that received a moderate dose, and one that received a high dose. The mice treated with genistein had prolonged estrous cycles with both dose- and age-related increases in severity. The female rats that had received the moderate and higher doses of genistein for only five days showed significant decreases in the number of live pups. For example, although 100 percent of the control group that received no genistein delivered live pups at 6 months, only 60 percent of the group that received low amounts of genistein did, 40 percent of the group that received the moderate dose did, and a shocking 0 percent of the group that received the higher dose delivered live pups at 6 months. Even though 60 percent of the mice that had received the higher dose of genistein were

determined to be fertile at 2 months, they were unable to maintain their pregnancies. The study stated in summary that "neonatal treatment with genistein caused abnormal estrous cycles, altered ovarian function, early reproductive senescence, and sub-fertility/ infertility at environmentally relevant doses."

Remember that this was after only five days of receiving genistein, and one of the things that makes this study so shocking is that many of the doses that affected fertility were relevant to what a baby on soy formula might receive. Doses of genistein are typically calculated based on the milligrams of genistein per kilogram of body weight. A baby receiving soy formula is estimated to receive between 6 and 9 mg of genistein per kg of body weight. This number is slightly higher than the amount given to the mice who received the moderate amount of genistein in the experiment mentioned previously, and only 40 percent of these mice delivered live pups at 6 months, compared to 100 percent of mice that received no genistein.

Research Study: "Neonatal Phytoestrogen Exposure Alters Oviduct Mucosal Immune Response to Pregnancy and Affects Preimplantation Embryo Development in the Mouse"
This study looked at the effect of treating neonatal mice with the phytoestrogen genistein. It demonstrated that "a brief neonatal exposure to the genistein causes substantial permanent changes in oviduct morphology, gene expression, and function in adulthood." The study found that treatment of neonatal mice with genistein "results in complete female infertility that is caused in part by preimplantation embryo loss in the oviduct between days 2 and 3 of pregnancy."

The potential reproductive effects of soy are one of the many reasons I cannot recommend it as part of the Four Seasons Diet until more studies are done to determine whether soy consumption is safe for human health.
There have been several studies done on women that tested the effects of longer-term consumption of isoflavones:

Research Study: "Endometrial Effects of Long-Term Treatment with Phytoestrogens: A Randomized, Double-Blind, Placebo-Controlled Study"
This study was conducted on 376 postmenopausal healthy women who were split into two groups. One group received 150 mg of isoflavones every day for five years, while the second group received

a placebo. The study concluded that "long-term treatment (up to 5 years) with soy phytoestrogens was associated with an increased occurrence of endometrial hyperplasia. These findings call into question the long-term safety of phytoestrogens with regard to the endometrium."

Isoflavones and Men's Health

Many men who have just read the last section are probably wondering how these isoflavone estrogens may be affecting their health. There has been much press about how soy may help lower a man's risk of prostate cancer; however, those press reports often fail to talk about what effect that same soy is having on a man's testosterone and estrogen levels. As mentioned earlier, clover disease is a fertility problem in male sheep that eat clover, which is high in isoflavones. The isoflavones actually make the sheep infertile, and many health experts have expressed concerns about isoflavones and men's sex drive and fertility. Studies show that both may be affected by consuming soy products. For example,

Research Study: "Effects of Replacing Meat with Soyabean in the Diet on Sex Hormone Concentrations in Healthy Adult Males"_
This study consisted of 42 healthy adult men between the ages of 35 and 62. They were placed on a diet of either lean meat or tofu for four weeks. The study found that men on the tofu diet had a testosterone:estradiol ratio that was 10 percent lower than the men on the meat diet. This ratio is very important to men's health. As men age, their estradiol levels gradually rise, while their testosterone levels gradually fall. This means that as men age, their testosterone:estradiol level gradually falls. So when this study found that men eating tofu had a lower testosterone:estradiol ratio, you can think of it as meaning that the men consuming tofu became hormonally more like men who were elderly. Of course, testosterone gives men many hormonal benefits, which most men prefer to keep. One of the few benefits of a lower testosterone ratio, however, may be a decreased risk of developing prostate cancer, so this is what most men often hear as being the advantage of eating soy. The soy industry spends $80 million a year on promoting soy, and they are not going to tell you about the Buddhist monks, their vows of celibacy, and how soy consumption helped keep their desires in check—something a man could also expect from a lower testosterone:estradiol ratio. Men deserve to have the complete picture, however, so although tofu may help lower your risk of

prostate cancer, it may come at a price that most men would not want pay, unless they have chosen the monastic lifestyle.

A short-term study conducted on rats that were fed isoflavones found a similar demasculinization effect:

Research Study: "Dietary Soy-Phytoestrogens Decrease Testosterone Levels and Prostate Weight without Altering LH, Prostate 5 Alpha-Reductase or Testicular Steroidogenic Acute Regulatory Peptide Levels in Adult Male Sprague-Dawley Rats"
This research study fed rats either an isoflavone-rich diet or an isoflavone-free diet. After five weeks on the diet, the rats fed the isoflavone-rich diet had significantly decreased body weights and prostate weights. They also had testosterone and androstenedione levels that were significantly lower than in the rats fed the isoflavone-free diet. Essentially, the rats that consumed the isoflavones for just five weeks had lower levels of important male hormones and lost size. Once again, this might be good for a Buddhist monk keeping a celibacy vow, but it's not exactly what most men are looking to accomplish. If your only goal as a man is to lower your risk of prostate cancer, however, then soy might make sense for you.

Other studies looked at what effect isoflavones might have on sperm count and quality.

Research Study: "Soy Food and Isoflavone Intake in Relation to Semen Quality Parameters among Men from an Infertility Clinic"
This study assessed the intake of 15 soy-based foods on 99 males. It found an inverse association between the consumption of soy foods and sperm concentration. The men with the highest soy intake had 41 million sperm/ml less than the men who did not consume soy foods. The study concluded that "these data suggest that higher intake of soy foods and soy isoflavones is associated with lower sperm concentration."

Remember that male sheep eating clover that was high in isoflavones became infertile, so it's not surprising that soy isoflavones appear to lower human sperm counts.

Isoflavones and Cognitive Function
There have also been concerns that soy consumption during midlife years might affect brain function later in life. For example,

Research Study: "Brain Aging and Midlife Tofu Consumption"

This study looked at the association between tofu consumption and how it affected brain function later in life. The original study conducted interviews from 1965 to 1967 and 1971 to 1974 and collected information on what foods people were consuming. Between 1991 and 1993, this same group of people had their cognitive function tested. The results showed that those who had consumed larger amounts of tofu in midlife had poorer cognitive performance and a lower brain weight later in life. The study concluded that "in this population, higher midlife tofu consumption was independently associated with indicators of cognitive impairment and brain atrophy."

Another study also showed a decrease in cognitive function from tofu consumption:

Research Study: "High Tofu Intake Is Associated with Worse Memory in Elderly Indonesian Men and Women"
This study measured the memories of 719 people between the ages of 52 and 98. It used a food frequency questionnaire to determine which foods the participants had regularly eaten. This study was conducted in Indonesia, a country where a fermented soy product called tempeh is often eaten. The study found that "high tofu consumption was associated with worse memory, while high tempeh consumption was independently related to better memory." The study concludes that "the results for tofu consumption as a risk factor for low memory function may tie in with the Honolulu Asia Aging Study data. It is unclear whether these negative associations could be attributed to potential toxins or to its phytoestrogen levels. Estrogen was found to increase dementia risk in women over 65 years of age."

People in the soy industry claim that soy isoflavones may enhance short-term memory in women. They cite the following study:

Research Study: "Cognitive Improvement after 6 Weeks of Soy Supplements in Postmenopausal Women Is Limited to Frontal Lobe Function"
This study assessed the effects of six weeks of treatment with soy supplements on mood, menopausal symptoms, and cognition in postmenopausal women who were not taking other forms of hormone therapy. The results showed that the women who received the soy supplements had better short-term nonverbal memory and better performance on two tests of frontal lobe function.

This is the study that the soy industry likes to cite when it claims that isoflavones may enhance short-term memory. What's important to keep in mind with this study, however, is that the researchers gave isoflavones to menopausal women who were not receiving hormone replacement therapy, and isoflavones are essentially like a natural form of hormone replacement. This study also gave them soy supplements for only six weeks. So, essentially, you can say that postmenopausal women not on hormone replacement who take isoflavones for six weeks will have better frontal lobe function.

Contrast this with the first study that looked at what foods people were consuming in the late 1960s and early 1970s and then followed up with those people in the early 1990s to see what effect isoflavone consumption in midlife had on cognitive function later in life. One study reveals what the long-term effects may be from eating tofu, while the other study states what the short-term effects may be for menopausal women who use isoflavones as a form of pseudo estrogen-replacement therapy.

Phytic Acid: An Anti-Nutrient That Impedes Mineral Absorption
Many foods, including grains and beans, contain a substance called *phytic acid,* also referred to as *phytate.* What makes soy unique is that it has an incredibly high level of phytic acid that is resistant to being broken down. The long, slow cooking of most grains will reduce the levels of phytic acid much more than the same type of cooking will do to soy. Fermentation is the most effective way to reduce these anti-nutrients in soy, which is the technique used historically in Asia for making miso, natto, soy sauce, and tempeh. When phytic acid is not destroyed by cooking, it can greatly impede the absorption of crucial minerals, such as calcium, iron, and zinc, from the foods we eat. Several studies have been conducted to determine the effect of this anti-nutrient on calcium absorption. For example,

Research Study: "Soybean Phytate Content: Effect on Calcium Absorption"
This study administered test meals to 16 healthy women between the ages of 20 and 45 to look at the effect of various levels of soy phytates on calcium absorption. The study says that "it is clear that phytate content had a definite and highly significant effect on calcium absorbability."

THE FOUR SEASONS DIET

Research Study: "Effects of Purified Phytate and Phytate-Rich Bread upon Metabolism of Zinc, Calcium, Phosphorous, and Nitrogen in Man"

This study looked at the effect of feeding people phytic acid, along with their bread. It found that the phytic acid increased the losses of zinc and upset calcium balances. The study states, "The results suggest that high-phytate intakes can cause the disturbances of zinc and calcium metabolism."

Research Study: "Soy Protein, Phytate, and Iron Absorption in Humans"

This study looked at the effect soy's phytic acid had on iron absorption in 32 human subjects. It found that "iron absorption increased four- to fivefold when phytic acid was reduced from its native amount of 4.9–8.4 to less than .01 mg/g of isolate." It found that "even after removal of virtually all the phytic acid, iron absorption from the soy-protein meal was still only half that of the egg white control."

Soy processors often claim that their processing techniques get rid of many of these harmful anti-nutrients; however, independent studies have found otherwise:

Research Study: "Compositional Changes in Trypsin Inhibitors, Phytic Acid, Saponins and Isoflavones Related to Soybean Processing"

This study analyzed raw soybeans and processed soybeans for a variety of anti-nutrients. It found that processed soybean products, such as textured vegetable protein and soy protein isolate, contain an amount of phytic acid that is comparable to that of raw soybeans. For example, fifteen different soy protein isolates were analyzed, and they were found to contain between 9.7 and 16.9 mg/g of phytic acid. The study mentioned before this one found that "even relatively small quantities of residual phytate were strongly inhibitory, and phytic acid had to be reduced to less than .3 mg/g of isolate before a meaningful increase in iron absorption." The analysis this study did on soy shows that processed soy has thirty times this amount of phytic acid.

The soy industry claims that phytic acid does not cause problems with mineral absorption when a person's diet is adequate in zinc, iron, and calcium. For example, the Soyfoods Association of North America website (May 12, 2012, http://www.soyfoods. org/soy-information/faq) made the following statements regarding phytic acid as question number 29 of its question-and-answer section.

29. Does phytic acid, which is found in soy, cause problems with mineral absorption?

Answer: No, when people's diets are adequate in zinc, iron, and calcium, phytates from soy or other vegetables and grains do not present a problem with mineral bioavailability. Phytic acid, a component of all plants, has benefits and detractions. Phytic acid affects mineral bioavailability, particularly zinc, iron, calcium and copper. It has the capability of forming complexes with these elements, making them less available. Possible beneficial effects of phytic acid include its antioxidant property, which reduces free radical formation. Phytic acid has been shown to have positive effects on lowering serum cholesterol and triglycerides, suppressing iron-mediated oxidation and preventing some cancers. (76 – 81)

At the end of the statement, the Soyfoods Association cites Research Studies 76–81, which stands for five sources being quoting when this claim was made. The average reader would most likely believe that based on this statement, phytic acid does not cause problems with mineral absorption and may actually be beneficial as an antioxidant. To many readers, it would appear that the Soyfoods Association has five sources that back up its claim that phytic acid does not cause problems with mineral absorption. Most readers will not bother to track down these sources. Yet I found it hard believe such sources existed, given what I know about phytic acid, so I decided to look up these sources. I will list them in order, from number 76 through number 81, with a brief summary of what the sources say about phytic acid.

Research Study # 76: "The Influence of Different Cereal Grains on Iron Absorption from Infant Cereal Foods"
This study states that "there was a strong inverse correlation between iron absorption and the phytate content of the different cereals." Basically, the higher the level of phytic acid, the lower the iron absorption. It goes on to state that reducing the amount of phytic acid is likely to improve iron availability significantly.

Research Study # 77: "Approaches to Improve Iron Bioavailability

from Complementary Foods"

This article states that "Different approaches to improve iron bioavailability from plant-based complementary foods, e.g., by enzymatic degradation of phytic acid and/or by increased consumption of ascorbic acid-rich foods, should be explored and adapted to local conditions." Basically, it is saying you can improve iron absorption if you lower the phytic acid content.

Research Study # 78: **"Degradation of Phytic Acid in Cereal Porridges Improves Iron Absorption by Human Subjects"**

This study states, "Phytic acid in cereal-based and legume-based complementary foods inhibits iron absorption. Low iron absorption from cereal porridges contributes to the high prevalence of iron deficiency in infants from developing countries." After conducting their study on removing phytic acid from food, the researchers conclude that "phytate degradation improves iron absorption from cereal porridges prepared with water but not with milk, except from high-tannin sorghum." Once again, you can improve iron absorption if you can get rid of the phytic acid.

Research Study # 79: **"Influence of Vegetable Protein Sources on Trace Element and Mineral Bioavailability"**

This study says, "Phytic acid is a strong inhibitor of iron absorption in both infants and adults," and that "decreasing phytic acid by 90% (100 mg/100g) would be expected to increase absorption about twofold and complete degradation perhaps fivefold or more." It is basically saying that reducing phytic acid levels to 100 mg per 100 g will double the iron absorption. Independent studies on fifteen samples of soy protein isolate show that the level of phytic acid is between 970 and 1,690 mg per 100 g. This current study claims that phytic acid should be reduced to one-tenth the amount present in soy protein isolate. The study goes on to state that "complete enzymatic degradation of phytic acid is recommended." Basically, it is recommending that no phytic acid at all is best.

Research Study #80: This reference is to a 773-page dietary intake manual, so there is no way of knowing which page they are referencing or how they are using this source material.

Research Study # 81: **"Phytic Acid in Health and Disease"**

This study states that "phytic acid has the strong ability to chelate multivalent metal ions, especially zinc, calcium, and iron. The binding can result in very insoluble salts that are poorly absorbed from the gastrointestinal tract, which results in poor bioavailability (BV) of minerals. Alternatively, the ability of phytic acid to chelate minerals has been reported to have some protective effects, such as decreasing iron-mediated colon cancer risk and lowering serum cholesterol and triglycerides in experimental animals. Data from human studies are still lacking. PA is also considered to be a natural antioxidant and is suggested to have potential functions of reducing lipid peroxidation and as a preservative in foods. "

This study states in no uncertain terms that phytic acid will inhibit mineral absorption. Although it says there might be some positive benefits, such as phytic acid acting as an antioxidant, why would you want to use an antioxidant that kept you from absorbing minerals? Just eat your vegetables and fruits, and you can get your antioxidants without having the negative impact from ingesting phytic acid.

Goitrogens: Anti-Nutrients That Target the Thyroid

Soy foods are particularly high in anti-nutrients called *goitrogens*, which block the synthesis of thyroid hormones. Many health experts claim that the isoflavones and the saponins in soybeans can act as goitrogens, and that these harmful anti-nutrients are generally not removed by most processing techniques. In fact, an analysis done on raw soybeans vs. processed soybean products shows that processed products often have a higher level of these anti-nutrients than raw soybeans do. For example, raw soybeans were found to contain between 2.2 and 3.3 mg/g of saponins. Soy protein isolate was found to contain 8.1 mg/g, soymilk had 3.9 mg/g, and tofu had from 3.0 to 3.3 mg/g of this potentially harmful anti-nutrient. This is because processing often eliminates the oil, while concentrating the protein, the nutrients, and the anti-nutrients.

According to many health experts, isoflavones inhibit the enzyme *thyroid peroxidase*, which is involved in the synthesis of the thyroid hormones T3 and T4. These hormones are crucial in enabling you to maintain energy and stay lean. Anything that affects our thyroid hormones has the potential to make us fat and lethargic. Several of the FDA's top experts on soy (Daniel Doerge and Daniel Sheehan) have also been sounding the alarm about soy and thyroid health and actually wrote a protest letter to their own agency, a rare and bold move for any scientist involved in the highly political world of government science to make.

These two scientists work for the FDA's national center for toxicological research, and one is the director of the estrogen base program. They were against giving soy any "health claim" because they felt there was abundant evidence that some of the isoflavones found in soy demonstrate toxicity in estrogen-sensitive tissues, as well as in the thyroid gland. They cited multiple research articles, in which the isoflavones present in soy are found to act as estrogenic endocrine disruptors during development. In the studies cited, these isoflavones were found to cause a variety of serious malformations and functional deficits in both animals and humans. The conclusion of these FDA estrogen experts was that no dose was without risk, and that the extent of risk was a function of the dose. They were very concerned that isoflavones cause problems with the thyroid gland, including inhibition of the thyroid hormones T3 and T4, along with goiter. They cited multiple studies documenting the goitrogenic effects from soy consumption in human infants. They also voiced concerns that soy isoflavones cause vascular dementia.

Research Study: "The Effects on the Thyroid Gland of Soybeans Administered Experimentally in Healthy Subjects"
The purpose of this study was to determine what effect dietary soybeans would have on thyroid function. They gave 30 grams a day of pickled soybeans to three separate groups for a period of one to three months. The study concluded that "these findings suggested that excessive soybean ingestion for a certain duration might suppress thyroid function and cause goiters in healthy people, especially elderly subjects."

Although studies done on rats suggest that these antithyroid effects from soy consumption occur only in conjunction with iodine deficiency, this study suggests otherwise. It posits that goiter and hypothyroid can occur in humans ingesting soy even in the absence of an iodine deficiency.

As mentioned earlier, soy isoflavones are thought to hinder thyroid function by inhibiting the key enzyme thyroid peroxidase. One study sought to determine the exact effect that soy isoflavones had on this essential thyroid enzyme:

Research Study: "Dietary Genistein Inactivates Rat Thyroid Peroxidase in Vivo without an Apparent Hypothyroid Effect"
This study gave rats various doses of the isoflavone genistein. It found that the activity of the enzyme thyroid peroxidase was

reduced by up to 80 percent, and the higher the dose of isoflavones, the more the thyroid peroxidase was reduced. Soy is now added to many types of animal feed, and these researchers found that rats consuming the standard soy-based rodent diet had thyroid peroxidase activity that was 50 percent lower than rats that consumed a soy-free diet.

As mentioned earlier, some studies suggest these antithyroid effects from soy occur only if a person is iodine deficient, while other studies say that even people with adequate iodine will experience antithyroid affects from consuming soy. Even if the studies are true in suggesting that an iodine deficiency is necessary in order for soy to have antithyroid effects, there are still major reasons for concern. First, it's been estimated that up to 25 percent of the U.S. population is iodine deficient, so these people may be especially vulnerable to the antithyroid effects of soy isoflavones. Second, up to 10 percent of elderly women are already thought to be in a subclinical thyroid state, so these women may also be affected more negatively when they consume soy.

Most Soy Foods in the United States Are Made from Genetically Modified (GM) Soy

It has been estimated that approximately 90 percent of all of the soy produced in the United States has been genetically modified. Later, I devote an entire section to genetically modified foods and why they should be avoided.

Soy History, Continued

The previously mentioned four major anti-nutrients in soy do not constitute all of the anti-nutrients believed to be in processed soy products. There is currently a fierce debate going on about whether soy foods are safe for human consumption. While some research articles suggest there are possible benefits from consuming soy, other research articles state that potentially serious negative effects occur from consuming soy.

Given the numerous scientific concerns about soy consumption, many readers are probably wondering why they have heard so many positive things about soy in magazines and television. Remember that historically, soy was not grown as a food crop, but as a cover crop that acted as a "green-manure" that put valuable nitrogen back into the soil. Small amounts of soy were historically fermented and eaten as condiments in many Asian countries. These time-consuming and expensive fermentation techniques helped reduce many of the harmful anti-nutrients in soy but did not completely eliminate them.

During the Great Depression, poor soil-conservation practices helped create the great "dust bowls" of the 1930s, in which hundreds of millions of acres of fertile soil were carried off into the wind, forming massive dust clouds. In 1935, Congress passed the Soil Conservation Act to encourage ways to help preserve valuable topsoil. In search of a method of preserving soil fertility, America finally discovered what the Chinese had known for thousands of years. Soy is a great crop for nurturing soil fertility after a food crop is grown. Its roots help keep valuable topsoil from being carried away by the wind, and it replenishes the nitrogen in soil. Soy was grown to nurture the soil; however, there was very little demand for soy products.

Soy got its next big boost during World War II. Prior to the war, America imported 40 percent of its edible fats and oils. When those supplies were cut off by the war, the U.S. government encouraged farmers to plant more soybeans in order to produce soybean oil, and production quickly doubled, leading to surpluses at the end of the war. In 1946, the Soybean Association (now known as the American Soybean Association) was incorporated in order to promote soybeans as a crop and to increase profit opportunities. Luckily for the soybean farmers, the American Soybean Association came to the rescue at the end of the war and fought many legislative battles to remove barriers that limited the sale of unhealthy hydrogenated soybean margarine and also opposed government efforts to reduce soybean production.

The U.S. government encouraged the planting of soybeans during the war so that soybean oil could be used to alleviate any potential war-time shortages. Farmers loved being able to plant soybeans, because soy helped restore soil fertility without farmers having to purchase expensive man-made fertilizer. Soy could also be planted after normal food crops were harvested in a rotational manner, giving farmers the potential for extra income during a time when soil would otherwise be producing no profits. All that was missing from this equation was a demand for soy products.

Soybean Associations and the "Soybean Checkoff"
During the 1960s, states began to form their own soybean associations, which affiliated themselves with the American Soybean

Association. Perhaps the biggest thing to happen for soybeans was the passage of legislation that allowed for the assessment of what is called the "soybean check-off." The soybean check-off is a fee each farmer pays in order to promote soybeans and amounts to half a percent of the market price per bushel received by farmers. The soybean check-off is directed by the United Soybean Board and receives a substantial amount of money. For example, in 2009, the soybean check-off totaled more than $73 million, and in 2010, the check-off was more than $83 million. This money was then spent to promote soybeans through marketing and lobbying efforts.

PR Campaigns Attack Tropical Oils and Promote Soybean Oil
In the late 1980s, the American Soybean Association launched a campaign to stop what it called "the hidden use of saturated tropical fats," such as healthy coconut oil, and to increase the market share for soybean oil, a vegetable oil high in processed omega-6 fats. You may recall hearing a lot of buzz in the media during this campaign about how coconut oil was supposedly unhealthy and how processed vegetable oils that were high in omega-6 fats were supposedly good for you. This campaign was so successful that most movie theaters stopped using healthy coconut oil to make popcorn. This huge $80 million-a-year war chest also gives the soybean association the means to hire lobbyists to influence the federal government and pay for massive marketing campaigns to promote soy. These lobbying efforts were rewarded with $1.5 billion' worth of soybean farm subsidies in 2010. By artificially inflating the price of soybeans with subsidies, farmers are encouraged to plant more soy, which otherwise might not be profitable to plant. Planting more soy gives the soybean check-off more money to lobby for more subsidies and favorable government regulations. These subsidies also give food producers a cheap source of protein to add to food, in the form of soy protein isolate.

FDA and the Soybean Industry Make Health Claims for Soy
You can hardly open a magazine or turn on the television these days without hearing something positive about soy. Although some research articles suggest there may be a few advantages from consuming soy, the reader needs to understand that many of those articles were paid for by the soy industry, conducted by researchers with ties to the soy industry, and then were taken by PR firms and turned into favorable newspaper articles and advertising copy that present only one side of the soy debate in

the most favorable way possible.

There are two sides to the soy debate, but one side is highly organized with lobbyists and vast sums of money to spend, and the other side consists of a handful of health experts armed with numerous research studies, very little money to get their word out, and no powerful friends in Congress and the FDA.

In 1999, the FDA even authorized a health claim for soy protein, saying that it may reduce the risk of heart disease, despite the fact that its own researchers were urging caution. The studies that were used to justify this health claim found that soy protein decreased blood cholesterol levels around 3 to 6 percent. The cholesterol-lowering effects of soy are believed to be due to its isoflavone phytoestrogens. Though it may be true that soy isoflavones can lower cholesterol levels 3 to 6 percent, I have cited many studies that point to potential negative effects from consuming these same isoflavones. In a span of twenty years, soy protein has gone from being a product that was barely considered safe enough to use in cardboard food packages to one that's actually allowed to make a "health claim." It's important to understand the history behind this health claim. Following is one of the earliest and most famous studies showing that soy lowered cholesterol levels.

Research Study: "Meta-Analysis of the Effects of Soy Protein Intake on Serum Lipids"
This study was paid for in part by Protein Technologies International, which is a Dupont business involved in the research, manufacture, and marketing of soy protein. The research study was conducted by a doctor who is a member of the Health and Nutrition Advisory Group of Protein Technologies.

Soybean growers and soy food manufacturers are behind many of the studies showing the possible benefits of consuming soy. Soy is very high in isoflavones, and earlier I presented many research articles showing the potential dangers of consuming these isoflavone phytoestrogens. If someone wanted to try to make soy's isoflavone estrogens appear good, instead of bad, the best way to achieve that would be to come up with research studies that showed some benefit from consuming isoflavones and then to spend millions marketing those studies. As many people are aware, estrogen offers some advantages when it comes to cholesterol levels. Estrogen increases HDL (good) cholesterol and decreases LDL (bad) cholesterol. This is one reason premenopausal women have less heart disease than men of the same age do, and why their risk suddenly sky-rockets after menopause. It's all about the estrogen. If the soy industry wanted to make soy look good, it would make sense to fund a bunch of studies to determine whether isoflavones did in fact protect against heart disease by lowering bad cholesterol levels and raising good cholesterol levels, as human estrogen does. It would be a pretty safe bet that plant estrogens would lower cholesterol the same way that human estrogen does. (Never mind the studies showing the potential harmful effects of isoflavones.) Once the soy industry paid for favorable studies, it could embark on a marketing and lobbying campaign, backed up by those studies. With that all-out effort, it would be pretty easy to get everyone in America to believe that soy was a healthy wonder-food.

Following are some other early studies showing benefits from consuming soy isoflavones:

Research Study: "Soy Consumption and Cholesterol Reduction: Review of Animal and Human Studies"
This review was published in 1995 and was supported in part by Protein Technologies International.

Research Study: "Soy Protein and Isoflavones: Their Effects on Blood Lipids and Bone Density in Postmenopausal Women"
This study was published in 1998 and was supported by the Illinois Soybean Program Operating Board and Protein Technologies International.

Research Study: "A Randomized Trial Comparing the Effect of Casein with That of Soy Protein Containing Varying Amounts of Isoflavones on Plasma Concentrations of Lipids and Lipoproteins"
This study was published in 1999 and was supported in part by a grant from Protein Technologies International.

Research Study: "Long-Term Intake of Soy Protein Improves Blood Lipid Profiles and Increases Mononuclear Cell Low-Density-Lipoprotein Receptor Messenger RNA in Hypercholesterolemic, Postmenopausal Women"
The study was published in 1998 and was supported by the Illinois Soybean Program Operating Board and Protein Technologies International.

Research Study: "The Effect of Dietary Soy Supplementation on

Hot Flushes"
This study was published in 1998 and was supported in part by
Protein Technologies International.

**Research Study: "Effects of Feeding 4 Levels of Soy Protein for
3 and 6 Wk on Blood lipids and Apolipoproteins in Moderately
Hypercholesterolemic men 1, 2, 3, 4"**
This study was published in 2000 and was supported in part by
Protein Technologies International.

**Research Study: "Bone-Sparing Effect of Soy Protein in Ovarian
Hormone-Deficient Rats Is Related to Its Isoflavone Content"**
This study was published in 1998 and was supported in part by a
grant from the Illinois Soybean Program Operating Board.

As you can see, many of the early research studies that showed
benefits from consuming soy isoflavones were paid for in part by
those with a financial interest in promoting soy. The results of these
studies would be fairly predictable, given what we know about the
effects of estrogen on cholesterol.

The soy industry has spent millions of dollars in advertising
every year in respectable newspapers, magazines, and television
shows. Those advertising dollars have often been rewarded with
positive magazine articles and television spots highlighting all the
positive benefits of soy, and discouraged those same magazines
and television stations from voicing anything negative about soy.
Newspapers and television stations are reluctant to talk negatively
about the advertisers who pay their salaries. In addition, the $80
million-a-year onslaught of marketing has created the belief that
soy is a miracle food for the heart, despite many studies to the
contrary. For example,

Research Study: "Soy Diet Worsens Heart Disease in Mice"
This study was published in 2006 and was funded by the National
Institutes of Health and the American Heart Association. It found
that a soy-based diet was actually worse for cardiac function. The
report states, "We report that dietary modification from a soy-based
diet to a casein-based diet radically improves disease indicators
and cardiac function in a transgenic mouse model of hypertrophic
cardiomyopathy. On a soy diet, males with a mutation in the
B-myosin heavy chain gene progress to dilation and heart failure.
However, males fed a casein diet no longer deteriorate to severe,

dilated cardiomyopathy. Remarkably, their LV size and contractile function are preserved. Further, this diet prevents a number of pathologic indicators in males, including fibrosis, induction of *B*-myosin heavy chain, inactivation of glycogen synthase kinase 3*B* (GSK3*B*), and caspase-3 activation."

So even though the estrogens in soy help lower your cholesterol levels a few percentage points, the previous study shows that mice on a soy diet progress to heart failure. The soy industry has convinced people that soy is a wonder food for the heart, yet it can actually worsen heart disease according to this study.

Use of Soy Protein Isolate Was Originally Restricted to Cardboard Boxes

As mentioned earlier, many soy opponents claim that soy protein isolate was never formally granted GRAS status by the government, and that it should not be allowed to be used in food. Although this view may sound a little extreme, there is some truth in it. In 1979, the government's "select committee on GRAS substances (SCOGS) looked into granting soy protein isolate GRAS status for use as a binder and sealer in cardboard boxes including boxes which might contain food." The committee stated that the

> data available to the Select Committee suggests that alkali-treated soy protein isolates account for less than 1 percent by weight of paper and paper board products in which they are used. Because of this relatively small concentration of soy protein and because only a small fraction of the coating from a food package would be expected to be transferred into the food by attrition or migration, the intake of alkali-treated soy protein entering the diet from food packaging material is assumed to be exceedingly small. . . . There is no evidence in the available information on soy protein isolates that demonstrates or suggests reasonable grounds to suspect a hazard when used in paper and paperboard products for food packaging at levels that are now current or that may reasonably be expected in the future. [My underlining for emphasis.]

Basically, the committee had concerns that some of the anti-nutrients in soy protein isolate might leach out of the cardboard and into the food but felt that those levels would be very small and would pose no risk. In 1979, the government's select committee on GRAS substances agreed to give soy protein isolate GRAS status for use in cardboard boxes but did not grant it GRAS status for use in food. The idea that this same soy protein isolate would actually be added to food and given a health claim would have been inconceivable to these original investigators. It's worth noting that at this time, the soybean check-off, which would ultimately give the soybean lobby an $80-million-a-year budget, had not yet been approved by Congress. Shortly after Congress approved the soybean check-off in 1990, massive marketing and lobbing efforts were able to be funded. Many soy opponents claim that this is when the soybean industry changed its tactics. These soy opponents claim that the industry had yet to find a way to remove all of the toxic anti-nutrients from soy, so it decided to fund studies that it thought would show benefits from consuming soy.

FDA: Consumer Watchdog or Industry Lapdog?

When you fast-forward twenty years, it appears as if these lobbying efforts paid off. After the soy industry funded studies favorable to soy, it petitioned the FDA to allow a health claim for soy on the basis that soy lowers cholesterol, something that seems obvious, given the high levels of plant estrogens in soy. During this process, many soy opponents claimed that soy protein isolate had never received GRAS status, and that not only was a health claim not warranted, but that it should not even be legal to add to food. The FDA, however, had changed its tune since 1979 and now claimed that soy protein isolate could be defined as soy flour. Products that were in use before January 1, 1958, are generally given GRAS status. Although soy flour was in use prior to 1958, soy protein isolate was not, so, according to soy opponents, the FDA simply changed the rules of the game as the result of the soy industry's expensive marketing and lobbying efforts and massive political clout at the state and federal levels.

If you read the FDA's own ruling in 1999, allowing for the health claim of soy protein, the soy opponents' belief that the "fix was in" at the FDA appears to have a lot of validity. At the very least, one has to wonder why in 1979 there were serious concerns about even allowing soy protein isolate to be used in cardboard boxes for fear that potential toxins might leach into the food, and then suddenly, in 1999, the FDA said that this same soy protein isolate was actually soy flour, and because soy flour had been around since before 1958, the FDA was no longer concerned about it, and, in fact, it was actually now good for you.

The FDA and Monsanto

Many health experts are troubled by the way that the FDA is often a revolving door between government and giant agribusinesses: that is, people work for the FDA for a while, then go to work for companies dependent on positive FDA rulings, and then go back to work for the FDA again.

In 2010, for example, Michael Taylor became deputy commissioner for foods at the FDA. He had been an attorney for the FDA during the 1970s, who went into private practice to represent Monsanto in the 1980s. Monsanto is an agricultural biotechnology company that owns the patents for genetically modified soybean seeds. It's estimated that at least 85 percent the soybeans in the United States are grown using genetically modified seeds. Despite serious concerns about their safety, the FDA, in one of the most controversial actions in its history, approved their use. According to OpenSecrets.org, Monsanto spent $8,831,120 for lobbying efforts in 2008. Monsanto also profits from the U.S. government's $1.5 billion-a-year subsidy of soybeans, because many farmers would lose money planting soybeans without the subsidy, meaning Monsanto would sell far less seeds. Monsanto also profits from favorable FDA actions that allow for health claims to be given for soy, despite all of the research showing serious potential consequences from consuming soy.

After representing Monsanto for approximately ten years, Michael Taylor left private practice in the early 1990s to return to the FDA as deputy commissioner for policy. The FDA approved the use of Monsanto's GM growth hormone for dairy cows during this time, without any requirements for labeling. Mr. Taylor's involvement in those decisions led to a federal investigation on conflict-of-interest charges, which ultimately led to his exoneration. He then spent a few years working for the U.S. Department of Agriculture as administrator for the Food Safety and Inspection Service. Mr. Taylor next returned to Monsanto, becoming vice president of public policy from 1998 to 2001. Finally, in 2009, he returned to the FDA and in 2010 became deputy commissioner for foods. The FDA is notorious for being a revolving door where people move back and forth between working for private companies that depend on favorable FDA treatment and then working for the FDA. Perhaps when making your decision about whether to consume soy, these issues will make a difference to you, or perhaps not, but I hope you will be aware of the full picture on how foods are often deemed safe, despite what seems like massive evidence to the contrary to many health experts. The other thing to keep in mind is that the Food and Drug Administration (FDA) has not had a very good track record lately when it comes to approving the safety of food and drugs.

The FDA and Big Pharma

The FDA approved the drug Vioxx in 1999, the same year it allowed a health claim for soy protein. After being prescribed to more than 20 million people in a six-year period, Vioxx was pulled from the market in 2004, the same year the *Wall Street Journal* cited unreleased governments reports stating that Vioxx was responsible for an estimated 27,000 heart attacks and cardiac deaths. In 1999, the FDA approved the drug Avandia to regulate blood sugar. The FDA is responsible for making sure drugs are actually safe before it approves them, the same way it is supposed to make sure foods such as processed soy products are safe. In 2007, an article in the *New England Journal of Medicine* showed that Avandia was linked to a 43 percent increase in heart attacks, when compared to placebos or other medications. Avandia has been the subject of more than 13,000 lawsuits against its maker, and in July 2010, Avandia's manufacturer agreed to settlements on more than 11,500 of these suits.

The FDA and the Toxin BPA

The FDA was also recently involved in a case regarding health concerns about another estrogenic substance called BPA, which is a chemical that has been added to many plastic bottles since the 1960s. BPA is an estrogen mimicker, similar to the way soy isoflavones are an estrogen mimicker. In fact, studies show that BPA lowers sperm count, testosterone levels, and fertility in male rodents. Keep in mind that studies show soy can do the same thing. Other studies done on female mice show that BPA causes decreased fertility and disruption of normal ovarian development, just as soy has been shown to cause the same effects in female mice. In addition, BPA is an endocrine disruptor, and many health experts claim that endocrine disruption also results from ingesting soy isoflavones. A recent study shows that BPA exposure changes gene expression in mice, and that even when BPA was removed from the diet, it continued to produce genetic changes into the fourth generation of mice.

Since 1997, research has shown many adverse health effects from BPA at exposure levels below those currently considered safe by the FDA. In 1998, Japanese scientists and industries, as well as Japan's government, began to have concerns about the toxic effects of BPA. Japanese industry responded by voluntarily and significantly reducing the use of BPA in food containers between 1998 and 2003. Japan also took the step of largely replacing polycarbonate (polycarbonate contains BPA) silverware in school lunches with safer alternatives. As a result of these efforts, the blood levels of BPA for people living in Japan are now 50 percent lower than they were before these voluntary industry efforts were adopted.

During the next ten years, hundreds of studies were published showing that BPA could potentially increase the risk for cancer, diabetes, and reproductive problems. Many health experts were especially concerned because BPA was used in making baby bottles and baby pacifiers and also lined the cans of many baby formulas. In April 2008, the Canadian government banned BPA from use in baby bottles. In August 2008, the FDA declared that BPA in baby bottles was not a health hazard. Many health experts were critical of that FDA decision, especially given the fact that the National Institutes of Heath had already issued a report expressing concerns. These FDA critics claimed that the FDA was ignoring relevant scientific reports showing the dangers of BPA, including research funded by the National Institutes of Health, while at the same time relying on what the critics considered flawed industry studies funded by the chemical industry. Two months later, the FDA's own science board, which is a group of outside experts, voted unanimously to endorse a report finding major flaws in the FDA's decision to declare BPA safe. The science board found that the FDA had based its decision on studies funded by the chemical industry, while excluding studies that suggested that BPA, which acts like the hormone estrogen, could pose harm to children. The report states that excluding the negative studies on the effect of estrogens in BPA "overlooks a wide range of potentially serious findings" and "creates a false sense of security" about the information that was used in the assessment.

These are the same types of accusations that soy opponents level against the FDA. In the case of BPA, 153 government-funded studies found adverse effects from BPA, while only 14 did not. There were 13 studies done by the chemical corporations, all of which showed no harm from BPA. The FDA chose to give consideration to the reports done by the chemical industry, while ignoring a far greater number of independent reports sponsored by the government, reports that a reasonable person would assume to have more scientific integrity than industry reports.

Although Japanese industries immediately made efforts to protect their consumers in 1998, one year after the first studies came out about BPA, American industry appears to have chosen a different route. According to an article in the *Washington Post* from May 31, 2009, "manufacturers of cans for beverages and foods and some of their biggest customers, including Coca-Cola, are trying to devise a public relations and lobbying strategy to block government bans of a controversial chemical used in the linings of metal cans and lids." According to the article, internal notes from a private meeting of industry executives showed that they were concerned about how to "tamp down public concerns" about BPA. The attendees at the meeting estimated it would cost $500,000 to craft a public relations campaign. The group appeared to be focusing on "legislative battles and befriending people that are able to manipulate the legislative process."

Have no fear, on July 26, 2011, the U.S. government responded to this issue by announcing that "the EPA and FDA are currently collaborating on research to better understand and assess the possible health consequences of BPA exposure." You almost have to wonder whether they are doing this in conjunction with the chemical industry's efforts to focus on "legislative battles and befriending people that are able to manipulate the legislative process," as part of a collaborative effort.

In June 2008, there was a controversy surrounding Martin Philbert, the FDA chair of the committee looking at the safety of BPA. He is also the founder and codirector of the Risk Science Center at the University of Michigan. Philbert's Science Center received a $15 million grant from Dow Chemical for research on dioxin. Dow also happens to be a major BPA manufacturer. In addition, Philbert's Science Center received $5 million from Charles Gelman, a retired businessman and the founder of Gelman Sciences, a maker of plastic filtration devices. Philbert did not disclose these donations to the FDA; however, the FDA learned about them when reporters began to ask questions. The FDA felt that there was no conflict of interest, due to the fact that Philbert's salary was not paid by the donation.

Similarities between the BPA and Soy Controversies

I mention the BPA controversy in detail because of its many similarities to the soy controversy in regard to the FDA's actions. For example,

1. Both BPA and soy contain estrogen mimickers that are believed by many scientists to act as endocrine disruptors.

2. Many studies show that both BPA and soy negatively affect male and female rodent fertility.

3. These negative studies on both BPA and soy existed for more than ten years, while the FDA took no apparent action to protect the public—in contrast to what Japan's government and industries did as soon as they learned about BPA.

4. Both BPA and soy have been the subject of multiple negative studies and multiple positive studies, with most of the positive studies funded by the BPA and soy industries. The negative studies on BPA and soy tend to be funded by researchers with no ties to the outcome of the studies.

5. In deliberating on the safety of both BPA and soy, the FDA appears to give credibility to industry studies, while ignoring the independent negative studies. For example, many concerns were raised about the safety of soy protein in infant formula. The FDA's response to this was "[the] FDA is aware of concerns raised about the safety of soy infant formulas, but notes that these are speculative at this time, pending the results of definitive research" and that "the New Zealand Ministry of Health have recently issued guidelines for the safe and suitable use of soy-based infant formulas." I hope you can see how disingenuous this is. Studies came out in 1997 showing BPA to be dangerous, Japan made efforts to eliminate BPA in consumer products in 1998, and Canada outlawed BPA in baby bottles in April 2008. Yet in August 2008, despite hundreds of studies showing the dangers of BPA, the FDA said it's safe in baby bottles and cited the New Zealand Ministry of Health's decision, while ignoring actions taken by countries such as Japan and Canada to protect children, babies, and consumers.

   The FDA's other reason for not being worried about soy protein in baby formula was: "In any case, concerns about effects of soy protein specific to infant formulas are beyond the scope of the current rule, which authorizes a health claim about the relationship of soy protein and CHD for foods intended for use by the general population." Basically, the FDA was there only to give soy the health claim the soy industry wanted.

When the FDA had concerns about soy protein isolate in 1979, these concerns mainly focused on the lysinoalanine that is formed when soy protein isolate is manufactured. In 1999, the FDA found "that the potential presence of lysinoalanine in soy protein isolates used for sizing and coating adhesives in paper and paperboard products is not relevant to the safe and lawful use of soy protein in food." Basically, the FDA was saying that the fact it had been concerned that lysinoalanine in tiny amounts of soy protein isolate used in cardboard food boxes could get into food had no relevance to whether large amounts of that same soy protein isolate was safe if it was actually put into the food.

When studies showed that soy was harmful to animals, the FDA found that "these dietary studies in animals do not provide evidence for detrimental developmental effects in humans." Then, when human studies were brought up, showing that the phytic acid in soy can affect mineral absorption, the FDA responded that "animal studies suggest that zinc status is a strong determinant of effects of phytate/soy on zinc absorption: zinc absorption is more impaired with zinc deficiency, in contrast to the effect of low iron status, which enhances iron absorption." When human studies show negative effects from consuming soy, the FDA instead relies on animal studies, which are more favorable to soy, yet when animal studies show negative effects from consuming soy, suddenly the FDA claims that animal studies are worthless.

When a study conducted on humans demonstrating negative effects from soy consumption was brought up, such as the one showing that tofu consumption in midlife caused more cognitive decline later in life, the FDA decided that "this abstract does not provide a sufficient basis to evaluate the merits and weaknesses of this study. As such, it is not useful in evaluating the safety concerns at issue."

In regard to the fact that soy protein can affect the thyroid hormones T3 and T4, the FDA says there is "lack of evidence of goiter in population[s] that eat a high amount of soy." The problem with this argument is that no culture, historically, has eaten a lot of soy, so long-term consequences cannot be measured. Consuming large quantities of soy foods is a recent U.S. phenomenon. Asian populations do not eat much soy; for example, the Japanese eat only about 2 teaspoons a day. Second, every day the Japanese eat large amounts of seaweed that is high in iodine, while up to 25 percent of Americans are iodine deficient. Soy's effects on the thyroid are especially pronounced when there is an iodine deficiency. This is just one example of the FDA making something up that sounds good, in order to dismiss credible studies. Remember, industries dealing with the FDA admit that they need to focus on "befriending people that are able to manipulate the legislative process."

6. Both the BPA industry and the soy industry appear to be focusing their efforts on counteracting any negative research studies by working on the legislative and public relations fronts.

7. Many concerns have been voiced about what appear to be potential serious conflicts of interest with FDA officials who are making decisions that affect both BPA and soy.

As you can see, the debate is far from settled. To recap, there is both negative and positive research about soy. The soy lobby spends millions of dollars a year on research studies, advertising, and lobbying efforts to promote soy through the soy check-off program, not to mention receiving additional support from large corporations with substantial soy interests. In addition, many farmers and farm states are now highly dependant on soy. Soy helps restore soil fertility, saves on fertilizer cost, and allows many farmers to grow an additional cash crop, rather than letting their fields "rest." Most farm states have their own soybean associations as well. These associations often have tremendous political clout. According to the United Soybean Board, there are 680,000 soybean farmers in the United States. They contribute more than $80 million a year to the United Soybean Board through the soybean check-off. They have tremendous political clout at the state and federal levels. They have the money necessary not only to sway, but to control the public debate about soy. If soy does turn out to be dangerous for human consumption, you have to wonder who is actually going to look out for the interests of the consumer.

Case Studies on Soy Consumption

A number of health experts claim soy is healthy, while many others say it's extremely unhealthy. Experience has taught me that in cases such as this, it's good to look at anecdotal evidence as well. Oftentimes, truths are obvious anecdotally long before science reaches a consensus.

There are many documented stories of people eating large amounts of soy who develop health problems that go away after they eliminate the soy. Often, they are in good health until they begin to consume large amounts of soy products. Following are a few examples of stories people have told about their soy experience.

Case Study #1: A woman begins to consume large quantities of soy foods, and her blood tests reveal high parathyroid hormone levels and low levels of the thyroid levels T3 and T4. She is told by her doctor to stop eating soy. When she is re-tested several months later, her thyroid tests are back to normal.

Case Study #2: A bodybuilder switches his protein source to pure soy protein isolate and begins to drink soy milk. His energy levels begin to plummet, along with his libido. He quits consuming soy, and his energy level and libido return.

Case Study #3: A young teenager who excels at football develops hay fever. A doctor tells him to eat a lot of soy products to help with his allergies. After a few months on the high soy diet, he gets asthma, gains excessive weight, and eventually cannot even run or climb stairs. He becomes temperamental and can no longer focus on his school work. Finally, after the teen spends a few years on the high soy diet, a new doctor takes him off soy products. Within a few weeks, the teenager's mind clears, and his physical problems begin to improve.

Although personal experiences such as these do not provide conclusive scientific proof that consuming soy is dangerous, they are yet another reason to have concerns about soy. I have gone over many studies that suggest there may be potentially serious health consequences from consuming soy. If these studies are valid, then you would expect to hear personal stories just like the ones I shared with you.

Now that you have more information about soy, the ultimate decision is up to you about how much soy you choose to consume. Keep in mind that the Japanese eat only a few teaspoons a day of fermented soy products. Also, many of the studies I presented show that the negative effects of soy are dose dependent, meaning the higher the soy consumption, the more negative the effects. Also, the personal stories I just shared with you have one thing in common; all three of these people began to consume large amounts of soy. Much of the research and anecdotal evidence suggests that consuming a little soy may be alright, and that eating soy in the form of fermented products, such as miso, tempeh, natto, and soy sauce, might be best, if you choose to eat soy foods. Although I cannot recommend eating large amounts of processed soy products as part of the Four Seasons Diet, I do feel that eating very small amounts of fermented soy products on occasion is probably alright. I encourage all of you to do your own research and make your own informed decisions.

9

Breathing

The science behind ancient yogic breathing and how breathing affects your health.

The breathing exercises described in this section should not be attempted by anyone with a medical condition without first consulting with his or her physician. The exercises are also not recommended for the very young or the very old.

Although it may appear that a chapter on breathing does not belong in a diet book, the truth is that oxygen and CO_2 are both vital nutrients that are needed by the human body. Because most people do not breathe correctly, they are not getting enough of these vital nutrients delivered to the various parts of their bodies where they are needed. Eating right for your season-type also means breathing right, because without the correct amount of oxygen and CO_2, your body cannot adequately produce energy or carry out a host of other crucial metabolic functions.

Most people think that the purpose of breathing is to inhale oxygen from the air and exhale the carbon dioxide (CO_2) produced by our bodies. Most people wrongly believe that the more air we breathe in, and the more oxygen we get into our lungs, the better. In reality, although both oxygen and CO_2 are required by the body, breathing too much causes us to exhale too much CO_2, which can cause a myriad of health problems. While oxygen is the energizer of the body, CO_2 is the source of life and serves to regenerate many functions in the body. One of the most important functions of CO_2 is its role in helping the body release oxygen into our tissues, and when we over-breathe, we actually reduce the amount of oxygen that gets into our bodies. As counterintuitive as this may seem, by the end of this chapter you should understand the science behind why this is so, you will be able to perform a simple test to make sure you have enough CO_2 in your body, and you will understand ways to increase your CO_2 to healthier levels.

Myths about Breathing

Breathing seems like such a simple act that, as the expression goes, "even a child can do it." The truth is, however, in our modern Western civilization, almost no one actually breathes correctly. This is exacerbated by several myths about proper breathing:

Myth #1: Deep breathing is good. In actuality, most deep breathing is the same as over-breathing, and over-breathing is one of the worst things you can do to your health.

Myth #2: The more oxygen you get into your lungs and blood, the better. This is another myth, and as you will soon learn, if you breathe too much oxygen into your lungs, you will actually help create a state of low brain and tissue oxygenation.

Myth #3: CO_2 (carbon dioxide) is a poisonous waste gas. The truth is that most people have too little CO_2 in their lungs and blood, and the key to keeping your brain and tissues oxygenated lies in keeping your CO_2 levels high.

Although the previous three statements may seem to totally contradict logic and common sense, by the end of the chapter you should understand not only why they are true, but also why over-breathing plays a role in many modern diseases, perhaps most notably in asthma. Low CO_2 levels cause constriction of the airways by overexciting the *cholinergic nerve*, which is responsible for keeping the smooth muscles in the bronchi relaxed.

Yoga and Reduced-Breathing

People with asthma are often chronic over-breathers and frequently are amazed that their asthma symptoms disappear when they begin to do reduced-breathing exercises to increase their CO_2 levels.

In fact, a comprehensive study conducted on asthma sufferers in the UK by Jill McGowan, an expert in reduced-breathing techniques, had amazing success. The final results showed that the 384 participants who finished the reduced-breathing study had their asthma symptoms lessen by 98 percent, and they were able to decrease their use of reliever inhalers by an average of 98 percent, as well as reduce their use of preventer inhalers by an average of 92 percent.

Years of using reduced-breathing to control asthma in countries such as Russia and Australia show that asthma disappears as what is called the "comfortable pause" (CP) increases. When the CP is around 5 seconds, a person may experience life-threatening episodes. A CP of 10 seconds usually means the asthmatic is on various drugs, in poor health, with a chronic state of asthma. Raising the CP to 20 seconds normally allows the asthmatic to control his or her symptoms with drugs. By the time the CP reaches 30, it has been found that asthma symptoms most often disappear, and no drugs are usually required.

Many people reading this chapter may practice yoga and are possibly thinking this contradicts everything they have been taught by their yoga instructors. Yet the ancient yoga texts all advocate exercises that create this high state of CO_2, by practicing "reduced-breathing." It wasn't until some time in the 1920s that many Western yoga practitioners first began to misinterpret the ancient texts. The result is that now roughly half of the yoga instructors in the United States teach the exact opposite of what the ancient texts taught. Many yoga instructors now teach deep and full breathing, which creates a low state of CO_2 in the body, rather than the proper reduced-breathing, which produces high levels of CO_2.

Where the confusion probably came from is that advanced yoga breathing techniques describe a method of deep breathing in which the practitioner may take only one breath every minute or even one breath every two minutes. This type of breathing does create a high level of CO_2 and is good for the body. It is meant for very advanced students, however. To attempt to deep breathe without being able to take only one breath a minute does not create a state of high CO_2 but rather creates just the opposite: a state of low CO_2. The secret to the ancient deep-breathing technique was not the "deep breathing" aspect, but rather the "reduced-breathing" aspect. Three of the most ancient yoga texts are the *Hatha Yoga Pradipika*, the *Gheranda Samhita*, and the *Shiva Samhita*. They all describe a type of breathing that creates this high level of CO_2 in the body. Following are some quotes from the ancient yogic texts, with the most relevant parts underlined:

> "So long as the Prana [breath] stays in the body it is
> called life. Death consists in the passing out of the
> Prana [breath]. It is therefore necessary to restrain

the Prana [breath]."

"The fully concentrated Yogi seated in Mahabandha should inhale. With the throat Mudra he should restrain the breath."

". . . through the Ida [the left nostril], and keep the air confined—suspend his breathing—as long as he can; and afterwards let him breathe out slowly, and not forcibly, through the right nostril."

"Again, let him draw breath through the right nostril, and stop breathing as long as his strength permits; then let him expel the air through the left nostril, not forcibly but slowly and gently."

"When the Yogi can, of his will, regulate the air and stop the breath (whenever and how long he likes), then certainly he gets success in *kumbhak* [the point between inhalation and exhalation], and from the success in *kumbhak* only, what things cannot the Yogi command?"

"Then gradually he should make himself able to practice for three *gharis* [one hour and a half] at a time, [he should be able to restrain breath for that period]. Through this, the Yogi undoubtedly obtains all the longed-for powers."

These ancient yogis had discovered the secret to health and mental clarity, which modern scientists would not "rediscover" until centuries later.

Soviet Research on Human Respiration

During the "space race" of the 1960s, a young Soviet doctor named Konstantin Buteyko, who had some unique theories on respiration, received his big break. He was chosen to head a respiration project, with the purpose of assisting the Soviets on their first manned space flights. Dr. Buteyko was given the funding and the equipment for what was probably the most advanced laboratory on human respiration in history, capable of recording the forty main parameters of the respiratory and cardiovascular process simultaneously in real time. Thousands of volunteers breathed air of varying composition, while parameters such as blood pressure, EKG, pulse, tidal volume, respiratory rate, minute ventilation, arterial and venous blood gases, and the composition of the expired air were measured.

As part of his research, he made two important discoveries, the significance of which cannot be overstated:

1. Sick people have low levels of CO2 in their lungs caused by chronic over-breathing. In fact, more than 90 percent of most people who suffer from modern chronic diseases over-breathe and suffer from low CO2.

and

2. If you teach sick people to normalize their breathing, their diseases and symptoms disappear.

What the yogis had discovered and practiced for thousands of years finally had a scientific explanation. The reason that proper "reduced-breathing" is good for a person's health is that it builds up his or her level of CO2, which actually oxygenates and relaxes the mind and the body.

The reason this seems illogical to the average person and even to most doctors is that until you understand a few important things about how respiration works, it's very easy to assume they work the opposite of how they actually do. Although the science is quite complicated, I'll do my best to give you a simplified version that's easy to understand. Remember that the first major finding of the Soviets was that "sick people have low levels of CO2 in their lungs caused by chronic over-breathing."

What Happens When We "Over-Breathe"

There are many reasons why low CO2 levels caused by over-breathing would cause a person to be sick.

Lack of CO_2 Leads to Low Levels of Oxygen in the Tissues

To understand why over-breathing is so detrimental to human health, the first thing you need to grasp is how oxygen and CO_2 are taken from the air we breathe into our blood and then are released back into the air we breathe. The air we breathe contains gases such as oxygen and CO_2, which will dissolve into a liquid (for example, water or blood) that they come in contact with and vice versa, depending on the concentration (technically, the partial pressure) of the gas in both the liquid and the air. Gases such as oxygen will go from areas of high concentration to areas of low concentration (low partial pressure), even if it means they are going from the air and dissolving into liquid or leaving a liquid and going into the air. For example, the air we inhale is relatively high in oxygen (20.9 percent) and low in CO_2 (.04 percent). This air comes into contact with the alveoli in our lungs, which are the tiny bubble-shaped structures that allow the gases in the air to be exchanged with the gases in our blood. This blood in the alveoli tends to be lower in oxygen and higher in CO_2 than the air in the lungs. As a result of the high level of CO_2 in our blood and the lower level in our lungs, much of the CO_2 in our blood exits into the air in our lungs. Similarly, due to the higher level of oxygen in our lungs and the low level of oxygen in our blood, much of the oxygen in our lungs enters our blood.

The blood then goes into our tissues, and this gas-exchange process continues. Remember that gases will go from areas where they have high concentrations (high partial pressure) into areas with lower concentrations of that gas. When the blood from the lungs reaches our tissues, our tissues have lower levels of oxygen and higher levels of CO_2 than the blood does. This is because the process of respiration inside the cells uses up oxygen and generates CO_2. As a result, the blood has more oxygen than the tissues, so some of the oxygen in the blood goes into the tissues. Similarly, the blood has lower levels of CO_2 than the tissues do, so some of the CO_2 from the tissues goes into the blood. This blood that is high in CO_2 and low in oxygen then goes back to the lungs, where the whole process is repeated again.

So far, it would seem that given what I have said, the more oxygen you could breathe in and the more CO_2 you could breathe out, the better. There are a few more facts, however, that actually make the opposite of this true.

First is the way in which the *hemoglobin* in our blood carries oxygen. Hemoglobin is the oxygen transporter in our blood cells, and each blood cell has a staggering 280 million of these transporters. Each of these hemoglobin oxygen transporters can carry up to four molecules of oxygen. The important thing to understand is that each hemoglobin molecule does not grab and release all four of these oxygen molecules equally. The first three are grabbed and released relatively easily; however, the hemoglobin molecule has trouble both grabbing and releasing a fourth molecule of oxygen.

This means that when we over-breathe, we make it easier for each of our hemoglobin molecules to grab four molecules of oxygen.

The problem is that when all of these molecules of hemoglobin reach our tissues, they have a hard time letting go of those fourth molecules of oxygen, and until they get rid of the fourth molecules, they cannot get rid of any of the others. What essentially happens to most chronic over-breathers is that the hemoglobin leaving their lungs is completely saturated with oxygen, and the hemoglobin molecules coming back to their lungs still have either three or four molecules of oxygen apiece.

Another way to think of it is that a chronic over-breather may have blood that is 98 percent saturated with oxygen leaving the lungs. In other words, the blood is carrying 98 percent of the maximum amount of oxygen it is capable of, which means almost every hemoglobin molecule is carrying four molecules of oxygen. This blood may very well leave the lungs and travel into the bloodstream 98 percent full of oxygen and return back to the lungs still 88 percent full of oxygen, meaning that only 10 percent of the oxygen being carried in our blood is actually released into our tissues. Although this may be adequate when we are at rest, when we begin to exercise and exert ourselves, our bodies need far more oxygen. While this unique property of hemoglobin is one of the reasons over-breathing can lead to a low state of oxygen in the tissues, it is not the most significant one. This is because the hemoglobin leaving the lungs is usually 96 to 98 percent saturated with oxygen, so over-breathing may increase it only a few percentage points above this, while reduced-breathing may reduce it only a little below this amount.

The most significant danger of over-breathing is that it causes us to lose too much CO_2. It's the body's CO_2 level that determines how much oxygen our hemoglobin ultimately releases. This is because hemoglobin has an easier time releasing oxygen when there is a high level of CO_2 present. This property of blood is known as "the Bohr effect" and is responsible for two of the benefits of reduced-breathing. First, if the level of CO_2 is higher in the lungs, the hemoglobin will be less likely to grab four molecules of oxygen, making it easier to release oxygen when it reaches the cells. For example, rather than having your blood 98 percent saturated with oxygen, high CO_2 levels may mean it's only 90 percent saturated with oxygen. This means less hemoglobin is carrying four molecules of oxygen, which means more oxygen will be released when it reaches the cells.

Second, reduced-breathing keeps a higher level of CO_2 in our tissues, which means that when the blood reaches our tissues, more oxygen is released for that reason as well. Someone using these properties to his or her advantage by practicing reduced-breathing would be able to deliver up to double or triple the amount of oxygen to the cells, when compared to someone who over-breathed. So over-breathing creates a state where your body has lower levels of CO_2, making it more difficult for your hemoglobin to release oxygen. As a result, your tissues are receiving less oxygen than they should.

The reason that over-breathing causes you to eliminate too much CO_2 has to do with the differences between the air outside our bodies and the air inside our lungs. Remember that the air we inhale is around 20.9 percent oxygen and .04 percent CO_2. Normally, the levels of oxygen and CO_2 in our lungs are between the levels in the outside air and the levels in our blood. For example,

CO_2 or Oxygen and Location	Normal	Over-Breathing
Oxygen in air	21%	21%
CO_2 in air	.04%	.04%
Oxygen in lungs	13.2%	Increased above 13.2%
CO_2 in lungs	5.3%	Decreased below 5.3%
Oxygen in arterial blood	11.6%	Increased above 11.6%
CO_2 in arterial blood	5.3%	Major decrease

When we over-breathe, the air inside our lungs becomes more like the air outside of our lungs. This will create a high level of oxygen and a low level of CO_2 inside our lungs, leading to a high level of oxygen and a low level of CO_2 in our blood.

When we breathe properly, however, the air inside our lungs becomes more of a mixture of the high oxygen, low CO_2 air that is outside our bodies and the low oxygen, high CO_2 in our blood. We are essentially creating an entirely different atmosphere inside our lungs, which has a different composition from the air outside. Ideally, this unique atmosphere in our lungs will have less oxygen and significantly more CO_2 than the air outside. Such an atmosphere will help keep our blood from grabbing too much oxygen. Both of these factors, but especially the higher level of CO_2, will allow the blood to release more oxygen into our tissues.

As odd as it may seem to create a separate atmosphere inside our lungs, there appears to be a scientific reason why this may be necessary. According to Professor John Manis, one of the foremost experts on the evolution of respiration, lungs evolved at a time when the earth had much lower oxygen levels and much higher

CO_2 levels. This is the atmosphere we were meant to breathe, and as our atmosphere has slowly changed, our bodies' needs have not. As a result, our health suffers when we over-breathe and create a situation where the air inside our lungs is too similar to the air outside. In fact, research shows that atmospheric levels of CO_2 were four time higher 60 million years ago than they are today, a relatively short period in the evolutionary time line.

Low oxygen levels play a significant role in the growth and development of cancer. Not surprisingly, studies show that cancer patients are chronic over-breathers. One study done in the Ukraine on breast cancer patients found that teaching them reduced-breathing techniques greatly increased their survival rates. In this study, women undergoing treatment for breast cancer were put into either a control group or a group that did reduced-breathing exercises similar to the ones I will describe to you later in this chapter. At the end of three years, the women in the group doing the breathing exercises increased the amount of CO_2 in their expired air by 65 percent, while those in the control group had no change in their CO_2 levels. What is striking is that after three years, the mortality rate of the women in the control group was 24.5 percent, while the women in the group doing the reduced-breathing exercises who had increased their CO_2 levels had a mortality rate of only 4.5 percent.

If the pharmaceutical companies ever invented a cancer drug that could match these results, it would be guaranteed to make them billions of dollars in profits, and every person with cancer would probably be given the drug as part of his or her cancer therapy. In fact, drugs are often approved because they are shown to have a very small increase in favorable outcomes of only a few percentage points.

The reason that cheap and easy solutions are not used in this country is that cheap and easy solutions usually cannot be patented by one company that would stand to make billions of dollars in profit, and therefore no company is willing to pay for expensive testing that will benefit other companies. In order to be "approved" by the FDA, any drug or therapy needs to undergo testing that often costs hundreds of millions of dollars. The only reason any company would pay for such testing would be if it had an exclusive patent on a drug or a therapy that could make billions of dollars in profit. As a result, cheap and better alternatives are usually excluded from medical use in the United States. In Chapter 13, you will learn how this corrupt system, which shortchanges the American people while it enriches the medical profession and pharmaceutical companies, was set up this way on purpose.

There are thousands of natural plants that often do a better, safer, and more effective job at treating disease than pharmaceutical drugs can do. In the United States, however, only patented drugs that have been "approved" by the FDA can be used to treat disease. So although the reduced-breathing techniques I am going to teach you have been proved to cure diseases in other countries, because these techniques cannot be patented, no U.S. company will spend the hundreds of millions of dollars necessary to gain FDA approval. For this reason, more than 99 percent of the doctors in the United States have never heard of these techniques, despite the fact that they have a greater than 98 percent success rate in curing diseases such as asthma. In fact, most U.S. doctors who specialize in treating asthma are unaware of reduced-breathing techniques, despite the fact that they have been proved in studies conducted in other countries to cure more than 98 percent of asthma patients.

In summary, the important points you should remember from this section are that

    a. Our blood leaving the lungs is normally almost fully saturated with oxygen, so inhaling more air will do little to help our hemoglobin molecules grab more of it. In addition, our blood has a difficult time letting go of oxygen when every hemoglobin molecule is carrying four molecules of oxygen.

    b. Our hemoglobin will release more oxygen when our CO_2 levels are high.

    c. Over-breathing will cause us to have low CO_2 levels, meaning our blood releases less oxygen.

    d. Over-breathing makes the air inside our lungs too similar to the outside air. It's important to think of the air in our lungs as a separate atmosphere, and our goal is keep the oxygen in our lungs lower than that in the outside air and the CO_2 in our lungs significantly higher than in the outside air.

Lack of CO_2 Leads to Low Levels of pH Buffers in the Blood

In Chapter 4, on how pH affects the season-types, I discussed blood buffers. Normally, we maintain a 20:1 ratio of alkaline bicarbonate to acidic carbonic acid, which is the dissolved form of CO_2 in our blood. Blood buffers help us maintain our blood pH, and when we have high levels of buffers, we feel good, and when our levels are low, we tend to feel bad. This is because when we have a high level of buffers, our bodies can easily keep our blood pH at perfect levels, but when our buffers are low, we have a tough time maintaining our ideal blood pH as the temperature and our exertion levels change.

When our CO2 levels begin to fall, our carbonic acid level falls, which means we are no longer maintaining a 20:1 ratio, but now our ratio begins to climb to, say, 22:1, 24:1, or higher. This makes our blood too alkaline, so our bodies respond by eliminating bicarbonate. Recall that bicarbonate is removed by the kidneys, and it happens very slowly. Ultimately, over-breathing creates a state where we have removed most of the bicarbonate from our blood. The body likes to maintain that 20:1 ratio, however, so it keeps our CO_2 levels low as well. As a result, our buffers are now at extremely low levels, and we have a tough time maintaining pH balance in our blood. People in this state would get super winded from simply walking up the stairs, they may cycle between being too hot or too cold, and meals might affect them significantly, due to the pH changes that various types of food are causing in the blood.

When we learn to keep our blood buffers high, we use the fast-acting carbonic acid as way to level our pH when we need to rapidly, such as when climbing up the stairs, and then we slowly build our buffers back up when we are able. Let me explain. Our lungs are able to quickly blow off excess CO_2 or retain excess CO_2 as a way of balancing our pH. If we purposely keep ourselves in a slight state of under-breathing, it means our blood is constantly in a slightly acidic state. As a result, our kidneys are always slowly increasing our bicarbonate levels, which keeps our bicarbonate levels high—this means we have super-high levels of both bicarbonate and carbonic acid. We may be slightly acidic, say, a 19:1 ratio at all times, but our buffers are now at super-human levels. This allows us to sprint up twenty flights of stairs without being overly winded, to go out in the cold or the heat and still be comfortable, and to eat various types of food without it causing negative pH effects.

Constantly increasing your blood buffers is like repeatedly putting money in the bank. People who constantly over-breathe are like those with $100 in the bank. When they need to cash a check for $200, which may be akin to walking up the stairs, they are going to have problems. People who correctly under-breathe and constantly increase their buffers are like individuals who keep putting money in their bank account. They may start at $100, may get to $250, may have a few large checks to cash, and might get down to $50, but as long as they keep increasing their "buffer bank account," they will eventually accumulate $1,000 and more. Now, when they have a $200 check to cash, they have no worries and a surplus to boot.

The Benefits of Reduced Breathing

In this chapter, you'll learn how to measure your "blood buffer bank account" and how to keep it high at all times. In addition to having the resiliency of a child again, you'll also be rewarded with incredible oxygen levels in the brain and the muscles, clarity of thought, and an abiding feeling of calm and relaxation.

CO_2 Increases Relaxation and Improves Brain Function

Keeping our CO_2 levels high helps us maintain an optimal degree of relaxation and brain function. First, higher CO_2 levels mean the blood can release more oxygen into our bodies. Getting more oxygen to the brain prevents us from getting "brain fog" and keeps us mentally sharp all day. In addition, CO_2 helps expand our blood vessels, which means that more blood actually gets to the brain as well. Experiments show that for every 2 percent drop in CO_2 (measured as mm Hg), blood flow to the brain is decreased by 1 percent.

High levels of CO_2 also help activate our parasympathetic nervous system, which is the rest-and-relax branch of our nervous system. This has a calming effect on the entire body. As a result, our brains become less agitated, and we have fewer irregular firings of our cortical neurons. This irregular firing is often the cause of many neurological issues, such as anxiety, panic attacks, and insomnia. When our CO_2 levels are low, the brain can get excited in an abnormal way, which allows the brain and our thoughts to race out of control.

How CO_2 influences Other Metabolic Functions

CO_2 affects other metabolic functions besides our oxygen levels and brain function. It also plays an important role in the regulation of the hormonal, cardiovascular, and digestive systems. As mentioned earlier, low CO_2 levels reduce the level of blood buffers. When this happens, we are very prone to electrolytic imbalances and the loss of magnesium, sodium, and potassium.

CO_2 also plays a part in the formation of proteins, amino acids, fats, and carbohydrates. Low CO_2 levels hinder *carboxylation reactions*, which are necessary to produce both "fast-sugar energy" and "slow-sugar energy" (glycolysis and Krebs cycle). All of this begins to affect the production of the thyroid hormone thyroxin, which causes further energy problems. In addition, hormones such as insulin, estrogen, epinephrine, norepinephrine, calcitonin, and other endocrine hormones are affected.

CO_2 increases our insulin sensitivity, so low levels of CO_2 can play a role in insulin resistance. CO_2 acts as a *vasodilator*, meaning it helps dilate the blood vessels of the brain, the heart, and other organs, allowing for more blood flow into those vital areas. In addition, CO_2 increases blood flow into the intestines and boosts hydrochloric acid production in the stomach, both of which help with the digestion and assimilation of food. CO_2 is also needed for our immune systems to function properly. Given all of the negative effects that low CO_2 levels cause in the body's metabolic functioning, it is not surprising that the Soviets found in their clinical experience with more than 200,000 patients that restoring proper CO_2 levels was able to dramatically improve 150 to 200 common health conditions.

What Causes Over-Breathing and the Development of Health Problems?

Many factors contribute to over-breathing, and a lot of them are related to our modern Western lifestyle. Stress and anxiety are two of the obvious things that can cause us to over-breathe. Our sedentary lifestyle also contributes to both over-breathing and less production of CO_2. Although many of us may spend an hour at the gym, a hundred years ago most people spent five to ten hours a day doing hard physical labor, usually on the farm. Tasks such as doing the laundry by hand and fetching water from the well or the stream were sources of exercise and helped produce CO_2. In addition, food is far more plentiful than it was a hundred years ago, and overeating and being overweight are both major contributors to over-breathing. When we overeat or are overweight (especially with belly fat), we are not able to breathe properly using our diaphragms, and we begin to use our chest muscles instead. Consciously deep breathing, in the mistaken belief that it's good for us, is another cause of over-breathing, along with breathing through the mouth, rather than through the nose. Excessive talking or talking in a loud voice also contributes to over-breathing. A hundred years ago, when most people lived on the family farm and there were no telephones, people probably talked a lot less than they do now, due to the minimal contact they had with other people. Imagine how much less you would talk without a phone and if you came into contact with only a handful of people every day. Finally, sleeping on your back causes over-breathing.

As we begin to over-breathe for any of these reasons, it usually leads to more over-breathing. When we first begin to over-breathe, we exhale CO_2 faster than our bodies can accumulate it, and our blood gets overly alkaline. In addition, over-breathing creates a state of oxygen deficiency, which keeps us from properly producing energy using oxygen. As a result, we begin to produce energy without oxygen, which creates acidic waste products in our cells. This causes our tissues to become too acidic, while our blood is slightly too alkaline. To compensate for the overly alkaline blood, the kidneys dump bicarbonate, which are a vital part of our buffer reserves. In this process, other electrolytes are also affected, especially magnesium. With low levels of CO_2 and low levels of blood buffers, many other metabolic processes are upset.

To make matters worse, we begin to feel short of breath, due to our lack of CO_2 causing an oxygen shortage. This makes us over-breathe to get more oxygen, which actually ends up having the opposite effect, leading to even less oxygen getting into our tissues. The body responds by trying to find a way to limit our breathing. Our noses respond by stuffing up, trying to get us to breathe less, so we end up breathing though our mouths, which makes the problem even worse. Oftentimes, as in the case of asthma, we begin to get bronchial spasms as the body attempts to find other ways to reduce our breathing. Of course, the panic caused by an asthma attack leads to further over-breathing once an inhaler is used to open up the airways.

Chronic over-breathing also contributes to the development of many diseases, and rather than treat the underlying cause of the disease, doctors often treat the symptoms. This often causes the CO_2 deficiency to get worse, making it difficult to achieve true healing and vitality. A good example of this is the role that low CO_2 levels play in cholesterol production. As CO_2 levels decrease, the body often responds by increasing cholesterol production as a way to protect the nerves. Simply increasing your CO_2 levels will get the body to stop producing as much cholesterol, often solving any cholesterol issues you may have. In addition, when your CO_2 levels are high, your appetite is usually less intense, making it easier to avoid health issues related to overeating.

How to Test Your CO_2 Levels

Remember that our goal is to create a second atmosphere inside our lungs, which has lower levels of oxygen and significantly higher levels of CO_2 than the air outside. There is a simple test you can perform any time, which will give you a good indication of the normal level of CO_2 inside your lungs, using the equation:

$$CO_2 \text{ at alveoli in lungs} = 3.5\% + (.05 \times CP \text{ [comfortable pause]})$$

There is no need to memorize this equation, because I'll provide you with a chart in just a bit. The beauty of this equation is that it shows that the higher the normal level of CO_2 is in our lungs, the longer we can comfortably hold our breath, due to the fact that our tissues have such a high level of oxygen and our blood contains more buffers. For those of you with a medical background, this equation works only if CO_2 is at least 27 mm Hg.

The most important thing to understand is what a "comfortable pause" (CP) is. A comfortable pause is the amount of time you can hold your breath comfortably, after taking a normal breath in and breath out. This contrasts with a "maximum pause" (MP), which is the maximum amount of time you can hold your breath after taking a breath in. The biggest mistake most people make when trying to test their CP is either taking too big a breath in or out or else holding their breath too long. Following are the correct instructions for testing your CP (comfortable pause).

> a. Sit down and relax for at least five minutes. Breathe normally, as if you were not paying any attention at all to your breathing. Pretend you are watching TV or reading a book, and just breathe without thinking about it. This is the level of breathing you want to have during the test. Most people think that because they are doing a breath-holding test, they need to breathe excessively or else take in a big breath right before they hold their breath. This is not what CP is testing, however. The CP tests how long you can <u>comfortably</u> hold your breath after taking a normal breath in and a normal breath out. Be prepared for the fact that you will be able to hold your breath for far less than if you took a big breath in and held your breath for as long as possible.

b. After inhaling and exhaling as described above for at least five minutes, take one last normal relaxed breath in and out. At the end of the normal breath out, pinch your nose and hold your breath. Begin timing how long you hold your breath on a stop watch. Fight the urge to take a bigger breath in or out for your last breath. Your last breath should be a normal breath, as if you were watching TV and not thinking about your breathing.

c. Hold your breath until you feel <u>the first sign of discomfort</u>. Often your diaphragm will begin to involuntarily push down or you may notice a swallowing movement in your throat at this point. At the first sign of discomfort, take note of how long you held your breath, using your stopwatch. The key to the CP (comfortable pause) is that when you are done with it and you start breathing again, you should be able to resume breathing at the same rate and intensity you were before you held your breath. IF YOU FIND THAT YOU NEED TO TAKE A BIGGER BREATH IN (MORE VOLUME OF AIR) THAN BEFORE YOU HELD YOUR BREATH OR YOU FIND YOURSELF BREATHING FASTER THAN BEFORE YOU HELD YOUR BREATH, YOU HELD YOUR BREATH FOR TOO LONG. The previous statement is the key to learning the CP. The first few times you take the test, you will probably hold your breath too long. When this happens, you will find yourself needing to take a few deep breaths and possibly breathing faster than before the test. These are both signs that you did the test incorrectly.

When the test is done correctly, you are breathing the same after the test as before the test, and this is why the pause is considered a "comfortable" pause. While you are resting for five minutes, preparing for the test, imagine that you are watching TV or reading a book, and notice your breathing. Notice both the rate at which you breathe, as well as how much volume of air you breathe in and out with each

breath. When you learn to do the test correctly, you
will breathe in and out at the same rate and volume
after the test that you did before the test.

The CP is a great indicator of both the level of CO_2 inside your
lungs and your general overall state of health. After conducting
measurements on more than 200,000 patients in a clinical setting,
the Soviets, led by Dr. Buteyko, came up with the "Buteyko Table
of Health Zones." This table provides a lot of information that will
help you interpret your own test results and how they relate to
your current state of health.

According to the table, normal CP should be 40 seconds.
Given that 90 percent of the people in industrialized Western
nations over-breathe, however, most of you will find that your CP
is much lower than this. The good news is that I will soon give you
some exercises you can do to increase your CP, which, as the table
shows, will also improve your state of health. People who breathe
normally should have a CP of 40, and multiple studies show that
people with various diseases have much lower CPs. For example,
people with severe heart disease usually have a CP of around 5. This
is not to say that if your CP is 5, you have heart disease. Rather,
it means that research shows that people with various diseases
also tend to have CPs that fall within a certain substandard range.
Although a 5-second CP does not necessarily mean you have heart
disease, it does mean that you are most likely in a very poor state
of health. People with disorders such as hypertension, moderate
heart disease, asthma (with symptoms), panic disorders, and
COPD tend to have CPs between 8 and 16 seconds. Your CP may
fall within this range, and you may appear healthy, but odds are,
you are heading for disease until you get your CP up to 40 seconds.
Following is the Buteyko Table of Health Zones, with a few changes
I made to make it easier to understand.

The main column to pay attention to is the second-to-the-
last one, titled "Comfortable Pause," which is the measure of your
CP in seconds.The first column, titled "State of Health," and the
third column, titled "Rating," tell you your overall state of health
and well-being based on your CP. For example, if you look at the
"Comfortable Pause (CP)" column and then go down to 40 seconds,
you can see that this row is listed as "normal" under the "State of
Health" column and is given a rating of "0" under that "rating."
This row has words and numbers in bold font, because this is the

CHART 9.1 BUTEYKO TABLE OF HEALTH ZONES

State of Health	Breathing	Rating	Pulse Rate per Minute	Breaths per Minute	% CO2 in Lungs	Automatic Breath Pause	Comfortable Pause (CP)	Maximum Pause (MP)
Superior Health	Shallow	+5	48	3	7.5%	16	180	210
Superior Health	Shallow	+4	50	4	7.4%	12	150	190
Superior Health	Shallow	+3	52	5	7.3%	9	120	170
Superior Health	Shallow	+2	55	6	7.1%	7	100	150
Superior Health	Shallow	+1	57	7	6.8%	5	80	120
Normal	Normal	0	60	8	6.5%	4	60	90
Disease	Deep	-1	65	10	6.0%	3	50	75
Disease	Deep	-2	70	12	5.5%	2	40	60
Disease	Deep	-3	75	15	5.0%	0	30	50
Disease	Deep	-4	80	20	4.5%	0	20	40
Disease	Deep	-5	90	26	4.0%	0	10	20
Disease	Deep	-6	100	30	3.5%	0	5	10

CP level that corresponds to normal health. You can further see that a 40 CP would correlate to 6.5 percent CO_2 in the lungs, with a pulse of 60 and eight breaths per minute. Furthermore, it correlates to an automatic pause of 4 seconds. This means that a person with a CP of 40 would normally and automatically pause for 4 seconds after each breath, even while he or she was sleeping. In fact, this natural pause is in large part what is responsible for keeping the CP at 40. Finally, a person with a CP of 40 would be expected to hold his or her breath for a maximum pause of 90 seconds after a normal inhalation and exhalation. When doing a maximum pause, you do not take a bigger breath in; however, you hold your breath as long as you can, and you should feel a need to breathe quickly and deeply when you are finished doing a maximum pause.

As you can see, when your CP gets below 40, you are considered to be in a diseased state of health, and because 90 percent of people living in the modern Western world over-breathe, 90 percent of people living in the Western world are in a state of disease. In fact, the studies show that people living in Western society usually have a CP of between 20 and 30 seconds. At the bottom of the chart are people with a CP of 5, which correlates to a health rating of –6. These people are in a serious state of poor health, and unless they bring up their CP, they are probably in for a very rough future, health-wise. It has been found that when people have a CP below 10 seconds, they often have a weak immune system, have malignant tumors, or are fighting death.

When the CP is below 20, the person is often in the grip

of a disease, and the diaphragm becomes locked and does not move properly, which helps keep the individual stuck with a low CP. When the diaphragm gets locked due to a low CP, it does not provide a gentle pumping action that helps keep the lymphatic system moving. As a result, a locked diaphragm often leads to lymphatic stagnation. A person with a CP below 20 also has an oxygen deficit in the tissues, which is disrupting his or her normal oxidative energy production, leading to elevated levels of metabolic acids and fatigue. This person also probably suffers from problems with temperature regulation and has poor heat tolerance but also gets cold easily. A person with a CP below 20 seconds usually feels best when he or she is slightly warm, without getting too hot.

When the CP is between 20 and 40 seconds, people may appear healthy, but they are often struggling with some disease, maybe without knowing it for many years. When people reach a CP of 40, their bodies will be able to repair, heal, and recover in a way that they cannot when the CP is below 40. A CP of over 60 usually means that people are in a superior state of health and completely free of disease and are very unlikely to suffer from disease as long as they keep their CP over 60.

The higher a person's CP, the more oxygen he or she is able to use in the blood. For example, people with a CP of 15 seconds use only 10 percent of the oxygen in their blood; their bodies are literally starving for oxygen. They are probably heavy breathers and struggle to find a way to get more oxygen. When people get to a normal CP of 40, they boost the amount of oxygen they are able to use to 25 percent. Beyond the "normal" levels are the "superior health" levels. These are people who are dedicated to making breathing exercises a part of their daily routines, such as hatha yoga masters. The 40-second CP can be a hard barrier to break, but once people do, they often quickly advance up to higher CPs. When people get to a CP of 60 seconds, they are using up to 35 percent of the oxygen in their blood. A true master, with a CP of 3 minutes, is able to use up to 60 percent of the oxygen in his or her blood.

In addition to an individual's using oxygen more efficiently, the higher the CP, the less water a person needs to drink and the less sleep he or she needs. For example, a person with a super-low CP of 5 to 8 seconds will often need 12 to 14 hours of sleep a night, while people with a CP of 15 seconds frequently need around 8 to10 hours of sleep a night. When the CP gets to a normal level of 40 seconds, the amount of sleep required usually goes down to

5 to 6 hours a night. People who push themselves into a state of "superior health" find that one of the many benefits of their hard work is that they need very little sleep. People with a CP of 60 seconds normally need only 4 hours of sleep, while those who attain a CP of 2 to 3 minutes often do well on 2 hours of sleep a night, with a high level of energy and vitality the remaining 22 hours of the day. People with a high CP also usually find that they need to drink much less water every day. This is believed to be largely due to the body's being able to maintain perfect pH balance more effectively, which reduces the person's need for water.

People with superior CPs of more than 60 seconds experience a variety of other health benefits as well. Women often undergo painless childbirth when the CP is more than 60. The Soviets also found that at high CPs, a person's saliva produces antibodies that prevent dental plaque and cavities. The higher a person's CP, the stronger his or her immune system is as well. When the CP reaches 60 seconds, the posture becomes perfect, and the spine becomes straight, without the person having to work at it or think about it. People with a 60-second CP move with grace, beauty, and ease that cannot be duplicated when the CP is low.

In fact, the only person who would want a low CP would be someone who was about to undergo an organ transplant. This is because a CP of 27 or lower means a person has a weak immune system, and his or her body is less likely to reject a transplanted organ.

How to Increase CO_2 Levels and Improve Your Health

After reading about all of the benefits about increasing your CO_2 levels, you are probably wondering how you can increase yours. The good news is that there are some very easy things you can do to immediately increase your CO_2 levels by small amounts. In addition, with hard work, dedication, and diligence, you can significantly increase your CO_2 levels and optimize your state of health.

The biggest challenge we have in changing the CO_2 levels is the body's own *chemoreceptors*. Chemoreceptors are sensors in our bodies that monitor things such as our blood pH and CO_2 levels. These chemoreceptors are very sensitive to changes in pH and CO_2 levels. The problem is that someone who chronically over-breathes has been in a state of low CO_2 for such a long time that the body has "reset" the level of CO_2 it considers normal. When your CO_2 levels begin to get higher than "your normal level," the body responds by making you feel uncomfortable and short of breath, which usually causes you to breathe. As you'll soon learn, the key to the exercises lies in consciously choosing to maintain this uncomfortable feeling of "air hunger" so that your body will eventually get used to higher levels of CO_2 and "reset" itself until this new higher level becomes the "normal level."

The first problem in raising your CO_2 levels is resetting your own chemoreceptors so that they get used to higher levels of CO_2. The main obstacle to this is your need for sleep. Hours spent on exercises to increase your CO_2 level can be undone by the body with a few hours of sleep, especially if you sleep on your back or with your mouth open. This is where daily practice and diligence pay off, because eventually the body will slowly begin to reset the level of CO_2 it considers normal. This is why it's important to practice the exercises I am going to give you in the morning, the afternoon, and the evening, because it will help get your body used to higher levels of CO_2 throughout the day. After practicing the exercises for a few weeks, you will begin to get used to feeling slightly "short of breath" and will find you can maintain a state of slight under-breathing for many parts of the day, which will help you attain a higher CP more quickly.

The next obstacle to increasing your CP has to do with the fact that as you initially raise the level of CO_2 in your blood, you also cause your blood to become more acidic. Chemoreceptors in the body respond to this by making you feel as if you need to breathe in order to help lower your CO_2 levels, which will help increase your blood pH.

I have stressed the importance of having a high level of blood buffers, namely, bicarbonate (alkaline buffer) and CO_2 (acidic buffer, CO_2 in form of carbonic acid) in a 20:1 ratio. The goal is to get levels of both as high as possible; however, one obstacle to achieving this is that although CO_2 levels are quickly raised and lowered with breathing, bicarbonate levels change much more slowly and rely on our kidneys. This is why it's necessary to maintain a slight feeling of "air hunger" for as much of the day as possible. This feeling means that your blood is most likely slightly acidic, and if you refuse to raise it by breathing, then your kidneys will raise it by increasing your level of bicarbonate. As a result, you now have higher levels of both bicarbonate and CO_2, meaning you have more buffering power in your blood and a higher CP, due to the overall increased level of CO_2 in the blood.

Of course, once you go to sleep, your body will respond

to overly acidic blood by increasing your breathing rate, which lowers your CO_2. When it comes to increasing your CP, your chemoreceptors often create a state similar to driving a car that veers sharply to the right. Unless you are diligent about keeping your breathing slightly restrained by paying constant attention to your breathing, so that you feel constant but slight "air hunger," your body will simply veer off the road that leads to perfect health and steer straight back into the ditch you have been in. Re-setting your chemoreceptors so that they are used to higher levels of CO_2 is a slow process and requires hard work and dedication.

Guidelines to Proper Breathing
You can help your body stay on course by following a few simple guidelines:

a. <u>Always breath through your nose</u>. One key to keeping your CO_2 levels higher is breathing through your nose. The amount of air contained between your nostrils and your lungs is much greater than the amount contained between your mouth and your lungs. This means that when you breathe through your nose, you are breathing in more air that you have already exhaled, air that is high in CO_2. When you breathe in this air, you breathe more CO_2 back into your lungs and help keep the air in your lungs higher in CO_2. The nose contains about 150 to 200 ml of this previously exhaled air, which is called "dead space" and which you re-inhale when you breathe through your nose. Normal breathing consists of breaths that are about 500 ml in volume (about 2 cups), so when you breathe through your nose, you breathe in 150 to 200 ml of the high CO_2 air in your nose first, followed by 300 to 350 ml of the low CO_2 air from the outside. This helps prevent the low CO_2 air from outside from suddenly rushing into the lungs, because it ends up getting mixed with the "dead-space" air, helping to keep the CO_2 in your lungs at a higher, healthier level.

      Many of you may not be able to breathe through your nose, and this is usually a sign that your CO_2 levels are too low. This is often the body's way of decreasing your rate of respiration; however, most over-breathers with clogged noses respond to this by simply breathing through their mouths, which makes their problems even worse.

      If your nose is clogged due to low CO_2 levels, you can usually unclog it quickly with the following trick. Simply take a normal breath in and a breath out, as you did in the breath-holding test, pinch your nose, and try to hold your breath until you feel a very strong urge to breathe. You will be holding your breath longer than you did during the CP, because you are waiting for a "strong urge to breathe," rather than the "first sign of discomfort." As you do this, gently bob your head up and down as though you are "agreeing" with someone or saying "yes" with a head bob. When you can't hold your breath any longer, let go of your nose, and <u>gently and slowly</u> breathe in through your nose. If this does not unclog your nose, you may need to wait 30 seconds and try it again. Usually, people with clogged noses experience relief after the first time they try this exercise. If you succeed in unclogging your nose, you now understand that your over-breathing has been the cause of your clogged nose, and if you just practice keeping your CO_2 levels high, you can keep your nose unclogged 24 hours a day.

b. <u>Sleep.</u> Sleeping on your back will quickly lower your CO_2 levels, because it has been found to often double the rate of respiration. The best position for sleeping is on your left side, followed by your right side, followed by your stomach, and finally on your back. Many people unknowingly mouth-breathe at night, and the Soviets found that "mouth-taping" was a quick and easy way to retrain a person to nose-breathe at night. Mouth-taping <u>should not be attempted</u> on children or on people with poor health, by someone who has drunk large amounts of alcohol, by someone who is sick, by individuals with gastrointestinal problems, or by people with sleep apnea or COPD. Mouth-taping consists of placing a small piece of tape, such as 3M micropour paper tape or paper tape (both can be purchased at a drugstore and are designed not to be very sticky and to come off easily), across the mouth at night to keep it closed. The tape is usually placed vertically from just under the nose to a little below the lower lip.

Usually, after people mouth-tape themselves for a few months, they will no longer have to continue doing so, because they get used to breathing through their noses at night. If you sleep with a partner, have this individual check your breathing at night if he or she wakes up, to see if your partner can notice you breathing out of your mouth at all. If he or she catches you breathing out of your mouth, continue mouth-taping again until you finally rid yourself of the habit.

Beds that are too soft, along with rooms that are too warm, will also cause over-breathing at night. It's best to sleep on a mattress that's on the firm side and in a room that is slightly cool.

c. <u>Meals.</u> Overeating leads to over-breathing. If you are serious about increasing your CP, keep your meals on the small side. The good news is that as you increase your CP, your appetite should diminish if you are overweight, which will also help you in your breathing exercises. Likewise, people with a large amount of belly fat tend to over-breathe, because the excess fat in their bellies hinders proper diaphragmatic breathing. This is especially true after a person with a lot of belly fat eats a large meal.

Heavier foods and foods that are more processed also increase our breathing rate, as do foods high in fat and animal protein. Fruits have the smallest impact on your breathing rate, followed in order by vegetables and leafy greens, grains, legumes, nuts, dairy, fats and oils, and, finally, meats and fish.

If you really want to increase your CP, focus on eating light vegetarian meals that also work for your season-type. Food preparation also affects your breathing rate. For example, eating your foods raw will have the least effect on your breathing rate. This is followed in order by frozen foods, then dried foods, steamed foods, cooked foods, baked foods, foods cooked for a long time, fried foods, grilled foods, and, finally, deep-fried foods.

Stop eating at the first sign that you are full or, better yet, learn to stop eating before you feel full. As you get used to practicing reduced-breathing, you will notice that it becomes very difficult for several hours after a large meal to do so. Do not feel as if you need to severely restrict your calories; simply stop overeating.

Breathe 2 Cups (Approximately 500 ml) of Air per Breath

Normal breathing volume should be approximately two cups (500 ml) of air per breath, which is an amount that would be considered extremely shallow breathing by most people. If you are unsure of what breathing in this volume of air equates to, there is a way to measure that amount of air as you breathe.

You will need a large bowl, a 4-cup glass measuring cup, and a two- to three-foot-long piece of vinyl tubing. Fill the bowl about half full of water, and put the measuring cup upside down in the water so that it is submerged to the 3-cup mark. When you submerge the cup, make sure the piece of vinyl tubing is inside the cup, with the end of the tube located at the bottom of the cup (the normal bottom of the cup, which will now be on top because the cup is submerged upside down); the vinyl tube will be above the water. During this entire process, the end of the tube should stay above the water and inside the cup in such a way that you can breathe through the tube. The other end of the tube should be between your lips as if you are sucking through a straw.

When you begin to breathe through the tube, the water inside the cup should be at the 3-cup mark. As you breathe in through the tube, the vacuum inside the cup will raise the water inside the cup. If you watch the water level while you slowly breathe in through the tube, you will see the water level rise as you breathe in. Slowly breathe in until the water level inside the cup reaches the 1-cup mark. You have now breathed in 2 cups of air.

Release your breath back into the vinyl tube, and watch the water level inside the cup fall back to the 3-cup mark. You can repeat this several times, until you get a good feeling for what breathing in 2 cups of air feels like. It will feel like a very shallow breath, and this is the volume of air you should be breathing at most times during the day, unless you engage in strenuous exercise.

Both men and women should try to maintain this 500 ml volume of breathing, even though the average man has a greater lung capacity than the average woman. The average man's lungs contain about 6 liters of air, compared to around 4.5 liters for the average woman. Breathing in 500 ml of air will feel like shallow breathing, and this is the volume that is recommended, regardless of your gender, size, or age.

Breathing Exercises

Now that you have the basics, you are ready to learn some exercises that you can perform, along with things you can do throughout the day while you are working. The most important advice to remember during the exercises and all day long is:

KEEP YOUR BREATHING SHALLOW AT ALL TIMES, IF POSSIBLE, TRYING TO INHALE ABOUT 500 ML (APPROXIMATELY 2 CUPS) OF AIR WITH EACH BREATH, AND BREATHE IN AND OUT ONLY THROUGH THE NOSE.

Many of the exercises involve holding your breath, and it's easy to put too much emphasis on the holding-the-breath part. The key to all of the exercises is to keep the amount of air you inhale and exhale at a constant 500 ml as much as possible. It's better to hold your breath for half as much time if that's what it takes to keep your breathing constant. If you hold your breath for too long, you'll end up breathing too much at the end, which defeats the whole purpose. The goal of the exercises is to maintain light "air hunger," which should feel similar to the comfortable-pause test you did earlier or similar to the way you might feel while walking up a hill. Many people describe the sensation as feeling slightly suffocated or smothered. You are not going for a maximum breath-hold, but rather are holding your breath a little past your comfort level. If you do it right, you will want to breathe more than 500 ml of air when you are finished, but if you try hard, you can maintain the 500 ml rate. You may feel very uncomfortable for many breaths, but as long as you can maintain this rate of breathing, you are doing it correctly.

So the first priority is to maintain a constant rate of breathing that consists of 2 cups (500 ml) of air per breath. The second priority is to maintain a slow, regular rate of breathing. If you hold your breath for too long, you may be able to maintain breathing 2 cups of air per breath by simply breathing more quickly. This is also incorrect. Push your breath-holding time in such a way as to allow you to return to the same volume and rate of breathing you had before the breath-hold after your breath-holding is over. You will experience some discomfort; however, you should be able to maintain your volume and rate of breathing with some effort.

If you do these exercises correctly, you should begin to feel your arms and feet get a bit warmer. You may also experience a warm fuzzy feeling in your stomach area the first few times you do them, which is a sign that your body is beginning to relax. Your nose may also become cold, while your nasal passages become moist. Some people may experience tearing in the eyes, similar to crying, but often with far more tears. This is simply a sign that you are increasing your level of CO_2.

The first exercise is the easiest for children to understand, so I'll explain it first. Children who are taught proper breathing can often accomplish increases in their CPs in a week that might take months for an adult to accomplish. This is because children have not spent the last twenty or thirty years of their lives stressed out and over-breathing, as most adults have.

Do not attempt any breathing exercises if you are currently being treated for cancer, type 1 diabetes, chest pains, blood pressure issues, heart issues, epilepsy, schizophrenia, sickle cell anemia, arterial aneurysm, hypothyroidism (unless it's being controlled), or kidney disease.

The following groups of people are also advised to keep their "air hunger" extremely slight, similar to what you might experience on a very gentle walk: people with emphysema, severe asthmatics, individuals with COPD, type 2 diabetics, women in their second to third trimester of pregnancy, people suffering from anxiety or depression, and people who get migraine headaches.

Exercise #1—Steps
1. Breathe in and out normally while walking.
2. After a normal exhalation, hold your breath while you continue to walk.
3. Initially, attempt to walk 5 to 20 steps while holding your breath for a slight breath-hold, or attempt 20 to 100 steps if you really want to push yourself.
4. Remember, the key is that when you begin to breathe again, you should resume your normal breathing and not be gasping for air or increasing your breathing volume. If you cannot resume your normal 500 ml breathing volume and normal slow breathing rate, you held your breath for too many steps. Hold your breath for fewer steps next time.
5. Continue to walk for 30 seconds to a minute while you breathe normally. If you are extremely healthy or you want to push yourself, you can experiment with lowering your rest time. For example, rather than resting for 30 seconds to a minute between breath-holds, you can try resting for a certain number of breaths. That is, after your breath-hold, you can try to breathe 2 to 10 normal breaths and then continue to hold your breath again. Rather than counting breaths, you can also count steps: breathe normally for 5 to 100 steps, and then go on to step 6 of this exercise. The key is to find something that works for you.
6. Go back and repeat steps 1 to 5 again.

Interestingly, it has been found that the number of "steps" a person can perform while doing a breath hold usually correlates to a person's CP in the following manner:

Steps	CP
20–40	10
40–60	20
60–80	30
80–100	40

Try to perform your "steps" for at least 15 minutes or longer, if you feel comfortable. The great thing about doing "steps" is that they help teach you what you should be striving to do most of the day: maintain a feeling of air hunger that you control. After doing "steps" for a while, you can begin to integrate the same concept into all of your physical activity. If you park your car somewhere, "step" your way to the store and through the store. If you're walking up the stairs at home, "step" yourself up. If you're raking the lawn, rake using "steps." That is, rake a certain number of times while holding your breath, then breathe normally again while you continue to rake.

For those of you who prefer to lift weights, use "steps" in your reps. Start by simply reducing your breathing to 500 ml per breath while you work out in your normal manner, making sure to breathe through your nose. If you find that you take one breath for every rep, try to push yourself to one breath for every other rep and then one breath for every three reps. You should find that you will be able to do more reps, as you begin to increase your oxygen levels by incorporating "steps" into your reps. I know people who struggled with breathing once every two reps and then quickly found they could breathe once every ten reps, while being able to do more reps than ever before. This is because what had been limiting their ability to work out was their low levels of oxygen. If you want to be an elite athlete, keep in mind that the higher your CP, the better athlete you will be.

If you do steps correctly, you should find that the number of steps you can perform gradually increases as your CP increases. Although performing steps takes a lot of concentration at first, eventually it will become second-nature, as long as you make an effort to push yourself. Once you get the hang of steps, you can incorporate them into all of your daily movements and routines.

Exercise #2—Breath-Holds

This exercise is similar to the comfortable-pause test we did earlier; however, rather than doing one comfortable pause to test your CP, you want to do a breath-hold after each breath and continue doing them for 30 minutes. Do not feel as if you need to push each breath-hold as long as possible. The goal is to keep yourself inhaling and exhaling at a constant 500 ml (2 cups), while you build up the amount of time you can hold your breath between each breath. At the same time, you want to focus on breathing in and out slowly. Your primary focus should be on maintaining shallow breathing of 500 ml of air, your secondary focus should be on maintaining a slow and steady breathing rate, and your third focus should be on the actual breath-hold. When you do them correctly, you will have a tough time maintaining the proper volume and rate of breathing but will be able to maintain it with a little struggle. If you are unable to maintain your volume and rate of breathing, you held your breath for a little too long. You also want to learn to unlock your diaphragm with this exercise, although this will not be fully possible until your CP gets to closer to 40 seconds.

1. Take a normal breath in, and hold your breath as long as you comfortably can. A normal breath in should take about 2 seconds and should consist of 500 ml or two cups' worth of air.
2. When you can no longer hold your breath, release it. Ideally, you want to learn to make your exhalation consist of nothing more than relaxing your muscles. This is because when you breathe in properly, only your very bottom ribs expand outward. While you hold your breath, they remain under tension, and when you release your breath by simply relaxing, they return back to where they were on their own. If your ribs return on their own without your having to exhale, it will take about three seconds. This is extremely hard for some people to learn, because many people chest-breathe using their middle and upper ribs, which is made worse by the fact that low CO_2 levels often "lock-up" their diaphragms. If you need to exhale, go ahead and do so.
3. After you relax, and your ribs return to their starting position, or after you exhale, if you needed to exhale, hold your breath again as long as you comfortably can. When you can no longer hold your breath, gently inhale.
4. Repeat steps 1 to 3 for another 30 minutes.

Ideally, you want to find a breath-holding time that works for you. It may be to breathe in for 2 seconds, hold for 2 seconds, breathe out for 3 seconds, and hold for 2 seconds. It can also be breathe in and hold for 4 seconds, breathe out and hold for 1 second. Find what works for you, so that you can maintain air hunger for a full 30 minutes. Then, try to push your hold times as your 30 minutes progress. You should find that if, when you first began, you could hold your breath for only 2 seconds, you might be able to hold your breath for 3 seconds at 15 minutes and 4 seconds at 30 minutes.

Try to push yourself as much as is comfortable to increase your breath-holding time as days and weeks pass. Remember, though, that the key for all of these exercises is to always have a controlled 500 ml breath in and a controlled 500 ml breath

out, lasting 2 to 3 seconds per breath. The breath-holding time
is secondary to keeping your air volume at 500 ml and a 2- to
3-second rate per breath. If you need to breathe more air or need
to take a faster breath in or out, you held your breath for too long.
If this happens, reduce your breath-holding time, and focus on
breathing 2 seconds in, 3 seconds out, with 500 ml of air for each
breath.

Another variation on this exercise is to hold your breath
only after the exhalation. For example, breathe in for 2 seconds,
relax your diaphragm to exhale (or forcibly exhale for 3 seconds if
your diaphragm is locked up) for 3 seconds, then hold your breath.
When you cannot hold your breath any longer, breathe in, and
start the process over again.

As you practice, you will begin to learn exactly what level
of "air hunger" pushes you to your limit, while still allowing you to
take a controlled breath in, lasting 2 seconds and consisting of 500
ml of air, when you resume your breathing. Hold your breath too
long, and you breathe in quickly or breathe in too much air. Hold
your breath for too short a time, so that you do not feel short of air
for a full 30 minutes, and you will not make any progress. If you
do the exercise correctly, your CP will be around 5 seconds higher
at the end of the exercise than it was at the beginning.

The more you increase your intensity levels while doing
this exercise, the less amount of time you will need to do it in
order to achieve results. The recommended 30-minute period is
based on maintaining a level of air hunger similar to what you
experience after the breath-holding test that measures your CP
and is considered a slight air hunger. Maintaining a medium air
hunger will allow you to reduce your exercise time to 20 to 25
minutes. You can cut your exercise time in half to 15 minutes by
maintain a high level of intensity; however, this is too extreme for
most people. A high level of intensity would be similar to what
you would experience after holding your breath for as long as you
possibly can. In addition, you can change the level of intensity
while you do the exercises. For example, you can do the exercise
for 5 minutes at light intensity, followed by 1 minute at high
intensity, followed by 5 minutes at light intensity. Once again,
find what works for you and allows you to make gains and progress
by pushing yourself in a way that makes you feel better, not worse.
Although actual exercises can be extremely tough mentally while
you are doing them, you should be rewarded afterward by feeling
better for the next few hours. As you progress from a 10 CP to a

20 CP, up to a 40 CP, you will begin to feel better than you have in years. Some people like to push themselves and make fast gains, while others prefer the slow and steady path.

Measure your CP every morning, afternoon, and evening. Your CP will usually be lowest in the morning and higher in the afternoon and evening. As long as you keep improving, keep doing what works for you. You may find when you get to a 40-second CP that you are happy staying there, and that is fine. Just continue to test your CP at least once a day, and, if necessary, do your exercises or practice reduced-breathing throughout the day in a way that helps you stay there. It's far easier to stay at a certain CP than to increase to a higher one.

Proper Diaphragmatic Breathing

Proper breathing uses the diaphragm muscle, which is a dome-shaped muscle inside the chest cavity. Very few people breathe properly using this muscle, because when the CP gets below 40 the body begins to lock this muscle and the lower ribs in a way that keeps a person from being able to breathe properly. Having excess belly fat or eating too much will also hinder a person's ability to properly use this muscle.

Usually, people say that when you breathe with your diaphragm, your stomach should move in and out, but this is incorrect. When you breathe properly, only your very lower ribs will expand outward. If you put your hands on your sides at your lower ribs, you should be able to feel them expand outward (toward your sides) on both sides when you breathe in, and then when you relax your muscles, those ribs should naturally return back into their starting position during a 3-second period. When you breathe properly, your stomach and chest should not move. Proper breathing is also very silent, and you should not hear any inhaling or exhaling.

Changes You Can Expect

As you begin to increase your CP time, you can expect to experience many positive reactions, along with some often unpleasant cleansing reactions. The unpleasant cleansing reactions often happen every time you double your CP and usually occur around 10, 20, 40, and 80 seconds. Common cleansing reactions include the following: increased mucus from the lungs, nervous excitement, frequent bathroom visits, insomnia, fatigue, loss of appetite, headaches, increased body temperature, tearing of the eyes, smells from the skin, irritability, hair loss, muscle pains, a metallic copper taste in the mouth, and peeling skin.

These reactions are a temporary part of the healing process and often involve a weak area of the body. For example, smokers may experience a dark discharge coming from their lungs. A person who has sinus trouble may have a mucus secretion from the nose. Often, people with cavities or oral problems may experience a worsening of their symptoms, due to increased blood and oxygen flow to the affected teeth, and they will need to visit the dentist. Most people normally lose their appetite during a cleansing reaction.

Some of the positive changes you can expect, such as increased oxygen and energy levels, along with a decreased need for sleep, have already been discussed. In addition, cravings for foods such as sugar, alcohol, and caffeine begin to go away. Your mood should also improve, and you should feel increased mental clarity.

Oftentimes, women who have been unable to conceive suddenly find themselves pregnant when their CP hits 40 seconds. The theory is that because pregnancy usually dramatically reduces CO_2 levels, it's nature's way of sometimes keeping a woman from getting pregnant who does not have the level of CO_2 necessary to maintain her health and the health of the baby during pregnancy.

Beyond 40 Seconds

If your initial CP is low, you can expect to increase it 3 to 4 seconds per week, if you work hard. As you begin to approach a 40-second CP, your gains may begin to slow down. As mentioned earlier, 40 seconds is a barrier that is frequently very difficult to break; however, once it's broken, people often progress very quickly. In order to break the 40-second barrier and get to 60 seconds, you are going to have to make a level of commitment that many people are not willing to make, which includes the following:

1. You will need to practice maintaining "air hunger" during all waking hours. At first, it is very difficult to practice maintain air hunger while you work and go about your normal business. Yet eventually, with practice, you'll find that your body gets used to maintaining a feeling of constant air hunger, and you'll notice when you are not doing so.

2. You will have to engage in 3 to 5 hours a day of physical activity, while breathing through your nose 100 percent of the time. If

you're stuck in an office all day and don't exercise, forget about trying to reach 60 seconds. You may be able to reach 30 or 40 seconds, however, and will benefit greatly by doing so.

3. As your CP gets close to 40, you will need to work in some long breath-holding that goes beyond the CP, in order to continue making improvements. This includes adding some "maximum pauses" (MPs), which consist of holding your breath past the "comfortable pause" mark, and holding it for as long as you can. Then, you will need to do your best to resume normal breathing without taking a big breath in. When your CP gets closer to 40 seconds, it's fairly safe to do an MP. If your CP is below 30 seconds, do not attempt to do an MP.

4. You will need to eat less, to enable yourself to maintain adequate air hunger all day. If you eat a large meal, you will usually not be able to maintain air hunger for a few hours after eating.

5. You will need to keep yourself on the slightly cool or cold side most of the day. Heat alkalizes your blood, which counteracts the effects of your breathing exercises. By keeping yourself slightly cool, you put pressure on your body to increase your bicarbonate buffers while you increase your CO_2 buffers with your breathing exercises. As silly as it might sound, experience shows that keeping cool includes things such as not wearing shoes or socks as much as possible and going for walks without shoes, if possible. We can lose a lot of heat through our feet, so not wearing shoes or socks is a great way to keep yourself cool.

6. You will have to sit as little as possible. Many people who want to increase their CP to 60 seconds will actually work on the computer or work in their offices standing up. Standing up provides a better position for the proper movement of the diaphragm than sitting does. I believe that you can achieve a similar effect if you sit in the half-lotus or lotus position, although this is not backed up by years of clinical experience the way that standing versus sitting in a chair is.

10
The Natural and Unprocessed Plant-Based Diet Advantage

Evidence shows that eating natural foods prevents most disease.

You now have almost all of the knowledge you need to maintain vibrant health, regardless of your age. You have learned how to eat according to your season-type, which tells you the proper ratio of protein, carbohydrates, and fat to include in your diet. You have learned about three foods that should be either avoided or strictly limited in your diet. This means limiting your fructose consumption to no more than 15 grams per day, limiting your soy consumption to a few servings a week of organic non-GMO traditional fermented soy foods such as miso and tempeh, and completely eliminating processed vegetable oils that are high in omega-6 fats, such as corn oil, vegetable oil, safflower oil, and canola oil from your diet. You have also learned how proper breathing and maintaining a high comfortable-pause time can virtually assure a disease-free life.

3 Principles of a Healthy Diet

This chapter is about another vital component necessary for optimum health. It is so basic that almost everyone knows it to be true, yet most people do not implement it into their daily lives. This vital component consists of the following three basic principles:

1. Eat foods that have not been processed.
2. Eat foods that are mostly plant-based.
3. Limit your consumption of meat.

The evidence is overwhelming that adhering to these three principles is one of the keys to disease-free longevity. Although many Americans live to see their eighties, they often suffer from multiple diseases, such as hypertension, diabetes, and obesity, for half of those eighty years. What I am talking about is living to your eighties and beyond, while maintaining your health and vitality. The advantage of a plant-based, unprocessed, organic diet has been proved by historical evidence, anecdotal evidence, and scientific evidence.

Benefits of a Vegetarian Diet

Numerous studies have been conducted to determine whether vegetarians are healthier than meat eaters. In 2003, many of these studies were analyzed, and the findings were reported in the *American Journal of Clinical Nutrition.* The conclusion from the review of these studies was that they raised the possibility that "a lifestyle pattern that includes a very low meat intake is associated with greater longevity." The review made note of that fact that during World Wars I and II, many Scandinavian countries were forced to eliminate most meat consumption. The mortality rate during this period actually decreased, and once the wars were over and meat consumption resumed to pre-war levels, mortality rates went up again.

Although saturated fat and cholesterol often get blamed for the negative health effects caused by eating meat, some season-types actually need saturated fat and cholesterol in their diets, while others do best restricting both. To their credit, rather than pointing the finger solely at saturated fat and cholesterol, as many medical professionals do, the authors of this review study looked at certain carcinogenic compounds in cooked meat, such as heterocyclic amines, polycyclic aromatic hydrocarbons, and n-nitroso compounds. They also found that the type of iron found in meat, called *heme iron*, produces oxidative stress and tissue damage, including in the tissues of the heart.

A large percentage of the increased cancer rates for meat eaters is due to cooking meat. For example, *heterocyclic amines* (HCAs) are cancer-causing compounds that are formed when meat is cooked, especially when it's grilled and fried. The longer the meat is cooked and the hotter the temperature, the more of these dangerous compounds are formed. Sadly, modern factory-farming practices produce meat that is so contaminated with bacteria that in response, the U.S. government was forced to change its cooking guidelines, and many restaurants now only serve meat that is well-cooked.

It has been estimated that more than 80 percent of the chicken in grocery stores is contaminated with salmonella. The

U.S. government's response was to tell consumers simply to cook meat to a high temperature until it's "well-done." Although this recommendation may kill the salmonella and the *e. coli* in meat, it also produces huge amounts of HCAs and causes a large portion of the protein in meat to become cross-linked, making it unusable by the body. Consumption of well-done meat, as the U.S. government recommends, has been associated with an increase in various types of cancer, such as breast cancer and colon cancer, so the choice seems to be either take the risk of getting infected with salmonella and *e. coli* or greatly increase your chance of developing breast and colon cancer by cooking your meat at high temperatures. A Harvard study found that men who eat red meat daily have 3.5 times the risk of developing colon cancer, when compared to men who ate red meat less than once per month. Another Harvard study done on male physicians showed that men who consume red meat at least five times a week had 2.5 times the risk of developing prostate cancer, compared to men who ate red meat less than once a week.

Grilling or broiling meat over a flame, which results in the fat dropping into the flame, produces *polycyclic aromatic hydrocarbons* (PAHs). The PAHs in the resulting smoke adhere to the surface of food and are also believed to play a significant role in human cancers. This may be one reason a study in Germany that tracked mortality rates of vegetarians found that they suffered from half the rate of cancer of the general population. One study that examined the effects of prenatal exposure to PAHs found that children who had been exposed to high levels of these toxic compounds in the womb had IQs that were about 5 points lower than other children and suffered from developmental delays and an increase in behavioral problems.

How the Modern Diet Causes Disease

Yet our high consumption of meat does not bear all of the blame for the increase in diseases such as cancer. It's really a combination of having a diet with too many processed foods and too much meat that is causing an explosion in age-related diseases, a diet that most people consider to be the modern "civilized" diet. The possibility that "civilized diets" lead to disease has been suspected since the time of the ancient Greeks. In fact, it was Hippocrates who said, "Let your food be your medicine," nearly 2,500 years ago.

Cancer Was Rare in Ancient Times

When researchers at Manchester University analyzed the remains of nearly a thousand individuals from Ancient Greece and Egypt, they found that diseases such as cancer were extremely rare. After an extensive examination of ancient mummies, only one isolated case of cancer was found. In ancient societies, which had no way to treat cancer, the evidence of cancer should have remained in 100 percent of the mummies who had the disease, and evidence shows that it was an extremely rare disease. Similar studies conducted on thousands of Neanderthal bones have found only one possible case of cancer among these primitive people as well. Professor Rosalie David, who led the study, concluded that since there is nothing in our natural environment that causes cancer, it has to be a man-made disease.

Essentially, it's the pollution of our environment from unnatural chemicals, along with adding unnatural foods to our diet, that is causing many of our modern diseases such as cancer. When researchers went back and examined the development of cancer during the last 3,000 years, they found that cancer had really only begun to emerge as a common disease about 250 years ago, and then the incidence of cancer rose dramatically during the last 100 years. The first reports of cancer concerned nasal cancer in snuff users, starting in 1761, and scrotal cancer in chimney sweeps in 1775. Researchers found that contrary to popular belief, ancient Egyptians had a long life expectancy and often lived long enough to develop diseases such as osteoporosis and atherosclerosis. The researchers concluded that cancer is mainly a "man-made" disease caused by our modern lifestyle and is totally preventable.

Tanchou and Price Discover That "Civilized" Food Causes Disease

In 1843, a French doctor named Stanislas Tanchou was able to prove that cancer deaths were increasing in urban areas such as Paris. He formulated what was called "Tanchou's Doctrine," which stated that cancer increases in direct proportion to the "civilization" of a people.

During the 1920s and the '30s, an American dentist named Weston Price spent his summers circling the globe to study the teeth and the overall state of health among "primitive" people. During his journeys, he visited native peoples, such as the Swiss, Eskimos, Polynesians, several African tribes, Australian Aborigines, and many other isolated cultures, who ate their traditional foods. His travels occurred at a time when many of these people were just beginning to be introduced to "civilized" foods, such as white flour and sugar. These "civilized" foods are really "unnatural" foods, because they do not exist in nature but need to be processed by man, while the so-called primitive foods are really "natural" foods, because they are eaten whole, the way they occur in nature. In many cases, Price was able to study multiple generations, in which the grandparents had been raised on natural foods ("primitive foods"), the children had been raised with a little "civilized" food ("unnatural foods"), and the grandchildren had been raised on large amounts of "civilized," unnatural, processed foods. The results were shocking and a huge boost in validating Tanchou's Doctrine that disease increases in direct proportion to the civilization of a people. Price's studies also showed that Hippocrates had been right, in that food can be our medicine, and that civilized food is our poison.

Part of what makes Price's work so amazing is that in addition to testing the nutrient values of the foods eaten by "primitive" peoples, he also took more than fifteen thousand photographs to document the physical changes that occurred as these people adopted a civilized, unnatural, processed diet. The photographs show that the people who ate the primitive natural foods had perfectly formed teeth with no cavities, well-formed dental arches, and well-formed faces, while those eating civilized, unnatural, processed foods suffered from cavities and crooked teeth, along with badly formed dental arches and poorly formed faces. In some cases, the older children in a family had eaten strictly primitive natural foods, while the younger children had eaten strictly civilized, unnatural, processed foods. This often occurred in primitive societies, because all it took was one new road into a village, which allowed civilized processed food to be imported into a culture that had relied on locally unprocessed natural foods for thousands of years. In cases where the youngest children received the civilized processed food, you could see the stark contrast between them and their older siblings who had eaten the primitive natural foods. Looking at the photographs, you would have to feel sorry for the children who were raised on the civilized foods—and angry, at the same time—yet sadly, this is how 99 percent of American children are being raised.

Price credited the overall good health of these "primitive" people to the fact that their diets did not contain processed foods, especially white flour and sugar. Price calculated that so-called primitive people, by eating unprocessed foods and whole grains, were receiving four times the amount of vitamins and minerals when compared to the standard American diet. The other foods that primitive diets did not contain, which I discussed earlier, were processed vegetable oils high in omega-6 fats, large amounts of fructose, and vast quantities of soy products. As a result of their natural diets, Price observed that primitive peoples were also free from most "diseases of civilization," such as cancer, heart disease, diabetes, asthma, arthritis, and obesity.

In some cases, Price visited groups of native people adhering to their native diet in a location that also happened to have a settlement of white people eating civilized, processed foods. For example, in the Torres Strait islands north of Australia, he visited a group of more than 4,000 natives eating primitive natural foods, along with a group of white people eating civilized processed foods. The doctor who oversaw the area reported that in his thirteen years there, he had suspected only one case of cancer among the native people who had a primitive diet. In stark contract, he had operated on several dozen cases of cancer in the much smaller population of white people who ate the foods of a civilized diet.

Another commonality among native people eating primitive natural foods was the ease and quickness of childbirth for women. When these "primitive" peoples adopted a civilized, unnatural, processed diet, childbirth suddenly became difficult, and labor became intense and prolonged. Price also observed the relationship between tooth decay and tuberculosis. Remember that native people eating primitive, natural, unprocessed foods had perfect dental arches and almost never had a cavity, while "civilized" people eating processed, unnatural foods had deformed dental arches and mouths full of cavities. Price found that people who had perfect dental arches appeared to be immune to tuberculosis, while among those who had tuberculosis almost 100 percent had deformed dental arches. It became clear to Price that our civilized diet was affecting the body's ability to grow properly and remain healthy.

Price even conducted several experiments to see what the effects would be of feeding "civilized" people a primitive diet of natural, unprocessed foods. The results were quite astounding, and he often saw a complete reversal of tooth decay and other health problems. Sometimes cavities healed themselves without the need for oral surgery.

Price's observations were similar to what Dr. Albert Schweitzer had found during his missionary years in Africa. When he first arrived in Africa, Schweitzer discovered that cancer was either nonexistent or else extremely rare in the native people. He noticed that over the years, as the natives began to adopt the dietary habits of the "whites," they began to suffer from an ever-increasing rate of cancer.

Szekely's "Great Experiment"

Another pioneer of the health benefits of natural, unprocessed foods named Edmund Szekely had results similar to Weston Price when he switched people suffering from disease off their civilized diet of processed, unnatural foods and put them on a natural, unprocessed diet. In 1940, he opened a spa named Rancho la Puerto in Mexico, which is currently considered one of the top spas in the world. During a 33-year period, Szekely conducted what he called "the Great Experiment," which consisted of placing more than 123,000 people on a natural, unprocessed, primitive-style diet that was very high in "live foods." Live foods are foods that have not been cooked at all, such as germinated seeds, nuts, sprouts, baby lettuce greens, and organic raw fruits and vegetables.

Although natural unprocessed foods are great at preventing disease, Szekely and others have found that when a person is already in a state of disease from eating civilized, processed, unnatural foods, healing happens fastest when large amounts of these "live foods" are eaten. The results were amazing, with a greater than 90 percent recovery rate from various diseases. What is particularly astonishing is that of the 123,000 participants in Szekely's Great Experiment, approximately 17 percent were considered to be "incurable" by medicine at the time.

Weston Price deserves credit for his travels around the world and twenty years of studying "primitive" peoples before the disappearance of many of their cultures due to modernization. Similarly, Szekely deserves credit for his 33-year commitment to his "Great Experiment" on more than 123,000 people.

The China Study

In stark contrast to the Price study, in which one man traveled the globe, and Szekely's "Great Experiment," which consisted of one man in one place treating 123,000 people, is the China-Cornell-Oxford Project, often called "The China Study." The China Study was heralded by the *New York Times* as "'the 'Grand Prix' . . . the most comprehensive large study ever undertaken of the relationship between diet and the risk of developing disease," and it found more than 8,000 statistically significant associations between lifestyles, diet, and disease variables.

The study found that in more affluent areas, people suffered from "diseases of affluence," such as cancer, diabetes, and heart disease. People from more impoverished areas, however, tended to get "diseases of poverty," such as parasitic diseases, pneumonia, and infectious diseases. Impoverished areas often lack clean water and proper sanitation, which are the causes of many diseases of poverty. As an area becomes more affluent, people are able to eliminate conditions that caused the diseases of poverty. The problem is that as people become more affluent, they are also able to afford the foods that cause diseases of affluence, and they adopt a more Western-style diet that is high in civilized, unnatural, processed foods. The China Study finally gave scientific validity to Tanchou's Doctrine, along with the findings of Weston Price and Edmund Szekely. The diseases that affect Western nations, such as cancer, heart disease, and diabetes, are a result of the poor dietary choices that people tend to make when they have the money to buy processed modern foods full of unnatural ingredients.

Health and Longevity in Blue Zones

It is clear that modern processed food has become our "poison." While many scientist have been busy proving this, others have been studying places where an unusually large number of people live to at least the age of a hundred, while maintaining high levels of physical and cognitive function throughout their lives. Places such as this have been given the name *Blue Zones*.

Okinawa, Japan—The Okinawan Miracle
Perhaps the most famous Blue Zone is the island of Okinawa. Okinawa is also probably the best modern validation of both Tanchou's Doctrine and the findings of Weston Price and Edmund Szekely. Okinawa is a Japanese island located 400 miles south of the main islands of Japan. Because of its relative isolation from the rest of Japan, prior to World War II most Okinawans grew their own food, and their diets centered around the consumption of sweet potatoes. Meat was eaten very infrequently, and there was no processed food or junk food available on the island. To supplement diets that consisted of approximately 80 percent sweet

potatoes, Okinawans ate other vegetables, along with a little fish and tofu. The climate in Okinawa is such that vegetables can be grown year round.

Okinawans currently have the world's highest life expectancy rate, and their odds of reaching one hundred are nearly 4.5 times greater than for someone living in the United States. What's most important, however, is that as Okinawans age, they remain active and healthy and maintain cognitive function. This contrasts with average Americans, who spend much of the later part of their lives being overweight, underactive, sick to some degree, and overmedicated.

What makes Okinawa such a great case study for Tanchou's Doctrine is that after World War II, America established a huge military presence on the island, taking up nearly 20 percent of the land mass of the main island. Okinawa was especially prone to "Americanization" because of its small population, along with the fact that the United States actually administered the island of Okinawa until 1972, when it turned full control back to over Japan. This period of U.S. control allowed for the rapid "Americanization" of Okinawa, which got its first American-style fast-food restaurant six years before Tokyo did. Okinawa currently has more fast-food restaurants per capita than anywhere else in Japan. Okinawans consume more hamburgers than any of Japan's forty-seven prefectures (similar to our states) and not surprisingly has the highest obesity rate in Japan among those born after World War II. In a matter of one generation, it was found that when Okinawa imported our food, it also imported our diseases of affluence.

If there ever was validation of Tanchou's Doctrine, Okinawa is it. The older generation never adopted the new Western diet, and they are overwhelmingly healthy and fit, with the greatest number of disability-free years for the elderly population of any country. When compared to older Americans, older Okinawans suffer from only one-fifth the rate of heart disease, one-fourth the rate of breast cancer, and one-third the rate of dementia. Given that the cost to treat heart disease and strokes in the United States was $432 billion in 2007, adopting the type of diet advocated in this chapter has the potential to save U.S. taxpayers more than $300 billion a year just for those two diseases. (This assumes that adopting a natural diet similar to the diet of older Okinawans would lower the rate of these two diseases to the same rate as that of older Okinawans.)

The problem is that disease is a big business in America,

and that $300 billion in savings would come out of the pockets of doctors and hospitals. If your doctors told you the truth about the connection between diet and disease, they would probably be out of business, which is one of the reasons doctors are never taught the whole truth in medical school. The processed food companies make billions selling food that makes us sick, while the medical community makes billions treating those illnesses. A large section of our economy has become totally dependent on U.S. residents eating foods that make us sick and on treating the sickness that results.

Meanwhile, the younger generation of Okinawans is less healthy than the older generation and suffers from obesity. In fact, among the younger Okinawans, 30 percent of men now die before reaching the age of sixty-five and nearly half of men in their forties are obese. Once the older generation is gone, the Okinawan longevity rate is expected to plummet. What Weston Price observed happening to countless "primitive" cultures is happening right now before the world's eyes in Okinawa. Much has been made about the "Okinawan miracle" or the "secret of the Okinawans," but there is no secret. The truth is so simple and basic that most "civilized" people refuse to accept it. Modern processed foods full of unnatural ingredients create modern diseases and states of poor health, and our medical system has no profit incentive to keep us from getting sick, but rather a huge profit incentive when we get sick by treating our sickness. The good news is that each individual has the power to take control of his or her health by eliminating the foods that cause all of the diseases. Although this sounds easy, many people remain in a detached state of denial about their dietary choices. In the same way that some smokers disregard their increased risk of lung cancer and emphysema that results from smoking, most Americans continue to ignore the fact that their diet gives them very high odds of getting cancer, diabetes, or heart disease.

Loma Linda, California, and the Seventh Day Adventists
If it sounds as if I'm picking on the modern Western diet, you're absolutely right, although not all places in the United States have adopted the standard American diet. The good news is that America does have a Blue Zone of its own: the town of Loma Linda, California. What makes Loma Linda unique is that it has the world's largest concentration of Seventh Day Adventists, with nearly half of the city's residents being members of that church. Historically, Seventh Day Adventists were vegetarians, although

many now eat meat in moderation. In addition to eating very little meat, Seventh Day Adventists tend to eat very little processed food. At the center of the town is the Loma Linda Market. The market's mission statement stresses "whole foods for the whole person," and it promotes natural fresh foods and whole-grain baked goods, along with "other healthful alternatives in keeping with the lacto-ovo vegetarian practices of the Adventist Church." The market is lined with more than eighty bins full of nuts, beans, and whole grains. If there is one place in this world that has succeeded in combining the best aspects of civilization, such as clean water and proper sanitation, with the best aspects of the "primitive" natural diet, Loma Linda may be it.

When you look at "diseases of civilization," Seventh Day Adventist men suffer from only 60 percent of the cancer and 66 percent of the heart disease that non-Adventist men do. Imagine if a miracle drug were invented that could reduce cancer and heart disease rates by 40 percent. It would make the front page of every newspaper, and the company producing it would earn countless billions of dollars. Nearly every person alive would probably take the drug, especially if there were no side effects. People would be willing to pay thousands of dollars a year for such a drug. That miracle drug already exists, and it's the type of natural diet that is free of processed foods and low in meat described in this chapter. What's even better is that rather than costing you thousands of dollars a year, you will save thousands of dollars a year in reduced food costs and thousands more in lower medical expenses.

Although organic fruits and vegetables are more expensive than conventional fruits and vegetables, which are usually loaded with toxic chemicals, the rest of the "primitive" diet is far less expensive than eating "civilized" food. When you buy foods such as whole grains, beans, and nuts in bulk, an entire meal becomes a fraction of the cost of most processed foods. When you factor in the improvement in well-being, which allows for increased productivity, along with the huge savings in money spent on health care, the natural unprocessed diet makes sense, both economically and for overall well-being.

Costa Rica and Sardinia

The two other Blue Zones are a region in Costa Rica called Nicoya and a region in Sardinia named Barbagia. Nicoyans who reach age sixty have twice the chance of reaching the age of ninety when compared to a sixty-year-old American. The rate of people living at least to the age of one hundred in Barbagia is more than 30 times the rate of people in America. Their recipes for longevity and health are very similar. People in both Blue Zones have mainly plant-based diets and eat meat only about once a week. They have active lifestyles that keep them lean and fit. Most important, however, is possibly the fact that they eat natural whole foods, with no processed foods, no processed vegetable oils, and no processed fructose or soy.

Kicking the Junk Food Habit

Just as a smoker needs to kick the tobacco addiction in order to stop smoking, a person eating processed foods needs to kick that addiction.

A study conducted on rats and reported in the journal *Nature Neuroscience* shows just how addictive civilized processed food is. Rats were given either a balanced diet or a balanced diet plus unlimited access to processed junk food, such as bacon, sausage, cheesecake, pound cake, and chocolate. In a very short time, the rats given access to the processed junk food began to eat compulsively and quickly became obese. The researchers believe that the rats' compulsive eating behavior was due to the processed junk food making their brains behave in a similar way to a drug addict's brain. The rats basically became obese and addicted to junk food, just as many Americans are.

Perhaps even more interesting is what happened when the processed junk food was removed. The rats that had become obese junk-food addicts actually refused to eat for two weeks, rather than eat the healthy food they were offered. Although the researchers believed this was due in large part to the rats' shifted dietary preferences for junk food, my experience in nutrition leads me to another conclusion. I have found that every person has an ideal weight that his or her body prefers to maintain. In my experience, when people are fed natural, unprocessed food according to the needs of their season-type, they will not be hungry and will tend to eat very little if they are above their ideal weight. Once their ideal weight is attained, they will regain their hunger and will resume eating larger amounts of natural foods again. In the same way that Weston Price did not encounter obesity among natives eating "primitive" natural diets, my experience has shown that when you eliminate processed foods, your body eats only what it feels it needs, and dieting to your ideal weight becomes effortless, as long as you also eat according to your season-type. Not surprisingly, Seventh Day Adventists who have a mostly natural, unprocessed diet have much lower rates of obesity than the general population, which is a major contributing factor to their superior health.

Studies show that thirty-year-old California Adventists will live more than seven years longer than an average thirty-year-old white California male, while an Adventist vegetarian will live almost ten years longer. Remember that even among Adventists who eat meat, they eat far less than the average American does, and they consume very little processed food. This is pretty convincing proof that if you're a man who lowers your consumption of meat and processed foods, you can add about seven years to your life, while if you choose to eliminate meat altogether, while limiting processed foods, you can add about ten years to your life. In addition to adding ten years, you can expect the last twenty to thirty years of your life to be relatively healthy, compared to average Americans who live their last twenty to thirty years sick and medicated, a state that I do not consider to be true "living." Another finding is that Adventist vegetarians have about half the risk of heart disease of Adventist nonvegetarians. When you look at the studies, much of this protection from heart disease is due to the fact that the vegetarians tend to have a lower body weight than the Adventists who consume meat.

The problem with many of these studies is that researchers did not realize the significance of a person's season-type when it comes to meat consumption and weight loss. Summers and Springs will tend to be leaner when they eliminate meat and saturated fat, so these season-types will see the most benefit from eliminating meat. As explained earlier, however, cooked meat also contains many other cancer-causing substances, so Winters and Autumns will benefit from reducing their consumption, as long as they learn how to do so while keeping their diets appropriate for their season-type.

A Diet for Optimal Health

Earlier, I discussed Tanchou's Doctrine, which states that cancer increases in direct proportion to the "civilization" of a people. Tanchou's research has been in large part validated by an organization called World Cancer Research Fund International, or WCRF International. It was created in 1982 and is a modern pioneer in research into the links between food, nutrition, physical activity, and the prevention of cancer. It focuses on cancer prevention, rather than on expensive treatments, as the true cure for cancer. WCRF International estimates that up to 40 percent of cancer is preventable through proper diet and physical activity, although I believe that number is much higher if you eliminate all processed foods, especially processed vegetable oils and processed soy, and limit your fructose consumption to less than 15 grams a day.

75 to 80 Percent of Cancer Is Avoidable

In 1981, two Oxford epidemiologists, Richard Doll and Richard Peto, published a 120-page report titled *The Causes of Cancer: Quantitative Estimates of Avoidable Risks of Cancer in the United Stated Today*, which concluded that about 75 to 80 percent of cancers in the United States might be avoidable with the proper dietary and lifestyle changes. In their report, they reviewed multiple factors, such as the changes in cancer over time and differences in cancer rates among various communities and nations. Keep in mind that early contact with native people who had a "primitive" diet of natural, unprocessed food consistently found that these people almost never had cancer. This suggests that the actual amount of cancer that could be prevented is at least 80 percent. During the last fifty years, our entire planet has become so polluted with cancer-causing chemicals that studies conducted on even the most isolated of peoples show that they have some amount of these toxic man-made chemicals in their bodies. So although getting rid of unnatural processed foods may reduce your risk of cancer by 80 to 90 percent, you still run a slight risk of getting cancer due to our polluted air, water, and soil.

True cancer prevention is beneficial for everyone, except for processed food companies, whose products contribute to most types of cancer, along with the doctors, the drug companies, and the hospitals that rake in almost $210 billion a year (National Institutes of Health, 2005 estimate) treating people with cancer. In American medicine, profits are made from sick people, not from well people, and as our food has become more and more processed, those profits have skyrocketed. For example, according to the Medicare and Medicaid Services, in 1965 approximately 5 percent of the U.S. gross domestic product was spent on health care. By 2004, health-care expenditures had grown to 16 percent of the gross domestic product, and they are soon projected to reach 20 percent of the GDP. During the forty-year period in which the consumption of processed foods, fructose, processed soy, and processed vegetable oils has skyrocketed, the amount that Americans spend on health care as a percentage of GDP has gone up 400 percent.

In the middle of this explosion in health-care costs, the World Cancer Research Fund International was created for the purpose of finding ways that lifestyle changes can prevent cancer. WCRF International published two major reports, one in 1997, and one in 2007 titled *Food, Nutrition, Physical Activity, and the Prevention of Cancer: A Global Perspective*. These are probably the most comprehensive scientific reports ever published on the relationships between food, nutrition, physical activity, and cancer prevention. The reports are based on an in-depth analysis of more than seven thousand studies that have been published in the last fifty years concerning cancer prevention. A panel of twenty-one world-renowned scientists reviewed the evidence and the research to compile the reports and their recommendations for cancer prevention.

Cancer-Prevention Guidelines from WCRF International
When you read the 2007 report and examine the recommendations, it seems to validate everything Tanchou, Weston Price, Edmund Szekely, and the Blue Zone studies on longevity have been saying.

1. Eat more whole grains, vegetables, beans, and fruits high in fiber.
This is the cornerstone of the Blue Zone diets, along with the Seventh Day Adventist diet. These foods tend to be high in nutrients and not very energy dense in terms of calories and are usually very filling. As a result, they help people maintain a lower body weight, which is one key to health and longevity. Sugary drinks are not recommended, because they contribute to weight gain. Nor are junk foods. For example, 100 grams of potato chips has 550 calories, while 100 grams of baked potato has only 100 calories. Grains should be eaten in their natural, unprocessed state, and consumption of refined starchy foods should be limited.

2. Limit your consumption of foods that are energy dense, such as high-fat and sugary foods that are low in fiber.
Energy-dense natural foods, such as nuts, that are high in nutrients have not been linked with weight gain when eaten in moderation. Processed fast foods, such as hamburgers, fried chicken, and pizza, tend to be energy dense and low in nutrients and contribute to obesity. Sugary drinks, even natural fruit juices, are often very

energy dense and should be avoided.

3. Be lean without being underweight.
This relates to the first two recommendations, because following the first two will help you achieve the third. Evidence shows that being overweight increases your risk of developing a number of cancers, including breast cancer. By eating according to your season-type and eliminating processed vegetable oils and soy, while keeping your fructose consumption to no more than 15 grams a day, you should have a relatively easy time maintaining a healthy weight.

4. Do some type of moderate physical activity for at least 30 minutes every day.
Physical activity is one of the keys to maintaining a healthy weight.

5. Drink alcohol only in moderation.
Limit your consumption of alcohol to one drink a day for women and two drinks a day for men. Evidence shows that excess alcohol consumption can increase your risk for developing a number of cancers, including colon and breast cancers.

6. Limit your consumption of salty foods and especially processed foods that are high in salt.
The recommended sodium consumption is no more than 2,000 mg a day.

7. Limit the amount of red meat you eat to no more than 18 ounces a week.
Also limit your consumption of processed meats, which includes foods that have been smoked, cured, salted, or have had chemicals added to them.

8. Supplements.
It's recommended that you try to meet your nutritional needs through your diet, without using any dietary supplements.

Vegetarians Live Longer, Healthier Lives
Vegetarians, in addition to living longer than meat eaters, also tend to age much better than meat eaters. The American Journal of Clinical Nutrition reported on a study in which vegetarians were compared to meat eaters in regard to bone loss later in life. The study found that both vegetarian men and vegetarian women

average about half the measurable bone loss later in life, when compared to their meat-eating counterparts. For example, elderly female vegetarians had a measurable bone loss of 18 percent, while the meat-eating women had a measurable bone loss of 35 percent. People have been led to believe that ingesting large amounts of calcium, especially dairy products, is the key to having strong bones. Another study in the American Journal of Clinical Nutrition, however, showed that the consumption of plenty of potassium and magnesium from vegetables and fruits is associated with greater bone mineral density later in life.

In an earlier chapter, I discussed acid and alkaline balance and how your body works to maintain pH balance. Two of the minerals that help your body maintain this balance are magnesium and potassium. When you do not eat enough foods that contain these minerals, your body begins to rob minerals from your bones when it needs to balance its pH.

Do Dairy Foods Build Strong Bones and Prevent Osteoporosis?

The milk industry has spent a lot of money trying to convince you to drink milk to get calcium and build strong bones. Yet most studies show that increasing your dietary calcium levels does not translate into better bone health later in life. One way in which milk may help contribute to greater bone density is that in the average American's diet, milk is the second leading source of both potassium and magnesium. Sadly, this is due less to milk being super high in these two minerals than it is to the fact that most Americans who eat processed foods get low levels of potassium and magnesium because these have been stripped out of the food by processing. For example, whole-grain wheat has 5½ times the amount of magnesium and nearly 3 times the amount of potassium as processed white flour. This is one of the many reasons that eating unprocessed natural food has been shown in study after study to be a key to superior health.

The Bantu tribe in Africa has a diet consisting mainly of a porridge made from corn, along with beans and vegetables. Corn is very low in calcium but has generous amounts of both potassium and magnesium. Due to their reliance on corn for a large portion of their calories, Bantu women ingest only about one-fourth of the calcium that is recommended for U.S. women. In addition to their low calcium intake, Bantu women often bear nine children during their lifetime and breast-feed each child for more than a year. Despite their low calcium intake and the large number of children they bear, Bantu women over the age of sixty rarely suffer from osteoporosis.

A twelve-year Harvard study of more than 75,000 women found that those drinking two or more glasses of milk a day had a greater chance of experiencing a hip fracture than did those who drank one glass or less per week. A study conducted in Australia found that a high consumption of dairy foods at age twenty was associated with an increased risk of hip fracture in old age. The exact reasons for this remain unclear, but I mention these two studies to help illuminate what does appear to increase bone strength: a natural, plant-based, unprocessed diet that is high in potassium and magnesium.

Potassium and Magnesium Strengthen Teeth and Bones

This is exactly the type of diet adhered to by those living in the Blue Zones, where people have a much greater chance of living to one hundred than in other places on the planet. Weston Price found many primitive people who had this kind of diet. He documented how their health changed when their natural diets were replaced by diets high in processed sugar and flour. When primitive people were given "civilized" foods that were stripped of their potassium, magnesium, fiber, and many other vitamins and minerals, their health rapidly deteriorated. A diet low in potassium and magnesium leads to a state of health where the body is forced to cannibalize calcium and other minerals from its bones. Not surprisingly, Weston Price rarely saw a cavity when looking at the teeth of a primitive person eating a primitive diet. Once the diet had been replaced by a civilized diet that was high in processed foods, however, Price found mouths full of cavities. I'm sure that if he had been able to measure bone density, he would have found that people with the civilized diet had bones that were far less dense than the bones of individuals with the primitive diet.

Personal Health = Planetary Health

Choosing a natural, plant-based organic diet is becoming increasingly more important in order to maintain health as mankind pollutes the planet with countless pesticides and toxic chemicals. Dioxins are just one of the many toxic chemicals that Americans are exposed to in the foods they eat.

Chemical Toxins in Meat, Fish, and Dairy

Dioxins are a class of chemicals, some of which are so toxic that the EPA has determined there are no safe levels of exposure. They are a known carcinogen and have been linked to birth defects, decreased fertility, immune system suppression, and many other health problems. A hundred years ago, when there were few chemicals in our environment, only 2 percent of the U.S. population died from cancer; now cancer is responsible for 20 percent of deaths, and that number continues to rise as we are exposed to ever-increasing amounts of chemicals in our environment.

Sadly, our environment has become so polluted with just this one class of chemicals that it's virtually impossible to avoid being exposed to them. Dioxins tend to accumulate higher up in the food chain, so the concentration in animals is much higher than in plants. Americans receive nearly 95 percent of their dietary dioxin load by eating foods such as meat and dairy products. Not surprisingly, vegans (people who consume no meat or dairy products) have much lower levels of dioxins than meat eaters do. Dioxins also cross the placenta barrier and get into breast milk, and meat-eating women expose their fetuses to higher levels of these chemicals in the womb and have much higher levels of these toxic chemicals in their breast milk than do vegetarians. Many experts attribute part of the rise in the number of children born with autism and attention deficit disorder to the chemicals they are exposed to in the womb, such as dioxins.

Because dioxins have also polluted the oceans, fish are a source of these toxic chemicals. Dioxins are just one class of chemicals that tends to work its way up the food chain. Other chemicals, such as mercury, PCBs, furans, and PDBEs, also work their way up the food chain and accumulate in the fat and the milk of animals. This means that the more meat and dairy you eat, the greater your consumption of all of these toxic chemicals.

Grain and Water Consumed by Livestock Could Feed Millions of People

Eating lower on the food chain by adopting a plant-based diet is also more environmentally friendly than eating meat. It's estimated that the amount of grain fed to livestock in the United States is enough to feed nearly 800 million people. U.S. livestock consume five times the amount of grain as people do in America. Worldwide, it's estimated that 40 percent of the world's grain is being fed to livestock. Producing protein by feeding grain to animals is very inefficient, in terms of energy and resources. It takes more than eight times as much fossil-fuel energy to produce animal protein as it does plant protein. Raising animals for meat also takes an inordinate amount of water resources, and in fact, animal agriculture is the largest consumer of water resources in the United States. It takes 900 liters of water to produce a kilogram of wheat, but a staggering 100,000 liters of water to produce a kilogram of grain-fed beef, when you factor in the water used to grow the grains that are fed to beef.

Destruction of Rain Forests for Cattle Ranching to Raise Cheap Beef

America's demand for cheap beef is also affecting the environment on a global scale and has caused massive destruction of the rain forests in Central and South America. Since the 1960s, 25 percent of Central American rain forests have been lost to beef production, and estimates are that for every quarter-pound fast-food hamburger made from Central American beef, 55 square feet of rain forests are destroyed. In many Central American countries, more than 90 percent of the rain-forest beef is exported to the United States and is used as a cheap source of meat, usually in fast-food restaurants. In 1994, the amount of Central American rain-forest beef imported into the United States was more than 200 million pounds, and by 2004, that figure was reported to be 300 million pounds a year. During one period in the 1980s, Costa Rica was losing about 4 percent of its rain forests per year to make way for cattle ranching, so that Americans could have cheap hamburgers. I am sure that if Americans were given the choice to pay an extra 5 to 10 cents for a quarter-pound hamburger so that 55 square feet of rain forest would not have to be destroyed, most of them would gladly pay a little extra to help save the planet. Unfortunately, low price has become king, and just as we buy cheap stuff made in China, while Chinese factories continue to dump huge amounts of toxins into their rivers, which end up in the oceans we all share, we continue to buy cheap food without ever asking what the real cost is.

Overfishing Will Cause Global Collapse of Ocean Fisheries

America's hunger for cheap meat is also causing the destruction of the world's oceans. More than one-third of all of the fish caught in the world's oceans end up becoming food to feed livestock and farmed fish. Nearly 50 percent of the fish used in feed goes to feed farmed fish. Basically, we have overfished species that humans prefer to eat, such as salmon, cod, and tilapia, to the point where there is no longer enough of those fish left in the wild to meet demand. Now we are overfishing species such as anchovies and sardines, called "forage fish," which play a key role low on the ocean's food chain and are eaten by larger fish. We are feeding these forage fish to farm-raised fish, such as farmed salmon, that people prefer to eat.

The world now uses so much of these fish to feed livestock that pigs and chickens alone consume six times the amount of fish every year as the entire U.S. population. Fishery experts are predicting that at the current pace of fishing, a "global collapse" of ocean fisheries is inevitable within the next thirty-five years.

The Moral Imperative to Eat Less Meat
It's clear that a growing world cannot continue to use grain and fish to feed livestock while people starve, rain forests are destroyed, and the oceans are near collapse. The only long-term solution to the massive environmental toll that meat production is taking on the planet is for people to eat less meat. Although this is relatively easy for Summers and Springs to do, it is a little more challenging for Winters, but it is possible to accomplish, as explained in the diet section. In addition to saving the environment, consuming less meat is also healthier because you won't be exposing yourself to all of the toxic chemicals that have worked their way up the food chain and found their way into meat. Remember that nearly 95 percent of the dietary dioxins that people consume come from animal products, and dioxins are just one of the cancer-causing chemicals you will eliminate from your diet when you stop eating meat. This is one of many reasons that vegetarians live longer, and that all of the people in the longevity-promoting Blue Zones were found to have a diet in which they ate no meat or ate meat only about once a week.

There was a time when women proudly wore their fur coats, but slowly people woke up and realized it was wrong, and attitudes about wearing fur changed. There was a time when diamond brokers had no issue with purchasing "blood diamonds," which are diamonds from war zones. Thousands of people have been killed and had their hands chopped off because of these diamonds, until people finally woke up and realized that in a way, they were guilty if they knew better and still purchased the diamonds that were causing so much harm and human suffering. Hopefully, the time is coming when people will wake up and realize that they cannot continue to eat as much meat, because it's causing the destruction of the planet we all call home.

It's time to take your health into your own hands and realize that most doctors are focused on treating disease, not on avoiding disease in the first place. The average doctor receives fewer than three hours of nutritional training during his or her four years of medical school. If Americans ever attained the same level of health as people living in the Blue Zones, the American medical system would go bankrupt, and most doctors would have to find a new line of work. Sickness is a business, an extremely profitable business. A person with cancer or some other disease will pay almost anything and endure almost any painful treatment to get better. The lessons from Tanchou's Doctrine, Weston Price, Edmund Szekely, and the Blue Zones are all the same. Choosing a mainly plant-based diet of foods in their natural state, with minimal processing, is the key to a long life free of disease. Although a lot of Americans live to be over eighty, many are not healthy for the last thirty or forty years of their lives. The lesson from the Blue Zones is that you can live to an old age and remain fit and active your entire life. There are plenty of stories of eighty- and ninety-year-olds in the Blue Zones who could physically out-perform the average forty-year-old American.

The Visionary Beliefs of Jack LaLanne

America had its own health food pioneer who advocated this type of natural, unprocessed foods diet: Jack LaLanne. As a teenager, LaLanne had a typical American diet of processed foods, and he was so sickly that he dropped out of school at the age of fourteen. He turned his life around by exercising and by adopting a natural plant-based diet, similar to that of people in the Blue Zones. LaLanne was ridiculed by medical doctors because he advocated that people to go to health clubs as a way to exercise and stay fit. He said, "The doctors were against me—they said that working out with weights would give people heart attacks and they would lose their sex drive." This was during the same time period when doctors claimed that cigarette smoking was not dangerous. I mention this because the medical establishment has a long history of making major blunders when it comes to the health effects of dietary and lifestyle choices. They were wrong about working out causing heart attacks, just as they were wrong in the 1970s and the '80s when they claimed trans fats were actually healthy, as they are currently wrong when they state that saturated fat causes heart disease and are also wrong when they say that processed vegetable oils and soy are healthy. Of course, when you listen to their bad advice, the result is that you get sick, and they get rich treating you.

What's amazing about LaLanne's story is that when he was a teenager, his health was similar to that of the average elderly person living in America, and when he became an elderly man, LaLanne's health was far better than that of the average American teenager. At the age of seventy, LaLanne towed seventy rowboats while swimming a distance of one mile through Long Beach Harbor while he was handcuffed, shackled, and fighting strong currents and winds. He turned his life around the same way that each and every one of you reading this book can turn yours around: by choosing a natural diet of unprocessed foods. I think LaLanne summed it up best when he said, *"If man made it, don't eat it."*

11
Unnatural Foods and Chemicals Lead to Sickness

If you say good-bye to unnatural foods,
you'll say good-bye to most forms of cancer and other diseases.

Jack LaLanne's advice mirrors Tanchou's Doctrine, Weston Price's findings, and the conclusions from studies conducted in the world's Blue Zones. Although many people know that processed foods are not as healthy for you as whole natural foods, what they are not aware of are the reasons why. While whole natural foods usually have more fiber, vitamins, and minerals than their processed counterparts, most processed foods have negative health consequences for reasons that go beyond simply the fiber and the vitamins being stripped out of them. In this chapter, you'll learn about some of the other reasons processed foods are less healthy than whole natural foods. Eating for your season-type means avoiding those foods that hurt your body and lead to disease, and this includes most highly processed foods. Hopefully, by the end of this chapter, you'll see that when in doubt, your best bet is to stick to whole natural foods and avoid processed foods altogether.

This includes avoiding all foods containing GMOs, as you'll read about in this chapter. It's worth mentioning a July 1, 2012, article in Vitality magazine titled "Dramatic Health Recoveries Reported by Patients Who Took Their Doctor's Advice and Stopped Using GMO Foods." According to the article, many doctors are now prescribing a non-GMO diet to their patients and are seeing remarkable recoveries as a result. The article states that thousands of physicians and nutritionists are reporting that "a wide variety of health conditions improve after people make the change" of eliminating GMOs from their diet. The article describes how many people have seen conditions such as irritable bowel syndrome, allergies, congestion, skin problems, migraines, and asthma disappear after they adopted a completely non-GMO diet, which also included eliminating corn oil, canola oil, and soy oil. Jack LaLanne clearly said it best: "If man made it, don't eat it."

376

Bleached and Bromated White Flour

When grain is first milled into flour for making bread or pasta, it is a light yellow color and not the white that we are used to when we buy flour at the grocery store. Historically, freshly milled flour, called "green flour," was stored for several months to properly age and oxidize. This aging improves its baking qualities, as well as its flavor.

Around a hundred years ago, flour makers abandoned this old method of aging flour and began to use chemicals to accelerate the aging process. This allowed them to sell flour to bakers a few days after it was made, rather than having to wait for it to age for several months. Bakers who still use the "old fashioned" and natural way of aging flour claim that it gives both good baking properties and a better flavor and a crumb that is creamier when compared to processed bleached flour. According to many experts, the key to a truly tasty artisan bread lies in using wheat that is unbleached, unbromated, and properly aged.

One step in making modern flour is to bleach it, using a bleaching agent such as chlorine dioxide. Another step is often to bromate the flour by adding potassium bromate, which improves the elasticity and allows bread to rise higher. Yet although these chemicals may help the millers sell their flour sooner, there are health concerns about the effects of the chemicals they use to avoid the natural aging process.

The chlorine dioxide that's used to bleach flour forms a substance called *alloxan* when it comes into contact with wheat. Alloxan is known to destroy the beta cells of the pancreas, putting a person at risk for developing diabetes. Alloxan is structurally very similar to glucose, which causes the cells of the pancreas to take it up very readily. Once inside the pancreas, alloxan causes free radical damage.

Chemical bleaching of flour is banned in the European Union and Australia, and even China recently banned the use of all wheat flour whiteners. They are still perfectly legal to use in the United States, however.

The other chemicals that are usually added to processed flour in the United States are bromates, which are a known cancer-causing agent. Bromates were first found to cause tumors in rats in 1982, and due to their ability to cause cancer, they have been banned in the European Union, Canada, China, Brazil, Peru, and even Sri Lanka but are still perfectly legal to use in the United States.

One of the many reasons that it's best to eat natural foods that have not been processed is that oftentimes the effects of the chemicals and the processing techniques used to make processed foods are not known for many years. In the case of bleaching agents and bromates, many countries decided to ban them to protect their citizens, while other countries, such as the United States, continue to allow their use. There are probably countless chemicals used in processed foods at this time that are assumed to be safe but will be proved to be unsafe at some time in the near future.

If you eat foods that contain wheat, such as bread or pasta, you should try to find products that are made with "unbleached" and "unbromated" flour.

Artificial Sweeteners

People who want to lose weight are a huge market for companies that produce artificial sweeteners made from chemicals. This section deals with two of the allegedly most dangerous ones that are currently on the market: aspartame and sucralose. I recommend that you avoid both of them. If you're looking for a zero-calorie natural sweetener that won't affect your blood-sugar levels and won't destroy your health, you might want to try stevia, which is made from the leaves of a South American plant. Stevia has been widely used for many years in Europe and Japan, with no apparent negative health effects.

Aspartame
Aspartame, also known as NutraSweet and AminoSweet, is the most consumed artificial sweetener in the United States. There has been a lot of controversy surrounding aspartame ever since its approval by the FDA, and I will highlight a few of the relevant issues. Despite the controversy, the FDA has stated that it is one of the most thoroughly tested and studied food additives the agency has ever approved. Citing more than a hundred toxicological and clinical studies, the FDA claims that it is safe for the general population.

How Aspartame Entered the U.S. Food Supply
According to an article titled "How Aspartame Became Legal—The Timeline," aspartame was discovered in 1965 by a scientist at G.D.

Searle, and the company began safety-testing it in 1967, in order to gain FDA approval for aspartame as a food additive. The article stated that safety testing was done on seven monkeys: one died, while five had grand mal seizures. There were also concerns that one of the ingredients in aspartame called *aspartic acid* produced holes in the brains of infant mice. Despite these drawbacks, the FDA granted aspartame approval for use in dry foods in 1974. In 1976, the FDA investigated the laboratory practices used by G.D. Searle in its aspartame studies and found its testing procedures "shoddy, full of inaccuracies and manipulated test data." In the article, the investigators reported that they "had never seen anything as bad as Searle's testing."

In 1977, the U.S. Attorney's office began a grand jury investigation to determine whether indictments should be filed against the company for "concealing material facts and making false statements" in its safety tests. During the investigation, the U.S. Attorney in charge of the investigation was hired away by the law firm that represented the maker of aspartame. His resignation as U.S. Attorney ended up stalling the grand jury investigation, which caused the statute of limitations on the case against G.D. Searle to run out, effectively ending the investigation. That same year, G.D. Searle hired Donald Rumsfeld as its new CEO, who at that time had been a former member of Congress and secretary of defense under President Ford. Meanwhile, the FDA released *The Bressler Report*, which found "that 98 out of 196 animals died during one of Searle's studies."

In 1979, the FDA established an inquiry board to rule on the safety issues surrounding aspartame, and in 1980, the board concluded that aspartame should not be approved until further investigations were conducted. According to the article, the new CEO of G.D. Searle, Donald Rumsfeld, stated in a sales meeting that he was going to "use his political pull in Washington, rather than scientific means," to get aspartame approved. In 1981, Ronald Reagan became the new U.S. president, and his transition team included Donald Rumsfeld, who hand-picked Arthur Hull Hayes Jr. to be the new FDA commissioner, replacing the old commissioner, who, in the belief of many, stood in the way of aspartame's approval. Even with the new friendly FDA chairman, the agency still rejected aspartame by a 3-2 vote. The solution was simply to add another member to the board, making the vote 3-3, with the new aspartame-friendly FDA chairman breaking the tie and approving aspartame.

Research Studies Confirm Health Concerns about Aspartame

In 1983, the FDA commissioner who helped get aspartame approved resigned over a controversy about his taking unauthorized rides on a private jet belonging to General Foods, a major customer of aspartame. He was quickly hired by the PR firm that represented J.D. Searle, the manufacturer of aspartame. That same year, the National Soft Drink Association urged the FDA to delay approving aspartame for carbonated beverages over concerns about its stability in liquid form when stored above 85 degrees. The concerns centered on the fact that at higher temperatures, aspartame breaks down into formaldehyde and DKP (diketopiperazine), which has been implicated in the occurrence of brain tumors and uterine polyps.

A review of the studies done on aspartame showed that 165 were believed to have relevance regarding its safety for human consumption. Of these, 74 were funded by people and companies with ties to the aspartame industry, and 91 were independently funded. Of the 74 industry-funded studies, 100 percent found that aspartame was safe for human consumption. Of the 91 independently funded studies, 92 percent found at least one potential concern for human health. Of the 7 nonindustry studies that found aspartame to be safe, 6 were done by the FDA, and many people questioned whether the FDA studies were truly independent, given that agency's history of often ignoring science and giving in to political pressure, then subsequently making decisions that were contrary to scientific findings.

One study on aspartame was conducted by a private citizen named Victoria Inness-Brown and was chronicled in her book *My Aspartame Experiment: Report from a Private Citizen*. Her two-and-a-half-year experiment consisted of raising more than a hundred rats, then giving some a regular diet and others the same diet supplemented with aspartame, equivalent to drinking about 13 cans of aspartame-sweetened soda a day. After thirty months on the aspartame-sweetened soda, 67 percent of the female rats fed aspartame had developed tumors the size of golf balls or larger, while only 21 percent of the control females not given aspartame developed tumors, and those tumors were usually smaller in size. The male rats were also negatively affected by aspartame, with 23 percent of the males fed aspartame developing tumors, while none of the control males who did not receive aspartame developed tumors. A large number of the tumors in the female rats appeared in the mammary glands, and other evidence suggests that aspartame has worse effects on women than on men. Of the complaints filed with the FDA concerning negative effects from consuming aspartame, more than 75 percent of them are from women, which lends further credence to the notion that aspartame affects women more negatively than it does men. The rats that had been fed aspartame also suffered from neurological problems, such as falling over or difficultly walking, eye disorders, skin disorders, obesity, and even paralysis.

Research on the long-term effects of consuming aspartame, conducted by Dr. Soffritti at the Cesare Maltoni Cancer Research Center, found that rats fed aspartame developed higher rates of lymphoma, leukemia, and other cancers, with the rates for cancer rising as the amount of aspartame in their diets was increased. Even at the lowest levels of aspartame exposure, there was a 62 percent increase in lymphomas and leukemia, compared to the control rats. The female rats that had been given aspartame also showed more abnormal lesions and carcinomas of the renal pelvis and ureter. Dr. Soffritti felt that the higher rates of lymphoma and leukemia in the aspartame-fed rats could be related to the fact that the methanol in aspartame is metabolized into formaldehyde in rats, similar to the way it is metabolized into formaldehyde in humans. This is further corroborated by research that shows that methanol administered in drinking water increases the rate of lymphoma and leukemia in female rats.

Adverse Reactions to Aspartame Reported to the FDA
Since its approval, aspartame has come under fire from natural health advocates as being a potentially dangerous food additive. Adverse aspartame reactions have accounted for roughly 75 percent of the complaints received by the FDA's Adverse Reaction Monitoring System (ARMS) for many of the years in which statistics have been kept, although this is often viewed only as anecdotal evidence that aspartame should be avoided. Following is a short list of other reasons to avoid consuming aspartame, given by many who have studied it.

The symptoms that are often reported from aspartame consumption include headaches, mood changes, fuzzy thinking, migraine headaches, nausea, muscle spasms, eye tics, dizziness, seizures, weight gain, depression, rashes, fatigue, irritability, insomnia, vision problems, anxiety, slurred speech, vertigo, memory loss, joint pain, and many others. There are numerous cases of people with these unexplained symptoms experiencing an end to their suffering shortly after eliminating aspartame from their diet. According to those studying aspartame, these symptoms can lead to a higher incidence of brain tumors, multiple sclerosis, epilepsy, Parkinson's disease, Alzheimer's, fibromyalgia, lymphoma, and other serious diseases.

Aspartame is composed of 50 percent phenylalanine, 40 percent aspartic acid, and 10 percent methanol. According to many experts, excessive levels of phenylalanine in the brain can cause a decrease in serotonin levels, leading to diseases such as depression. Furthermore, the aspartic acid is considered an excitotoxin by many experts, which can overstimulate the neurons in the brain until they die. The most dangerous part of aspartame is often said to be the methanol, which is claimed to be metabolized into formaldehyde, a known neurotoxin and carcinogen. The EPA's recommended limit of methanol consumption is less than 8 mg per day, and a 1-liter bottle of soda sweetened with aspartame can contain more than 50 mg of methanol.

Although many people consume aspartame in an attempt to lose weight, some studies show that those who drink aspartame-sweetened beverages actually gain more weight than do individuals who drink calorically sweetened beverages. While the reasons for this are still being debated, the theory is that artificial sweeteners actually perpetuate the craving for sweets, leading to increased calorie consumption. A study done at Purdue University suggests that artificial sweeteners may interfere with the body's natural ability to regulate calories. The study found that rats that drank artificially sweetened liquids consumed more high-calorie foods than did those that drank high-caloric sweetened liquids.

Sucralose
Sucralose, also known as Splenda, is an artificial noncaloric sweetener that was approved for use in the United States in 1998 and is currently contained in more than four thousand food products. Despite its approval by the FDA, many natural health experts caution against the use of sucralose.

Negative Health Effects from Consuming Sucralose
A study conducted at Duke University found that sucralose had a negative effect on the beneficial bacteria contained in the colons of rats, decreasing helpful bifisobacteria, lactobacilli, bacteroids, clostridia, and total bacteria. At even the lowest doses administered in the study, beneficial bacteria began to decrease immediately on

oral administration of Splenda, and at the end of twelve weeks at the lowest dose, intestinal microflora was reduced by nearly 50 percent, when compared to the control rats that did not receive Splenda. The higher doses of Splenda in this study reduced healthy microflora levels by nearly 68 percent.

In addition, sucralose also increased fecal pH and levels of proteins that are known to limit the bioavailability of ingested nutrients and drugs. According to the study, "adverse consequences from the elevated presence of sucralose have been reported in animal models, which included gastrointestinal tract DNA damage. . . . Unabsorbed sucralose in the gut may affect the intestinal microbial milieu." The microflora in our gut carry out numerous important functions, with the study citing such benefits as: "(1) Fermentation of dietary carbohydrates, (2) Salvage of energy as short-chain fatty acids, (3) Production of vitamins, (4) Maintenance of normal immune system functioning, (5) Gastrointestinal tract mobility, (6) Inhibition of pathogens, (7) Metabolism of drug[s]."

Splenda Causes Weight Gain in Rats
Although people often consume sucralose in the belief that it will help them lose weight, this study showed that rats given "the lowest Splenda dose showed a significant increase in body weight gain during and after Splenda supplementation." In fact, even twelve weeks after the end of all sucralose supplementation, the rats still showed a decrease in beneficial microflora, along with a continued increase in fecal pH. In addition, after the twelve weeks of "treatment with Splenda, numerous alterations were observed that did not occur in control animals, including lymphocytic infiltrates into epithelium, epithelial scarring, mild depletion of goblet cells, glandular disorganization, and focally dilated vessels stuffed with intravascular lymphocytes."

The study concludes that "intake of Splenda for 12-wks exerted several adverse effects on the intestines of rats, including a significant decrease in beneficial intestinal bacteria, elevated fecal pH, histopathological changes in the colon, increased body weight, and enhanced intestinal expression of proteins that inhibit absorption of drugs and nutrients."

Does Sucralose Contribute to Skyrocketing Rates of IBD?
Due to sucralose's apparent ability to alter healthy gut microflora and pH, many experts speculate that sucralose consumption may

be connected to the increase in inflammatory bowel disease (IBD) in the United States. Canada was the first country to approve the use of sucralose in 1991, a full seven years before the United States approved it. Since this time, Canada has seen its rate of Crohn's disease (CD), a form of IBD, skyrocket from being one of the lowest in the industrialized world to the highest. In 1981, for example, prior to the introduction of sucralose into Canada, the reported rate of CD in Alberta was only 44 per 100,000 people; however, by 2000, it had increased more than 600 percent to 283 cases per 100,000 people. An article in the *Canadian Journal of Gastroenterology* theorizes that sucralose may be to blame for this sudden and rapid increase in IBD in Canada.

Other Adverse Symptoms Reported by Sucralose Users
There have been many cases of sucralose users complaining of symptoms such as feeling a general malaise, feeling foggy-headed, being unable to concentrate, and having a general bad mood, which they later attributed to having consumed sucralose. Some of the symptoms commonly reported within twenty-four hours of consuming sucralose included achy joints, stuffy or runny nose, headaches, shortness of breath, heart palpitations, anxiety, dizziness, stomach bloating, nausea, and itchy or watery eyes.

Dr. Mercola has posted a list of testimonials on his website, Mercola.com, which highlights some real-world experiences of numerous sucralose users. In many of the testimonials, shortly after beginning sucralose consumption, sucralose users describe the onset of symptoms similar to those in the previous paragraph. Oftentimes, the symptoms were not at first attributed to the consumption of sucralose, and visits to doctors and the ER resulted. Eventually, sucralose was found to be the culprit that caused the symptoms, according to the testimonials, and once it was eliminated from the diet, the symptoms subsided. In several cases, once the symptoms disappeared, the people in the testimonial accidentally consumed sucralose again, and their symptoms quickly returned.

Genetically Modified Organisms (GMOs)

A genetically modified organism (GMO) is a plant or any other organism whose genetic DNA has been artificially altered using genetic engineering. Oftentimes, the DNA of two completely different species is combined in a way that would be impossible in nature. For example, one GMO was created by combining the DNA of a tomato and a winter flounder, in the hope that the tomato would be better able to tolerate freezing temperatures. In other cases, DNA is altered so that plants produce pesticides or are able to withstand large doses of herbicides that would kill natural plants.

An Attempt to Control the World's Seed Supply

Unfortunately, the science used to create these new unnatural GMOs is not very precise, and inserting genes from one organism into another can have profound consequences that may not be readily apparent. Although GMOs have been marketed as the solution to feeding the world, the evidence does not support the marketing spin that GMOs will solve world's food problems. The real purpose of GMOs is to allow corporations to patent seeds, with the eventual goal of all seeds being controlled by a few large corporations. In the world envisioned by these companies, they control the food supply and reap enormous profits in the process. To achieve this goal, the companies that make GMOs have been buying up many of the independent seed companies, while lobbying for "The Food Safety and Modernization Act," which was passed in 2010 and which puts rules in place that could ultimately prohibit farmers from saving their seeds from their current year's crops to plant the following year. Although this is what farmers have done for thousands of years, "seed saving" is a threat to those who wish to patent and control the world's seed supply, so the U.S. Congress passed this law, which will help the GMO companies, while hurting the small farmer and the U.S. consumer.

To achieve their goal of controlling the world's seed supply, the GMO companies have resorted to a series of tactics that have no place in a free, civilized, and open society. To understand how GMOs have been allowed to enter the food supply in America, you need to learn about some of the tactics that have been used by the companies that sell them. Following that explanation, I will provide a brief history of GM (genetically modified) foods, with a special emphasis on describing how these tactics have been used to force GMOs on a public that overwhelmingly has indicated it does not want these foods in its food supply.

Tactics Used by Many GMO Companies

Influencing people in high places: At the top of the list of tactics is influencing those who have the most power to make decisions that affect the rest of us. Oftentimes, these people are unelected officials with no accountability to the electorate, and more often than not, they have ties to the companies that produce GMOs.

Bribes: The GMO industry has made an extraordinary effort to reward friends and punish those they see as enemies. During my discussion of GMOs, I will provide many examples where individuals were offered incentives to help change their minds about GMOs. These incentives included cash payments or, in the case of a job, either job security or a promotion.

Threats: When bribes do not work, threats are often made. Threats often entail the threat of job demotion or even of being fired. In many cases, individuals have been met at their homes by what they describe as very large and intimidating men who work for the GMO companies, and oftentimes phrases such as "we know where your children go to school" are used.

Discrediting: When bribes and threats do not work, an all-out effort is often made to ruin a person's reputation.

Silence: Along with the campaign to discredit, there is frequently a campaign to silence those who disagree, usually in the form of some type of "gag order" to prevent people from talking about what they know.

Retaliation: This can take the form of a job demotion, a loss of job duties, or loss of an actual job. It sends a message to others who work for the government that standing in the way of GMO approvals could mean the end of your job and your hard-earned pension.

Questionable science: To promote GMOs, scientific standards are used that are often contrary to normally acceptable scientific procedures. In many cases, these questionable scientific practices are so absurd that they go beyond the term *questionable science* and become *junk science* or, really, fake science.

Misinformation: To keep the public from revolting against GMOs, an extensive misinformation campaign is often waged.

Dissenters and the media silenced: As part of this misinformation campaign, those in the media who dare to offer another viewpoint are frequently targeted and silenced.

Lawsuits and threats of lawsuits: The companies that make GMOs have very deep pockets, and people who attempt to disseminate information unfavorable to the GMO industry are often threatened with lawsuits. In several documented cases, publishers who were about to publish information the GMO companies did not want published were threatened with lawsuits for simply publishing factual books or magazine articles or running news stories on television.

Offices ransacked, files stolen: In many documented cases, offices of individuals who discovered research that might make GMOs look bad had their offices broken into and files stolen.

Real research halted: Because the GMO companies control the seeds they have patented, when research begins to show unfavorable facts about GM foods, the companies can simply refuse to supply researchers with the seeds they need to finish their research.

Failure of GMO industry suppression techniques: Although these tactics have worked quite well in keeping the American public largely in the dark about GMOs, they have not been as successful overseas, especially in Europe. It is mostly thanks to a few failures of GMO company tactics to silence those who might hurt their industry that the public has been made aware of some of the potential dangers of GM foods.

GM Foods Are Unnatural Foods

By combining the DNA of species that would never mate in nature, science is creating food that would never exist in nature, and as such, these foods should be considered "unnatural." Because the FDA in America is largely controlled by the GMO and pharmaceutical industries, however, the U.S. government actually allows GMO companies to use the term *natural* on the labels of foods that contain GM ingredients.

Many Animals Would Rather Starve Than Eat GM Foods

There are numerous reports of animals in nature recognizing the "unnatural" nature of these foods. Farmers tell stories about wild elk and deer that will eat natural organic soy and corn growing in the fields but avoid unnatural GM corn and soy growing in adjacent fields. One farmer experimented with feeding his cows a mix of natural corn and artificial GM corn. He filled up half of their feed troughs with the natural corn and the other half of the feed troughs with artificial GM corn. Normally, cows will eat all of the corn they are fed, but in this case, they ate only the natural corn. They nibbled slightly on the artificial GM corn and then simply walked away. One farmer would leave some of his corncobs each winter for the squirrels to eat, and when he replaced the natural corncobs he had been feeding them with artificial GM corncobs, the squirrels stopped eating the corncobs. As soon as he replaced the artificial GM corncobs with natural corncobs again, the squirrels resumed eating his corncobs. One farmer even went so far as to leave out corn for the mice in his mouse-infested barn. He left both natural corn and artificial GM corn. To his surprise, the mice ate the natural corn but left the GM corn alone.

It appears that the animals in these cases would rather starve than eat the artificial GM food. Perhaps their taste buds are more sensitive than ours, or maybe they can sense that something is "not right" with the artificial GM food that we cannot sense. Experts on GMOs have voiced numerous concerns about these genetically altered substances being put into our food supply without adequate safety testing.

Dangerous Unintended Results of Genetic Modification

One of the main concerns is that due to the imprecise method of creating GMOs, the foreign genes inserted into GM crops could potentially create unintended proteins that would have negative effects on animal and human health. Perhaps the animals tasted and sensed this, and this was the reason they avoided GM foods.

Another major concern is that GM foods can transform a perfectly healthy and harmless food into a food that contains a dangerous allergen that science is unable to detect. This appears to be exactly what happened in at least a few cases. If these new artificial GM foods are able to produce a completely new protein that has never been part of our food supply, there could be disastrous consequences. In fact, neither the GMO industry nor government officials are 100 percent certain which genes have been inserted from one organism into another. In the process of trying to insert a single gene, additional gene fragments are often inserted by accident and go undetected.

Whatever the animals are sensing in these artificial GM foods could be serious cause for human alarm. If this were the case, you would expect to hear of problems arising from these foods being in our food supply. In fact, that is just what has happened. Remember that the industry has worked very hard to silence the opposition to its artificial GM foods. The industry has also successfully infiltrated the highest levels of the U.S. government, and despite serious concerns from scientists at the FDA, these officials allowed artificial GM foods into our food supply without proper safety testing. It was largely accomplished by rigging the system and not requiring GMO companies to conduct any FDA safety testing on their foods. This is allowed, because in 1992 the FDA issued a policy that stated,

"The agency is not aware of any information showing

*that foods derived by these new methods differ in
any meaningful or uniform way."*

The history of GM foods, however, clearly shows that these
foods must differ in some meaningful and uniform way, and this is
the reason the GMO companies resort to extreme tactics to silence
the opposition. As I review the history of these foods in our food
supply, I will pay special attention to the tactics that I described
earlier, and when I give an example of one of them being used, I will
use bold and italics type to point out a fact, such as officials were
offered a **bribe** to change their position on GMOs.

History of GMOs
Following is a brief time line showing some tragic milestones
and significant evelopments regarding the release of genetically
modified organisms (GMOs) into the world's food supply.

1989: Use of GM Bacteria to Produce Vitamin Supplements
The first major noteworthy GMO was not a food, in the traditional
sense, but was a genetically modified bacteria that was used to
produce a vitamin supplement called L-tryptophan. L-tryptophan
is an amino acid that had been taken in supplement form, due
to its ability to increase serotonin levels naturally. It was found
to help with insomnia, anxiety, depression, and panic disorders,
and many people considered it more effective than pharmaceutical
drugs such as Prozac, Paxil, and Zoloft. Manufacturers in Japan
had long employed a method of producing l-tryptophan using a
combination of natural bacteria, enzymes, and fermentation.
Between 1984 and 1989, a company in Japan called Showa
Denko began to produce l-tryptophan using bacteria that had been
genetically modified. The company modified its GM bacteria to
produce successively higher amounts of l-tryptophan, starting
with strain II and ending with strain V.
In 1989, doctors discovered a new disease that would
later be called *eosinophilia-myalgia syndrome* (EMS), which is an
incurable neurological condition that is sometimes fatal. Although
it was discovered in 1989, it is believed to have been around for at
least a few years before its discovery. The disease was ultimately
linked to l-tryptophan produced by Showa Denko, using the
company's GM bacteria. With up to ten thousand suspected cases
and forty deaths attributed to the disease, this should have been
the end of GM foods and GM supplements in the United States.

Using **questionable science**, however, the U.S. government chose to blame a change in the filtration techniques, rather than the GM bacteria, for the problem. Many people with serious concerns about GMOs believe this was done to save the fledgling GMO industry from destruction at its very infancy.

Although Showa Denko had changed its filtration process, the real question should have been, how were the toxic substances created that produced EMS in the first place? It's been theorized that by genetically altering the bacteria to produce higher and higher levels of l-tryptophan, levels of other toxic substances were also increased, and perhaps new substances were created that would not be created by natural non-GM bacteria. *Newsday* even ran a story titled "Genetic Engineering Flaw Blamed for Toxic Deaths."

The U.S. government appears to have blamed the filtration process to help save the GMO industry, but it seems that the GMOs were really to blame. This is because Showa Denko changed the filtration process only after it began to produce its fifth and last strain, and it had used conventional filtration for strains II through IV. There were approximately 350 to 700 cases of EMS, which, in fact, had occurred before the introduction of strain V. At least three studies done by the CDC showed that Showa Denko's product was associated with cases of EMS prior to the introduction of strain V, and that no other manufacturer's products were implicated.

The pre-1998 cases of EMS appear to be the result of the GM strains II through IV. Each successive stain had been modified by Showa Denko to produce higher and higher levels of l-tryptophan, which would also increase the chance for larger amounts of the dangerous toxins being created. In fact, the evidence shows that cases of EMS gradually increased as Showa Denko tweaked each successive strain of GM bacteria.

Even though the FDA knew about the successive strains of GM bacteria used by Showa Denko at the time of the EMS outbreak, most people believed that it was only strain V that had been genetically engineered and did not have knowledge that three other strains had also been genetically engineered. In a classic **misinformation** campaign, the FDA stated that GMOs could not be to blame for EMS because the FDA falsely claimed that the disease had not existed before the introduction of strain V, the only strain that used the new filtration technique.

Subsequent testing done on l-tryptophan pills that were produced using strains III and IV clearly showed that they also contained the toxins that caused EMS. So even though the evidence showed that GM strains II through V created successively higher levels of toxins, resulting in a greater numbers of EMS cases, the FDA's spin was that the EMS was due to the filters used in strain V. The FDA falsely claimed that EMS had not existed before strain V and the filters; therefore, GMOs were not the cause, the filters were. Even though strains II through IV were GMOs and used the old filtration process and produced cases of EMS, the American public sadly believes what the FDA tells them, even when it's not supported by the facts.

The FDA used this tragedy, which was most likely caused by GMOs, to further the case of several of its other pet projects. One was to attack the vitamin supplement industry by outlawing l-tryptophan in America, even though it was only Showa Denko's GMO-produced l-tryptophan that caused the problem. This helped further the FDA's other pet project, which is to help support costly pharmaceutical drugs at the expense of cheap, natural, and healthy alternatives. Natural l-tryptophan acts to increase serotonin levels, much as the drugs known as serotonin reuptake inhibitors do. This class of drugs accounts for $7 billion' worth of sales in the United States alone, and natural l-tryptophan was a threat to the entire industry. In hearings before Congress regarding the EMS incident, the FDA representative stated that the tragedy "demonstrated the dangers inherent in the various health fraud schemes that are being perpetrated upon segments of the American public," ostensibly categorizing all natural vitamin supplements as "health fraud schemes." I'll leave it up the reader to decide what the real "health fraud scheme" is when it comes to GMOs.

By outlawing all l-tryptophan, while exonerating the Showa Denko GM bacteria that produced the dangerous toxins that caused EMS, the FDA was able to help its cronies in the pharmaceutical companies and the GMO companies, while at the same time tightening its control over the natural supplement industry. Even though the GM bacteria had clearly appeared to produce the toxins that caused EMS, and not a single case of EMS was blamed on l-tryptophan produced from natural non-GM bacteria, two years later the FDA allowed the quick entry of GMOs into the U.S. food supply.

In the end, Showa Denko paid more than $2 billion in claims to the victims of the l-tryptophan produced from its GM bacteria, but the FDA, with the help of some *questionable science* and slick *misinformation*, was able to save the GMO industry from what should have been its demise.

The only reason the problem with the GM bacteria even came to light was that it caused a brand-new disease. What if, instead of causing EMS, the GMO had simply caused cancer, diabetes, or some other common disease? In that case, to this day you would probably still have Showa Denko l-tryptophan on the market, and this is what worries many experts the most. If GMOs are simply increasing the rate of common diseases, and no adequate testing is being done before they are added to the food supply, how are we ever going to know if one GMO is increasing breast cancer, while another is making diabetes more widespread, and a third is lowering women's fertility rate?

1994: The GM FlavrSavr Tomato

In 1994, a company named Calgene began selling a GM tomato called the FlavrSavr tomato. Because the FDA had already issued a ruling highly favorable to the GMO companies, stating that GM foods were essentially the same as natural foods, companies were not required to do any FDA testing or seek any special approval from the U.S. government before introducing new GM foods into the market. Due to the fact that GM foods were new, Calgene decided to voluntarily conduct testing and submit it to the FDA for the FDA's "blessing." Given that these tomatoes were the first major GM food to enter the marketplace, perhaps Calgene was a little uneasy about introducing them without any conducting tests, or perhaps Calgene felt that the public would accept the tomato more readily if the company conducted testing that the FDA "blessed." For whatever reason, Calgene conducted tests on its GM tomato, even though the company could have begun selling it in the United States without testing or any FDA approvals.

Calgene conducted feeding tests on rats to determine the safety of its tomatoes. Calgene's first problem, as reported in the *Washington Post*, was the fact that although rodents are usually happy to eat natural tomatoes, they turned their noses up at the artificial GM tomatoes. Calgene overcame this problem by eventually force-feeding the rats through gastric tubes. No one ever bothered to ask why the rats would not eat the artificial GM tomatoes.

In one study, of the forty rats that were fed a line of GM tomatoes, seven rats died, compared to only one death in the control group that ate natural tomatoes. In a different study, none of the rats eating natural, non-GM tomatoes developed lesions, while seven out of twenty rats eating the artificial GM tomatoes developed lesions in their stomachs. FDA documents show that scientists within the agency were concerned about the presence of stomach lesions in the rats that were fed GM tomatoes.

Despite numerous other concerns by FDA scientists, the FlavrSavr tomato was allowed to enter the market for human consumption.
Yet one has to wonder why:

1. Rats would eat natural tomatoes but not artificial GM tomatoes.
2. In one study, rats that ate the GM tomatoes developed stomach lesions, while those eating natural tomatoes did not.
3. In another study, seven of forty rats eating GM tomatoes died, while only one of the control rats eating natural tomatoes did.

All three of these facts would suggest that GMO foods must differ in some meaningful way from natural foods; otherwise, you would expect rats to freely eat GM tomatoes and not to develop stomach lesions and have higher mortality rates.

1994: rbGH, the Cow Hormone Banned in Most Countries, except in the United States

A cow growth hormone called rbGH, produced using GM *e. coli* bacteria, is given to many cows in the United States to increase their milk production. It has been banned in Europe, Canada, New Zealand, Japan, and most other industrialized nations. Giving this hormone to cows has been shown to adversely affect their health. While 95 percent of cows not treated with rbGH became pregnant during one trial, only 52 percent of the cows that received rbGH became pregnant. Note that rbGH also increases the amount of a substance in milk called IGF-1, with one study showing that milk from cows given rbGH had 360 percent more IGF-1 than milk from cows not given the hormone. IGF-1 has been shown to increase human cancer rates, with one study conducted on premenopausal women showing that those with the highest levels of IGF-1 had up to a seven times greater risk of developing breast cancer, when compared to women with the lowest levels of IGF-1. Men with high levels of IGF-1 are four times more likely to get prostate cancer. Even though milk from cows given rbGH has been shown to significantly increase the amount of IGF-1 in milk, and even though IGF-1 has been shown to significantly increase a women's risk for breast cancer and a man's risk for prostate cancer, the FDA still claims that

> *"The agency is not aware of any information showing that foods derived by these new methods differ in any meaningful or uniform way."*

Despite the many reservations scientists have about letting cows be given rbGH to increase milk production, the reason it is allowed to be used in the United States but not in other countries is a story with the same plot and themes of most other GMO approvals. Although the story is long and complex and could fill an entire book by itself, I'll give you some of the highlights.

Three of the main scientists involved in studying the safety of rbGH in the United States were Joseph Settepani, who worked for the Center of Veterinary Medicine (CVM); Alexander Apostolou, the director of the Division of Toxicology; and Richard Burrows, who had a leading role in the review process concerning rbGH. Numerous scientists in the United States had serious concerns about rbGH, but many were punished with **retaliation** for trying to make sure the proper scientific and safety standards were met.

When Settepani spoke at a public hearing about the "systemic human food safety breakdown" at the CVM, he had his duties as supervisor taken away, received a reprimand for insubordination, and was threatened with job termination. His reward for trying to speak out to protect the American public was that he was sent off to work in an isolated trailer at an experimental farm, effectively isolating him and neutralizing any threat he might pose to rbGH's chance of gaining approval in the United States.

Apostolou stated in an affidavit that scientific procedures for evaluating human food safety had been disregarded, that he had faced constant pressure from supervisors to reach conclusions that favored the companies making rbGH, and that he had personally witnessed the makers of rbGH improperly influencing the agency's decision making and scientific analysis. For expressing his concerns, Apostolou was assigned an impossible task to perform, then was put on notice for "poor performance" for allegedly failing to complete it, and was pressured to leave.

Burroughs, who had experience with dairy herds, expressed

his concerns about what he saw as unacceptable compromises made on safety. He insisted that cows in the study be given rbGH for two years, so that he could determine the long-term effects of the hormone. He was told that he was slowing down the approval process, and a month after he called for toxicology and immunology tests to be performed to ensure human safety, he was fired. After his firing, the toxicology tests he had ordered were canceled.

Other employees were fully aware of the **retaliation** that was unleashed on employees such as Burroughs, Apostolou, and Settepani, who tried to do their job to protect the public. Certain employees were so terrified at what was happening that they wrote an anonymous letter to Congress. In this letter, they mentioned that people with *influence in high places* in their agency had close ties to Monsanto, the main maker of rbGH. The letter expressed outrage over numerous apparent cases of conflict of interest, as well as the way in which employees ended up in trouble when they pointed out fraud and abuse perpetrated by senior management that threatened public safety.

Although rbGH was approved for use in the United States, it was only with the help of some extremely *questionable science*. After the approval of rbGH, an independent analysis of the science used in the approval process found many serious problems. On dairy farms, cows receiving rbGH are usually injected every two weeks with large doses of the hormone. Originally, the FDA had ruled that the milk could not be sold until at least five days after these injections, ostensibly due to concerns over spikes in hormone levels in the milk. Because this certainly would have hurt, if not destroyed, the sales of rbGH to the dairy industry, the GMO industry was quick to come up with a study that showed that hormone levels would not be elevated. The GMO industry accomplished this by giving the cows 10.6 mg of the hormone every day, rather than the 500 mg given every two weeks in most dairies that use rbGH. Even by using procedures that they knew would not be replicated in the real world, hormone levels in the milk still went up more than 25 percent, but the study simply claimed this was not significant.

GMO companies also made the case that pasteurization would destroy the hormones in the milk. Normally, in the real world, milk is pasteurized for 15 seconds at 162 degrees. In an attempt to show that pasteurization would destroy the hormone, GMO companies pasteurized the milk for 30 minutes, but this reduced the growth hormone levels by only 19 percent. They finally got the result they wanted when they simply added powdered hormone to the milk and increased the level to 146 times that normally found in milk. When they did this, and they pasteurized it for 30 minutes, 90 percent of the hormone was destroyed, and the FDA was satisfied by what is at best very *questionable science*.

Cows that are given rbGH have a much higher incidence of developing serious infections and as a result need to be given large doses of antibiotics. This posed a serious problem for the approval of rbGH, because at the time in the approval process, the FDA allowed milk to contain only one part per 100 million of antibiotics. It always seems as if the GMO companies have *influence over those in high places*, however, and in this case, an FDA employee named Margaret Miller, who had worked for Monsanto and was still publishing papers with Monsanto scientists concerning rbGH, came to the rescue. She arbitrarily changed the allowable level of antibiotics in milk from one part per 100 million to one part per million, effectively allowing 100 times as much antibiotics in milk than had previously been allowed and solving a huge potential problem for the GMO industry. Her subordinates accused her of picking an arbitrary number with no scientific basis or any consumer safety testing.

Although the preceding three examples are *questionable science* and these techniques would probably earn you a failing mark in a high school science fair, they were enough to make the FDA happy and approve the use of rbGH in the United States. The FDA even issued labeling guidelines to prohibit dairies from notifying the public that their milk was free of these hormones. These guidelines were written and implemented by former Monsanto attorney Michael Taylor, who was now deputy commissioner of FDA policy. He stated that the

> FDA is concerned that the term "rbST-free" [rbST is another term for rbGH] free" may imply a compositional difference between milk from treated and untreated cows rather than a difference in the way the milk is produced. Without proper context, such statements could be misleading. Such unqualified statements may imply that milk from untreated cows is safer or of higher quality than milk from treated cows. Such an implication would be false and misleading.

In 2010, a U.S. appeals court found that there is a difference between milk from cows treated with rbGH and milk from untreated cows. The court found that the milk from cows given rbGH had lower nutritional quality at certain times in the cows' cycles; larger amounts of IGF-1, which has been shown to increase human cancer rates; and a higher somatic cell count.

A Dutch high school student conducted and presented the following experiments to the Dutch Parliament. Hinze Hogendoorn devised laboratory tests that have exceeded anything the FDA has yet to conduct. Hinze fed one group of mice organic corn and soy and another group GM corn and soy. Hinze observed profound behavioral differences between the two groups of mice. The mice that ate the GM food seemed less active and more "distressed" and nervous than the mice eating natural, organic corn and soy. Later I will discuss actual scientists who have done similar experiments, but I mention this to illustrate that high-school age students are conducting the type of research that the FDA should be conducting, which makes you wonder what has happened to real science at the FDA.

Once rbGH received approval in the United States, the GMO companies headed north to Canada to get it approved there. It appears as if the GMO companies also had *influence over those in high places* at Health Canada, Canada's equivalent of the FDA. Senior officials there tried to get rbGH approved without normal review, under the premise that it had already been approved in the United States. Health Canada's rank-and-file employees had serious concerns about rbGH, similar to the concerns that FDA employees had voiced. When these Health Canada employees reviewed all of the data concerning rbGH, they wrote the "GAPS report," which was extremely critical of the FDA's approval process. At least six employees at Health Canada felt that milk from cows given rbGH was not safe for human consumption. Recall that Richard Burroughs, who was a lead reviewer for rbGH in the United States, was fired shortly after calling for toxicology tests to ensure the safety of rbGH. He had also asked for two years of testing, rather than the short-term 28-day test that ended up being conducted. Health Canada employees seemed to vindicate Richard Burroughs, by citing the lack of toxicology testing and lack of long-term studies as two of the many serious flaws in the FDA's approval process.

When Health Canada's rank-and-file employees issued this scathing report about the FDA's approval process, their department head insisted that changes be made, and they were silenced and told they were not allowed to talk about the parts of the report that he insisted be omitted. Although this tactic almost worked, every now and then the public gets lucky and the GMO industry suppression techniques fail. In this case, scientists at Health Canada had made allegations of harassment to the Canadian labor board, and as part of the harassment claim, they submitted a copy of the original GAPS report, which they had later been told to alter and not talk about. This report made its way into the press, and when the media reported on it, the Canadian Senate demanded to see the report. It then became an international news story, which was instrumental in causing the European Union to ban rbGH in all European countries. New Zealand, Australia, Japan, and other industrialized countries also decided to ban rbGH. Sadly, many of the employees who had testified claimed they experienced retaliation for their truthful testimony, including threats, harassment, denial of promotions, and even job suspension. In addition to threats and harassment, Dr. Margaret Haydon testified that at a meeting with Health Canada officials and Monsanto, officials at Monsanto had made an offer of $1 million to $2 million to the Health Canada scientists, which she stated in her testimony she had interpreted as a bribe. Monsanto claimed that Dr. Haydon misunderstood its offer for research money; however, Monsanto paid a $1.5 million fine to the Justice Department and the SEC and admitted that a Monsanto employee paid a senior Indonesian official $50,000 to avoid an environmental impact statement on its GM cotton. Monsanto further admitted to paying bribes to a number of other high-ranking officials from 1997 to 2002. The Asia Times reported that according to U.S. authorities, Monsanto made payments to at least 140 current and former Indonesian government officials and their family members. The total amount of illicit payments was reported to be around $700,000.

In addition to testifying that she felt Monsanto had offered Health Canada scientists a $1 million to $2 million bribe to approve rbGH, Dr. Haydon also testified that files were stolen from her office, which were critical of data that had been supplied by Monsanto. When she refused what she thought was a bribe and refused to approve rbGH, due to her concerns, she was simply taken off the case. Her testimony before the Canadian Senate was reminiscent of the anonymous letter that was sent to the U.S. Congress from FDA employees. She stated that Health Canada employees felt that their jobs were in danger if they voiced safety concerns that might jeopardize the approval process of rbGH. Another Health Canada employee claimed that his manager told him that if he and his coworkers did not hurry up with favorable evaluations for rbGH, they would face retaliation, such as being shipped to other departments where they would never be heard from again. His reward for truthful testimony before the Canadian Senate was a five-day suspension without pay.

A subsequent analysis of the rbGH approval process in Canada showed that senior management at Health Canada has already prepared a plan to get it approved, despite the objections of employees. Under Health Canada rules, outside panels can be convened to approve or reject new drugs when their own scientists cannot reach a consensus, although in this case it appears scientists had reached the consensus that they did not want rbGH approved. When these outside panels are convened, they are supposed to be free any conflict of interest; however, the panel that was going to be assembled apparently had strong ties to the GMO industry. One member actually worked for Monsanto, another received funding from a company that had a profit-sharing agreement with Monsanto regarding the sale of products related to rbGH, and a third member had a spouse who worked for G.D. Searle, which was a subsidiary of Monsanto. Only because the Canadian GAPS report was made public, due to an employee of Health Canada sending a copy to the labor board as part of a harassment complaint, did Canada deny approval to rbGH in 1999. Otherwise, it probably would have been approved by the outside panel that Health Canada had already assembled, which was composed of many people with ties to the GMO industry. This could have led to the widespread use of rbGH in Canada and perhaps the rest of the industrialized world.

Although other countries saw fit to ban rbGH to protect their citizens, people living in the United States were not so lucky. Part of the rationale for approving rbGH in the first place was that it would increase milk production and make prices go down for the consumer. Milk production did go up, but now there was too much milk, so the government paid farmers to kill 1.5 million dairy cows in order to boost prices. So although rbGH may have been profitable for the GMO companies, it was bad for cows, it increased the amount of potentially cancer-causing IGF-1 in the milk, and it lowered the milk's nutritional content at certain times of the cow's cycle. Consumers became confused, as many scrambled to find ways to avoid milk with rbGH but had a difficult time, due to the FDA's labeling policy, which was meant to protect the GMO companies. Furthermore, GMO companies began to sue dairies that dared to label their milk with the pledge that they did not use artificial growth hormones. One dairy finally settled by agreeing to add the FDA's statement that no differences were found in milk from rbGH-treated cows, even though studies have shown that there are differences in milk from rbGH-treated cows. In addition to suing dairies, the GMO companies sought to keep the media from informing the public about rbGH by *silencing* news stories.

For example, in 1997, a television station in Florida, WTVT Fox 13 Florida, was going to run an investigative documentary about rbGH, but right before it was to air, Monsanto sent a fax to the head of Fox News, Roger Ailes. The letter threatened that "there was a lot at stake" in Florida for both Monsanto and Fox. Fox was the owner of the station in Florida, and Fox was owned by Rupert Murdoch. Rupert Murdoch also owns Actmedia, which is an advertising agency. Monsanto is both a major advertiser on Fox television stations nationwide and a client of Actmedia. If Monsanto withdrew its business from Fox nationwide, along with its business from Actmedia, this could be very costly to Fox. The Florida station pulled the story from being aired and reviewed it with attorneys. The station manager insisted that the story was completely accurate, and Monsanto sent a second letter that indicated that if the story ran, it could lead to serious damage to Monsanto, as well as dire consequences for Fox News. Soon after this, both the station manager and the manager of the news were fired. The reporters were adamant that the story run, and the new station manager offered to pay them $150,000, plus the full amount remaining on their contract, along with allowing them to leave the station for new employment on the condition that they agree never to talk about rbGH again. The reporters refused to go but agreed to attempt to rewrite the story to make it less offensive to Monsanto. During a six-month period in 1997, the story was rewritten eighty-three times. One of the things Monsanto insisted on was that this statement be aired: that the milk from cows that got rbGH was no different from other milk. This statement was even contradicted by Monsanto's studies, but Monsanto insisted it be included. The couple refused to cooperate in what they felt was falsification of the news, and they were suspended for insubordination and then fired.

GMO companies also went after newspaper reporters who wrote stories about rbGH. The *L.A. Times* ran a story on July 27, 1989, titled "Growth Hormones Would Endanger Milk," which explained many of the health risks that rbGH posed to consumers.

Soon after the op-ed piece ran, Monsanto representatives visited the *L.A. Times* and urged the paper to refuse any more stories from the reporter. The GMO companies then created a new group called the Dairy Coalition, which, according to some people, served the GMO industry by seeking to **silence** reporters and stories that were critical of rbGH and effectively squelched most media coverage of rbGH.

Silencing the opposition appears to be a major strategy of GMO companies. For example, when the *Ecologist* magazine in the United Kingdom created a special Monsanto issue of the magazine in 1998 that was very critical of the GMO company, the printer shredded all fourteen thousand copies of the already printed magazine, rather than send them out. At first, workers at the printing company denied they had been contacted by Monsanto prior to shredding the magazines, but later they admitted they had spoken with Monsanto before they destroyed the copies.

That same year, the book *Against the Grain, Biotechnology and the Corporate Takeover of Your Food*, which was critical of the GMO industry, was going to be published. Three days before the book was scheduled to leave the printer, the publisher received a letter from Monsanto attorneys. The letter claimed that an excerpt of the book that had been published in a magazine was potentially libelous and defamatory against the herbicide Roundup, which was produced by Monsanto. The publisher decided to cancel the book, fearing Monsanto's deep pockets.

Although the GMO companies are largely successful at stopping dissent and controlling the highest echelons of power, every now and then the truth is able to escape, and the public is actually made aware about the truth concerning GMOs. Remember the accidental release of the GAPS report in Canada, which thwarted Health Canada's plan to approve rbGH.

In the United States, the truth about rbGH has spread largely through natural health websites on the Internet, which led many consumers to question their grocers and dairy companies about whether rbGH was being given to the cows that produced the milk they were drinking. Luckily for consumers, many large grocers have pledged not to sell milk from rbGH-treated cows, along with national trend-setting companies such as Starbuck's and Ben and Jerry's ice cream, which have also pledged not to use milk from cows given rbGH.

1995: The Soybean Combined with DNA from the Brazil Nut

Soy and corn are often used as animal feed, and because they are low in sulfur-containing amino acids, animal feed containing soy and corn is often supplemented with amino acids that contain sulfur. In an attempt to create soy that was high in sulfur-containing amino acids, a GMO company combined some DNA from the Brazil nut with the DNA from a soybean. When they tested the new artificial GM soy, it was in fact high in sulfur-containing amino acids, but to everyone's surprise, it was also high in an allergen found in Brazil nuts, which can be fatal to a person with that known allergy.

The testing done by the company was not required by the FDA, and luckily the company thought to test for allergens, for had it not, the results could have been deadly. The implications of this one case of genetic engineering gone awry are quite profound. Although this example of unnaturally mated DNA was from a Brazil nut and a soybean, many other genetically engineered foods used DNA from bacteria and viruses. No one really knows what the effects are going to be from combining DNA from viruses and bacteria to engineer food products, and no real legitimate independent testing is being done to find out.

Remember that the FDA has taken the position that

"The agency is not aware of any information showing that foods derived by these new methods differ in any meaningful or uniform way."

Yet in this case, the GM soy derived from these new methods did differ in a meaningful way because it had the ability to kill someone with an allergy to Brazil nuts, whereas natural soybeans do not have this ability. When the manufacturer discovered the deadly potential of its new soybean, the company scrapped its plans to bring the soybean to the market.

What's amazing is that the testing the manufacturer did was not required by the FDA but was totally voluntary, and the testing just happened to catch the allergen that had been created with the new unnatural GM food. The company could have chosen to bring it to market without testing, and we could have had another disaster on our hands, as in the case with l-tryptophan. In DNA-recombining experiments where bacteria and viruses are used instead of nut protein, however, it's not as simple as testing for nut allergens. In these cases, who knows what the potential effects could be and how to even fully test for them? Yet luckily for the GMO companies, in the United States, FDA testing is voluntary, and if the GMO companies say their products are safe, then the FDA assumes they are safe and allows them to be sold to U.S. consumers.

1996: GM Corn Causes Chicken Fatalities

In 1996, testing was done on a type of corn called Chardon LL, which was genetically engineered to withstand the herbicide glyphosate. The growing of Chardon LL was approved in the UK, based on animal-feeding experiments where the investigators concluded that the tested animals gained weight normally. Yet what they seem to have overlooked in granting this GM corn approval is that twice as many chickens that ate the GM Chardon LL corn died in the experiment, compared to chickens that ate natural, non-GM corn. In this experiment, 3.57 percent of the chickens eating natural corn died, compared to a mortality rate of 7.14 percent for the chickens eating the GM corn. Using what many describe as **questionable science**, the researchers trivialized the doubling of the mortality rate for the GMO-fed chickens by stating that "mortality was normal for this fast-growing strain of bird, where at our research facility we normally see values of 5 to 8 percent in male broilers."

An independent review of the research by independent reviewers found that the entire study had major flaws in its design. In addition, they found that average mortality for chickens in the UK, where the study was conducted, is approximately 4 percent. So, in actuality, the mortality of the chickens eating natural corn was normal, while the mortality rate of the chickens eating the GM corn was double the normal rate in the UK.

Stating that the value of 5 to 8 percent is normal is a prime example of **questionable science** for several reasons. First, this assertion was not supported by any data in the study. Second, data cannot be used from one study to justify data in another study. Studies are designed to stand on their own, and in this study, the chickens eating the GM corn had double the mortality rate of the chickens eating the natural corn.

1998: First Real Independent Government GMO Study Is Halted

Although the U.S. government decided to let the GMO companies regulate themselves and declared that GM foods were essentially the same as natural foods, the GMO industry was not able to completely corrupt the political process in Europe as it had in its home country. European officials decided to actually conduct independent tests on GMOs before allowing them to enter Europe, and the man they chose to lead the research was Arpad Pusztai. Pusztai was one of the top researchers in biology in Europe, having authored or edited twelve books and having almost three hundred published research articles to his credit. At the time, he was also a believer in GMOs, and it was his job to create a true scientific model for testing GMOs in Europe. He began this task in 1995 by researching GM potatoes.

While conducting his research, he also evaluated the **questionable science** that had been submitted previously by the GMO industry. His evaluation found that the industry research had poor research design, with missing data, and tests that were very superficial in nature. He concluded that the industry research was not adequate for demonstrating that GMOs were safe for either human or animal consumption.

In 1998, he ignited a firestorm in the middle of his research, when he stated that his preliminary results showed that rats eating the GM potatoes had suffered damage to their immune systems, intestines, and other organs. The structural changes he has observed in the cells lining their stomachs and intestines showed a potential increase for cancer. This is one of the concerns many scientists have had about GMOs since their inception. For example, some "insect-resistant" GM crops are designed to punch holes in the intestines of insects and kill them. Scientists have been concerned that if GM crops can "punch holes" into the intestines of insects, what would they do to beneficial insects such as ladybugs and to humans themselves?

The negative changes that occurred in the rats were a result of the rats eating the GM potatoes for only ten days; however, Pusztai knew that it would take years in humans for problems to develop. Even more troublesome was that if the food was already on the market, the problems would develop and no one would be able to associate the problem with a certain GMO. If Pusztai had conducted the same type of **questionable scientific** research that was carried out by the GMO industry, the GM potato probably would have passed through the study with flying colors. The ramifications were enormous; there could already be GMOs in the food supply capable of causing serious heath problems that no one was aware of.

What's perhaps most shocking is that his research team was the only one in the world at the time that was actually conducting true scientific feeding experiments on GMOs. Remember that the

U.S. government allows GMO companies to police themselves and does not even require that they do feeding experiments. The potato in question could have easily entered the U.S. food supply.

Another alarming part of Pusztai's study was that the lectin that the potatoes had been engineered to produce was harmless to humans and rats. For this reason, Pusztai, who was a renowned expert in lectins, was confident that the study would show the potatoes to be harmless. The fact that the potatoes were shown to have serious health consequences means that the problem was not with the lectin the potato was designed to produce but with the GM process itself. It appeared that in designing the potato to produce a certain lectin, other unforeseen changes had occurred in the potatoes, and it was these unforeseen changes that caused health problems in the rats that ate them.

You would think that as Pusztai's preliminary results became known, a worldwide ban would have been issued on GMOs. What happened was quite the opposite, and the GMO industry, sensing a potential catastrophe, sprang into action. What followed could be the subject of an entire book. Remember that the GMO companies have *influence on those in high places*, so Pusztai was suspended from his job and then forced to retire. His entire research team was dismantled, and their computers, notes, data, and files were all confiscated. This research had been paid for by the UK taxpayer to the tune of 1.6 million pounds for the purpose of protecting the citizens of the UK. As soon as the first bad signs incriminating GMOs showed up, the entire study was canceled permanently. At the time of this entire episode, it was no secret that the British government and especially Tony Blair were huge supporters of the biotech industry.

Per his employment contract, Pusztai was not allowed to talk about the incident and was told he would be taken to court if he did anything to harm the research institute. With *real research halted*, and the *dissenters silenced* with *threats of lawsuits*, it was time to begin the *misinformation campaign*. Because Pusztai could not defend himself, his research was accused of being deficient, and there were allegations that he fabricated his findings. The press was fed a story about Pusztai's "mistakes," and this is the story that people were led to believe. The *Times* even wrote an article on August 13, 1998, titled "Scientist's Potato Alert Was False, Laboratory Admits," while the *Scottish Daily Record and Sunday Mail* headline read "Doctor's Monster Mistake." Pusztai had not only been thoroughly *discredited*, but his entire reputation was now ruined, and he was unable to speak to defend himself.

The next step in the *misinformation* campaign involved creating a panel of scientists to audit Pusztai's work. The panel was handpicked by the institute that had fired Pusztai, and its members were not even given all of Pusztai's data and they reviewed what they were given for less than a day. Although the full audit report was not released to the public, a summary of the audit claimed that there were "important deficiencies" in Pusztai's study.

Despite all of the efforts to *silence* and *discredit* Pusztai, there was a major *failure of the GMO industry suppression techniques*. It turned out that Pusztai's employment contract did not prohibit him from sharing unpublished research with other scientists. Pusztai had also been called to testify before the British Parliament, and even though his data had been seized, he would have to be given that data back in order to testify before Parliament. Once Pusztai gained access to some of his data, he was able to send it to other scientists, and when they received it, twenty-three scientists from thirteen countries formed their own independent panel to formally review his research and send a report to Parliament.

The report exonerated Dr. Pusztai and showed that the GM potato had significant effects on immune function. The panel even went so far as to call for a moratorium on the sale of GMOs on February 12, 1998. A few days later, it was exposed that Monsanto, the main GMO company, had given 140,000 pounds to the institute Pusztai had worked for. With all of the new media coverage, Parliament invited Pusztai to present evidence in front of a House of Commons committee, and the institute Pusztai had worked for was forced to release its gag order, which had kept Pusztai from speaking. That month alone, the British press wrote more than seven hundred articles on GMOs, and the public's view of them began to get increasingly negative. Brits and Europeans began to call GMOs "Frankenfoods." This led to consumer demands to remove GMOs from the food supply, and the food manufacturers, always wanting to please their consumers, complied, followed by the grocery stores and even the fast-food restaurants. The European Union responded by placing a moratorium on any new GM crop approvals in 1998, and on July 2, 2003,the EU began to require that all foods that contain greater than .9 percent GMOs to be labeled, so that consumers could make an informed decision.

Yet GMO companies have effectively lobbied to keep consumers from being informed in this manner in the United States.

Following all of this, Pusztai's home was **burglarized and papers were stolen**, and his old office at the institute was also **burglarized**, as was the home of a colleague who had been following up on Pusztai's work. It appeared as if the GMO industry had not given up in the UK yet, because these companies still had **influence over those in high places**. During Pusztai's testimony in Parliament, he was not allowed to go into scientific details about his research, and when the committee issued its report, it appeared that the committee had twisted much of his testimony in an attempt to protect GMOs. The Royal Society, breaking with 350 years of tradition, went so far as to conduct the first peer review in its history, choosing Pusztai's work to review, even though the society lacked all of his data and did not meet with Pusztai or even reveal the names of the scientists conducting the review. This anonymous committee reviewing only part of Pusztai's data declared that Pusztai's research was "flawed." There is a reason the GMO companies like to have **influence over those in high places**. If Parliament holds a hearing, for example, and allows Pusztai to speak and then issues a report favorable to the GMO industry, the public perception is that Parliament is there to protect UK citizens, and it must have been fair in its report.

After the report from Parliament and the Royal Society came out in June of 1999, ministers "handpicked" scientists to engage the British media, in an attempt to salvage the GMO industry. This tactic might have worked, if not for the fact that the very same week the British Medical Association "called for a moratorium on planting GM crops commercially" and "warned that such food crops might have a cumulative and irreversible effect on the environment and food chain." Even the prestigious *Lancet* medical journal chimed in on May 29, 1999, declaring its astonishment that the U.S. FDA had not changed its 1992 policy, which announced,

> *"The agency is not aware of any information showing that foods derived by these new methods differ in any meaningful or uniform way."*

The *Lancet* stated that the FDA took this position despite the fact that there were good reasons to believe that specific risks may exist. The *Lancet* also reported that governments should not have allowed GMOs into the food chain without "insisting on rigorous testing" on the health effects of GMOs. That same week, Cornell University issued a news story in *Cornell News* titled "Toxic Pollen from Widely Planted, Genetically Modified Corn Can Kill Monarch Butterflies," which was based on a study done at Cornell University. This study described how in laboratory tests, pollen from GM corn kills monarch butterfly larvae. This GM corn pollen is dispersed by the wind and lands on plants such as milkweed, which is the exclusive food of monarch caterpillars and commonly grows around corn fields. The primary investigator stated that "pollen from Bt-corn could represent a serious risk to populations of monarchs and other butterflies." The article went on to say that "Monarchs are considered to be a flagship species for conservation. This is a warning bell."

In the Cornell study, monarchs were fed milkweed dusted with both GM corn pollen and natural corn pollen. All of those that fed on leaves dusted with natural corn pollen survived the study. In contrast, those that ate the milkweed dusted with GM corn pollen grew more slowly and suffered a higher mortality rate. The researchers found that the GM corn pollen goes into the gut of the caterpillar, where it binds to the gut wall and changes the protective layer, allowing pathogens normally kept inside the gut to be released into the monarch's body, causing the caterpillar to quickly sicken and die. This sounds a little similar to what happened to the rats that ate the GM potatoes in Pusztai's study.

As all of this was happening, the GMO industry was scrambling to contain the damage by having the UK's agriculture minister make a statement claiming, "There is no spin-doctoring exercise with scientists." A mere week after making those statements, the *Independent* ran a story on May 23, 1999, titled "Exposed: Labour's Real Aim on GM Food." The *Independent* had been passed a confidential document from the offices of that very same agricultural minister that laid out "an astonishingly detailed strategy for spinning, and mobilizing support for the Government's announcement of new measures." These "new measures" included the creation of new agencies and guidelines that would have allowed the GMO companies a framework under which "to begin to gain acceptance to the view that the industry should be given time to develop and demonstrate possible benefits from GM products." No doubt, these guidelines would have allowed the entry of GMOs into Europe, while assuring the public that the government was there to protect them. Fortunately for the citizens of Europe, the GMO industry's standard campaign tactics of ***discrediting, silencing,*** *misinforming, threatening with lawsuits*, enlisting the help of top government officials, and halting the only credible research ever done on GMOs did not work this time. The GMO industry was losing control of the message fast.

The *Lancet* was now considering publishing Pusztai's work, and the *Lancet*'s editor received a telephone call he described as very aggressive. The editor was told that if he published the paper, it would "have implications for his personal position as editor." The *Guardian* later identified the caller as the president of the Academy of Medical Sciences, who had also been the former vice president and biological secretary of the Royal Society and had several ties to the biotech industry. It seems the GMO industry was still trying to rely on its old strategy of *having influence on those in high places* and attempting to use those people in high places to *threaten* the editor of the prestigious *Lancet* not to publish credible science.

The UK government had originally been convinced, as had Pusztai, that the GM potato research would show results favorable to the GMO industry. When things did not turn out to be favorable, the UK government, rather than spending its energy to protect the public, tried every conceivable way to help the GMOs gain entry into the UK. Because the scientific research was not working out the way it was supposed to, the UK government ended all funding to test the safety of GMOs.

By this time, the entire population of Europe realized what was going on, and they were opposed to GMOs in their food supply. When you go over all of the facts in the Pusztai story, it's really quite amazing how close the GMO industry was to victory, which would have most likely led to GMOs making their way into Europe the way they did in the United States. If Pusztai's contract had not allowed him to share unpublished research, and if he had not been called to testify before the British Parliament, which gained him access to his seized data, the entire controversy would have been contained, due to the fact that Pusztai would had been effectively silenced, while his research was being discredited without his being able to defend himself. The two favorable government reports would have been enough to assure the public of the safety of GMOs, if not for the fact that the truth was able to get out in this case.

1999: Soy Allergens in UK Double the Same Year That GM Soy Is Introduced

What made the deaths and disabilities caused by the GM l-tryptophan bacteria unique was that the toxins produced by the GMOs created a new and novel disease, which ultimately led doctors to discover that it was the GMO-produced 1-tryptophan that caused the disease. If the 1-tryptophan had caused a drastic increase in cancer, diabetes, or some other common disease, chances are doctors never would have attributed these diseases to the 1-tryptophan. Many scientists are concerned that because GMOs are not being adequately tested by the government, they could be causing health consequences that no one is aware of, including allergies.

If allergies were to rise as a result of GMOs, most countries would not be aware of it, because they do not do yearly testing of a sample of their populations. In 1998 and 1999, however, York Nutritional Laboratory did an allergy survey in conjunction with the University of York and the British Allergy Foundation. The survey was conducted on a random sample of 4,200 individuals. In 1999, the UK began to import soy from the United States, and because most soy grown in the United States is GM soy, much of the imported soy was GM. The researchers discovered that in 1999, the year when GM soy began to be imported, soy allergies increased 50 percent. People also suffered from other problems, such chronic fatigue syndrome, headaches, lethargy, and neurological problems, and scientists found increased antibodies in their blood that showed there was a link to soy.

The timing of the jump in soy allergies and other problems the same year that GM soy was introduced into the UK led the *Daily Express* to report that "their findings provide real evidence that GM food could have a tangible, harmful impact on the human body."

One allergen in soy is known as a trypsin inhibitor, and testing suggests that GM soybeans are higher in this allergen, and that the trypsin inhibitor in GM soy does not break down as easily when heated as in natural soy. There could, of course, be other allergens in the GM soybeans that have not been tested for yet, because the U.S. government does not test for such things but rather trusts that GMO companies will do their job. Soybeans and peanuts also have what's called a *cross-reactivity*. If you are allergic to one, your allergy could be triggered by eating the other. Another concern of scientists is that if GM soybeans had some new allergen or higher levels of existing allergens such as trypsin inhibitors, then allergies to other foods, such as peanuts, could increase. GM soy was introduced into the U.S. food supply in 1996, and from 1997 to 2002 the number of peanut allergies in the United States has doubled.

2000: The StarLink Corn Fiasco

StarLink is a type of GM corn that was intended for animal feed but not for human consumption. This is because StarLink was engineered to create its own pesticide, and the form of pesticide StarLink manufactured was highly resistant to heat and stomach acid. This had the potential to cause serious allergic reactions in some people, including the possibility of fatal anaphylactic shock. It was actually the EPA that prohibited the use of StarLink corn for human consumption, because the corn makes its own pesticide, and that pesticide could potentially do serious harm to human health.

StarLink corn that was intended for animal consumption ended up getting mixed in with corn destined for human consumption at grain silos around the United States. When the corn entered the food supply, some people did in fact go into anaphylactic shock and had to be rushed to the hospital. A massive recall was issued for foods that might contain StarLink corn, and the GMO industry feared a public backlash against its foods.

Luckily for the GMO industry, the FDA stepped in and conducted some tests to determine whether StarLink was to blame for the allergic reactions that people had experienced. The FDA claimed that its tests showed that StarLink was not the cause of the allergies. When the results of the FDA's "tests" became public, scientists once again claimed it was *questionable science* on the part of the FDA, such as a lack of failure to follow standard scientific protocols.

Even worse, rather than testing StarLink corn itself for an allergic response in individuals, the FDA chose to test the response to a single protein in the corn called Cry9C and relied on samples from the corn maker, while not even bothering to test whether the sample did in fact contain Cry9C. Remember that one concern about GMOs is that the plants could produce a toxin that no one is even aware of, such as occurred with the GM l-tryptophan or as was apparently the case with Pusztai's potato experiment. The Cry9C protein that the corn's maker supplied did not even come from StarLink corn, and StarLink corn was known to add a sugar chain to its version of the Cry9C protein, which increased its allergic potential when compared to the type of Cry9C supplied to the FDA.

So the FDA did not test the Cry9C from StarLink or even

bother to test StarLink itself, but rather tested an isolated Cry9C protein from a different source. When the people who were believed to have had an allergic reaction to StarLink were tested with this isolated form of Cry9C, they did not react, so the FDA concluded that StarLink could not be to blame. Of course, this type of science would be laughed at during peer review if a scientist tried to publish it in a scientific journal, and many were critical of the FDA's *questionable scientific methods*.

The easiest thing would have been for the FDA to gather together the people who had a suspected allergic reaction to StarLink and give them some corn to eat, with the proper medical professionals on hand in case of an adverse reaction, to see whether StarLink actually caused the reaction. This would have been a very simple and honest test to conduct, but the results could have been disastrous to the GMO industry.

One of the individuals who had experienced a severe reaction was a doctor, who actually volunteered to eat some StarLink corn as a guinea pig. That simple test on the part of the FDA never happened, and when the doctor went public with that information, he received some StarLink corn in the mail from an anonymous source. He then had the corn tested to make sure it was StarLink, and when that test concluded it was, he ate some of the corn. Needless to say, when the doctor ate the StarLink corn, he ended up in the hospital, with rapidly rising blood pressure and itchy rashes all over his body.

The corn recall and the ensuing lawsuits are estimated to have cost the maker of StarLink corn more than $1 billion. This included damages to farmers from the GM corn, damages to consumers from the GM corn, and damages to the companies that had to recall more than three hundred products containing the GM corn, but to this day, the FDA still insists that

> "The agency is not aware of any information showing that foods derived by these new methods differ in any meaningful or uniform way."

2001: Farmers Report Lowered Animal Fertility

In 2001, more than twenty-five farmers in five states reported fertility issues with pigs that were fed GM corn. The fertility issues included lowered conception rates, sterility of both male and female pigs, and reports of pigs essentially giving birth to "bags of water." The biggest concern to farmers was the fact that the sows were not getting pregnant, with fertility rates dropping from the normal 80 percent down to 20 percent. When the farmers who were having all of the problems spoke to one another, it turns out they were all feeding their pigs the same GM seed corn. The farmers reported that when they stopped feeding the GM corn, their problems went away.

There are many other reports about lowered animal fertility as a result of eating GMOs. GMO expert Dr. Huber recently wrote a letter to the USDA secretary, informing him of a new microfungal organism associated with something called sudden death syndrome (SDS) in soy. This new microorganism was first identified in 1998, just two years after glyphosate-tolerant soybeans were first introduced. At first, the vets could not figure out what was causing such high reproductive failures in animals, with some dairies experiencing 70 percent abortion rates. The cause of the high abortion rate has now been linked to this new microorganism, which is believed to be an entirely new entity and is found in GM corn and soybeans, according to Dr. Huber. Dr. Huber also points out that in the last ten years, there has been an increase in human infertility and miscarriage rates.

2001: Cows in Germany Die after Eating GM Corn

In 2001, some dairy cows died in Germany, and according to a report, it was suspected they had eaten a form of GM corn called Bt 176. The rate of milk production also dropped in the cows eating the Bt 176, and some had to be slaughtered, due to unknown illnesses. The U.S. license for Bt 176 corn expired in 2001 and was not renewed, while Austria, Luxembourg, and Italy banned its cultivation.

According to an article in *QW Magazine* titled "Syngenta Charged for Covering up Livestock Deaths from GM Corn," the biotech company Syngenta "has been criminally charged with denying knowledge that its genetically modified (GM) Bt corn kills livestock during a civil court case that ended in 2007." The article stated that the charges stem from a civil lawsuit brought by the German farmers against Syngenta, during which Syngenta claimed it had no knowledge that its GM corn caused harm to cows. Based on Syngenta's testimony, the civil case against it was dropped, and subsequently a farmer learned of a 1996 study Syngenta had conducted in which four cows died within days of eating its GM corn. That feeding trial was quickly terminated by Syngenta, and the German head of Syngenta "is charged for withholding knowledge of the U.S. study from the judge and from Gloecker [the farmer whose cows allegedly died from eating the GM corn] in the original civil court case.

The suspected cause of the deaths was from a protein contained in the GM Bt 176 corn called Cry1Ab. A 2003 study done in Japan showed that after calves ate another corn with the same protein, undigested Bt toxin Cry1Ab was found in their stomachs, intestines, and dung.

In 2011, a study was conducted in one township in Canada to determine the blood levels of Cry1Ab in women, and the results were reported in the journal *Reproductive Toxicology*. According to that study, the blood of 93 percent of pregnant women, 69 percent of nonpregnant women, and 80 percent of fetal blood samples tested positive for the protein Cry1Ab. The study states that "trace amounts of the Cry1Ab toxin were detected in the gastrointestinal contents of livestock fed GM corn raising concerns about this toxin in insect resistant GM crops; (1) that these toxins may not be effectively eliminated in humans and (2) there may be a high risk of exposure through consumption of contaminated meat. . . . Given the potential toxicity of these environmental pollutants and the fragility of the fetus, more studies are needed."

When GM foods were first introduced into the United States, the GMO companies and the EPA assured everyone that the Bt-toxin would be completely destroyed in the human digestive system and therefore would have no impact on human health. The fact that the previously mentioned study showed that Bt toxin was present in the blood of 93 percent of pregnant women clearly shows that the EPA's claims that Bt toxins would hurt only insects and would be completely destroyed in the human digestive system cannot be relied on.

A study done in Italy showed that mice fed one type of Bt corn had a wide range of immune responses, including elevated levels of certain interleukins. The interleukins that were elevated in the mice fed Bt corn are also elevated in humans suffering from diseases such as rheumatoid arthritis, inflammatory bowel disease, multiple sclerosis, autoimmune disease, osteoporosis, allergies, and various forms of cancer.

2002: BBC Reports Doubling of Mortality Rates from GM Corn

In 2002, the BBC reported that twice as many chickens died when fed Chardon LL corn as did chickens that ate natural corn. Although the corn had been approved in 1996 as the first UK

GM crop, somehow the doubling of the mortality rate had been overlooked in the approval process.

2002: Mexican Corn Biodiversity Tragedy

Scientists believe that people in Mexico have been cultivating corn for at least seven thousand years. Although ancient corn did not resemble modern corn, for thousands of years farmers have selectively bred corn to produce the most desirable traits for each specific region in Mexico. There are more than twenty thousand traditional varieties of corn, which are specific to each region of Mexico and which do best for that region's soil, climate, and other factors.

One of the biggest fears of those who caution against GMOs is that the pollen from GM corn and from other crops, for that matter, could blow into fields with natural crops and cross-pollinate with them. This means that the GM DNA would essentially change the DNA of the natural plants DNA, very likely forever. This type of cross-pollination is often called *genetic-pollution*.

Corn is a significant source of food in the Mexican diet, and about twenty years ago, Mexico produced enough corn to meet its needs. Today, Mexico is a major importer of corn, with much of it coming from the United States. The reason this has happened is that thanks to U.S. subsidies to farmers who grow corn, the United States can produce corn cheaper than Mexican farmers can. The U.S. export market was also affected when Europe and other nations began to reject U.S. GM corn shipments into their countries, which lowered the price that farmers could get for their GM corn.

Due to Mexico's incredible corn biodiversity and the potential that GMOs have for ruining it though cross-pollination, scientists have warned for years that Mexico should not allow GM corn to be grown there. Scientists feared that the threat of genetic-pollution from GM corn could be disastrous to Mexico. It's been estimated that nearly a million small farmers, who are the growers and stewards of these diverse varieties of corn, have already been driven out of farming, due to the cheap subsidized imports.

In 2001, Mexican officials admitted that they had detected an alarming number of GM corn plants growing next to traditional natural varieties. Although Mexican officials had proclaimed a moratorium on growing GM corn in Mexico, this was very hard to enforce, due to the dumping of millions of tons of cheap U.S. taxpayer–subsidized corn into Mexico. Although that corn was supposed to be used for food only, given that it was so much cheaper than traditional natural Mexican corn, which received no subsidies, many poor farmers planted this corn that was never supposed to be planted.

As a result, in 2001, the Mexican government discovered that some of the country's native corn varieties had been contaminated with GM corn DNA. The presence of GM genetic pollution in natural Mexican corn was first discovered by a microbial ecologist from the University of California—Berkeley named Ignacio Chapela.

Chapela tells of a meeting with Mexico's top official in charge of biotechnology that seems to be right out an episode of *The Sopranos*. According to Chapela, he was taken to meet with this official in a taxi that first drove him through a very rough part of Mexico to what he thought was a government office building. He was taken up to the twelfth floor, into a makeshift office that consisted of desk that had been created by laying an office door on top of two cardboard boxes. Chapela was attacked verbally for more than an hour, being told that his information was damaging and problematic and was going to create problems.

No one else was present in the building, and things got so tense for Chapela that at one point he asked if they were going to take a gun out and shoot him. Chapela was not shot, but he was being pressured to withdraw his evidence of corn contamination from publication. Chapela refused, and when they got back outside, he was asked questions about where his kids went to school. He was driven back to were he was staying, and the comment was made that they now knew where his children went to school.

A few days before Chapela's article was to be published, he received a fax from the underminister of agriculture that stated that Chapela would be held personally responsible for all damages caused to agriculture and to the Mexican economy that might result from the publication of his article.

As soon as the paper was published, the smear campaign started against Chapela. He was accused of being biased, it was falsely claimed that his paper had not been peer-reviewed, he was labeled an activist, and even the magazine that published the article was inundated with a campaign to retract the article. Although there were questions about one of Chapela's findings, the main point of his article, which was that natural Mexican corn had been contaminated with GMO corn DNA, was found to be true.

2002: Italian Study Shows Damage to Mice Livers

A study was conducted at the University of Urbino in Italy in 2002. Researchers fed mice GM soybeans and then studied the livers of the mice to determine whether the GM soybeans had affected them in some adverse way. The study concluded that the GM soybeans could influence the liver nuclear features in both young and adult mice. They found irregularly shaped nuclei and a higher number of nuclear pores.

2004: Filipinos Get Sick

As reported in the *Guardian* in 2004, Filipino islanders are blaming GM corn for a mysterious illness that has caused up to a hundred villagers to fall ill. Villagers say their problems began when the GM corn plants that were engineered to produce their own pesticide began to flower and produce pollen. They claim there was a very pungent smell that got into their throats and that "it was like we were breathing in pesticides." Their symptoms included coughing, vomiting, dizziness, headaches, and stomach aches. At first, the people living closest to the GM corn fields were the ones who got sick, but within a few days, those living a little farther away also became ill.

One villager also reported that his horse ate some of the GM corn plants, and its belly swelled, while it started to froth at the mouth and slowly died. Up to four other horse deaths were also blamed on the GM corn.

Other reports have been made around the world of animals getting sick or dying from eating GMOs. According to an article at Mercola.com titled "10 Reasons to Avoid Genetically Modified Foods," "in one small feeding study, all the sheep that consumed GM Bt Plants died within a month. Those that ate natural plants remained healthy." The article goes on to state that "in addition, thousands of sheep, goats, and buffalo have died after grazing on Bt cotton plants."

According to an article in *BusinessWorld*, a Norwegian scientist found that "farmers developed three antibodies to IgG, IgA, and IgM, which indicate the farmers were exposed to an antigen which could possibly be the Bt toxin," which is the toxin the GM corn is engineered to produce.

It was alleged that when one concerned Filipino farmer began traveling around the country, speaking about the plight of those struck by the strange new illness, a Monsanto representative arrived and started to look for the farmer. According to the allegation, the Monsanto employee was accompanied by what were described as "three large men" on motorcycles, which had no license plates, and they wanted to "negotiate" with him. The neighbors reported feeling intimidated and said the man was not home.

2005: Australian Snow Peas Cause Allergic Reactions in Mice

The Australian Commonwealth Scientific and Industrial Research Organization created a pea that would be resistant to the pea weevil. They did this by combining pea DNA with some kidney bean DNA, because kidney beans produce an anti-nutrient that interferes with the weevils' digestion, effectively starving them to death.

The peas were tested by feeding mice both natural peas and these new GM peas. The mice that ate the GM peas developed allergic reactions to the GM pea and also began to exhibit allergic reactions to other foods. If the pea had entered the human food supply, it could have caused deadly allergic reactions. After $2 million was spent developing the pea, it had to be pulled from production, due to health concerns.

It turned out that DNA from the kidney bean had caused the protein that ended up being expressed in the pea to be different from what is expressed in the kidney bean. Essentially, the GMO process created a new protein, and this is one of the biggest concerns scientists have had about GMOs.

Even more worrisome is that the type of testing done on the peas is normally used to test medicines and is almost never used to test GMOs. Had the pea been tested the way GMOs normally are in the United States, the pea would probably have been put on the market for human consumption.

2005: Russian Scientist's Findings: 55 Percent of Rats Fed GM Soy Die

In 2005, a Russian scientist named Irina Ermakova, who works for the Russian Academy of Sciences, published the results of her experiment feeding rats GM soy and natural soy. This is similar to the experiment done by the Dutch high school student, a simple type of study that the U.S. FDA has yet to conduct.

In Ermakova's experiment, some rats had GM soy flour added to their food, while other rats had natural soy flour added to their food. When the pregnant rats started to give birth, the GM soy–fed rats had pups that were smaller. When the pups had reached the age of two weeks, the GM soy–fed pups were six times more likely to weigh less than 20 grams than the natural-fed pups were.

The most shocking part of her experiment concerned the mortality rates of the rats fed the GM soy. After only three weeks of being supplemented with GM soy flour, 55.6 percent of the GM soy-fed rats had died, compared with only 9 percent of the rats being supplemented with natural soy flour.

Although this type of research seems pretty basic, the researchers doing these types of studies may actually be breaking the law. This is because they are performing research on a patented product. The agreement that farmers have to sign when they plant most GMOs states that the farmer cannot do their own research on the crops they grow, and the GMO companies have refused to supply their seeds to countless legitimate researchers around the world.

Other Russian scientists have also documented potentially serious health risks to animals fed GM feed, according to a June 19, 2012, article in *GM Watch* titled "GM-Feed May Harm the Reproductive System of Animals." The article stated, "Russian scientists have proven the existence of very serious health risks for animals given genetically modified (GM) feed," which included "a ban on reproduction," making it almost impossible to obtain a third generation of animals." The article further said that the Russian parliament is considering a new law to address the issue, with many experts advising a total ban on the use of GM feed for farm animals.

2005: Monsanto Tries to Keep Its 90-Day GM Corn Study Secret

Monsanto developed a type of GM corn known as MON863, which was intended to protect itself against the corn rootworm by creating its own pesticide. In attempting to gain approval in Europe, Monsanto was required to submit a study to the governing bodies.

In 2005, Greenpeace requested access to the study from the German agriculture ministry. Monsanto claimed that the study was "confidential business information" and began to fight Greenpeace in court. Monsanto lost several rounds in court, including a number of appeals. The German court ultimately ruled that Monsanto could not keep the data confidential.

When the study was released, the results showed some "meaningful" differences between the rats fed the natural corn and those that had been fed GM MON863 corn. These included significant differences in white blood cells, which are often indicative of abnormalities such as inflammation or infection. The female rats also experienced a reduction in immature red blood cells and a significant increase in blood sugar. The male rats experienced physical irregularities in their kidneys, which included inflammation and a reduction in weight.

MON863 corn had already been approved for use in the United States, because the FDA does not require any safety testing, due to its policy that states that

> *"The agency is not aware of any information showing that foods derived by these new methods differ in any meaningful or uniform way."*

Monsanto also took the FDA's position that these differences were not "meaningful." In its report, Monsanto concluded that these facts were irrelevant and should not be attributed to its GM corn, even though the animals that ate the natural corn did not experience the same problems.

The Committee of Independent Research and Information on Genetic Engineering at Caen University and the University of Rouen analyzed Monsanto's research data. According to an article in *Z Magazine*, the independent analysis of the data "clearly underlines adverse impacts on kidneys and liver, the dietary detoxifying organs, as well as different levels of damages to heart, adrenal glands, spleen, and haemotopoietic system."

Numerous scientists and experts criticized Monsanto's study as being **questionable science**, stating that the design of the experiment was poor, and Monsanto's conclusions were "laughable." A renowned professor stated that "the set-up for the experiments was inadequate and evaluation of the data was incorrect." According to Pusztai, the scientist who had found problems with GMOs in the UK, the quality of Monsanto's study was well below that normally required for a peer-reviewed publication. According to an article by GMO expert Jeffrey M. Smith, "several features of the study appear to have been rigged to avoid finding problems."

Many scientists have accused GMO companies of "rigging" scientific experiments to help them reach favorable conclusions. The most common accusations are that

- Animals are used with varying starting weights to make it

harder to detect food-related changes.

- The studies are kept very short term in order to avoid any potential long-term effects from GMO food.
- Rather than feed animals actual GMO crops, animals are often fed GM protein produced from GM bacteria. This would limit the ability to find adverse reactions from unknown toxins.
- Very few test animals are used as subjects, in order to avoid finding a statistical significance.
- Inappropriate statistical methods are used.
- Older animals, rather than young animals, are used, to avoid finding effects in more sensitive growing juveniles.

2006: Sheep Die in India after Eating GM Cotton

As reported in an ISIS press release titled "Mass Deaths in Sheep Grazing on Bt Cotton": "At least 1,800 sheep reported dead from severe toxicity after grazing on Bt cotton fields in just four villages Andhra Pradesh India." The article goes on to say that "the shepherds said that the Assistant Director of Animal Health Centre in Warangal, told them these deaths appeared to be due to grazing on Bt cotton fields, as she has earlier seen such cases."

In India, goats and sheep are often allowed to graze on fields after crops are harvested. Sheep and goats grazing on leftover cotton residue usually eat the tender leaves and pods that are still left in the fields. In 2006, reports began to come in that sheep and goats were dying after grazing on GM Bt cotton. According to the farmers, the mortality occurred within a week of the animals' continuous grazing on the residue of GM Bt cotton crops.

Farmers said that within two to three days of grazing on the GM cotton, the sheep became dull and depressed, along with developing a cough, a nasal discharge, reddish lesions on their mouths, bloat, and diarrhea, and they were dead within five to seven days. Some of the shepherds who examined their own sheep noticed black patches in the intestines and the livers. In one village, of 2,601 sheep that belonged to 42 shepherds, the mortality rate was found to be 25 percent from grazing on GM cotton residue. In another village, of 2,168 sheep owned by 29 shepherds, the mortality rate was also 25 percent.

A team was assembled to assess the situation, and the team members concluded that "the preliminary information gathered from meeting shepherds across 3 mandals, strongly suggests that the sheep mortality was due to a toxin, and most likely Bt toxin from the foliage."

2011: Study Review of Mammals Fed GMOs

In 2011, a study titled "Genetically Modified Crops Safety Assessments: Present Limits and Possible Improvements" was published in France, which reviewed nineteen studies of mammals that had been fed GM soybeans and corn. The study also looked at the raw data from several studies that the researchers were able to obtain by court order, which included blood and urine parameters of mammals eating GMOs, along with organ weights.

The study claims that "several convergent data appear to indicate liver and kidney problems as end points of GMO diet effects in the above-mentioned experiments . . . the kidneys were particularly affected, concentrating 43.5% of all disrupted parameters in males, whereas the liver was more specifically disrupted in females."

The study also states that in order to protect large populations from the unintended effects of GMOs, it's crucial to do two-year testing. This is because, as the study rightly points out, the ninety-day feeding experiments done by GMO companies are an insufficient time period to evaluate chromic toxicity.

Following are some of the statements made in this study:

"Some GMOs (Roundup tolerant and MON863) affect the body weight increase at least in one sex."

"Several convergent factors appear to indicate liver and kidney problems as end points of GMO diet effects in these experiments . . . the kidneys in particular are affected. . . however other organs may be affected too, such as the heart and spleen or blood cells."

"The Roundup residues have been also shown to be toxic for human placental, embryonic, and umbilical cord cells. . . . Roundup adjuvants even stabilize glyphosate and allow its penetration into cells, which in turn inhibit estrogen syntheses as a side effect."

The U.S. Government's Role

After reading all of these stories about GMOs, you may wonder why they were allowed to enter the U.S. food supply without any independent testing from the U.S. government. In Chapter 8 on soy, I mentioned a former Monsanto attorney named Michael Taylor. In 2010, Michael Taylor became deputy commissioner for foods at the FDA, a position that was newly created for him. Prior to that, he had gone back and forth several times, between working for the FDA in various capacities and representing Monsanto as an attorney in the law firm of King and Spalding. As Monsanto's attorney, he helped draft many of the favorable GMO regulations that the industry would lobby for. Then, while working at the FDA, he helped implement many of those same favorable regulations.

Mr. Taylor's tenure as the FDA's deputy commissioner for policy from 1998 to 2001 ushered in extremely favorable policies toward GMO companies. His new position at the FDA made him the government official with the greatest influence over GMO food regulations and the development of government policy concerning them. One of the policies most favorable to the GMO industry was the one that stated,

> *"The agency is not aware of any information showing that foods derived by these new methods differ in any meaningful or uniform way."*

It is largely due to this policy that GMO companies would not be required to submit any independent testing to the FDA before bringing new GMOs into the U.S. food supply. Although this was the policy the FDA adopted, many of its scientists felt that there was in fact a "meaningful" difference between GM foods and natural foods. The predominant view among FDA scientists was that the risks posed by GMOs could not be determined without proper feeding studies.

FDA Scientists Protest Lack of GMO Safety Testing

Many documents obtained from lawsuits and the Freedom of Information Act show that the FDA's rank-and-file scientists were extremely concerned about GMOs and wanted serious testing, while those at the highest levels of government wanted a more lax policy. As the FDA developed its lax policy on GMOs, the FDA, overseen by former Monsanto attorney Michael Taylor, deleted more and more of the scientists' input as the final policy was drafted. Following are just a few of the many concerns of the FDA's own scientists.

Dr. Linda Kahl, an FDA compliance officer, stated that

"genetically modified plants could also contain high concentrations of plant toxicants. . . . in addition, plant toxicant genes which were normally inactive could be expressed in the modified plant gene as a result of insertion of new genetic material." In an internal memo she sent to James Maryanski, the FDA's biotechnology coordinator, concerning the Biotechnology Draft: "I believe there are at least two situations, relative to this document in which it (FDA) is trying to fit a square peg into a round hole. The first square peg in the round hole is that the document is trying to force an ultimate conclusion that there is no difference between food modified by genetic engineering and foods modified by traditional breeding practices. The process of GE and traditional breeding are different, and according to the technical experts in the agency, they lead to different risks."

Dr. Louis Pribyl, of the FDA's Microbiology Group, made the following comments in an internal memo regarding the department's Biotechnology Draft Document: "What has happened to the scientific elements of this document? . . . It reads very pro-industry, especially in the area of unintended effects. . . . This document reads like a biotech REDBOOK!! . . . there is a profound difference between the types of unexpected effects from traditional breeding and genetic engineering." Dr. Pribyl was also concerned that the GMO companies would not be able to pick up potentially dangerous effects from their foods that might not be obvious. He stated that "This is the industry's pet idea, namely that there are no unintended effects that will raise the FDA's level of concern. But time and time again, there is no data to back up their contention. . . . It reads very pro-industry, especially in the area of unintended effects. There is a profound difference between the types of unexpected effects from traditional breeding and genetic engineering, which is just glanced over in this document. . . . If there is no difference between traditional foods and genetically engineered foods, then why would the FDA even bother to challenge them: unless it is really saying that they are in fact different."

Dr. Edwin Matthews, the FDA director of Toxicology Review and Evaluation, stated in an internal memo, "At this time it is unlikely that molecular and compositional analysis can reasonably detect or predict all possible changes in toxicant levels or the development of new toxic metabolites as a result of genetic modifications introduced by the new methods or biotechnology." He further said, "We cannot assume that all gene products, particularly those encoded by genes from non-food sources, will be digestible. For example, there is evidence that certain types of proteins (e.g., plant lectins and protein allergens) are resistant to digestion and can be absorbed in biologically active form." He also expressed concerns over the possibility of toxins in GMOs and stated that a GMO "plant may contain an identical profile of expected plant toxicant levels (i.e., expected toxicants) as is normally found in a closely related, natural plant. However, genetically modified plants could also contain unexpected high concentrations of plant toxicants. The presence of high levels of toxicants could be amplified through enhancement of toxicant gene transcription and translation. This might occur as a result of up-stream or down stream promotion of gene activities in the modified plant DNA. In addition, plant toxicant genes, which were normally inactive, could be expressed in the modified plant gene as a result of insertion of the new genetic material (i.e., positional mutagenesis). Thus, the task of analysis of all major toxins in GE plants food include[s] the assessment of both expected toxicants and unexpected toxicants that could occur in the modified plant food. The unexpected toxicant could be closely related chemicals produced by common metabolic pathways in the same plant genus/species; however, unexpected toxicants could also be uniquely different chemicals that are usually expressed in unrelated plants."

Dr. Gerald Guest, the director of the CVM, stated in a memo that "some undesirable effects such as increased levels of known naturally occurring toxicants, appearance of new, not previously identified toxicants, increased capability of concentrating toxic substances from the environment (e.g., pesticides or heavy metals), and undesirable alterations in the levels of nutrients may escape breeder' attention unless genetically engineered plants are evaluated specifically for these changes." He sent a letter to the FDA that stated that scientists at the CVM concluded there was "ample scientific justification" to require that each new GMO food be tested before being allowed to be eaten by the public. He stated in his letter that "CVM believes that animal feeds derived from genetically modified plants present unique animal and food safety concerns. . . . it has always been our position that the sponsor needs to generate appropriate scientific information to demonstrate product safety to humans, animals and the environment. . . . I would urge you to eliminate statements that suggest the lack of information can be used as evidence for no regulatory concern. . . . We believe that animal feeds derived from GM plants present unique animal and food safety concerns. . . . it is important to determine if significant concentrations of harmful plant constitutes or toxicants are present in the transgenic plant byproducts. . . . Sponsors with products to be incorporated into animal feeds should conduct appropriately controlled feeding studies in the target animal comparing the new plant variety to the conventional plant. The study should be of sufficient size and duration to provide adequate statistical power to detect adverse effects should they occur."

Dr. Mitchell Smith made the following comments in an internal memo to James Maryanski at the FDA concerning the Biotechnology Draft. "The statement 'organisms modified by modern molecular and cellular methods are governed by the same physical and biological laws as are organisms produced by classical methods' is somewhat erroneous because in the former, natural biological barriers to breeding have been breached. . . . The statement 'to the extent that it is known' begs the question as to what degree of identification and toxicological evaluation is sought and prudent. In this instance, ignorance is not bliss."

U.S. Politicians Push GMOs, Favoring Economics Over Public Safety

While many of the FDA's own scientists were calling for proper safety testing of GMOs before they were allowed to be consumed by the public, those at the top levels of power in government wanted the opposite approach. In a memo from the Bush White House from 1992, the White House council issued a statement that read: "The policy statement needs to stress the role of decentralized safety reviews by producers; with informal FDA consultation only if significant safety or nutritional concerns arise. It should avoid emphasizing obligatory FDA review and oversight."

Melinda Kimble at the State Department, which was negotiating trade policy concerning GMOs, issued a statement that said, "I want to make very clear that it is the position of the United States government that we do not believe there is a difference between GMO commodities and non-GMO commodities."

In 2003, Speaker of the House Dennis Hastert stated, "There is a general consensus among the scientific community that genetically modified food is no different from conventional food."

The record shows that the FDA scientists whose job it was to evaluate the safety of GMOs based on science, and not on politics, had numerous concerns about GMOs and were advocating that each new GMO be tested for toxins prior to being allowed into the U.S. food supply. Meanwhile, politicians were urging that GMOs be approved without any testing, making it more of an "economic" issue than a safety issue. In the middle between the scientists and the politicians, the FDA's top man with regard to the GMO industry was Michael Taylor, Monsanto's former attorney. This is the system in which the concerns of scientists were silenced by the politicians.

It appears as though the government ignores not only its own scientists, but common sense as well. For example, when Monsanto produced a corn with a high lysine content, there was concern about a GM protein produced by the corn. Monsanto told government regulators that the protein should be considered safe, because the protein is found in the soil, and people consume small amounts of it from the residue on many vegetables. A simple calculation, however, shows that in order to consume the amount of that protein a person could realistically get from eating the high-lysine corn, he or she would need to eat as much as 22,000 pounds of soil every second of every day.

Royal Society of Canada Report Echoes Scientists' GMO Warnings

When credible scientific organizations look at GMOs, free of the "politics," their conclusions often mirror those of the FDA's own scientists. For example, in 2001, the Royal Society of Canada issued a list of recommendations for the regulation of food biotechnology in Canada. The report was prepared at the request of Health Canada, which is Canada's equivalent of the FDA, the Canadian Food Inspection Agency, and Environment Canada. Although Canada chose to have an independent respected scientific organization come up with its guidelines for GMO regulations, here in the United States we created a new position at the FDA for Monsanto's former attorney, giving him the power to direct our GMO policy. The Canadian Royal Society starts its report by quoting a statement made in the journal *Nature Biotechnology*:

> *The risks in biotechnology are undeniable, and they stem from the unknowable in science and commerce. It is prudent to recognize and address those risks, not compound them by overly optimistic or foolhardy behavior.*

When you compare its statement with the policy of the FDA in the United States, you almost have to wonder whether "overly optimistic and foolhardy behavior" is referring to the FDA's policy that states, *"The agency is not aware of any information showing that foods derived by these new methods differ in any meaningful or uniform way."*

The Royal Society of Canada also issued a list of recommendations concerning the regulation of GMOs that makes the FDA policy look like a complete joke. The list of recommendations from the Royal Society seems to be rooted in basic common sense and is a far cry from the FDA's policy, which is essentially "whatever the GMO companies say about their products we will accept, and we won't even require any testing." While the list is extensive, a highlight of some of the recommendations includes passages such as

> *The Panel recommends that approval of new transgenic organisms for environmental release, and for use as food or feed, should be based on rigorous scientific assessment of their potential for causing harm to the environment or to human health. Such testing should replace the current regulatory reliance on "substantial equivalence" as a decision threshold.*

In contrast, the current U.S. FDA policy does not require any FDA testing of GMOs and accepts whatever the GMO companies say about their products.

The Royal Society of Canada stated,

> *The Panel recommends that analysis of the outcomes of all tests on new transgenic organisms should be monitored by an appropriately configured panel of "arms-length" experts from all sectors, who report their decisions and rationale in a public forum.*

Yet in the United States, the entire scientific process concerning GMOs has been corrupted by politicians and insiders.

The Royal Society of Canada further said,

> *The Panel recommends the precautionary regulatory assumption that, in general, new technologies should not be presumed safe unless there is a reliable scientific basis for considering them safe. The Panel rejects the use of "substantial equivalence" as a decision threshold to exempt new GM products*

*from rigorous safety assessments on the basis of
superficial similarities because such a regulatory
procedure is not a precautionary assignment of the
burden of proof.*

The U.S. FDA policy, however, is that GM products are presumed
safe and are no different from those made from natural plants and
animals.

The Royal Society of Canada stated,

*As a precautionary measure, the Panel recommends
that the prospect of serious risks to human health,
of extensive, irremediable disruptions to the natural
ecosystems, or of serious diminution of biodiversity,
demand that the best scientific methods be employed
to reduce the uncertainties with respect to these
risks. Approval of products with these potentially
serious risks should await the reduction of scientific
uncertainty to minimum levels.*

The U.S. FDA's position, though, is essentially that no risks are
posed by GMOs. As reports about their negative effects continue
to come in, year after year, only the future will tell whether the
environment and biodiversity have been irreparably harmed by
GMOs.

The Royal Society of Canada advised,

*The Panel recommends that Canadian regulatory
agencies and officials exercise great care to maintain
an objective and neutral stance with respect to
the public debate about the risks and benefits
of biotechnology in their public statements and
interpretations of the regulatory process.*

Yet rather than being neutral, the U.S. government has attempted
to bully the entire world into taking the FDA's position, which is
essentially that GMOs present no risks and are no different from
natural foods.

The Royal Society of Canada stated,

*The Panel recommends that the Canadian regulatory
agencies implement a system of regular peer review*

of the risk assessments upon which the approvals of genetically engineered products are based. This peer review should be conducted by an external (nongovernmental) and independent panel of experts. The data and the rationales upon which the risk assessment and the regulatory decision are based should be available to public review.

Not only did the U.S. FDA not seek an independent review from independent experts, it even ignored its own scientists, and many government scientists who attempted to protect the public were fired or threatened with termination or demotion.

The Royal Society of Canada said,

The Panel recommends that companies applying for permission to release a GM organism into the environment should be required to provide experimental data (using ecologically meaningful experimental protocols) on all aspects of potential environmental impact.

Yet as pollen from GMO plants continues to cross-pollinate with natural plants and forever change their DNA, the U.S. government does not appear to be concerned about the loss of natural biodiversity.

The Failure of GMOs
GMOs were sold to the world through a slick marketing campaign that promised to feed the world, increase yields, reduce pesticide use, and make farming more profitable. According to many experts, GMOs have failed to achieve any of these goals. Because many countries, such as those in Europe, chose not to accept GMO foods, U.S. farmers who are growing corn and soy, two crops that are usually GMO, have seen their markets shrink and prices fall. U.S. corn exports to Europe were down more than 99 percent after European food manufacturers and grocers decided to stop using most GM foods. The American Corn Growers Association estimates that as a result, corn prices for U.S. farmers dropped 13 to 20 percent, and the farmers have been kept profitable only through an increase in subsidies. It has been estimated that the U.S. government's subsidies to farmers have increased $3 to 5 billion per year, due to the economic damage caused by GMOs,

which is paid for by the American taxpayer, most of whom do not even want GMOs in the food supply.

Meanwhile, Monsanto has been lobbying for food crops to be used as biofuels, which takes food out of the food supply to be made into fuels, leading to increased food prices and more hunger throughout the world. Because so many countries do not want U.S. corn, however, you have to wonder whether making it into fuel and food for the U.S. market are about the only things left to do with it.

Farmers were also told that GMO crops would have increased yields; however, studies of the most widely grown GMO crops show that they actually have decreased yields.

GMO Crops Produce Super-Pests and Super-Weeds
Farmers were told they would save money because they could use fewer chemicals on their crops, but GM crops have caused chemical use to increase, not decrease.

A recent article in the St. Louis newspaper *STLtoday* suggests that GM corn that was engineered to kill a pest called the rootworm is now being damaged by that pest instead. According to the article, titled "Pests Damaging Biotech Corn: Getting an Early Start," the GM corn, which was grown on 23 million acres in the United States last year, could be losing its efficacy. The article cites a study conducted at Iowa State University stating that "rootworms were becoming resistant to the product, creating so-called superbugs in Iowa fields.

Many GM crops are engineered so that they can withstand large doses of the herbicides produced by the GMO companies. This was supposed to help farmers control weeds, but all it has really accomplished is help create "super weeds." Due to the ability of some GMOs to withstand being sprayed by herbicides such as glyphosate, there are now twenty-one weed species resistant to that herbicide, whereas in 1996 there were no weeds with resistance.

This has caused farmers to have to spray more herbicides on their crops in an attempt to control the new super-weed problem. Although the slick marketing campaign promised that planting GMOs would mean less toxic chemical use, it appears that just the opposite is happening, and because GMO companies own the companies that make the toxic chemicals, this means more profits for them. According to one estimate, by 2004 farmers used 86 percent more herbicides on GM soy fields than on natural soy fields. All of these chemicals ultimately find their way into the air, soil, and water, leading to environmental consequences for both beneficial soil bacteria and animal life.

GMOs Kill Beneficial Human Gut Flora and Soil Microbes
According to an article at <u>Mercola.com</u> titled "The Hidden Epidemic Destroying Your Gut Flora," GMOs are wreaking havoc on the microorganisms that are crucial for proper plant growth, as well as on the flora in our own guts that are essential for our health. The article interviewed Dr. Donald Huber, an agricultural scientist and an expert in microbial ecology. According to Dr. Huber, the herbicides and the pesticides that are commonly used on GMOs are metal chelators, which immobilize vital nutrients and render them unavailable to both the plant and people who consume the plant. According to the article, the nutrients in GM plants such as iron and zinc can be reduced by as much as 80 to 90 percent. Furthermore, the high use of glyphosate herbicides in GMOs is dramatically affecting the microbes in soil, which are crucial for proper plant health. According to Dr. Huber, once this herbicide is sprayed on crops, it cannot be washed off. He claims, "It's going to be in your root tips, your shoot tips, your legume nodules, and in the food that you eat." In addition to harming the beneficial soil microbes, Dr. Huber states that it also harms the beneficial gut bacteria in humans and other animals when they eat food that has been sprayed with glyphosate.

According to a 2011 study conducted in France, the "GM plants exposed to glyphosate-based herbicides such as Roundup do not specifically degrade glyphosate. They can even accumulate Roundup residues throughout their life. . . . glyphosate and its main metabolite AMPA (with its own toxicity) are found in GMOs on a regular and regulatory basis. Therefore, such residues are absorbed by people eating most GM plants (as 80 percent of these plants are Roundup tolerant)."

A report sponsored by the UN and the World Bank and compiled by four hundred scientists came to the conclusion that GMO crops are not the answer when it comes to solving the world's poverty, hunger, and climate change issues. This is because better alternatives are already available that work with nature, such as integrated pest management and new low-input organic methods that both control pests and increase yields.

GMOs Lead to "GM Genocide" of Impoverished Farmers
There are methods that can be taught to impoverished farmers

without forcing them to buy expensive patented GM seeds and chemicals they cannot afford. Compare the GMO companies' promises with reality in the following true story happening in India.

According to a November 2, 2008, article in *MailOnline* titled "The GM Genocide: Thousands of Indian Farmers Are Committing Suicide after using Genetically Modified Crops." The article stated that farmers in India were told by GMO salespeople and government officials that GM seeds were "magic seeds" that would produce better crops, free of parasites and insects. Even though the seeds were a thousand times more expensive than traditional seeds, farmers were promised unheard of harvests and income if they switched to the GM seeds.

To help promote the GM seeds, the government even banned traditional varieties from many government seed banks. It seems that India was granted loans from the International Monetary Fund in the 1980s and the 1990s, and as part of those loans the IMF had agreed to allow the new GMO companies, such as Monsanto, to sell their seeds in the world's second most populous country.

With the promise of future riches, farmers borrowed money to buy the GM seeds, rather than using either the cheap natural seeds they used to buy or the free seeds they had simply saved from the previous year's harvest. It turns out that the seeds were far from "magic," however. Farmers had not been told that the GM seeds would need twice as much water as the natural seeds, and it turns out that the seeds were not "pest-proof" as promised and were devastated by a voracious parasite called the bollworm.

When the normal amount of rain did not come, the GM crops withered and died, leaving the farmers with a huge debt they were unable to pay off. To make matters worse, they had to purchase more GM seeds from more borrowed money for the next year's crops, because they did not have the free saved seeds from their own crops to use as before.

Ultimately, the farmers faced debt that they simply could not repay and resorted to mass suicide as their only way out. It has been estimated that 125,000 farmers have ended their own lives, many by drinking the toxic pesticides and herbicides intended for their own crops. This mass tragedy has been called the "GM Genocide."

Most of these farmers left behind wives and children, who, having lost their land, will now become part of India's lowest caste, with the children facing a future as "slave labor," working for a few pennies a day. For them, the failed promises of GMO companies mean that they will become the lowest of the low, India's homeless and penniless.

If these same farmers had simply been taught a few natural organic techniques for their farms and had grown more food crops for their families, they would still own their land and have a way to feed their families. Clearly, GMOs do not appear to be the solution for the world's poor farmers.

Is This the End of "Organic"?

Many people fear that GMOs could be the end of truly organic food, due to cross-pollination of GM crops with natural crops. According to an article in *GM Watch* titled "10 Reasons Why We Don't Need GM Foods," GMOs and natural crops cannot coexist. The article cites examples of GM crops contaminating natural crops through cross-pollination. For example, GM rice that was grown for only a year in field trials "was found to have extensively contaminated the US rice supply and seed stocks." The article also states that the organic oilseed rape industry, from which canola oil is made, had been destroyed due to contamination from the GM rape.

This problem of the GMO contamination of organic crops has made headlines in Australia, a country that has very strict organic standards. One organic farmer is suing his neighbor who was growing GM canola. It seems the GM pollen blew into his natural organic farm, and because of the GM contamination, the farmer was stripped of his organic certification. About 70 percent of his land is no longer usable for organic farming, and the farmer has lost the ten years of work it took to build his farm up to organic status.

What You Can Do about GMOs

If you are concerned about GMOs in your diet and the potential hazards they pose, there are some simple things you can do to eliminate most of them from your diet.

First, be aware of what the major GM foods are. They include canola, cotton, corn, and soy, along with milk from cows that get rbGH and meat from animals fed GM grains. Other foods that may be GM include yellow squash, zucchini, and papaya. While most corn in the United States is GM corn, only about 3 to 5 percent of sweet corn is estimated to be GM, so you are usually safe if you buy nonorganic sweet corn.

If you buy certified "100% Organic" foods, you are assured to be getting foods free of GMOs, because GMOs cannot be used in "100% Organic" foods. If a food is simply "Organic," as opposed to "100% Organic," it means that at least 95 percent of the food is organic and the other 5 percent can contain GMOs. If a label says "Made with Organic Ingredients," at least 70 percent of the ingredients must be organic, but up to 30 percent can contain GMOs. Because nonorganic corn and soy have the highest chances of being GM, your best bet is to try to purchase 100 percent organic foods if the product contains either corn or soy. If you cannot afford organic foods all of the time and want to avoid GMOs, it's best to buy organic when you think there is a high chance the food could contain GMOs.

For example, most processed vegetable oil, which is not recommended on the Four Seasons Diet anyway, is made from corn, canola, soy, or cottonseed. All of these, if they are not organic, most likely contain GMOs.

Most processed foods in the United States contain soy or corn in one form or another, and if they are not organic, they most likely contain GMOs. The soy and the corn can be found as soy or corn on the ingredient label but can also be found as soy protein, soy flour, soy lecithin, textured vegetable protein, corn meal, corn syrup, dextrose, maltodextrin, soy oil, or corn oil.

When buying dairy products, either purchase organic products or buy products that state that the milk comes from cows that did not receive rbGH. If you eat meat, unless the meat is organic, you have to assume the animal was fed GM grain.

Eating out can pose more of a challenge when you're trying to avoid GMOs. The first rule is to avoid corn and soy unless you know they are organic. The other source of GMOs is usually in the oil used for cooking. If a restaurant uses vegetable oil, it's most likely soy, canola, or corn oil, all of which are usually made from GMOs.

The other thing you can do is stop accepting the status quo in the United States, where the tail is allowed to wag the dog. In the United States, the consumer has let the GMO companies and the FDA allow the entry of GMO products into the food supply without the type of protests we saw from European consumers when governments in Europe attempted the same thing. If consumers demand non-GMO foods from their grocers and food makers, the food makers will ultimately comply. They will tell the farmers who grow the foods they purchase that they will only purchase non-GMO foods, and the farmers will go back to growing the natural foods they have grown for thousands of years. This is what happened in

Europe, and this is what can happen here as well, if enough people demand it.

Why Natural Foods Are Best

There are many reasons to eliminate highly processed foods that are full of artificial chemicals from your diet. Recall that in 1843, "Tanchou's Doctrine" found that cancer increases in direct proportion to the "civilization" of a people. This doctrine was validated when Weston Price found disease to be virtually nonexistent in native peoples who consumed natural foods and discovered that their state of health quickly deteriorated when Western processed and artificial foods were introduced into their diets. Tanchou and Price were further validated in 1981 when two Oxford epidemiologists published a 120-page report that concluded that up to 80 percent of the cancer in the United States could be avoidable with proper dietary and lifestyle changes, mainly through limiting our exposure to processed foods and artificial chemicals. The Blue Zone studies added more validity to how beneficial natural foods are and how detrimental processed foods are to a person's health.

Artificial Chemicals and Preservatives in Food

Many things are ruining the health and well-being of the average American, and processed food, full of artificial chemicals, may be at the top of the list. Most Americans rely on the FDA to protect them, but the FDA has become highly political in nature, with top managers who usually have strong ties to industry often overruling the findings of their own scientists and physicians who claim specific harms from various foods, food additives, and pharmaceutical drugs. The FDA usually gives credibility to industry-funded science, which is often severely biased, while ignoring neutral science.

University studies frequently rely on industry for funding, and that funding may be threatened if a particular research institution publishes any studies that could hurt industry profits. Even at the FDA, scientists are often pressured to change their findings by managers with ties to industry.

The solutions to our health problems are clear: <u>eliminate the artificial and processed foods that are causing poor health and replace them with natural foods that contribute to good health</u>. Needless to say, countless other artificial foods are currently being eaten by Americans that are not safe for consumption. In some cases, science has yet to evolve to the point where it can ascertain that some additives are toxic. In other cases, industry science shows a certain additive to be safe, while objective science raises concerns. This is the reason it's always best to choose foods that are as natural as possible.

Sodium Benzoate Damages DNA

A common preservative used in foods, especially in soft drinks, is *sodium benzoate*. One study done in 1999 by Peter Piper at Sheffield University found that sodium benzoate (aka benzoic acid) may potentially damage the DNA in the mitochondria of our cells. The mitochondria are the power stations of our cells, which help produce the energy that keeps us going. In 2007, it was discovered that sodium benzoate may also cause a type of DNA damage that has been linked to cirrhosis of the liver and Parkinson's disease. According to the newspaper the *Independent*, Piper stated, "These chemicals have the ability to cause severe damage to DNA in the mitochondria to the point that they totally inactivate it—they knock it out altogether."

It has also been found that when sodium benzoate combines with vitamin C, it creates cancer-causing benzene. Many soft drinks contain both sodium benzoate and vitamin C. Sodium benzoate was approved as a food additive approximately fifty years ago, and since that time, science is now able to detect harmful effects that could not be detected previously. Although benzoic acid occurs in some foods naturally, when used as a food preservative the amount used is often fifty times higher by food weight than what is found in natural foods. Several soda manufacturers in the UK, where the story made the most news, have pledged to take sodium benzoate out of their products.

Brominated Vegetable Oil Causes Memory Loss and Nerve Disorders

Another additive called brominated vegetable oil (BVO) found in many sodas and sports drinks in the United States has also made the news lately. According to a December 12, 2011, article in Environmental Health News titled "Brominated Battle: Soda Chemical Has Cloudy Health History," BVO was patented as a flame retardant for plastics and has been banned throughout Europe and Japan for use in foods. The article states that a few extreme soda bingers have needed medical attention for memory loss and nerve disorders, both of which are symptoms of overexposure to bromine. A study done in 1972 titled "Toxic

Effects of Brominated Vegetable Oils in Rats" studied the effects of feeding rats .5 percent BVO for 105 days. It found that the rats fed BVO had "degenerative myocardial lesions." Another study published in 1983 titled "Behavioral and Reproductive Effects of Chronic Developmental Exposure to Brominated Vegetable Oil in Rats" studied the effects of feeding BVO to rats two weeks prior to mating. The study found that as little as 1 percent BVO in the diet "severely impaired conception," while a diet consisting of 2 percent BVO "completely blocked reproduction." Lower doses of .5 percent did not affect reproduction as much; however, a 1 percent dose produced "severe behavioral impairments" in offspring.

Although these doses are considered high, they were given for only a short duration, and it has been suggested that BVO builds up in tissues over time. Another study titled "Bromism from Excessive Cola Consumption" reported that excessive consumption of sodas had caused what is called bromism. Bromism is a neurological condition caused by bromide ingestion. Bromide has a very long half-life in the human body of nine to twelve days, which means that people who consume large amounts of soda containing BVO often have a high concentration in their tissues. According to the research article, a hospital patient had consumed 2 to 4 liters of soda containing BVO per day. His symptoms included "headache, fatigue, ataxia, and memory loss which progressed over 30 days." The patient's condition deteriorated until he was no longer able to walk. Although BVO was banned in Europe and Japan, the FDA considers BVO safe as an additive in sodas. In European sodas, a natural product that is slightly more expensive is used in place of the BVO that the United States uses in sodas.

I mention sodium benzoate and brominated vegetable oil because they are two additives that are currently allowed in foods in the United States that have some safety concerns. The United States allows many other artificial additives that have been banned in other countries to be put into food and cosmetics. This is one reason it's important to eat only natural foods and eliminate artificial foods, if you want optimal health.

Artificial Food Colorings and Dyes Banned in EU Are Legal in USA

Other artificial additives that are considered perfectly safe today are likely to be found toxic sometime in the future. This is because history has shown that artificial additives and chemicals once considered perfectly safe were later shown to be harmful. Consider the case of artificial food colorings, most of which are synthesized from coal tar and petroleum. Between 1950 and 1973, at least seven food dyes were banned when they were found to cause various potential health effects, such as cancer, organ damage, and heart damage.

There are currently seven remaining food dyes used in the United States, all of which were shown to have potential toxicity in at least one study. For example, two genotoxicity studies showed potentially negative effects (such as damage to DNA and chromosomes) from consuming Blue No. 1, while six studies demonstrated potential negative effects from consuming Yellow No. 5. Note that Yellow No. 5 was connected to childhood hyperactivity in a British study in 2007, so in Europe foods must carry a warning label if they contain Yellow No. 5. Sadly, many products made by U.S. companies, such as McDonald's, Mars, Kraft, and Pepsi, often contain these dyes in the U.S. version of their products but not in the European version. Meanwhile, other companies such as Starbucks deserve credit for eliminating artificial dyes from their U.S. products.

According to an article by Dr. Mercola, the EPA considers 60 percent of herbicides, 90 percent of fungicides, and 30 percent of insecticides to be carcinogenic. Recall that an epidemiological study conducted at Oxford showed that at least 80 percent of cancer cases could be prevented by dietary and lifestyle changes. One of the many changes you can make to minimize your risk of getting cancer is to eat organic fruits and vegetables and eliminate processed foods that have artificial ingredients. If Americans begin to demand natural foods, food companies will replace many of the artificial ingredients with natural ones. Food manufacturers have already done this in Europe with many artificial ingredients because they have no choice if they want to stay in business.

The FDA Mammography Scandal

As of the writing of this book, the FDA is involved in yet another scandal, this time involving mammography. It appears as though the FDA installed secret spy software on the computers of certain employees and then used that software to gain the passwords to private e-mail accounts. The FDA then used that information to monitor the private e-mails of nine "whistle-blowers" during a two-year period. If any of us hacked into someone's private e-mail, especially if it concerned confidential communications to Congress, we would quickly find ourselves in jail. In 2010, the college student who hacked into Sarah Palin's e-mail account was sentenced to more than a year in prison. In this case, according to reports, FDA managers were secretly hacking into the private e-mail accounts of their own doctors and scientists and monitoring their private communications.

These doctors and scientists worked in the office that reviewed medical devices, including devices used for cancer screenings. It seems that they had expressed some concerns over several devices, which may have included the dangers of mammography. According to news accounts, these whistle-blowers, using their personal e-mail accounts, had warned congressional members that the FDA was approving medical devices that the doctors and the scientists felt posed unacceptable risks to patients. Six of those employees are currently suing the FDA, claiming that the information gathered from their personal e-mail accounts led to their harassment or dismissal.

The concerns started in 2007, when FDA employees began to complain internally that radiological devices were being approved, despite a lack of proof of their effectiveness. They even recommended against approving one breast cancer imaging device three times, but a senior FDA manager overruled them after the third rejection. You wonder why the taxpayers are even paying for scientists at the FDA, because the top managers, who are industry insiders, completely ignore the scientists when they can't get the scientists to change their findings.

Things are so bad at the FDA that a letter sent from FDA employees stated that the FDA is in need of a total overhaul, due to deep-rooted and systemic corruption at the highest levels. The letter said, "Currently there is an atmosphere at FDA in which the honest employee fears the dishonest employee, and not the other way around. Disturbingly, the atmosphere does not yet exist at FDA where honest employees committed to integrity and the FDA mission can act without fear of reprisal. . . . America urgently needs change at FDA because FDA is fundamentally broken, failing to fulfill its mission, and because re-establishing a proper and effectively functioning FDA is vital to the physical and economic health of the nation." The letter further stated that "FDA's top leaders at the Center for Drug Evaluation and Research (CDER) testified that they 'didn't have a choice, and . . . [weren't] sure that [they] would be allowed to remain [in their positions if they] didn't agree' to ignore the science and the law." The judge ruled that there was "unrebutted evidence that the FDA's [decision] stemmed from political pressure rather than permissible health and science and safety concerns." The "improper political influence" and the many "departures from its own policies" reveal that such FDA officials are "incapable of ensuring integrity and science at FDA."

The signatures on the letter have been blacked out to protect the signers, but they are ostensibly current FDA employees. The letter mentions how, in 2005, "Dr Daniel Schultz approved a medical device against the unanimous opinion of his scientific staff . . . overruling more than twenty FDA scientists, medical officers and management staff."

A second letter sent to HHS secretary Tom Daschle and nine members of Congress stated that "In the case of an April 2008 approval of a computer-aided detection device for mammography," the scientists specifically charged (by title, but not by name) ODE director Donna-Bea Tillman "and her subordinates" with the "most outrageous misconduct by ordering, coercing, and intimidating FDA physicians and scientists to recommend approval, and then retaliating when the physicians and scientists refused to go along." That letter, which is also signed by FDA physicians and scientists, claimed that "the scientific review process for medical devices at FDA has been corrupted and distorted by current FDA managers, thereby placing the American people at risk. . . . managers at CDRH have ignored the law and ordered physicians and scientists to assess medical devices employing unsound evaluation methods, and to accept non-scientific, or clinically validated, safety and effectiveness evidence and conclusions, as the basis of device clearance and approval. . . . Managers have ordered, intimidated, and coerced FDA experts to modify scientific evaluations, conclusions and recommendations in violation of the laws, rules and regulations. . . . the long-standing FDA practice of secret meetings and secret communications between FDA managers and regulated industry must be strictly prohibited."

I feel compelled to share large portions of these two letters, because they were signed by multiple FDA employees and reaffirm many of the things I have stated about how the FDA reaches decisions.

12
Fluoride, the Toxin in Your Drinking Water

Studies show that fluoride lowers IQ, causes cancer, and weakens bones.

When it comes to avoiding unnatural foods and chemicals, it's usually a matter of not purchasing and eating foods that are highly processed or that contain added chemicals. One of the most harmful toxins Americans are exposed to, however, may be hiding in our water. Despite all of the current research that shows how toxic fluoride is, doctors and dentist continue to cling to flimsy junk science from the 1950s in their defense of fluoridation, despite the fact that all of the valid studies conducted since the 1980s show that fluoride has numerous negative effects on our health.

The United States, along with several other countries, currently advocates adding fluoride to water for the alleged reduction in cavities it is said to provide. Most countries have outlawed the practice of adding fluoride to public water, due to a substantial amount of evidence that suggests it can cause serious health problems, such as lowering a child's IQ by up to 10 percent when given in the same quantities currently allowed in water by the U.S. EPA.

The History of Fluoride

To understand why the United States allows fluoride to be put in the public water supply but most other nations do not, you'll need to learn about the history of fluoride, both as a pollutant and as a water additive. Although early studies done in the 1950s showed that fluoridated water reduced cavities in children, a subsequent analysis of those studies reveals that they were seriously flawed and suffered from bias. Some newer studies show a very slight reduction in cavities from water fluoridation; however, most recent studies demonstrate that water fluoridation actually causes cavity rates to increase. In the 1950s, when fluoride was first added to public water, the belief was that fluoride reduced cavities, and that

442

this benefit was achieved by ingesting fluoride. Since then, science has gained new information about fluoride, and the consensus now is that fluoride works topically and not by ingestion. The Centers for Disease Control finally acknowledged this fact in 1999 and 2001, and that should have put an end to water fluoridation. Fluoride's ability to reduce cavities when applied topically is the reason it is added to most toothpastes currently on the market. Yet many scientists say that the potential health dangers of fluoride are so serious that they far outweigh any benefit we might gain from a slight reduction in cavities.

Following is a brief history of how water came to be fluoridated in the United States, followed by an examination of many of the new studies conducted on the health effects of fluoridated water and fluoride in general.

1850–1899
During this time, there were many lawsuits resulting from the health problems caused by emissions from aluminum plants, metal smelters, and phosphate fertilizer plants. By the 1930s, fluoride was suspected as the cause of the most serious health problems near these industrial plants.

1900–1919
In this time period, "mottling" of tooth enamel was first observed and studied. Mottling of tooth enamel is when white or brown patches appear on the tooth. Scientists eventually discovered that water that contains natural fluoride is responsible for this staining of teeth, and the condition was renamed "dental fluorosis." A few places in the United States, such as areas of Colorado and Texas, have high levels of natural fluoride in their water, and a large percentage of the people living there suffered from dental fluorosis. It was also noticed in published reports that people who had dental fluorosis from ingesting fluoride had unusually coarse hair, similar to horse hair; that their fingernails did not appear to be normal; and that they suffered from an unusually large number of skin disorders.

1920–1929
During this decade, doctors treated patients suffering from overactive thyroid glands (hyperthyroidism) with fluoride, because it was found that fluoride lowered thyroid function. A study done on fluoride at Johns Hopkins and published in 1925 found that

fluoride disturbs the structure of teeth. The study's scientists found that contrary to their expectations, "the ingestion of fluorine, in amounts but little above those which have been reported to occur in natural foods, markedly disturbs the structure of the teeth." The study further mentioned that the animals fed fluorine were stunted in growth, and that the bones of the animals fed fluoride did not seem to be as good in quality as the normal animals' bones. The teeth of the animals given fluoride were found to be of inferior quality, with a dull opaque white color that lacked the natural polish of a well-formed tooth. Essentially, the 1925 Johns Hopkins study discovered what the studies conducted from the 1980s onward found, which is that fluoridated water actually damages teeth and causes other health problems. As you will learn, however, the scientific studies produced by industry and the U.S. government to protect fluoride would soon falsely claim that fluoride was actually good for you.

1930–1939
Kettering Lab's Dr. Kehoe Vouched for the Safety of Leaded Gasoline and Fluoridated Water

In 1930, the Kettering lab was founded with donations from the Ethyl Corporation and Frigidaire and was headed by Dr. Kehoe, who had been the Ethyl Corporation's chief medical consultant. Critics of the early work of the Kettering lab contend that its real purpose was to conduct scientific investigations that aided industry in its defense against lawsuits. The Ethyl Corporation was founded in 1923 by General Motors and Standard Oil and held the main patents to produce anti-knock gasoline using tetraethyl lead, a lead-based additive.

Even though there were serious health concerns about lead in the 1930s, Dr. Kehoe advocated the position that leaded fuels did not pose any health threat. As head of the prestigious Kettering lab, Kehoe became the chief safety spokesman for adding lead to gasoline, and he was able to convince many key government officials to believe that leaded gasoline was safe. Not until overwhelming evidence in the 1970s began to show the harmful effects of lead, especially on the IQs of children, did lead begin to be phased out of gasoline, with the final U.S. ban occurring in 1995. Leaded gasoline was shown to reduce the IQs of children in a dose-dependent fashion, much in the same way that fluoride has been shown to. For example, a blood lead level of 30 μg/dL was associated with a 6.9 point reduction in IQ, while a blood level of under 10 μg/dL reduced IQ by about 3.9 points. The eventual ban on lead would lower the average level of lead in children's blood from 16 µg/dL to only 3 µg/dL.

This is an important point, because the same scientist and lab that had vouched for the safety of lead for nearly fifty years, even though it damaged the brains of children, also vouched for the safety of fluoride. As of the writing of this book, at least twenty-five studies show that fluoride negatively affects the IQs of children; however, just as it took many years for the new scientific discoveries about lead to change years of pro-lead propaganda and flimsy old lead science, the new findings on fluoride are also taking a long time to change the pro-fluoride propaganda and spurious fluoride science. Keep in mind that the first clinical research articles about the toxicity of lead were published in the 1960s; however, it was not until 1995 that the United States finally banned leaded gasoline. Although most people prefer to believe that the U.S. government would quickly ban any product shown to adversely affect the IQs of children, the truth is that politics and bad science usually dictate that this process may take twenty to thirty years. We are currently in the middle of this time frame when it comes to fluoride. Despite numerous studies showing adverse health effects from consuming fluoride, the politics and bad science involved mean that it will probably be at least another ten to twenty years before fluoride is finally eliminated from the public water supply in the United States.

The Influence of Pro-Industry Junk Science

It's hard to underestimate the effect that pro-industry science has had on the addition of lead to gasoline, as well as on the addition of fluoride to our water. From 1930 until about 1970, nearly all of the scientific research concerning the health effects of leaded gasoline was controlled and financed by companies such as GM, Standard Oil, and DuPont. Not surprisingly, this research usually favored the pro-lead industry that paid for the scientific research and helped sway those in power politically. Even though most of this pro-lead research was fatally flawed, it would take nearly fifty years for independent research to finally debunk the pro-lead junk science. History appears to be repeating itself with fluoride.

Keep in mind that both lead and fluoride were known poisons back in the 1930s. In fact, lead has been recognized as a poison for nearly three thousand years, and in 1922, a few months before leaded gasoline was about to be unleashed on the developing brains of children in the United States, a lab director at the U.S. Public Health Service named William Mansfield Clark warned that leaded gasoline was a "serious menace to public health." He cited emerging reports that "several very serious cases of lead poisoning have resulted." The Public Health Service director responded that the trials Clark suggested to determine the health effects of leaded gasoline would be too time consuming, and he decided to instead have the Public Health Service rely on industry to supply the relevant data. Dr. Kehoe at the Kettering lab handled the job of proving the safety of lead for nearly fifty years, and he did the same thing for fluoride. This is the man who testified before Congress that he and his colleagues at Kettering lab "had been looking for thirty years for evidence of bad effects from leaded gasoline in the general population and had found none"; suffice to say, as with lead, so with fluoride. These industries have taken the same stance as the tobacco companies, the asbestos companies, and others. First, they claim that their products are safe. When scientific studies emerge showing they are not safe, the industries attack the science and the scientists behind those studies. Eventually, the public realizes it has been conned, by which time the industries that have misled the public have often made billions of dollars in profit at the expense of the health of American citizens.

Fluoride Pollution and Fluorosis

It happens that 1930 and 1931 were very bad years for industries that produced fluoride pollution, and the events of these two years would be instrumental in the history of water fluoridation. In 1930, the world's first major documented air pollution disaster occurred in Belgium's Meuse Valley. Weather conditions allowed smog from factories to become trapped in the valley, resulting in sixty deaths. A scientist named Kaj Roholm determined that the fluoride in the factory emissions was ultimately responsible for the deaths.

In 1931, Union Carbide was facing $4 million in lawsuits from more than 500 plaintiffs over an epidemic of silicosis among workers at the Hawk's Nest Tunnel. Out of a workforce of around 5,000, an estimated 764 men eventually died from silicosis. That same year, scientists at ALCOA discovered that dental fluorosis was occurring near their aluminum smelter in New York.

That region of New York naturally has very low levels of water fluoride; recall that fluorosis was discovered to occur only in regions with high levels of fluoride in their water. Although the ALCOA scientists kept this discovery secret, they were very worried.

The fluorosis could help prove that ALCOA's plant was poisoning people with fluoride, and given the well-publicized Union Carbide lawsuits and the Meuse Valley disaster, they had to be terrified by the potential of literally thousands of lawsuits, which could dwarf even the Union Carbide lawsuits that were going on at the time.

To make matters worse, this was the same year that three independent studies finally proved that the cause of dental fluorosis was fluoride. The U.S. Public Health Service dispatched a dentist named Trendley Dean to towns in states such as Colorado and Texas that had high levels of fluoride in their water. His supposed mission was to determine how much fluoride people could tolerate without obvious damage to their teeth.

An Unholy Partnership: Andrew Mellon, ALCOA, and the Public Health Service

During this time period, the U.S. Public Health Service (PHS) was run by the U.S. Treasury Department, and Andrew Mellon was secretary of the treasury from 1921 to 1932. Andrew Mellon was also the founder of ALCOA, the Aluminum Company of America, and was its largest stockholder. This was the same Public Health Service that a year later, in 1932, began a syphilis study in Tuskegee to study syphilis in black men without treating them for the disease or even telling them they had syphilis. It seems as if scientific ethics were a bit different back then, so when the Public Health Service, run by Mellon, the founder of ALCOA, sent Trendley Dean out to study the effects of fluoride, a known toxin and industrial pollutant, you are forced to question what the real purpose was behind Dean's mission. At the time that Dean was dispatched by Andrew Mellon, ALCOA was very possibly the largest fluoride polluter in the nation. Dean's research concluded in 1934 that the natural fluoride in drinking water that caused the staining known as dental fluorosis resulted in lower cavity rates. Dean was rewarded for his findings by being placed in charge of dental research at the PHS and was named the first director of the National Institute of Dental Research in 1948.

What was not known at the time about dental fluorosis was that although fluoride does make teeth more resistant to acid attack, it also makes teeth far more brittle, so that when cavities do occur, the teeth are much more prone to serious damage. Fluoride does this by replacing the hydroxyl ions in tooth enamel by reacting with calcium hydroxypatite, which makes enamel and bones harder, yet more brittle at the same time. Recall that the

1925 Johns Hopkins study had already found that fluoride made teeth weaker. The Dean study looked only at cavities in children, and although children living in areas with high levels of fluoride in the water did have lower cavity rates, they also had much higher rates of dental fluorosis. In Pueblo, Colorado, which had a low water fluoride content of .6 parts per million, 37 percent of children were cavity-free and only 2.4 percent had dental fluorosis. In Colorado Springs, which had a high water fluoride content of 2.5 parts per million, only 41 percent of children were cavity-free, while an astounding 67.6 percent suffered from dental fluorosis. Dental fluorosis is a marker for other potential health problems, such as weak bones, and even though young kids with dental fluorosis might have fewer cavities early in life, when they get older that same fluorosis could cause their teeth and bones to be far weaker. That same fluorosis, which is a marker for high fluoride content in the diet, has also been shown in at least twenty-five later studies to lower a child's IQ.

Warnings about Fluoride in the Media
Meanwhile, prior to Dean's announcement in 1934 that fluoride in water helped prevent cavities, fluoride continued to get bad press. In 1932, a study published in Denmark by Moller and Gunjonsson found that workers in the cryolite industry who were exposed to fluoride dust suffered from bone disorders. In 1933, a Department of Agriculture toxicologist began to warn people about the growing risk caused by industrial fluoride. In 1934, Dean would claim that fluoride offered protection for cavities; however, doctors living in areas with high fluoride levels in their water often reported negative effects from drinking fluoridated water. For example, a pediatrician in Amarillo, Texas, reported that babies who received large doses of fluoride had defective development of their long bones, with a greater tendency to bowing legs.

Mellon Institute and Industry Scientists Contrive to Promote Fluoride as "Good for Teeth"
In 1935, the Mellon Institute got involved in fluoride research. The Mellon Institute was founded by the same Andrew Mellon who founded ALCOA and was the secretary of treasury who sent Dean out to research fluoride. The Mellon Institute was originally established as a research institute for American industry. Industry would contract with the institute to solve a specific problem. Interestingly, the Mellon Institute's first announcement concerning

fluoride did not really mention fluoride by name. The Mellon Institute simply stated that there was some "mysterious" factor that seemed to protect teeth, and the institute was going to find out what it was. It is alleged that a researcher at ALCOA named Francis Frary approached Gerald Cox at the Mellon Institute and questioned him on whether he had ever considered that good teeth might be the result of exposure to fluoride. That same year, the Mellon Institute founded the Air Hygiene Foundation, which would later become the Industrial Hygiene Foundation. This was done in response to the Hawk's Nest Tunnel disaster in 1931, mentioned earlier. The foundation was heavily involved in defending corporations when they violated safety and environmental regulations. For example, even though asbestos had been linked to serious health issues since 1918, in 1967 Dr. Paul Gross, who was director of research at the Industrial Hygiene Foundation, helped publish a report that disputed the allegedly dangerous nature of asbestos fibers.

In 1936, researchers at the Mellon Institute gave rats some fluoride and announced that fluoride was the "mysterious" factor that protected teeth from cavities. If we look back at all of the facts, it appears that when the Mellon Institute announced that there was a "mysterious" factor protecting teeth, it had already planned to conduct a study that would allow it to announce that fluoride just happened to be the "mysterious" factor. That same year, Charles Kettering, the inventor of leaded gasoline and the founder of the Kettering Foundation, met with officials at the American Dental Association and is alleged to have been very generous in helping to fund their activities. He ended up becoming a member of the ADA's three-person committee in charge of researching dental cavities. Up until that time, the American Dental Association appears to have had quite a different view of fluoride. An article published in the *Journal of the American Dental Association* in 1936 titled "Fluorine in Relation to Bone and Tooth Development" stated that "fluorine is a general protoplasmic poison, but the most important symptoms of chronic fluorine poisoning known at present are mottling of the teeth and interference with bone formation."

Independent Scientists Warn of Fluoride's Toxicity
During this time, while industry scientists were beginning to form a strategy to protect fluoride, independent scientists were finding serious health problems from fluoride exposure. In 1937, Kaj Roholm published a 364-page study called *Fluorine Intoxication*, which contained references to 893 scientific articles on fluoride. He

was a Danish doctor who studied the health problems of workers in the cryolite industry, of which fluoride is the main pollutant. He found that fluoride compounds were far more toxic than other compounds that were part of industrial emissions. He fed fluoride to rats, pigs, and dogs to study the toxic effects and noted that fluoride was very harmful to the central nervous system. That same year, Shortt et al. published an article on fluorosis in India, which noted that fluoride damages the central nervous system. The work of both Roholm and Shortt would later be validated by a 1970 U.S. Department of Agriculture study, which claimed that "airborne fluorides have caused more worldwide damage to domestic animals than any other air pollutant."

To Avoid Lawsuits, ALCOA and the Mellon Institute Ramp up the "Spin" on Fluoride

Objective scientists were quickly beginning to demonstrate that fluoride was a dangerous pollutant that negatively affected the central nervous system, as well as teeth and bones. ALCOA had a potentially serious problem on its hands, given that residents downwind of its New York plant were showing signs of dental fluorosis, despite the lack of fluoride in their water. It was only a matter of time before people realized that they were being poisoned by the fluoride emissions from the plant and a major lawsuit would be filed.

In 1938, Gerald Cox at the Mellon Institute declared that "the case for fluoride should be regarded as proved." What he meant was it should be considered proved that fluoride was the "miracle" factor that protected teeth. Most mainstream Americans would not have been aware of the negative fluoride science piling up in the late 1930s, so calling fluoride a miracle factor that prevented cavities was simply a way of putting a positive spin on the greatest industrial poison being released into the atmosphere at the time.

Legitimate science was not buying the spin. In 1939, the *Yearbook in Agriculture* published an article that stated, "Fluorine interferes with the normal calcification of the teeth during the process of their formation so that affected teeth, in addition to being usually discolored and ugly in appearance, are structurally weak and deteriorate early in life. For this reason, it is especially important that fluorine be avoided during the period of tooth formation, that is, from birth to the age of 12 years." It was well understood even in 1939 that dental fluorosis created weak teeth. Sure, these teeth may have been a bit more cavity resistant very early in a child's life, but it was understood that later in life the child's teeth would deteriorate, due to the fact that fluoride had made them weaker.

1940–1949
Dean's 21-City Study Falsely Claims Fluoride Lowers Tooth Decay

In 1941, Trendley Dean released a 21-city study claiming that fluoride in the water at one part per million lowers tooth decay without causing fluorosis. Remember that Dean was the dentist who worked for the PHS and was sent out to study fluorosis while the PHS was under control of Andrew Mellon, the founder and a major stockholder of ALCOA, a company that was arguably the worst fluoride polluter at the time. Subsequent reviews of Dean's study, decades later, found that it was based on highly selective data, and that when Dean's study data was combined with data from 23 other studies that followed, it turned out that there was no apparent reduction in cavities when people consumed fluoride. This would not be discovered until water fluoridation was a generally accepted practice in the United States, however, and just as it took almost fifty years to remove lead from gasoline, the fight to get fluoride out of water has been a slow and steady battle.

Regardless of industry's attempt to put a smiling face on fluoride, independent science was painting a far more accurate picture. A 1943 study in the *Journal of the American Medical Association* titled "Chronic Fluoride Intoxication" has this to say about fluoride: "Fluorides are general protoplasmic poisons, probably because of their capacity to modify the metabolism of cells by changing the permeability of the cell membrane and by inhibiting certain enzyme systems." That same year the *Journal of the American Medical Association* published another article titled "Acute Sodium Fluoride Poisoning," which detailed how forty-seven hospital patients had been accidentally killed when a worker put sodium fluoride in the form of roach powder into scrambled eggs by mistake.

Fluoride, a Vital Bomb-Making Component in the Manhattan Project

Prior to World War II, fluoride was a known poison and toxin, which negatively affected teeth and bones, and efforts were made to remove it from water, not add it to water. Yet even though objective scientific studies showed fluoride to be toxic, World War II was about to get the government involved in the fluoride controversy. Fluoride was a vital ingredient in making the first atomic bombs as part of the Manhattan Project. Newly declassified documents have shed a lot of light on just how crucial fluoride was to making the first atomic bombs and the lengths to which the U.S. government went to hide this fact.

Millions of tons of fluoride-containing compounds were needed to manufacture the bomb-grade uranium and plutonium necessary for the nuclear weapons built from World War II through the early Cold War. During World War II, the race was on to beat the Germans and the Japanese in developing the first atomic bomb, and war-time urgency meant that many safety short-cuts were allowed by the government. These included exposing thousands of workers to toxic doses of fluoride and releasing countless tons of fluoride into the atmosphere, usually in the middle of night to avoid detection. The Manhattan Project was so top secret that even the role fluoride played was a closely guarded secret. Even when workers began to get sick, along with residents downwind of where the fluoride had been released into the atmosphere, the U.S. government considered information regarding fluoride to be top secret and vital to national security.

Code Name: "Program F"

The government knew this opened it up to potential lawsuits after the war, due to the adverse health effects caused by fluoride, so government officials began to gather the evidence they would need after the war to protect themselves. Much of the original "proof" that fluoride was safe for humans consisted of studies conducted by the U.S. government as part of the Manhattan Project and by the Atomic Energy Commission, under the code name "Program F." In 1948, when "Program F" discovered adverse effects from fluoride, that information was censored by the U.S. Atomic Energy Commission (AEC), arguably the most powerful government agency during the Cold War.

This was during the time that government researchers at the University of Rochester secretly injected hospital patients with toxic doses of plutonium simply to test the effects on the human body. That was the mind-set under which the government operated during this time. Secretly injecting hospital patients with plutonium, exposing thousands of workers to toxic doses of fluoride compounds, and releasing tons of these compounds into the environment were considered vital to national security, and nothing would be allowed to get in the way.

Farmers Downwind of the Deepwater Chemical Plant Initiate Lawsuit

Given the amount of toxic fluoride the government had released into the atmosphere, officials had been 100 percent correct in their belief that the U.S. government would be sued after the war. The first lawsuits were initiated by farmers in Gloucester and Salem counties in New Jersey. Farms downwind of a chemical plant located in Deepwater, New Jersey, which had produced millions of pounds of fluoride for the atomic bomb program, had been severely damaged by fluoride. Beginning in 1943, farmers began to notice that something was burning up their crops and that farm workers who ate those crops were getting very sick. Farm horses also got sick and seemed to be too stiff to work. There were reports of cows that had become so crippled, they could not even stand up, and they were reduced to grazing the grass by crawling on their bellies.

Declassified documents have revealed that the government was aware of the potential damage that fluoride had done to crops, and that people living in those parts of New Jersey had unusually high levels of fluoride in their blood. Documents reveal how, rather than attempting to help the farmers, the government began a well-coordinated plan to downplay any connection fluoride might have had to the damage to farmers' health and their crops. The farmers' lawsuit could have caused a serious setback for the U.S. atomic bomb program, and for national security reasons an all-out effort was made to derail the lawsuit. According to declassified documents, secret meetings were held that were attended by officials from the FDA, the War Department, the Manhattan Project, the Department of Agriculture, and the Department of Justice— even DuPont lawyers were present. The alleged purpose of the meeting was to use the full force of the U.S. government to derail the lawsuit.

U.S. Government's Strategy to Derail the Farmers' Lawsuit

If the farmers had won their lawsuit against the government, it would have invited other lawsuits, which could have ultimately slowed the bomb program by impeding the government's use of fluoride and limiting its ability to dump toxic fluoride waste into the environment. Part of the strategy used to derail the lawsuit included attempts to counter the public's fears about fluoride, a known toxin and roach poison. Harold Hodge, the bomb program's chief fluoride toxicologist, came up with the idea of giving lectures about the usefulness about fluoride in dental health.

The only scientists up until this time who had claimed any benefit from fluoride exposure had ties to industry or to Andrew Mellon, the founder of ALCOA, while he served as secretary of the treasury. The farmers' lawsuit against the government suffered a serious blow when the government refused to reveal how much fluoride had been released into the atmosphere. Without this key piece of evidence, the farmers were forced to accept token settlements. Then the government began to give pro-fluoride lectures to control the public's perception of fluoride. ALCOA had already discovered fluorosis near its plants in New York before the war, and with the government dumping tons of fluoride into the atmosphere during the Cold War, there was sure to be a dental fluorosis epidemic in areas that did not contain natural fluoride in their water. In these areas, which included many parts of the United States, the coming fluorosis epidemic would be 100 percent proof that local industry was poisoning its citizens with toxic fluoride.

Water Fluoridation Plan to Protect the Atomic Bomb Program
The only solution seemed to be to explain away the fluorosis, and the only way that could happen was if there actually was fluoride in the public water that everyone was exposed to. Industry had generated some very flimsy science that has since been disproved, which claimed that fluoride helped reduce cavities, so this seemed to be an answer to a very serious Cold War problem. In 1943, a special New York State Health Department committee was appointed to study the advisability of adding fluoride to the drinking water in Newburgh. The chairman of that committee was Harold Hodge, the chief fluoride toxicologist with the Manhattan Project. The man who had been in charge of secretly injecting plutonium into innocent hospital patients would now be in charge of the committee that would administer a known toxin, fluoride, to an entire city. Other members of the committee that planned to fluoridate Newburgh also had ties to the Manhattan Project, and these members, along with Harold Hodge, were given new credentials that served to conceal their involvement with the government's atomic bomb program. Harold Hodge was described as a pharmacologist, while a committee member who was a captain with the Manhattan Project's medical section was described as a pediatrician. Clearly, the plan to add fluoride to an entire city had very little to do with protecting children's teeth and everything to do

with protecting the atomic bomb program from lawsuits. Why else would the Manhattan Project's top scientists be on the advisory panel to consider the pros and cons of fluoridating public water?

The Newburgh Study and How the Government Misled the Public

In 1945, the city of Newburgh had its water fluoridated, and the residents were studied by the State Health Department, along with secretly being studied by scientists involved with the atomic bomb program at the University of Rochester. At the time, the American public never knew that the atomic bomb program was the driving force behind water fluoridation. Although numerous documents concerning fluoride and the atomic bomb program have been declassified, many others are either still classified or have disappeared from government files for other reasons.

What is clear is that during the early Cold War, the U.S. government repeatedly lied to and misled the American public about fluoride. In 1948, a fluoride safety study conducted by atomic bomb program scientists was published in the *Journal of the American Dental Association*. In addition to the published study, a secret version of the same study was later discovered by investigative reporters. The study concerned the dental and physical health of factory workers who had worked with fluoride as part of the atomic bomb program. The published study reported that the men had very few cavities, while the top-secret study reported that the men had very few teeth left and admitted that it was probably due to their exposure to fluoride at the factory. Keep this in mind later when you read about how the original Newburgh study claimed that fluoridation helped protect children from cavities, while the most current studies done on Newburgh show no such protection from fluoridation. Clearly, the U.S. government has very little credibility when it comes to truthful reporting about fluoride during the Cold War.

Study of Fluoride Health Effects in Bartlett and Cameron, Texas

While the government was beginning its Newburgh fluoridation study in 1945, another study that had been completed in 1944 nearly ended the Newburgh study before it even started. This study was done in Texas in the communities of Bartlett and Cameron and is very different from the study that was to be done in Newburgh. The study in Bartlett and Cameron looked at the health effects on people from drinking fluoridated water for at least twenty years.

The pro-fluoride study that was going to be conducted in Newburgh would look only at the cavity rates of children. The government scientists obviously understood that adding fluoride to Newburgh's water would cause fluorosis, which would offer cavity protection to young children, while making teeth and bones more brittle when those children aged. The Newburgh study clearly appears to have been rigged, by being designed to find the one benefit fluoride has to offer, namely, some cavity protection at a very young age. The Newburgh study did not consider all of the effects fluoride exposure early in life causes as people age. The Bartlett and Cameron study was the first study that actually tried to answer this question.

Bartlett, Texas, has a naturally high level of fluoride in its water, while nearby Cameron has naturally low levels of fluoride in its water. People in high-fluoride Bartlett were found to have some bony changes in their lumbar and pelvic regions. It also appeared that fluoride was affecting their blood hemoglobin. Those living in high-fluoride Bartlett had more than four times the incidence of cataracts over the age of fifty than did people in low-fluoride Cameron. It was also noted that younger people living in high-fluoride Bartlett appeared to have an unusual structure to their nails.

Although the committee considering the fluoridation of Newburgh heard about the Texas study, many of those members were secretly working for the atomic bomb program and had an ulterior motive for fluoridating Newburgh's water as part of their bomb research. If the committee had been composed of impartial scientists who looked at all of the fluoride data from the 1920s to the 1940s, there probably would have been a unanimous vote not to fluoridate Newburgh's water. In October 1944, the *Journal of the American Dental Association* even published the following editorial statement about fluoride:

> We do know that the use of drinking water containing as little as 1.2 to 3.0 parts per million of fluoride will cause such developmental disturbances as osteosclerosis, spondylosis, and asteropetrosis, as well as goiter, and we cannot afford to run the risk of producing such serious systemic disturbances.

Scientists with the Manhattan Project misled the public during the Newburgh water fluoridation trials. For example, it was stated that all of the fluoride ingested, up to 4 to 5 mg, would be excreted in the urine, and that none would be retained in the bones. The truth is that at least half of the fluoride ingested is retained in the bones, and fluoride has been shown in multiple studies to increase bone fractures, hip fractures, and bone cancer rates. The Newburgh study was not going to look at these health effects, however, or at the fact that fluoride lowers children's IQs. The scientists were going to focus on the one positive thing they knew their study would prove: that fluoride lowers cavity rates in very young children. Essentially, fluoride lowers cavities in temporary teeth (baby teeth) and causes permanent teeth to be far weaker. The logic of protecting temporary teeth, while causing harm to permanent teeth, is obviously absurd. Yet the purpose of water fluoridation was not to protect teeth from cavities, but rather to protect the government and industry from lawsuits in response to all of their fluoride pollution.

PHS and the Head of FSA Spearhead a National Fluoridation Program

Right after the Newburgh water fluoridation trial began, the fluoride industry got a new ally at the U.S. Public Health Service, the agency that had previously been under the control of Andrew Mellon of ALCOA for more than ten years while he was treasury secretary. In 1947, Oscar Ewing, who had been the lead council for ALCOA, was named the new head of the Federal Security Agency. While the Public Health Service had been under the control of the treasury secretary, in 1939 the Federal Security Agency was created, and it was put in charge of the Public Health Service.

In 1944, Oscar Ewing had gone on the payroll of ALCOA as its lead attorney for an unheard of salary at that time of $750,000 a year. As ALCOA's lead attorney, he had to be intimately aware of the huge potential for lawsuits ALCOA faced when it was discovered that children downwind of ALCOA's plants were getting fluorosis. With the Public Health Service once again under the control of a key ALCOA insider, the PHS quickly helped spearhead a national fluoridation program. Keep in mind that at this time, the vast majority of studies showed negative effects from fluoride ingestion, and the Newburgh fluoridation trial would not be completed for another ten years. Essentially, there was no science in 1947 that would even begin to suggest that the fluoridation of water was warranted.

Given what was sure to be a huge backlash from the very notion of adding a known toxin to water, Ewing hired Edward

Bernays, perhaps the greatest propagandist of all time, to run the public relations campaign advocating the fluoridation of water. Bernays was such a good propagandist that he is even responsible for changing the name of "propaganda" to "public relations" and hence is known as the "father of public relations." He had written books with titles such as Propaganda (1928), in which he described society as irrational and dangerous and in need of manipulation by the corporate elite for economic benefit. Bernays understood that the key to combating what was sure to be heavy resistance to adding fluoride, a known bug and rat poison at the time, to the water supply would be to get doctors and dentists on board. He also had fluoridation opponents viciously attacked as being cultists, food faddists, and ignorant people. Doctors and dentists who were critical of fluoride were often expelled from their professional organizations and ridiculed in the press. The message to doctors and dentists was that if you did not support fluoridation, you were not a professional and hence your career might not be safe, while the message to the public was that doctors and dentists supported fluoridation, so it must be safe. Little did the public know that doctors and dentists had a proverbial gun to their heads. To stifle public debate, Bernays went so far as to contact the TV network bosses and tell them that debating fluoride is like presenting two sides for anti-Semitism or anti-Catholicism.

Release of Fluoride Gas in Lethal Industrial Accident—Donora, PA

In 1948, the pro-fluoridation campaign was in full swing, even though the Newburgh study, which was going to be used as the scientific justification, was still almost seven years away from being completed. That same year, a major industrial accident happened in the town of Donora, Pennsylvania, resulting in one of the most deadly air pollution catastrophes in U.S. history. This accident was almost identical to the one that had occurred in 1930 in the Meuse Valley in Germany. A temperature inversion in Donora trapped pollution from the zinc smelter in the valley floor, killing more than twenty people and sickening approximately five thousand. Early evidence collected by neutral scientists clearly showed that it was primarily the fluoride emissions that had caused most of the deaths and other illnesses. Autopsy results of the victims showed that their bodies contained lethal levels of fluoride, often twenty-five times above what is normal, and fluorine gas is known to be the most toxic gas generated in the process of smelting zinc.

Philip Sadtler was one of the first chemists who conducted research into the disaster, and he concluded that fluoride was responsible for the deaths and debilitating illnesses that would follow. Sadtler's father had served as the first president of the American Institute of Chemical Engineers, and Philip was one of the most respected chemists in the nation and an expert in fluoride pollution. He had been involved in investigating the fluoride pollution of New Jersey farmers caused by the Manhattan Project. According to Sadtler, the U.S. Public Health Service conspired with U.S. Steel to cover up the role that fluoride had played in the Donora tragedy. ALCOA's former top attorney, Oscar Ewing, was now in charge of the Public Health Service, and ALCOA had its own potential fluoride poisoning lawsuit to worry about. According to Sadtler, the cost for companies such as ALCOA to clean up all of the pollution that had been caused by fluoride would have been in the billions. Sadtler had claimed that Public Health Service workers conducting tests in Donora had admitted to him that they knew fluoride had been the primary culprit in the disaster; however, they were not allowed to say so. In addition to ALCOA's former top attorney running the Public Health Service, also recall that as part of the fluoride lawsuit filed by the New Jersey farmers, the U.S. government had pledged to put the full force of the government behind exonerating fluoride in that disaster.

Sadtler's account of the Donora disaster was published in 1948 in an issue of *Chemical Engineering News*. He cited blood fluoride levels that were twelve to twenty-five times above normal, as well as hundreds of cases of symptoms that were typical for acute fluoride poisoning. Sadtler claims that industry quickly moved to have him silenced, which included influential members of industry and research telling the editor of *Chemical Engineering News* not to publish any more articles from Sadtler. When the official government report came out, not surprisingly, the report did not place any blame on fluoride or on any other single substance, for that matter. The report placed most of the blame on the temperature inversion and said that the disaster was an "act of God." Since the disaster, the Public Health Service documents concerning site visits, interviews, and draft reports have vanished. The Public Health Service's report helped insulate industry from lawsuits, and despite all of the dead in Donora and thousands of others who would suffer for decades from lung and respiratory ailments, U.S. Steel was able to settle with the victims for a mere $235,000. Had the PHS report not blamed the weather, but instead placed the blame on fluoride, where it belonged, the lawsuit would most likely have gone to court and could have yielded what might have been the largest damage award ever, up to that time.

Sugar Industry Claims Cavities Are Caused by Fluoride Deficiency

In 1949, fluoride gained another ally, the sugar industry. The Sugar Research Foundation funded research into how cavities could be controlled without restricting sugar intake. Rather than blaming sugar for cavities, the spin became that fluoride was an essential nutrient, and cavities were caused by a fluoride deficiency. As silly as it sounds now, this was a rather shameless time in America when it came to advertising. The soda manufacturers back then went so far as to advocate soda for babies. For example, one ad featured a large headline that stated, "For a better start in life, start COLA earlier." The ad featured a picture of a mother and her baby and explained that "laboratory tests over the last few years have proven that babies who start drinking soda during that early formative period have a much higher chance of gaining acceptance and 'fitting in' during those awkward pre-teen years. So do yourself a favor. Do your child a favor. Start them on a strict regimen of sodas and other sugary carbonated beverages right now, for a lifetime of guaranteed happiness."

1950–1959
Dentists and the Public Health Service Endorse Fluoride

In 1950, the U.S. Public Health Service endorsed fluoride, and the American Dental Association and other professional organizations quickly followed suit. This endorsement came before the results of the Newburgh/Kingston were completed and was simply based on several limited and highly selective earlier studies. Remember that at this time, most of the evidence showed toxic effects from fluoride exposure. One study that was used to advocate water fluoridation was McClure's study, conducted in 1945, which claimed that fluoride did not accumulate in bones when ingestion is less than 5 mg a day. This would later be proved to be false. The truth is that about 98 percent of ingested fluoride from water is absorbed by the gastrointestinal tract, and 50 percent of that gets excreted through the kidneys, while the remainder accumulates in the teeth, the bones, the pineal gland, and other tissues. The endorsement of fluoride was also based on very preliminary unpublished results from the Newburgh study. Keep in mind that the Newburgh study never looked at the long-term health effects of adding fluoride to water. It simply looked at cavity rates in young children.

As the propaganda expert Bernays, who was running the fluoride PR campaign, had rightly surmised, fluoride would need the endorsement of dentists and doctors if it was to have any chance of gaining acceptance. In 1952, a pamphlet of the American Dental Association advised dentists that "at no time should the dentist be placed in the position of defending himself, his profession, or the fluoridation process. Fluoride should not be submitted to voters, who cannot sift through and comprehend the scientific evidence."

Public Efforts against Water Fluoridation
At this time, there were no studies on how the addition of fluoride to water might affect pregnant women, the elderly, or people suffering from diseases. A huge movement then erupted to ban water fluoridation, which peaked in the mid 1950s. In 1954, national legislation was proposed to prohibit the fluoridation of public water. HR 2341, titled "A Bill to Protect the Public Health from the Dangers of Fluoridation of Water," would have forbidden any government agency from adding fluoride to water.

In 1955, a doctor named George Waldbott published three articles about the dangers of water fluoridation in respected scientific journals. His most famous one was titled "Chronic Fluorine Intoxication from Drinking Water." The public was becoming wary about adding roach poison to water, and by 1955, 231 communities had left the decision of fluoridation up to the voters, with 127 communities rejecting fluoridation.

Newburgh/Kingston Study Ignores Negative Health Effects and Concludes Fluoride Is Safe in Small Doses
In 1956, the results of the Newburgh/Kingston water fluoridation trials were published and concluded that fluoride in small concentrations was safe for U.S. citizens. This was despite the fact that the Newburgh/Kingston study discovered that fluoride increased cortical bone defects by 100 percent, caused girls to reach menstruation earlier, and resulted in some blood abnormalities. At the time that it was published, the Newburgh study seemed to usher in a turning of the tide in the fluoride debate in favor of fluoride, even though the study did not look at long-term health effects and focused primarily on cavities in young children.

A combination of the U.S. government's efforts to protect fluoride, due to the vital part it played in the atomic bomb program, and the industry research that had been conducted at the Mellon

462

Institute, along with the brilliant strategy of the world's foremost propagandist to gain the endorsement of dentists, seemed to win out over mountains of evidence that indicated fluoride was a serious toxin and warranted further study. If medial professionals had voiced their concerns about fluoride, it most certainly would never have been allowed in the water supply. The professional organizations that had only a decade earlier cautioned against fluoride had suddenly become its staunchest advocates. The attitude of the professional organizations can best be summed up in a 1979 white paper issued by the American Dental Association, which stated that "individual dentists must be convinced that they need not be familiar with scientific reports of laboratory and field investigations on fluoridation to be effective participants in the promotion program and that nonparticipation is an overt neglect of professional responsibility."

The most troubling aspect of this statement is the last part, which states that nonparticipation in the promotion of fluoridation is considered to be neglecting one's professional responsibility, and the implication is that one could lose one's professional membership or even one's license for daring to speak up against fluoridation. This was exactly the strategy envisioned by Bernays, the propagandist, and it has succeeded in working for the last fifty years in the United States.

1980s–Present

Things rapidly started to change in the 1980s, however, when better studies and research began to prove that fluoridation not only was ineffective at preventing cavities, but also appeared to be downright dangerous. For example, during the 1980s, all five- and twelve-year-old children in New Zealand were required to have their teeth examined for tooth decay. The results showed that there was no difference in tooth decay between children living in fluoridated cities and those who lived in nonfluoridated cities.

Large U.S. Survey States Fluoride Does Not Reduce Dental Decay

In 1986 and 1987, the National Institute of Dental Research conducted the largest survey of dental decay ever done in the United States, and the data was published by John Yiamouyiannis under the title "Water Fluoridation and Tooth Decay: Results from the 1966–1987 National Survey of U.S. Schoolchildren." The study examined the teeth of nearly forty-thousand children who lived in eight-four communities. The survey found that there was no statistical difference in the tooth decay of permanent teeth between children living in fluoridated communities vs. those who lived in nonfluoridated communities. The children living in the fluoridated communities did suffer from higher rates of dental fluorosis, however; meaning they probably also had lower IQs and more fragile bones.

Harvard Toxicologist Proves Fluoride Causes Brain Damage

In 1995, the antifluoridation forces finally got the smoking gun they were looking for. That year, a toxicologist named Phyllis Mullenix published a study that showed that fluoride actually accumulates in the brain and causes brain damage. Mullenix was a renowned toxicologist at Harvard who developed a new technology known as the Computer Pattern Recognition System. At the time, it was perhaps the most powerful tool in the world for analyzing the effects of various chemicals on the brain and the central nervous system.

Mullenix was hired by Forsythe Dental Center to help establish its toxicology department, the first of its kind for a dental research institution. Her work was to focus on investigating the impact of various substances used in dentistry. One of her studies was designed to test the effects of fluoride on the brain, using her powerful new computer system. Everyone working on the study felt confident that there would not be any problems in the rats fed fluoride, because the scientists working on the project believed what the government and professional associations had been saying for more than thirty years: that fluoride is safe.

Rats were given fluoridated water in a quantity necessary to raise their blood fluoride to the same level that caused dental fluorosis in children who drank fluoridated water. Her study, titled "Neurotoxicity of Sodium Fluoride in Rats," showed that fluoride was a very serious neurotoxin that caused brain damage and behavioral problems similar to what a person undergoing radiation or chemotherapy for cancer might experience. Her study showed that fluoride caused a marked reduction in the IQs of rats that had been fed fluoride, when compared to the rats that had not received fluoride. This drop in IQ from ingesting fluoride, often in doses considered perfectly legal in the United States, has now been shown in at least twenty-five different studies. At the time, Mullenix's work seemed to support everything the antifluoride people had been saying for more than thirty years, which is that fluoride is a dangerous toxin to the brain and the nervous system. Remember that this fact had been well documented in the 1930s.

In Mullenix's study, the rats fed fluoride after birth also exhibited what she called "couch potato syndrome." They suffered from malaise, often lacking initiative and energy. While feeding fluoride after birth seemed to damage one part of the brain, feeding it to pregnant mother rats seemed to damage a different part of the developing fetal brain. The rat pups that had received fluoride in the womb often suffered from hyperactivity. When scientists dissected the brains of the rats that had been fed fluoride, they found major fluoride accumulation in all regions of their brains.

Mullenix Is Fired from Her Job amid Suspicious Circumstances

Mullenix's superiors were certain that she had to be incorrect. In fact, they tried to stop her from publishing her study. This is a very typical response of people who believe in the validity of fluoride. Despite hundreds of research articles showing the dangers of fluoride, they refuse to believe anything that shows fluoride to be dangerous. Mullenix was also told that her study was jeopardizing funding for other studies.

Mullenix's study had been thoroughly peer-reviewed, and she knew the results were valid. She stuck to her guns, and the study was published in the *Journal of Neurotoxicology and Teratology.* Three days later, Mullenix was dismissed from her job, and almost immediately after that, the institute received a $250,000 grant from the Colgate Company, the makers of fluoridated toothpaste. Following her departure, a mysterious water leak destroyed the equipment and the computers that had been designed for the study.

More Studies Show Fluoride Offers Little Protection against Cavities

The same year that Mullenix's study came out, an updated Newburgh/Kingston study, titled "Changes in Dental Fluorosis and Dental Caries in Newburgh and Kingston, New York," was published. This study looked at the rates of tooth decay and dental fluorosis in children in the cities of Newburgh and Kingston. Remember that the Newburgh/Kingston study was supposed to be the one that proved fluoride helped reduce cavities. Newburgh received fluoride, while Kingston did not. This new study looked at the current rates of tooth decay and fluorosis in both fluoridated Newburgh and nonfluoridated Kingston. The study showed that when the dental decay rates between poor and nonpoor residents were averaged, the overall rate of dental decay was actually less in nonfluoridated Kingston than in fluoridated Newburgh. Children in fluoridated Newburgh also suffered from nearly twice the incidence of dental fluorosis, a known marker for many potentially serious health conditions.

Also that same year, another study titled "A Bayesian Analysis of Multivariate Doubly-Interval-Censored Dental Data" was made public. This large longitudinal study analyzed the oral health data of more than four thousand Flemish schoolchildren and concluded that "The results show that the protective effect of fluoride-ingestion is not convincing."

Suddenly, study after study seemed to be saying that fluoride offered little to no protection against cavities. This is a far cry from what the American public had been promised when they were told fluoridation would reduce tooth decay by 66 percent, with no harmful effects. Back in 1951, the U.S. surgeon general Leonard Scheele had stated before a congressional subcommittee, in regard to the Newburgh/Kingston study, that "During the past year, our studies progressed to the point where we could announce an unqualified endorsement of the fluoridation of the public water supplies as a mass procedure for reducing tooth decay by two thirds."

Bone Defects, Heart Disease, and Lower IQs Are Linked to Fluoride

When the original Newburgh study was completed, bone defects likely linked to fluoride that were very similar to bone cancer had been noticed by Dr. John Caffey of Columbia University. The bone defects were detected on X-rays, and boys in fluoridated Newburgh were twice as likely to suffer from the defects as were boys in nonfluoridated Kingston. All that the public was told about fluoridation, however, was that there would be a miraculous 66 percent reduction in cavities.

An article in the *Newburgh Times*, dated 1954 and titled "Local Heart Deaths Top U.S. Average," stated that heart disease accounted for 58.3 percent of all local deaths. The article noted that the average death rate in the United States from heart disease was 507 per 100,000, while the rate in Newburgh, an early city to receive fluoridated water, was 882 deaths per 100,000, one of the highest rates in the country. Another early city to receive fluoridated water, Grand Rapids, Michigan, saw heart disease double only five years into the fluoridation experiment. It was also noticed during the Newburgh fluoridation experiment that girls in fluoridated Newburgh reached puberty faster than did girls in nonfluoridated Kingston.

Perhaps the most troubling studies about fluoride are the ones that concern fluoride's effect on a child's IQ. Remember that the surgeon general told Congress that fluoride would reduce cavities 66 percent without causing any negative health effects. If the real truth had been told, which is that fluoridated water has little to no ability to prevent cavities and it lowers a child's IQ, fluoride would never have been allowed in the water. In the 1950s, people opposed to fluoridation were labeled "lunatics" by the propaganda specialist who was hired to help promote fluoride. One such "lunatic" was Dr. Waldbott, mentioned earlier, who published three studies in 1955 critical of fluoride. Back in the 1950s, Dr. Waldbott had warned about the diminished mental acuity that could occur from ingesting fluoride.

The new studies prove that Waldbott the "lunatic" was right. In fact, many scientists over the years have understood this fact. For example, in 1978, a neuropharmacologist in Sweden named Dr. Arvid Carlsson cited the fact that fluoride can cross the blood-brain barrier as one of the reasons not to fluoridate water; Sweden subsequently decided not to fluoride its water supply. Carlsson was awarded the Nobel Prize in Medicine in 2000 and claims that water fluoridation is "obsolete." He has stated that countries that still fluoridate their water "should feel ashamed of themselves." At least twenty-five studies show an association between fluoride exposure and lowered IQ in children. Following is a brief synopsis of some of the current studies concerning fluoride and IQ. The full reference to each study can be found in the back of this book.

Research Study: Effect of Fluoride in Drinking Water on Children's Intelligence
This Chinese study measured the IQs of children between the ages of eight and thirteen living in two separate villages in the same region. One village had a high level of natural fluoride in the water at 2.47 parts per million, while another village had a low concentration of .57 parts per million. The U.S. government allows water to have up to 4 parts per million of fluoride. The study showed that children in the high-fluoride village had an average IQ of 92, while those in the low-fluoride village had an average IQ of 100, which is 8 points higher than the fluoridated children. The study also found that greater levels of fluoride in the water were also significantly associated with higher rates of mental retardation (an IQ of less

than 70) and borderline intelligence (an IQ of 70–79). There was an "inverse concentration-response relationship between the fluoride level in drinking water and the IQ of children. As the fluoride level in drinking water increased the IQ of children fell and the rates of mental retardation and borderline intelligence increased." China stopped fluoridating its water in 1983.

This study also puts fluoride's effect on intelligence into historical perspective. It acknowledges the work of Kaj Roholm in 1937, which showed that skeletal fluorosis is associated with neurological symptoms. In addition, it cites the work of Shortt, also conducted in 1937, which associated fluoride with damage to the central nervous system, and the work of Singh and Jolly, done in 1961, which reported that 10 percent of patients with skeletal fluorosis had nervous system damage. I mention this because it's important to understand that the unbiased scientific studies have been very consistent in determining that fluoride damages the central nervous system and lowers IQ. Only the science generated by industry and the U.S. government has put a positive spin on fluoride's ability to reduce cavities in temporary teeth.

The Newburgh study, which was used to rationalize the fluoridation of water in the United States, never looked at the effects on adults or on the intelligence of children. The Chinese do not allow fluoride to be added to their drinking water, and their children consistently score higher on IQ tests than U.S. children do. Their national standard of less than one part per million of fluoride in drinking water is believed to be low enough to protect 90 percent of children from the intelligence-lowering effects of fluoride. The United States currently allows up to four times that amount of fluoride in water. Prior to the atomic bomb program, the U.S. government officially regarded fluoride as a pollutant, and the Public Health Service had stated that fluoride concentrations in water greater than one part per million were the maximum permissible level of fluoride in drinking water.

Research Study: Effect of Fluoride Exposure on Intelligence in Children

This Chinese study measured the intelligence of children in different areas, based on the level of fluorosis in an area. Remember that the higher the level of fluoride in the water, the greater the general rate of fluorosis will be in a given area. The study found the "the IQ of children living in areas with a medium or severe prevalence of fluorosis was lower than that of children living in areas with only slight fluorosis or no fluorosis." The study concluded that "the development of intelligence appeared to be adversely affected by fluoride in the areas with medium or severe prevalence of fluorosis. A high fluoride intake was associated with a lower intelligence."

Research Study: Effect of Excessive Fluoride Intake on Mental Work Capacity of Children and Preliminary Study of Its Mechanism

This Chinese study both investigated children in an area high in fluorosis and experimented on the fluoride intake of rats, in an attempt to discover the mechanism that causes fluoride to lower IQ. The scientists discovered that fluoride intake in early childhood reduces mental work capacity by three different possible mechanisms. First, it affects zinc metabolism; second, it causes a decrease in 5-hydrosy indole acetic acid (the main metabolite of the neurotransmitter serotonin); and third; it increases norepinephrine in the rat brain.

Research Study: Effect of High-Fluoride Water on Intelligence in Children

This Chinese study measured the IQs of children in two different villages, with the primary difference between the villages being the level of fluoride in the water. The average IQ of the children in the high-fluoride village (3.15 parts per million in water) was 92, while the average IQ of children in the low-fluoride village (.37 parts per million in water) was 103. The scientists also found that 21.6 percent of the children in the high-fluoride village suffered from retardation (an IQ less than 70) or borderline retardation (an IQ of 70–79), while only 3.4 percent of children from the low-fluoride village suffered from either form of retardation. Essentially, the children's average IQ in the high-fluoride village was 11 points lower than the average IQ of children in the low-fluoride village and had more than a six times greater rate of some form of mental retardation.

Research Study: Influence of Fluoride Exposure on Reaction Time and Visuospatial Organization in Children

This Mexican study evaluated the neuropsychological development of children in correlation to the fluoride concentration in tap water. Higher fluoride levels were correlated with lower scores in visuospatial organization, which could be affecting the reading and writing abilities in those children.

Research Study: Effects of High-Fluoride Drinking Water on the Cerebral Functions of Mice
This Chinese study measured the effects of high fluoride concentration in drinking water and concluded that "high fluoride concentration in drinking water can decrease the cerebral functions of mice. Fluoride is a neurotoxicant."

Research Study: The Effect of Fluorine on the Developing Human Brain
This Chinese study was very unique, in that it studied the brains of fetuses that had been aborted in the fifth through eighth month of gestation. The study compared the brains of aborted fetuses from high-fluoride areas with the brains of aborted fetuses from low-fluoride areas. The study concluded, "The results showed that chronic fluorosis in the course of intrauterine fetal life may produce certain harmful effects on the developing brain of the fetus."

Research Study: Association of Silicofluoride Treated Water with Elevated Blood Lead
This study, conducted on more than 150,000 children in the United States, showed that silicofluorides, which is the form of fluoride most often added to water in the United States, raised the level of blood lead in children. The study concluded that "there was a consistently significant association of silicofluoride treated community water and elevated blood lead." Elevated levels of blood lead are associated with lower IQs and brain damage in children.
The following study came to the same conclusion.

Research Study: Water Treatment with Silicofluorides and Lead Toxicity
This study done in the United States looked at data from more than 280,000 children in Massachusetts that screened for levels of blood lead. The study concluded that "silicofluoride usage is associated with significant increases in average lead in children's blood, as well as [with the] percentage of children with blood lead in excess of 10 ug/dL." The study stated that lead is a "highly significant risk factor in predicting higher rates of crime, attention deficit disorder or hyperactivity, and learning disabilities." The study found that fluoride in the water "apparently functions to increase the cellular uptake of lead." The scientists also pointed to studies done in both Massachusetts and Georgia and stated that "behaviors associated with lead neurotoxicity are more frequent in communities using

silicofluorides than in comparable localities that do not use these chemicals."

In addition to increasing the uptake of lead, silicofluorides appear to boost the uptake of aluminum into the brain, a problem I will discuss further in the section on Alzheimer's disease.

Research done in Germany by Johannes Westendorf shows that silicofluorides inhibit cholinesterase, an enzyme that plays a vital role in the regulation of neurotransmitters. According to Roger Masters, a research professor at Dartmouth College, "if silicofluorides are cholinesterase inhibitors, this means that silicofluorides have effects like the chemical agents linked to Gulf War Syndrome, chronic fatigue syndrome and other puzzling conditions that plague millions of Americans." The disruption of enzymes is the process by which fluoride causes fluorosis, so if people have visible signs of fluorosis, you have to question what other important enzymes have been disrupted in their bodies by fluoride.

As mentioned previously, fluorosis occurs when an individual is exposed to excess fluoride during childhood; it consists of a staining or "mottling" of the teeth. It is essentially a marker for "fluoride poisoning" during childhood, and besides indicating a lowered IQ, it also foretells a host of other physical problems that may develop later in life, such as an increase in hip fractures. Fluorosis can be very unsightly and can lower a child's self-esteem. There have actually been several studies on the way in which fluorosis can affect the self-esteem of children, with one study noting that oftentimes children with fluorosis are teased to such an extent that they go into a "severe psychological depression."

The staining of teeth is just a marker that fluoride has negatively affected the formation of teeth and bones. Although these teeth may be more resistant to acid attack early in life, both the teeth and the bones will be more brittle later in life, with the bones being more susceptible to fracture.

Multiple studies show that fluoride ingestion from water can increase the rate of hip fractures in the elderly. The following article was published in the *Journal of the American Medical Association*.

Research Study: Hip Fractures and Fluoridation in Utah's Elderly Population
This study looked at hip fracture rates in people over sixty-five

years of age, and the researchers concluded that "we found a small but significant increase in the risk of hip fracture in both men and women exposed to artificial fluoridation at 1 part per million, suggesting that low levels of fluoride may increase the risk of hip fracture in the elderly." This study found that women in fluoridated areas were 27 percent more likely to suffer from hip fractures when compared to women in nonfluoridated areas.

Keep in mind that studies show that the risk of death in the year following a hip fracture is between 20 and 25 percent. There are approximately 300,000 hip fractures every year in the United States, and fluoridated water has been shown to increase the rate of hip fractures by 27 percent, while two-thirds of people in the United States consume fluoridated water. Doing the math, you get approximately an additional 46,000 hip fractures attributed to fluoridated water every year, and assuming that 22.5 percent of those fractures will be fatal within a year, you can say that water fluoridation may be responsible for approximately 10,000 additional deaths a year in the United States just from hip fractures alone. Those additional 46,000 hip fractures will increase the costs to the U.S. taxpayer via Medicare by more than $1 billion. Given that the United States has one of the highest rates of water fluoridation in the world, it is not surprising that the this country also has one of the highest rates of hip fractures in the world.

Research Study: The Association between Water Fluoridation and Hip Fracture among White Women and Men Aged 65 Years and Older. A National Ecologic Study.
This study, conducted in the United States, looked at 129 counties with fluoridated water and compared them to 194 counties without fluoridated water. It concluded that "there was a small, statistically significant positive association between fracture rates and fluoridation."

Research Study: Summary of Workshop on Drinking Water Fluoride Influence on Hip Fracture on Bone Health
This study, done in the United States, compared hip fracture rates in 216 counties that had natural fluoride levels greater than .7 parts per million with 95 counties that had fluoride levels of less than .4 parts per million. Remember that the U.S. government allows up to 4 parts per million of natural fluoride in water and 2 parts per million if the fluoride is added fluoride. The study found that as the level of fluoride rose in the drinking water, so did the

hip fracture rate. It concluded that if 100 percent of the water in the United States was fluoridated, as many medical professionals advocate, hip fracture rates would increase another 5.3 percent.

Fluoride has also been shown to increase the rate of bone fractures for other bones besides the hip bone.

Research Study: Well Water Fluoride, Dental Fluorosis, and Bone Fractures in the Guadiana Valley in Mexico
This study, conducted in Mexico, looked bone-fracture rates in relation to dental fluorosis. It found a linear correlation between the severity of dental fluorosis and the frequency of bone fractures among children and adults. Basically, it determined that the more fluoride a person is exposed to, the greater his or her chance of suffering a bone fracture.

Research Study: High Fluoride Intakes Cause Osteomalacia and Diminished Bone Strength in Rats with Renal Deficiency
This study, done in the United States, found that "fluoridated water in concentrations equivalent to 3 and 10 parts per million in humans, caused osteomalacia and reduced bone strength in rats with surgically-induced renal deficiency." One of the many concerns people have about fluoridating water is that people with weakened kidney function cannot eliminate as much of the fluoride from their systems and are more susceptible to its toxic effects.

Research Study: Effect of Fluoride Treatment on the Fracture Rate in Postmenopausal Women with Osteoporosis
This study, published in the *New England Journal of Medicine*, looked at the effect of administering fluoride to postmenopausal women with osteoporosis. It concluded that "fluoride therapy increases cancellous [the inner soft portion of the bone] but decreases cortical [the outer hard layer of the bone] bone mineral density and increased skeletal fragility."

In addition to increasing bone fracture rates, fluoride has also been found to raise the rate of bone cancer (osteosarcoma) in young boys. Osteosarcoma is one of the most common cancers of childhood, and under the age of twenty, it affects more males than females. As mentioned earlier, the original Newburgh study detected bone abnormalities in boys, but that data was largely ignored and fluoridation was called a success. The rate of cortical defects in bones in fluoridated Newburgh was nearly twice the rate in unfluoridated Kingston, and it was noted that the defects had many similarities to bone cancer. In 1977, it was realized that the original Newburgh fluoridation study had shown a potential risk for bone cancer in boys, and the National Academy of Sciences expressed its concerns, prompting Congress to request animal studies to determine whether fluoride actually causes cancer. You'd think that should have been done before they started dumping fluoride into everyone's water, but, as you've learned, the fluoridation of water had everything to do with protecting the atomic bomb program and industry from liability and very little to do with real science. Current research shows that fluoridated water does in fact increase the rates of bone cancer among young boys.

Research Study: An Epidemiologic Report on Drinking Water and Fluoridation
This report was published by the New Jersey Department of Health and looked at the incidence of osteosarcoma between 1979 and 1987 in seven counties in New Jersey. The study found that all of the cases of osteosarcoma occurred in the three-county area with the greatest prevalence of fluoridation. When those three counties were examined, the rate of osteosarcoma was more than five times higher in fluoridated municipalities than in nonfluoridated ones. Among ten- to nineteen-year-old males, the ones living in fluoridated municipalities had nearly seven times the rate of bone cancer, compared to those living in nonfluoridated municipalities.

Research Study: Age-Specific Fluoride Exposure in Drinking Water and Osteosarcoma
This study, conducted at Harvard, explored the effects of fluoride levels in drinking water and the incidence of osteosarcoma based on gender and age data. It "found an association between fluoride exposure in drinking water during childhood and the incidence of osteosarcoma among males." The study also discovered that the osteosarcoma rate in teenage boys who had been exposed to fluoride between the ages of six and eight was five times higher than the rate for boys who had not been exposed to fluoride.

Research Study: Regression Analysis of Cancer Incidence Rates and Water Fluoride in the U.S.A. Based on IACR/IARC (WHO) Data (1978–1992). International Agency for Research on Cancer.
This study looked at data on nearly 22 million people in the United States and compared it with water fluoridation information from

the Fluoridation Census, to determine whether fluoridated water increased cancer rates. In addition to showing an increase in bone cancer rates from drinking fluoridated water, the study also showed an increase in twenty-three other types of cancer. Some of the types of cancer correlated with fluoridated water include "brain tumors and T-cell system Hodgkin's disease, non-Hodgkin's lymphoma, multiple myeloma, melanoma of the skin and monocytic leukaemia."

There have been other studies that show a correlation between drinking fluoridated water and cancer.

Research Study: Relationship between Fluorine Concentration in Drinking Water and Mortality Rate from Uterine Cancer in Okinawa Prefecture, Japan

Remember from an earlier chapter that when the United States took over Okinawa Island in Japan, we quickly "Americanized" it? Okinawa received fluoride in its public water from 1945 to 1972, while it was under U.S. control. This study analyzed the mortality rates in twenty municipalities in Okinawa and concluded that "a significant positive correlation was found between fluoride concentration in drinking water and uterine cancer mortality in 20 municipalities."

The early studies that were conducted to justify fluoridation of the water supply in the United States essentially looked only at the cavity rates of young children. By limiting early studies to this one finding, this research essentially proved the one possible benefit of adding fluoride to water: fluoride causes temporary teeth to be more resistant to acid attack early in life, even though it causes permanent teeth to become weaker and more brittle later in life and lowers IQ by about 10 percent.

Many studies have now shown that fluoride increases the risk for developing Alzheimer's disease later in life. Fluoride also appears to boost the cellular uptake of aluminum in the human body, similar to the way it raises the uptake of lead. A higher aluminum uptake has been associated with a greater incidence of Alzheimer's disease, although, just as there is a fluoride controversy, there is also an aluminum/Alzheimer's controversy. Some people argue that there is no connection between the two, while others claim there is a strong connection.

Research Study: Chronic Administration of Aluminum-Fluoride or Sodium-Fluoride to Rats in Drinking Water: Alteration in

Neuronal and Cerebrovascular Integrity

This study, done in the United States, looked into the suggestion that when fluoride was added to drinking water, it would form fluoroaluminum complexes that could be transported more easily into the bloodstream and across the blood-brain barrier. Aluminum is often used as a clarifying agent in municipal water, so the concern is that adding fluoride to that same water could significantly increase the uptake of the aluminum.

This study found that the group of rats given sodium-fluoride had increased levels of aluminum in their brains, when compared to the controls. It concluded that "sodium fluoride in the drinking water of rats resulted in distinct morphological alterations in the brain, including effects on neurons and the cerebrovasculature."

Research Study: Enhancement of Aluminum Digestive Absorption by Fluoride in Rats

This study, conducted in France, found that fluoride increased the levels of aluminum in plasma and concluded that it could be a result of the ability of aluminum and fluoride to form complexes when combined together, which increases the absorption of aluminum into the human body.

The *Wall Street Journal* reported on the results of one study in 1992, in an article titled "Rat Studies Link Brain Cell Damage with Aluminum and Fluoride in Water." The article mentions that studies had "found that Alzheimer's disease seemed more prevalent in areas that added aluminum sulfate (alum) to the drinking water to clarify it."

Research Study: Toxin-Induced Blood Vessel Inclusions Caused by the Chronic Administration of Aluminum and Sodium Fluoride and Their Implications for Dementia

This study, done in the United States, found that prolonged administration of low levels of sodium fluoride caused elevated levels of aluminum in the brain. The kidneys of rats that drank water containing sodium fluoride also exhibited pathological changes. In addition, immune deficiencies were found in the animals, which suggests that dementia is a microvascular immune disease that begins as an attack on the capillaries that line the brain and other organs. The damaged areas could provide for the deposit of harmful compounds, such as aluminum, cholesterol, or amyloid. The immune response from the brain to such foreign matter could reduce the brain's metabolic activity. In 2006, the

National Research Council conducted a review titled "Fluoride in Drinking Water: A Scientific Review of EPA's Standards" and in the report stated that "it is apparent that fluorides have the ability to interfere with the functions of the brain. . . . Fluorides also increase the production of free radicals in the brain through several different biological pathways. These changes have a bearing on the possibility that fluorides act to increase the risk of developing Alzheimer's disease."

Research Study: Fluoride Deposition in the Aged Human Pineal Gland
This research, conducted in the UK, sought to discover the extent to which fluoride accumulates in the human pineal gland. The pineal gland is a rice-size gland in the brain that produces melatonin, a hormone that helps regulate our sleep/wake cycle. The human pineal gland lies outside the blood/brain barrier, which helps protect the brain from dangerous toxins. The researchers dissected the pineal glands from the cadavers of people who were over the age of seventy when they passed away. This study showed that "fluoride readily accumulates in the human pineal gland." It also cited studies that suggested fluoride may accumulate in the pineal glands of young children, which could affect pineal metabolism.

The concern of many experts is that fluoride deposits in the pineal gland have been associated with lower levels of melatonin, which could lead to a host of problems, including accelerated sexual maturation. Recall that the original Newburgh/Kingston study showed that girls in fluoridated Newburgh reached menstruation earlier than did girls in nonfluoridated Kingston.

In addition to affecting the pineal gland, fluoride appears to affect the other glands that are part of the endocrine system. Recall that doctors used to prescribe fluoride for overactive thyroid glands, because it was shown to lower thyroid function. In patients suffering from overactive thyroid glands, it was found that fluoride doses as low 1 to 4 mg a day were enough to reduce the basal metabolic rate. It has been estimated that the average American living in a fluoridated community ingests between 1.6 and 6.6 mg of fluoride a day, an amount that has been shown to be more than enough to reduce thyroid function. The real question is that if 1 to 4 mg of fluoride a day can reduce thyroid function in a person with an overactive thyroid, what does ingesting 1.6 to 6.6 mg a day do to a person with normal thyroid function? Symptoms of an underactive thyroid include fatigue, weakness, difficulty losing weight, depression, and decreased libido. The following study, done in Russia in 1985, reaffirmed what doctors already knew in the 1920s through the 1950s, which is that low doses of fluoride could be used to lower thyroid function.

Research Study: Action of the Body Fluorine of Healthy Persons and Thyroidopathy Patients on the Function of Hypophyseal-Thyroid the [sic] System
This study, conducted in Russia, examined people with normal thyroid function, low thyroid function, and high thyroid function. It determined that prolonged consumption of water with a high fluoride content of around 2.3 parts per million by healthy people "caused tension of function of the pituitary-thyroid system that was expressed in TSH elevated production, a decrease in the T3 concentration.... The results led to a conclusion that excess fluorine in drinking water was a risk factor of more rapid development of thyroid pathology."

Research Study: Effects of High Iodine and High Fluorine on Children's Intelligence and the Metabolism of Iodine and Fluorine
This research, done in China, showed that in areas with high fluoride content in the water, the rate of thyroid enlargement was nearly 30 percent.

Research Study: Effect of Fluoride on Thyroid Function and Cerebellar Development in Mice
This study looked at the effect that sodium fluoride had on young mice by giving their mothers fluoride from the fifteenth day of pregnancy until the fourteenth day after delivery. The study found that at fourteen days of age, the mice whose mothers had been given fluoride had 35 percent less body weight, a 75 percent decrease in the free plasma level of the thyroid hormone T4, a 27 percent reduction in cerebellar protein, and a 17 percent reduction in cerebral protein.

Other Diseases Associated with Fluoridated Water

Diabetes
Fluoride is also suspected of contributing to other diseases, such as diabetes. In 2006, the National Research Council issued a report

on fluoride in drinking water. Concerning fluoride and diabetes, the report states, "The conclusion from the available studies is that sufficient fluoride exposure appears to bring about increases in blood glucose or impaired glucose tolerance in some individuals and to increase the severity of some types of diabetes. In general, impaired glucose metabolism appears to be associated with serum or plasma fluoride concentrations of about 0.1 mg/L or greater in both animals and humans. In addition, diabetic individuals will often have higher than normal water intake, and consequently, will have higher than normal fluoride intake for a given concentration of fluoride in drinking water. An estimated 16–20 million people in the U.S. have diabetes mellitus; therefore, any role of fluoride exposure in the development of impaired glucose metabolism or diabetes is potentially significant."

Cardiovascular Disease
Several studies have shown that fluoride negatively affects cardiovascular function. A research study titled "Impact of Chronic Fluorosis on Left Ventricular Diastolic and Global Functions" found that "chronic fluorosis patients had left ventricular diastolic and global dysfunctions." Another study titled "Aortic Elasticity Is Impaired in Patients with Endemic Fluorosis" found that the "elastic properties of ascending aorta are impaired in patients with endemic fluorosis."

Kidney Malfunction
Fluoride has been found to negatively affect kidney function. A study titled "The Dose-Effect Relationship of Water Fluoride Levels and Renal Damage in Children" found that "over 2 mg/liter (over 2 parts per million) fluoride in drinking water can cause renal damage in children, and the degree of damage increases with the drinking water fluoride content." Doctors with the Department of Nephrology at the Mayo Clinic studied the role that fluoride plays in kidney disease and wrote a report titled "Renal Failure and Fluorosis," which was published in the *Journal of the American Medical Association*. The report stated that "therapeutic measures included the elimination of fluoride from the drinking water." The report concluded that "the available evidence suggests that some patients with long-term renal failure are being affected by drinking water with as little as 2 parts per million [of] fluoride." A study done in 2007 titled "Dose-Effect Relationship between Drinking Water Fluoride Levels and Damage to Liver and Kidney Functions

in Children" concluded that "our results suggest that drinking water [with] fluoride levels over 2.0 mg/L (2 parts per million) can cause damage to liver and kidney functions in children and that the dental fluorosis was independent of damage to the liver but not the kidney."

Another study titled "Effect of Sodium Fluoride Administration on Body Changes in Old Rats" studied the effects of feeding low levels of sodium fluoride to rats from conception until later in life. They found hypertrophy and hyperplasia in the kidney tubules of the rats that had received sodium fluoride and no kidney damage in the rats that had not received fluoride. In the rats whose kidneys were damaged by fluoride, it was found that "the severity increased in proportion to the level of the sodium fluoride in the drinking water."

Reproductive Health Problems
A study done in the United States titled "Exposure to High Fluoride Concentrations in Drinking Water is Associated with Decreased Birth Rates" looked at regions in the United States with high levels of fluoride to determine any correlation with fertility rates. It found that "most regions showed an association of decreasing TFR (total fertility rate) with increasing fluoride levels." A study conducted in India titled "Circulating Testosterone Levels in Skeletal Fluorosis Patients" compared males with skeletal fluorosis to males who drank water with low fluoride levels. It concluded that the evidence suggested that "fluoride toxicity may cause adverse effects in the reproductive system of males living in fluorosis endemic areas." India does not fluoridate its water and does not allow natural fluoride levels to go above 1.2 parts per million, about one-fourth the level allowed in the United States. Essentially, Indian law requires that fluoride be removed from water, to reduce its concentration to below 1.2 parts per million. Recall that it used to be a common practice in the United States to remove fluoride from the water as well, not to add it.

A study done in Japan titled "Fluoride-Linked Down's Syndrome Births and Their Estimated Occurrence Due to Water Fluoridation" found that "it appears that the dose-response line of Down's Syndrome birth rates for daily fluoride intake may have no allowable level that does not induce fluoride-linked Down's Syndrome births. Therefore, fluoride may be one of the major causes of Down's syndrome of aging mothers. The number of excess Down's Syndrome births due to fluoridation is estimated to be several thousand cases annually throughout the world." Remember that because most of the world does not fluoridate its water, those several thousand Down's syndrome births will occur in one of the few countries that does fluoridate, such as the United States. Because Japan does not fluoridate its water, it had to look at data from Atlanta, Georgia, and compare fluoridated areas to nonfluoridated areas. When more than forty thousand births from mothers under the age of nineteen were compared, it was found that mothers living in fluoridated areas had more than twice the rate of Down's syndrome births compared to mothers in nonfluoridated areas.

An endocrinologist named Dr. Ionel Rapaport who worked at the Psychiatric Institute of the University of Wisconsin in the 1950s and the 1960s was the first to notice the association between Down's syndrome and fluoride. He noticed that many of the Down's syndrome children had mottled teeth from dental fluorosis, along with very low levels of cavities. Rapport found that the cities in Wisconsin with a high fluoride content in their water had a significantly higher rate of premature stillbirths.

Fluoride has been found to damage human DNA, and this is part of the mechanism that is believed to increase the rate of Down's syndrome in areas that fluoridate their water. A study conducted in China titled "Micronucleus and Sister Chromatid Exchange Frequency in Endemic Fluorosis" studied inhabitants of a region in Inner Mongolia who drank water high in fluoride. The study concluded that the data "showed that the DNA of the patients with fluorosis was seriously damaged, and that the DNA of the healthy people in the endemic regions was also damaged in varying degrees."

In addition to damaging DNA, fluoride harms many of the enzymes necessary for a variety of cellular and physiological functions, which can lead to metabolic problems such as low levels of blood calcium and high levels of blood potassium.

New Studies Show Fluoride Does Not Prevent Tooth Decay

The early studies done on water fluoridation looked only at the cavity rates of young children. They did not try to determine whether more children were being born with Down's syndrome or had higher levels of lead in their blood. They did not look to see whether the elderly suffered from more hip fractures, higher rates of Alzheimer's disease, or cancer. This work would have to wait for the next generation of scientists.

A New Generation of Scientists

In addition to looking at the health effects of fluoride, this new generation of scientists has also examined whether the fluoridation of water actually helps reduce cavity rates. Although some studies suggest a slight reduction in cavities from fluoridated water, the majority of studies show no reduction in cavities from drinking fluoridated water and some even found higher cavity rates.

New Zealand's National Fluoridation Committee Chairman Exposes Selective Science of Earlier Studies

While John Colquhoun was the chairman of the National Fluoridation Committee in New Zealand, he analyzed the fluoridation of water in New Zealand. A staunch fluoridation advocate at the time, he was shocked when he looked at the results of the data. In 1981, the data showed that in most of the Health Districts in New Zealand, the percentage of twelve- to thirteen-year-old children free of tooth decay was higher in nonfluoridated areas than in fluoridated areas. During the next few years, the statistics continued to show that the dental health of children in nonfluoridated areas was slightly better than that of children in fluoridated areas. He was warned not to make the data public, but eventually the facts about fluoridation forced him to drop his support of fluoridation, and he published an article titled "New Evidence on Fluoridation." In his article, he explained how fluoride's benefits are from topical application and not from ingesting it. He also exposed the "selective science" that was used to validate fluoridation in New Zealand, much as had happened in the United States. For example, when researchers in one study in New Zealand chose to compare fluoridated vs. nonfluoridated areas, they specifically chose the one nonfluoridated community with the highest decay rate among nonfluoridated communities, while choosing the two fluoridated communities that had the lowest decay rates among fluoridated communities.

When that highly biased study was made public, the media reported how fluoridation resulted in 50 percent less tooth decay. John Colquhoun deserves credit for coming forward with all of the data he was privy to. He showed that when all of the data was considered, not only the "selected data," decay rates were lower overall in nonfluoridated communities. Another New Zealand study, called the Hastings Fluoridation Experiment, was rigged by changing the way tooth decay was diagnosed, so that much less decay would be diagnosed once fluoridation began. Many teeth that had been classified as "decayed" before the experiment began would be classified as "normal" after the experiment began; the only thing that changed was the method of classifying decay, ensuring that the fluoridation trial would be successful. The same type of "selective science" was used in the early trials in the United States, such as the Newburgh and Grand Rapids trials, according to experts who have analyzed the scientific methods that were used.

U.S. Study of 40,000 Schoolchildren Finds No Statistical Difference between Fluoridated and Nonfluoridated Areas

Similar studies done in the United States show essentially the same thing as the New Zealand data. A study conducted in the United States titled "Water Fluoridation and Tooth Decay: Results from the 1966–1987 National Survey of U.S. Schoolchildren," examined the data of nearly 40,000 children between the ages of 5 and 17, in 84 areas of the United States. The study stated that "no statically significant differences were found in the percentages of decay rates of permanent teeth or the percentages of decay-free children in the fluoridated, non-fluoridated, and partially fluoridated areas." It did find that five-year-old children in fluoridated areas had lower decay rates of temporary teeth (baby teeth). This, of course, is what the Kingston study was designed to prove: that very young children receiving fluoride will have less decay of temporary teeth, due to the fluoride. When they get older, there will be no real difference in decay rates, although the children who received fluoride may suffer from lower IQs and later in life may have higher cancer rates, higher rates of bone and hip fractures, and an increased risk of Alzheimer's disease, along with a host of other diseases. This is quite a price to pay for reducing the cavities in your temporary teeth when you are young.

Studies of Schoolchildren in Missouri and Arizona

Other studies done in the United States have come to the same conclusion. A study that looked at data on more than 6,500 schoolchildren in Missouri titled "Caries Prevalences among Geochemical Regions of Missouri" found that "there were no significant differences between those children drinking optimally fluoridated water and those drinking sub-optimally fluoridated water."

A similar study done in Arizona by Professor Steelink was based on the dental screenings of 26,000 elementary schoolchildren. When the incidence of tooth decay was plotted, based on the fluoride content in a child's neighborhood (at the time the city relied on multiple neighborhood wells, with all of them having varying amounts of fluoride), a positive correlation was found between the level of fluoride and tooth decay. The higher the level of fluoride in a child's drinking water, the higher the level of tooth decay and the more cavities the children's teeth had.

Australian Study of Ten-Year-Olds between 1977 and 1987
Studies in other countries have also come to the same conclusion. An article titled "Have the Benefits of Water Fluoridation Been Overestimated?" looked at the average levels of tooth decay of Australian ten-year-olds between 1977 and 1987. The article states that "it is clear that tooth decay in unfluoridated Brisbane is now the same as in fluoridated Adelaide and Perth, and is less than in fluoridated Melbourne." The article notes that tooth decay had gone down in both fluoridated and unfluoridated cities and gives credit to improved diet and nutrition, including the consumption of more cheese, and better oral hygiene, such as brushing and flossing. Other experts also credit the increased consumption of fruits and vegetables, and the introduction of refrigeration in the 1930s as factors that allowed for better overall nutrition.

Canada Claims Decay Rates in Children Are Falling for Other Reasons
An article in the *Journal of the Canadian Dental Association* titled "Fluoridation: Time for a New a Base Line?" reviewed the findings from British Columbia and other localities. The article states that tooth decay "rates in children are falling drastically in non-fluoridated areas as well as fluoridated areas." In fact, dental decay rates have been falling all over the world, even in countries that do not fluoridate. What has essentially happened is that countries and cities that fluoridate have looked at their falling rates of tooth decay during the last thirty years and claimed that fluoride was responsible. When data is examined from neighboring cities or countries that have never fluoridated, however, it becomes clear that tooth decay has been decreasing over the world, and countries that have never fluoridated their water have seen just as much decline in tooth decay as countries that do. A better measure of

success might be to measure the IQs of children in fluoridated areas vs. nonfluoridated areas, which has already been done many times and has shown that fluoridation decreases the IQs of children by around 10 percent.

World Health Organization Data Reviews Global Decay Rates

An article published in 1993 titled "WHO Data on Dental Caries and Natural Fluoride Levels" examined data collected by the World Health Organization in 1987. The article states that "it can be seen that dental caries (cavities) prevalence does not change significantly with variation in water fluoride content. In most countries the relationship tends to be direct rather than inverse: dental caries increases as water fluoride increases. . . . The belief in an inverse caries-fluoride relationship was reinforced by the numerous 'fluoridation trials.' But they too have been shown to be based upon highly selected data." The WHO data shows that the rate of "decayed, missing, and filled teeth" for twelve-year-olds in the United States was 1.4 per child. Many countries that have outlawed fluoridation have much lower rates of decay than the United States. In the Netherlands the rate is .9, in Sweden it's .9, and in Denmark it's .9. Other countries that do not fluoridate have slightly higher rates than the United States, such as Belgium, where the rate is 1.6, and Germany, where it's 1.7. The bottom line is that when all of the data is examined, overall tooth decay rates are slightly lower in most countries that do not fluoridate vs. countries that do.

Randomized, Double-Blind India Study of More Than 400,000 Children

One of the largest studies concerning fluoride and cavities occurred in India. It was a randomized study involving more than 400,000 ten-year old children titled "Dental Caries: A Disorder of High Fluoride and Low Dietary Calcium Interactions." Keep in mind that not a single study conducted in the United States to justify fluoridation of the water supply has been a randomized, double-blind study. The study in India looked at children living in areas where the fluoride content of the water was less than one part per million and compared them to children living in areas with a fluoride content greater than one part per million. Among children getting adequate calcium, only 2 percent in the low-fluoride area had cavities, while 10 percent of the children living in higher-fluoride areas had cavities. Among children who were not getting adequate calcium, a little more than 31 percent of the children living in low-fluoride areas had cavities, while 74 percent in high-fluoride areas had cavities. Even more disturbing was the fact that among children getting enough calcium, 7 percent in low-fluoride areas had fluorosis, while 59 percent of the children in higher-fluoride areas had fluorosis. Among children not getting enough calcium, 59 percent of the children in low-fluoride areas had fluorosis, while 100 percent of the children in higher-fluoride areas had fluorosis.

Put another way, children getting adequate calcium and higher levels of fluoride have more than three times the rate of cavities and are more than eight times more likely to suffer from fluorosis. Remember, fluorosis is a marker that you have been exposed to too much fluoride, and according to all of the research I have read, it puts people at a greater risk for a lowered IQ, weak bones, cancer, Alzheimer's disease, and many other diseases.

The study in India concluded that "our findings indicate that dental caries (cavities) was caused by high fluoride and low dietary calcium intakes, separately and through their interactions. . . . The only practical and effective public health measure for the prevention and control of dental caries is the limitation of the fluoride content of drinking water to less that ½ part per million and adequate calcium nutrition." This recommendation is eight times lower than the level of fluoride allowed in water in the United States.

Conclusions

Recall that the main study that was used to force fluoridation on the American people was the Newburgh/Kingston study. The latest study on those two cities shows that the decay rates are about the same but are slightly lower in nonfluoridated Kingston vs. fluoridated Newburgh. The other study used in the United States to justify fluoridation was the 21-city Dean study, mentioned earlier, which has since been found to be based on highly "selected data."

The World Health Organization data has made it clear that cavity rates are slightly higher in areas with higher fluoride levels. The WHO data concurred with the findings of the "York Review," which was a 2000 study sponsored by the UK government and published in the *BMJ*, formerly called the *British Journal of Medicine*. The study, titled "Systematic Review of Water Fluoridation," reviewed 214 studies that pertained to the safety and efficacy of the fluoridation of drinking water. The review found that not a single one of the studies that examined the effectiveness of water fluoridation at preventing cavities was considered a "Grade A" study. "Grade A" means that the study is of high quality and that bias is unlikely. Another way to put it is that of the 214 studies that examined the effectiveness of fluoridation at reducing tooth decay, every single one of them is of marginal quality and very possibly suffers from bias. For example, the Grand Rapids, Michigan, study, which was one of the main studies used to validate fluoridation, dropped the control city six years into the study. Based on the results that both industry and the government wanted at the time, you really have to question whether the control city was dropped because the study was not producing the desired results. This is similar to what happened in the Hastings, New Zealand, study, where the control city was dropped after two years, and the method of diagnosing tooth decay was changed so that less decay would be diagnosed once fluoridation started.

Silicofluoride, an Industrial Pollutant, Has Never Been Safety Tested
There is even serious debate over whether the type of fluoride added to most water is legal. There is no such thing as simple "fluoride" that is found in nature. Fluoride is an extremely "reactive" element, which is part of what makes it so toxic to the human system. It must be combined with another element to make it stable. In nature, it combines with calcium, forming calcium-fluoride, which is not very soluble and therefore difficult for the body to absorb. All of the early studies done on fluoridation in the United States used pharmaceutical-grade sodium-fluoride, which is the type of fluoride used in many toothpastes and is absorbed to a greater degree by the body than is natural calcium-fluoride, making it more toxic, according to many fluoride experts. Sodium-fluoride is expensive, however, so most municipalities use industrial-grade silicofluoride (about 90 percent of fluoridated water is from silicofluoride). Much of this silicofluoride comes from the industrial smokestacks of the phosphate fertilizer industry. Some is even being imported from China now. According to press reports, certain water departments have had problems with this Chinese fluoride not dissolving properly in their water systems, and it creates an unknown sludge. Silicofluoride is an industrial pollutant, and if you were to dump it into a river or into the ocean, you would face serious fines and jail time. Even though this type of fluoride has never gone through one double-blind, randomized study for safety, it's perfectly legal

to dump it into the public water supply in the United States. As mentioned earlier, this type of fluoride has been shown to increase the absorption of lead and aluminum in the human body.

Fluoride, the Most Commonly Prescribed Drug

Even if fluoride prevented cavities, and the most credible science shows it does not, and even if pharmaceutical-grade fluoride was used in water, instead of industrial waste by-products, there would still be many reasons not to fluoridate the water supply. First of all, in the United States, any substance used to treat or prevent a disease is a drug subject to FDA regulation, and the FDA has declared that fluoride is a drug. Given that more than 180 million Americans drink fluoridated water, it is essentially the most prescribed drug in America. Yet the FDA has never subjected fluoride to the same clinical trials required of other drugs.

Shouldn't Mass Dosing of Fluoride Be Illegal?

Any drug given to any person in the United States is supposed to be given with his or her "informed consent," which means that the individual is informed of the dangers and risks that could be associated with the taking of the drug. Most Americans have never been informed by their local water departments or dentists that fluoride may lower the IQs of children 10 percent, raise the level of lead in their blood, increase the rate of more than twenty different cancers, or increase the risk of hip and bone fractures, so, from this standpoint alone, fluoridation appears to be illegal. Fluoride is the only drug that is added to the water as a way to medicate large portions of the population. Second, there has never been any safety testing on the silicofluorides used to fluoridate 90 percent of the fluoridated water in the United States, so once again it is questionable whether it's even legal to add it to the public water supply. Remember, it's against the law to dump silicofluorides into a stream, a lake, or the ocean.

At-Risk Populations in Danger of Fluoride Toxicity

Another serious reason not to add fluoride into the water as a drug to prevent cavities is that it's impossible to control the dose. People drink different amounts of water. A laborer working in a hot climate might drink three to four liters of water a day, while a more sedentary person might drink half a liter. In this case, one person is getting up to eight times the dose of the drug, compared

THE FOUR SEASONS DIET

to the other person. It has been shown that people with impaired kidney function do not eliminate as much fluoride from their bodies as normal people do, and fluoride begins to accumulate in their bones at a much faster rate. Diabetics are also prone to drinking more water than nondiabetics and may suffer more ill effects from consuming excess fluoride.

There is concern that babies who are fed formula made with tap water containing fluoride may be especially vulnerable to fluoride's health effects. In 2006, the American Dental Association recommended that its dentists advise patients not to use fluoridated tap water to make baby formula. Unfortunately, poor Americans are least able to afford to buy bottled water to make baby formula. Poor children often grow up in homes that contain more lead, and given fluoride's ability to increase lead absorption, parents should worry about what happens to babies who are exposed to fluoridated formula and lead. Formula made with fluoridated water usually contains 250 times more fluoride than breast milk, and a baby's developing brain may be far more affected by fluoride's IQ-lowering effects than a fully developed brain is.

In the United States, potentially toxic substances are supposed to operate under a margin of safety. This means that the lowest dose that is considered toxic is usually divided by 10, to arrive at a safe exposure level. Given that people with kidney problems, diabetics, babies, the very old, and those with a poor diet may be especially prone to fluoride's toxic effects, the margin of safety dose for fluoridated water is estimated to be .1 part per million, which is 40 times less that the 4 parts per million allowed by the EPA. At the current level allowed by the EPA of 4 parts per million, many people in parts of Texas and South Carolina, which have high levels of fluoride in their water, and those living in hot climates who consume up to 4 liters of water a day could be exposed to as much as 16 mg of fluoride per day just from the water they drink. When the EPA set the maximum level of fluoride in water at 4 parts per million, that organization considered only crippling skeletal fluorosis to be the main health effect from fluoride, yet the EPA's allowed level has been shown to lower IQs in children, increase hip and bone fractures, and raise cancer rates, along with causing all of the other health problems mentioned in this section.

Furthermore, some people are especially sensitive to even moderate doses of fluoride, and they may have no idea that they have a "fluoride allergy." It has been found that about 1 percent of the population can react negatively to even 1 mg of fluoride, exhibiting skin problems, such as eczema and dermatitis; gastrointestinal problems, such as alternating constipation and diarrhea; neurological problems that may include headaches and depression; excessive tiredness and weakness; bone and joint pain; and stiffness in the back and the legs. Many people who are sensitive to fluoride develop lesions in their mouths from using fluoridated toothpaste. People who suffer from fluoride sensitivity have reported that their symptoms, which often have plagued them for decades, disappear very quickly after they stop drinking fluoridated water and using fluoridated toothpaste. Other sensitive people who have lived their entire lives in unfluoridated areas experienced a rapid onset of symptoms when they moved to fluoridate areas. Tea is also very high in fluoride, and many people with arthritis have reported that their pain stops within several months after they quit drinking tea.

In addition to the margin of safety, there is also the precautionary principle. The precautionary principle states that if an action or a policy has a suspected risk of harm, despite the absence of a scientific consensus, the burden of proof that the action or the policy is not harmful falls on those taking the action. In the case of fluoride, the studies and the evidence I have presented make it more than clear that there is a strong indication of harm and therefore a lack of scientific evidence regarding fluoride's safety.

Recent Public Efforts to Ban Water Fluoridation
Fortunately, people are starting to become aware of the dangers posed by fluoridated water. In 2011, the city council of Calgary, Canada, voted 10 to 3 to stop fluoridating its water. Every month, multiple cities in the United States and Canada are voting to end fluoridation. Some of the larger cities to end fluoridation in just the last year alone include the following:

CITY	POPULATION	DATE
Moncton, New Brunswick	140,000	December, 2011
College Station, Texas	100,000	September, 2011
Lakeshore, Ontario	33'000	October, 2011
New Plymouth, New Zealand	50,000	October, 2011
Spring Hill, Tennessee	30,000	August, 2011
Fairbanks, Alaska	30,500	June, 2011
Calgary, Alberta	1,300,000	February, 2011

Most Americans would probably be shocked to learn that

the United States is one of only eight countries that fluoridates more than 50 percent of its public water. The other seven countries are Australia, Colombia, Ireland, Israel, Malaysia, New Zealand, and Singapore. Most of the world has rejected fluoridation of the public water supply. Countries such as Denmark and Sweden made fluoridation illegal, on the grounds that the long-term effects were unknown. Sweden became one of the first European countries to allow fluoridation in 1952, but in 1971, the Swedish parliament outlawed the practice, citing lack of knowledge. Other countries have also banned the use of fluoride in drinking water, citing many of the reasons I outlined in this section. Germany, France, Belgium, and Luxembourg banned water fluoridation over concerns about the ethics of requiring the compulsory medication of an entire population via the drinking water. Fluoridation was banned in the Netherlands in 1973 after its Supreme Court ruled that there was no legal basis for fluoridation. The Czech Republic stopped fluoridating water in 1993, citing the unethical nature of forced medication, along with the inability to control the dosage, especially in certain "at risk" populations.

While almost every nation that has looked at fluoridating its water has decided to ban the practice for various moral, ethical, and health reasons, the U.S. government advocates the use of water fluoridation. The dogmatic belief of those who support fluoridation in the United States is that the science has been 100 percent settled and that anyone who opposes it is ignorant and mentally deficient. In actuality, the science is about 90 percent settled against fluoridation. At least fourteen Nobel Prize winners in Chemistry and Medicine have either opposed fluoridation or expressed serious reservations about it. According to National Fluoridation News, these include Dr. James Summer, Giulio Natta, Nikolai Semenov, Sir Cyril Norman Hinshelwood, Hugo Theorell, Walter Rudolf Hess, Sir Robert Robinson, James B. Summer, Artturi Virtanen, Adolf Butenandt, Corneille Jean-Francois Heymans, William P. Murphy, Hans Euler-Chelpin, Arvid Carlsson, and Joshua Lederberg.

The Greatest Advance in Dental Health or the Greatest Scientific Fraud?
So the question is, who do you believe? Do you believe more than fourteen Nobel Prize winners, most of the scientific research conducted since the 1980s, and the majority of countries that have studied fluoridation and now oppose it? Or do you believe a few studies from the 1940s and the 1950s that used highly selective

data and your doctor and your dentist, who probably don't know the truth and, even if they do, may be afraid to go against the stance of their professional organizations out of fear of retaliation? The good news is that many health-care professionals are beginning to feel less threatened about speaking the truth, and, to date, more than four thousand have signed a petition with Fluoride Action Network, calling for an end to water fluoridation. In their petition, they cite many of the same reasons I do for ending water fluoridation.

The two sides in the fluoridation debate can best be summed up in two quotes, one from a fluoridation advocate, and another from a fluoridation opponent. Former surgeon general Thomas Parran, a fluoridation advocate, once stated, "I consider water fluoridation to be the greatest single advance in dental health made in our generation." A former EPA scientist named Dr. Robert Carton, who became a fluoridation opponent after examining the evidence, stated, "Fluoridation is a scientific fraud, probably the greatest fraud of the century." Now that you've read all of the evidence, I'll leave it up to you to decide which is true.

If you want to limit your exposure to fluoride, you should be aware that many dental products contain up 12,300 parts per million of fluoride. A study conducted in the UK titled "Fluoride Ingestion from Toothpaste by Young Children" measured the amount of fluoride that was retained in the mouth after brushing. It found that the average amount of toothpaste applied to a brush was .36 grams, of which .27 grams was retained in the mouth after rinsing. This means that using toothpaste that contains 1,500 parts per million fluoride, a child will retain .42 mg of fluoride per brushing. When combined with fluoride from water and food, it is very easy for a child to get far too much fluoride. This study concluded that "it is essential that parents of children less than 7 years apply a small (pea-sized) amount of fluoride toothpaste on the toothbrush and discourage swallowing." A study done in Japan titled "Re-Examination of Acute Toxicity of Fluoride" found that "fluoride retention is said to be around 15 to 30% in fluoride mouth rinsing." The study states that "fluoride poisoning has also occurred from recommended use of fluoride," and regarding the increase in fluorosis, it says that "this increase may be attributable to increased daily fluoride intake from fluoride-containing toothpaste."

All-Natural Xylitol Prevents Cavities

A natural sweetener called xylitol has been found to be highly effective at preventing cavities without the toxic effects of fluoride. Several toothpastes and mouth rinses that use xylitol are currently on the market in the United States. A study conducted in Estonia titled "Xylitol Candies in Caries Prevention: Results of a Field Study in Estonian Children" found that children chewing gum with xylitol showed a 35 to 60 percent reduction in cavities. Remember that most current studies on fluoride show either no cavity protection from ingesting fluoride or actually more cavities from ingesting fluoride. Also, xylitol will not lower your child's IQ, so if the studies showing reduced IQ from fluoride ingestion are correct, you can instead reduce cavities in your children without lowering their IQs by switching your children from fluoride to xylitol.

Finland has conducted several studies on the effectiveness of xylitol chewing gum at preventing cavities, and in Finland, oral health professionals often recommend the use of xylitol chewing gum. One study showed a 30 percent reduction in cavities from chewing two pieces of xylitol gum a day and a 60 percent reduction from chewing three pieces of gum a day. This is similar to the results of a study in the Soviet Union, in which half of a child's normal sucrose confections were replaced with xylitol, resulting in a 73 percent reduction in cavities. Because Finland does not have an FDA that restricts freedom of health speech, as we do in the United States, companies there are able to advertise their xylitol products by emphasizing their effectiveness at preventing cavities. In the United States, this would be illegal because of the way the FDA is allowed to censor even truthful health information about the effectiveness of natural healthy products with no harmful side effects that often outperform patented and highly profitable artificial products.

Tests on xylitol were started in the United States at the National Institute of Dental Research, but that trial was canceled after only three days. A dentist can charge considerable amounts of money for sealants and topical fluoride application at his or her office, and that lucrative business could end if the public was aware that simply chewing xylitol-sweetened gum was far more effective at preventing cavities and without any toxic side effects.

The World Health Organization has even gotten involved in xylitol research and has conducted a study in Hungary titled "Collaborative WHO Xylitol Field Studies in Hungary. VII Two-year

Caries Incidence in 976 Institutionalized Children." In that study, children were given either xylitol or fluoride for two years. The children receiving fluoride had 26 percent more tooth decay than the children who received xylitol.

13
The Current "Medical Dark Age"

*The second "Dark Age," courtesy of Rockefeller, the FDA, and the
American Medical Association and the need for reformation.*

Hopefully, by now you are starting to realize that most disease is
caused by eating processed foods, and that by eating right for your
season-type, which includes eliminating most processed foods from
your diet, you can prevent most disease. The connection between
natural foods and health and processed foods and disease is so
profound and obvious, many of you may be wondering why doctors
don't simply advocate this type of diet to all of their patients as way
of eliminating most diseases in America. In fact, most doctors say
very little to their patients about preventing illness.

I have cited many research studies that show that natural
foods and proper vitamin and mineral supplementation can
eliminate 80 to 90 percent of all disease. Proper vitamin D levels
have been shown to prevent up to 77 percent of breast cancer
in women; reducing fructose consumption gets rid of the main
cause of insulin resistance, which is the root of many diseases in
America; and avoiding processed vegetable oils high in omega-6
fats has been shown in multiple studies to reduce the rates of
breast cancer, insulin resistance, diabetes, and osteoporosis.

A 2009 study titled "Healthy Living Is the Best Revenge:
Findings from the European Prospective Investigation into Cancer
and Nutrition—Potsdam Study" reported the findings of a study
conducted on 23,153 German participants during a nearly eight-
year period. The study looked at four factors that can prevent
disease, which included never smoking, having a body mass index
lower than 30, performing at least 3.5 hours of physical activity
per week, and adhering to healthy dietary principles, such as
consuming plenty of fruits, vegetables, and whole grains, while
limiting meat consumption. When participants who had included
all four prevention factors into their lifestyle were compared to
those who had included none, the results were astounding. The
group that had included all four prevention factors had a 93 percent

494

lower incidence of diabetes, an 81 percent lower incidence of heart attack, a 50 percent lower incidence of stroke, and a 36 percent lower incidence of cancer during the eight-year study period.

When was the last time your doctor told you that incorporating four simple prevention factors into your lifestyle could prevent 81 percent of heart attacks and 93 percent of diabetes, while maintaining proper vitamin D levels could reduce your breast cancer risk by 77 percent, or explained that if you stopped eating most types of fructose and omega-6 oils, you could eliminate two of the other major causes of many diseases? Sadly, not only will most doctors never tell you these things, but for years many of them have actually told their patients that omega-6 oils are the "healthy" oil and have told many diabetics that fructose is the "good" sugar.

Although most medical professionals in the United States believe that Western medicine is at the forefront of science, the truth is that we have entered a second "Dark Age," courtesy of J. D. Rockefeller, the FDA, and the American Medical Association. In the original religious Dark Ages more than a thousand years ago, the church ruled supreme, and the masses were kept illiterate and in the dark. It was illegal for a common person to own even a page of the Bible. Under this system, all power came from the Vatican and flowed down though the priests, who presided over the people.

In the modern "Medical Dark Ages," we have slowly been losing the right to make our own health-care choices and are being kept in the dark about the truth of powerful natural herbal and plant-based cures. Under this new system, the FDA acts as the Vatican, and doctors are the new priesthood. While this may sound a little far-fetched at first, by the end of this chapter you may come to realize the extent to which a lot of modern Western medicine is not really based on science and that we have lost most of our health freedoms in the United States. What little freedom we do have is under vicious attack, and unless enough Americans stand up within the next decade and demand their rights back, even our right to purchase natural herbs and vitamin supplements is likely to be taken away.

Under the current medical monopoly system, only expensive patented artificial pharmaceutical drugs can be used to treat illness, and cheaper, safer, and more effective natural herbal treatments are not allowed or tolerated. The ultimate goal, which is closer to being put in place than most people realize, is to ban all vitamins and herbal supplements that can currently be purchased at health food stores and make them available only with a doctor's prescription. Thanks largely to the Internet, people are waking up to the superior medical advantages that natural herbs provide, when compared to toxic and artificial patented pharmaceutical medicines. In order to understand how we got to such a sorry state of medical freedom in the United States, you'll need to learn a little about the history of medicine in this country, along with how J. D. Rockefeller played a major role in creating current practices and institutions.

The Corrupt Legacy of J. D. Rockefeller

When you adjust the net worth of various people throughout history, J. D. Rockefeller is probably the richest person ever to have lived. He was the world's first billionaire, and at the time of his death, his net worth, adjusted for inflation, is estimated to have been as high as the equivalent of nearly $700 billion today. To put this into perspective, the combined net worth of the ten richest people today, a list that includes Bill Gates and Warren Buffett, is only around $400 billion. Stated in another way, at the time of his death and adjusted for inflation, J. D. Rockefeller was worth about seven times the current wealth of Bill Gates and Warren Buffett combined.

Rockefeller attained much of his wealth through what have been described as the most ruthless business practices ever known to mankind. He hated competition and realized that great wealth was easiest to accumulate when you had no competition. At one time, he controlled 90 percent of the entire world's oil-refining capability, and his goal was to control 100 percent. This is an important fact to remember, because he applied some of those same business tactics to controlling medicine.

In 1911, the U.S. government broke up Rockefeller's illegal oil monopoly into many smaller companies. Although this fact is well known, what is not well known is that he learned many lessons from the government breakup of his oil monopoly. He next set his sights on creating a monopoly in medicine, in the United States and the entire world.

This was the next logical monopoly for Rockefeller to create, because many patented pharmaceutical medicines at the time were made from oil derivatives, and they had a huge profit potential, if it were not for one major obstacle: cheap, effective, and safe herbal medicines.

In the late 1800s, being a doctor was a rather low-paying profession, and doctors had low social standing. During this time, many different independent medical schools taught diverse ways of healing. Probably the most popular schools were the homeopathic schools, which were built around natural herbal medicines. Because medical schools were truly independent, they made their money by teaching doctors to become doctors and were in competition with other medical schools. This is in large part what helped keep doctors' wages low and medical care very affordable. With a surplus of doctors and cheap herbs for medicine, even the poorest people could afford adequate medical care.

In order for Rockefeller to create a monopoly with the patented pharmaceutical drugs he controlled, he had to find a way to get rid of any medicines that could not be patented. Rockefeller found a very willing partner in this endeavor in the American Medical Association. The AMA was interested in raising the incomes of doctors who were part of that association. The only way to accomplish this goal was to close as many medical schools as possible, thereby reducing the number of doctors practicing medicine, which would drive up the amount of money each doctor could charge, due to lack of competition. This would ultimately mean that poor people and minorities, who had been able to afford medical care before Rockefeller and the AMA hatched their plot to close as many medical schools as possible, would no longer be able to afford medical care once this plan was successful.

With Rockefeller's help, this was accomplished in a very short time period. It's important to get a good picture of medicine in the United States a hundred years ago. In 1904, medical schools were free to compete under the various forms of medicine, and 166 medical schools existed in the United States. By 1929, the number of medical schools had been reduced by more than 50 percent, to only 76, and only medical schools that taught the type of medicine the Rockefeller Foundation dictated had survived. In the oil business, Rockefeller demolished the competition with his ruthless business practices. The U.S. government and the American people were on to his ways, however, so to destroy the competition in medicine, he would have to use a combination of merciless stealth and cunning.

The way he accomplished this was by giving away approximately half a billion dollars to college universities that would agree to teach only the type of medicine he dictated. For example, Harvard received more than $8 million, Johns Hopkins more than $10 million, and Yale more than $7 million, enormous sums at the time. Rockefeller and the universities that aligned with him set up a new type of medicine they called "scientific medicine." Yet this type of medicine had very little to do with real science. So-called scientific medicine required expensive teaching hospitals, teaching clinics, and costly laboratories. At the time, doctors and medical schools were very poor, and the only way medical schools could hope to pay for these new additions to their programs was through Rockefeller grants.

A man who was richer than anyone who had ever lived could afford to purchase pretty much anything he wanted. Rockefeller had learned from his mistakes in the oil business. In 1913, the Rockefeller Foundation was formed, along with the FDA and the American Cancer Society. According to many people, this was not a mere coincidence. There are those who believe that Rockefeller was instrumental in helping to create both the FDA and the American Cancer Society, and although this may be hard to prove, we do know that Rockefeller contributed more than $100,000 to the American Cancer Society during its infancy. With Rockefeller's new medical monopoly, he was determined to have the government working for him, not against him, as it had done when it broke up his oil monopoly. The theory of many people is that by allegedly controlling medical schools, the FDA, medical associations such as the AMA, and charities such as the American Cancer Society, Rockefeller could fully control medicine.

Once he bought the most prestigious medical schools, such as Harvard and Johns Hopkins, with his money, he was able to control the state licensing boards. The cunning part of the scheme was that rather than go after the homeopathic schools directly, he had the state licensing boards refuse to license doctors from schools that were not "modern" and that did not have expensive teaching hospitals and labs. The only schools that could afford these amenities were the ones that he gave money to, and the condition for receiving Rockefeller money was that the schools could teach only medicine that used expensive patented drugs and excluded cheap, effective, and safe natural herbs. Rockefeller donated (actually, invested) nearly $500 million in this endeavor, which forced medical schools that taught natural-based medicine to close. These efforts also extended overseas. Rockefeller invested $45 million in China to help "Westernize" Chinese medicine. China had been an extremely lucrative market for Standard Oil's kerosene, which was used in lamps throughout China during the early 1900s, and Rockefeller felt that it could be a lucrative market for patented medicines as well.

The other thing Rockefeller did after the breakup of his oil monopoly was to hide much of his money in trust funds. Part of the reason for this was so that only his family and his attorneys would know how many trust funds there were and which trust funds were Rockefeller's. Rockefeller had been livid when the U.S. government broke up his oil monopoly, and by hiding his fortune in various trusts, he made it impossible for the government to know about all of his business dealings, because only Rockefeller and his attorneys would know what companies he controlled. One Rockefeller trust is said to own part of Chase Manhattan Bank, and Chase Manhattan Bank is allegedly among the largest shareholders of Exxon, Mobile Oil, and Standard Oil. According to some experts, such Rockefeller trusts could number in the hundreds or even the thousands, making the true extent of the current Rockefeller family fortune known only to the family.

This system of hiding things in various trust funds has made the full extent of Rockefeller family holdings in the various pharmaceutical companies hard to gauge. According to an article in *Newsweek*, dated September 2, 1974, much of the Rockefeller family fortune is distributed in "well over 100 and perhaps 200 individual Rockefeller trusts." According to some reports, Sterling Drug, a single Rockefeller holding company, had sixty-eight subsidiaries that often made profits on its investments of more than 50 percent each year. Estimates are that early on in the pharmaceutical industry, various Rockefeller companies and trusts owned the majority of pharmaceutical companies. Monopolies can be extremely profitable, and, according to many experts, this was the reason Rockefeller was willing to invest $500 million in medical schools, as long as they agreed to teach the type of medicine he dictated, because he would control the expensive patented medicines. Without a doubt, were it not for Rockefeller's intervention in the field of medicine in this country, we would probably have a medical system today that relied far more on safe, natural herbal cures than our current system does. In addition, there would be far more doctors practicing medicine, earning much smaller salaries, which would make health care far more affordable.

Fuel from Hemp: Did Henry Ford Have a Solution to the Energy Crisis?

Besides forever changing health care in our country, Rockefeller also changed energy in the United States. Remember that at one point he controlled more than 90 percent of the entire world's oil-refining capability. Central to his control over oil refining was his control over crude oil. The biggest threat to this monopoly was Henry Ford's plan to run his automobiles on clean and renewable ethanol made from hemp. Hemp is a plant that is related to cannabis (marijuana) but is not grown or smoked as a recreational drug; the THC content in hemp is too low for that. What makes hemp unique is that it grows extremely quickly and can yield four times as much biofuel per acre as corn.

Henry Ford built cars to run on this hemp biofuel, a fuel he told the *New York Times* in 1925 was "the fuel of the future," and he was teaching farmers how to make their own fuel in backyard stills. Hemp is easy to grow and needs almost no pesticides or herbicides. In fact, hemp is such a good source of biofuel that its been estimated the United States could meet its entire current demand for gasoline of 140 billion gallons a year by simply growing 6 million acres' worth of hemp. Hemp is the only plant that is fully capable of quickly replacing fossil fuels for energy.

Henry Ford's plan included building distilleries all over the United States to produce his hemp fuel. Hemp was effectively outlawed in 1937, however, along with cannabis (marijuana). As you will soon learn, cannabis was outlawed because it was a huge threat to the Rockefeller drug empire, while hemp, cannabis's cousin, was the single biggest threat to Rockefeller's fossil fuel empire.

Many people believe that Rockefeller was instrumental in helping to get Prohibition passed. Prohibition made it illegal to distill alcohol from 1919 through 1933. When the distilleries were forced to close, Henry Ford tried to get the federal government to allow him to use those closed distilleries to produce hemp fuel; the government said no. Ford's dream of running cars on hemp fuel was stopped by the government at every turn. Eventually, when Prohibition was repealed, it was replaced by a prohibition on growing hemp, ensuring U.S. dependence on fossil fuels.

Currently, it is legal to grow hemp in nearly every country on the planet, except the United States. Hemp was an extremely important plant in colonial America, and George Washington stated, "Make the most you can of the Indian Hemp seed and sow it everywhere." It can be used to make paper that is superior to paper made from wood pulp and clothes that offer many advantages over other fibers. In fact, I'll state that without a doubt, growing hemp to replace fossil fuels and wood pulp paper would do more to help the environment than any other measure currently being proposed. The problem is that hemp could bankrupt the oil companies, and the U.S. government will not allow this to happen, so it must keep the cultivation of hemp illegal.

Cannabis: A Threat to the Pharmaceutical Drug Monopoly

Rockefeller used his enormous wealth to control politics in America and was instrumental in pushing for legislation such as the Harrison Narcotic Act and the creation of federal agencies such as the FDA. The real purpose of many of the laws and the agencies Rockefeller helped create was to protect his newest monopoly: the pharmaceutical drug trust. The biggest threats to Rockefeller's drug and medical monopolies were natural herbal cures, and one of these threats was cannabis. For most of U.S. history, medical marijuana was known as cannabis. From 1842 through the early 1900s, cannabis was contained in approximately half of all medicines sold in the United States, and there were no fears over the "high" it created. In fact, from 1850 to 1937, when it was outlawed, the U.S. Pharmacopoeia listed cannabis as the primary "medicine" for more than a hundred different illnesses and diseases, and it had no known side effects. This is the reason Rockefeller had to have it outlawed.

Cannabis was outlawed though a combination of laws and deceptive PR campaigns. The first thing that had to be done was to change the name of cannabis to marijuana, because everyone in the United States at the time knew that cannabis was the best and safest drug available. The Mexican word marijuana was chosen for several reasons. It allowed the government to deceive people into believing marijuana was a new drug and not the trusted cannabis they had used for nearly a hundred years. When the word marijuana was used in newsreel films of the day, it was spoken with a strong Hispanic accent, and its use was tied to Mexican immigrants and black jazz musicians. In the year prior to its ban, the U.S. government released a film called *Reefer Madness* (1936), which is about how high school students who smoked the Mexican drug "mareeeeewaaaaaaaanaa" all went crazy and either committed suicide or had to be locked away in insane asylums.

In addition to creating movies such as *Reefer Madness*,

the U.S. government began a newspaper campaign to spread false stories to scare parents about this new drug called marijuana. There were stories of a teenage boy who smoked a single marijuana cigarette and then went home and murdered his family with an axe. He later woke up in jail, perfectly normal and oblivious to what had happened. There was even a Movietone newsreel on marijuana during this time. Movietone newsreels were news stories shown in movie theaters before the main movie and were very popular before the advent of television. The Movietone newsreel on marijuana said that when marijuana was smoked, it caused more nightmares than opium. Then followed scenes of kids smoking marijuana and driving a car while running over pedestrians, unaware of what they are doing. In the next scene, a girl in a high-rise building runs down the hall and then jumps out a window to her death for no apparent reason, other than the fact that she has gone insane from smoking marijuana. The last scene is of girls smoking marijuana at a party, who take off all of their clothes and then run around naked outside. The message was that smoking marijuana made you crazy, and you would eventually kill yourself, kill someone else, or end up in the insane asylum. After World War II, when more people began smoking cannabis without killing their families or jumping out of high-rise windows, the government changed its tune. Before World War II, the government said that cannabis would make people violent and crazy, but after World War II, it claimed that cannabis was a communist plot, and smoking it made you a zombie peace activist who would lose any will to fight or harm another person. It had to be eradicated after the war so that Americans would have the will to fight the commies!

In 1938, the mayor of New York, Fiorella LaGuardia, commissioned the New York Academy of Medicine to study the effects of marijuana. In 1944, the academy issued its report, which completely contradicted the federal government's ludicrous claims. The report concluded that marijuana is not a factor in crime or other social problems, and that there were actually some benefits associated with it. When the report came out, it infuriated Harry Anslinger, who was the commissioner of the Federal Bureau of Narcotics. Anslinger's response was akin to something you might expect in a totalitarian communist country. He used the full force of the government to halt any more research into the positive health effects of cannabis, threatened AMA doctors with jail if the AMA did not get on board with his anti-cannabis plan, and even forced Hollywood to give him control over any movie scripts that mentioned marijuana. The evidence suggests that Anslinger may have had ties to the Rockefeller family prior to becoming the man in charge of destroying cannabis because of its threat to the pharmaceutical industry.

Anslinger also had ties to Andrew Mellon, the founder of ALCOA mentioned earlier, who was also the U.S. treasury secretary. In addition to being a founder and a large stockholder of ALCOA, Mellon owned a significant portion of the Gulf Oil Company and was a major investor in the DuPont Petrochemical Company. DuPont was working on creating synthetic fabrics, rubber, and plastics, and hemp posed a threat to these industries, as well as to the oil industry. Mellon had an important reason, along with Rockefeller, to stop Ford's plan to produce fuel using hemp, and it was ultimately Mellon's man Anslinger who would be instrumental in making both hemp and cannabis illegal.

The AMA and Our Modern Health-Care System

The current medical monopoly has rigged the U.S. health-care system, as well as health care in most of the industrialized world, to reject using natural herbs for medicine in favor of pharmaceutical drugs. In addition, medical school enrollment should not be controlled by medical associations, but by the needs of the American people. Currently, only a small number of students are allowed to attend medical school, in order to graduate very few doctors.

Having More Doctors Would Mean Affordable Health Care

Medical schools and professional organizations would like you to believe that the number of students allowed to attend medical school is limited because medical school is so hard to get into, the reason being that it accepts only "qualified" applicants. The truth is that medical school has been made extremely hard to get into because the number of "qualified" students allowed to attend is far lower than the number of "qualified" students who would like to attend. Make no mistake, this is done as a way to limit the number of doctors in the United States so that each individual doctor earns far more than doctors in other countries do. This is a simple matter of supply-and-demand economics. By keeping the supply of doctors artificially low through limited medical school enrollments, doctors' wages go up. Yet for American consumers, the exorbitant amount of money they pay for health care as a result of this artificial manipulation of the marketplace is very real.

The world's most famous economist, Nobel Prize–winner Milton Friedman, understood how professional organizations were limiting medical school enrollments as a way to keep doctors' salaries high, and he often spoke against this corrupt system. He gave a speech at the Mayo Clinic in 1978, in which he stated,

> The key to the control of medicine starts with who is admitted to practice, . . . don't make any mistake about this, the evidence is overwhelming, that there was a deliberate policy on the part of the medical association in the 1930s to keep down the number of physicians. . . . that point is included because of the necessity of reducing and eliminating the monopoly power of the American Medical Association. . . . control over that licensure procedure is what enabled the American Medical Association to exercise its monopoly power for these many decades.

In an article written by Milton Friedman in 1994, titled "Medical Licensure," he stated that

> The American Medical Association is perhaps the strongest trade union in the United States. The essence of the power of a trade union is its power to restrict the number who may engage in a particular occupation. . . . The American Medical Association is in this position. It is a trade union that can limit the number of people who can enter. How can it do this? The essential control is at the stage of admission to medical school.

I mention Milton Friedman's comments because, as an economist, he understood that a large part of the reason medical care is so expensive in the United States is that the supply of doctors has been kept artificially low as a way to keep doctors' salaries artificially high. Like much of the rest of the U.S. medical system, this benefits doctors to the great detriment of the American people.

The United States has only around 2.2 doctors per 1,000 people, while countries such as Germany, Sweden, and France have around 3.4 doctors per 1,000 people, nearly 50 percent more per capita than in the United States. The result is that in Germany, Sweden, and France, doctors earn less than half of what doctors in the United States make.

The current medical monopoly of permitting only artificial patented drugs to be used to treat disease, while limiting the number of doctors who can practice medicine, makes the pharmaceutical companies and the doctors very rich, at the expense of the American people. If the system were not rigged, we would have around 50 percent more doctors in the United States than we currently do, similar to the number of doctors per capita in Germany, France, and Sweden, In addition, many diseases would be treated with natural herbal medicines that cannot be patented and sold for enormous profits. Imagine how ridiculous it would be if we allowed plumbers to artificially limit the number of plumbers who were licensed or electricians to dictate how many electricians there could be. They would obviously restrict the entry of new plumbers and electricians into the marketplace, to drive up their own salaries. We would not tolerate this if plumbers or electricians did this, yet we tolerate the fact that the number of students allowed to attend medical school is essentially limited in order to keep doctors' salaries high, when the number should instead be increased to keep doctors' salaries low and medical care affordable.

Under a fair system of medicine, health care would probably cost less than half of what it does today. Under a truly enlightened system of medical care, medicine would focus on prevention and not on treatment, in which case there would actually be very little need for most doctors. Remember that all of the evidence I have presented shows that disease is being caused mainly by the processed and artificial foods we eat and the artificial chemicals in our environment, including fluoridated water. In an enlightened system of medicine, doctors would be mainly used for accidents and trauma. Food would cost a little more, and we would buy from smaller family farmers who raised healthier organic foods, while GMOs would be banned unless it could be proved that they did not harm humans, animals, or the environment. Cancer and other diseases would be reduced by 80 to 90 percent, and people would lead more productive and healthy lives. The current system needs cancer, needs cardiovascular disease, needs diabetes, needs illness, needs suffering, needs people to be sick; in fact, the sicker people are, the better off the pharmaceutical companies and the doctors are. The healthier the American people become, the less prosperous the pharmaceutical companies and doctors will be.

The AMA's Vendetta against Chiropractors

In addition to limiting medical school enrollment, medical associations have also attacked other forms of health care that alleviate suffering, and efforts have been made to put them out of business. The early code of ethics of the American Medical Association considered it unprofessional for its white male doctors to confer with female doctors or black doctors. This rule was later changed, but over the years, the AMA has sought to discredit other professionals who challenge the current medical monopoly, such as chiropractors. Until 1983, the AMA's position was that it was unethical for medical doctors to associate with "unscientific practitioners," such as chiropractors, whom the AMA had labeled "an unscientific cult." Finally, chiropractors had had enough, and in 1976, four chiropractors filed an antitrust suit against the AMA. The case was called Wilk v. American Medical Association, and the judge ruled that the American Medical Association had engaged in an unlawful conspiracy in violation of the Sherman Antitrust Act, in restraint of trade in order to attempt to contain and eliminate the chiropractic profession. The judge further stated that the American Medical Association "had entered into a long history of illegal behavior" and issued a permanent injunction against the AMA to prevent such future behavior.

The ironic thing is that studies actually show chiropractic to be nearly three times as effective at eliminating neck pain as the pain-medication approach advocated by most doctors. A research study titled "Spinal Manipulation, Medication, or Home Exercise with Advice for Acute and Subacute Neck Pain: A Randomized Trial" found that chiropractic "was more effective than medication in both the short and long term." Yet despite chiropractic's effectiveness at eliminating neck pain, without the harmful side effects and the potential for addiction patented pharmaceutical drugs, the AMA disparaged chiropractic for many years. Now that scientific studies have determined that chiropractic is a valid method of pain relief, you would expect the AMA to instruct all of its physicians that it would be unprofessional to treat their patients with drugs for neck pain, and that they should instead refer these patients to a chiropractor. If the AMA had been successful in its crusade against chiropractic, that form of treatment would have been outlawed, and the millions of people who are helped by it would instead be medicated by a doctor, and most of them would still be in pain. Clearly, this is about power, control, and money and not about what is best for the American people.

The Medical Monopoly's Campaign against Natural Cures

Although the illegal campaign to destroy chiropractic was not successful, the campaign to destroy safe, cheap, and effective natural cures has been extremely effective. It's been estimated that between 25 and 33 percent of modern drugs were originally obtained from plants and then slightly changed chemically so that they could be patented and sold for huge profits. Both the government and the pharmaceutical industry study thousands of plants every year, looking for ones that cure disease, and then work on changing a drug's healing component in some artificial way so that it can be patented and sold for huge markups. Natural cures cannot be patented, so they are cheap, and the medical monopoly will not allow cheap natural cures.

Taxol, an Anti-Cancer Drug Made from the Pacific Yew Tree

From 1960 to 1982 alone, the National Cancer Institute collected and screened approximately thirty-five thousand plant species for anticancer activity. Following is an example of how one cancer drug was approved.

In the early 1960s, the National Cancer Institute commissioned USDA botanists to collect thousands of plant samples per year and began testing them for anticancer activity. In 1964, one of those plants, the Pacific yew tree, was found to have tremendous anticancer potential, and in 1966, the active natural ingredient was named taxol. In an enlightened world, farmers would be encouraged to grow trees, plants, and herbs that cured disease, so that doctors could use them to heal people. In the world Rockefeller created, things do not work this way. In the case of Taxol, once the active ingredient had been isolated, the taxpayer-funded National Cancer Institute spent a small fortune developing a manufacturing process that could be patented, along with conducting the clinical trials that were necessary to prove Taxol's effectiveness. Because taxpayer money was used to discover the natural cure and then develop the process to manufacture and test it, the drug should be owned by the American people and should be a cheap cancer therapy. Instead, the government gave away all of the rights to Taxol to Bristol-Myers Squibb, which proceeded to charge the American people $4.87 per milligram, or twenty times what it cost the company to make. Of course, the pharmaceutical companies reward the politicians who continue to grant them such favorable deals, so the medical monopoly appears to serve politicians as well. Only the American people keep getting the short end of the stick.

Taxol is just one example of a cheap, natural, safe, and effective plant cure that was turned into an expensive, artificial, toxic, and not as effective patentable cure. Aspirin was originally obtained from a plant called spirea. The natural form does not have the side effects of aspirin and can actually help treat stomach disorders, rather than upsetting the stomach, as aspirin often does.

Cannabis versus Marinol

The drug Marinol, which is used to treat nausea and vomiting caused by chemotherapy, was derived from cannabis (marijuana). Marinol has been found to be as effective as cannabis in only 13 percent of patients. Although cannabis does not have any negative side effects for chemotherapy patients, the list of potential side effects for Marinol include weakness, stomach pain, nausea, vomiting, memory loss, anxiety, confusion, dizziness, elevated blood pressure, seizures, hallucinations, and many others. Marinol is also more expensive than cannabis. So if Marinol is only 13 percent as effective, is more expensive, and has potential serious side effects that you would not experience from using cannabis, you would expect doctors to prescribe cannabis. In fact, you would figure that any doctor who prescribed Marinol, instead of cannabis, would be guilty of malpractice and would potentially lose his or her license over it. The FDA has not approved cannabis to treat cancer patients suffering from chemotherapy, however, so doctors could actually risk malpractice if they did prescribe it, instead of Marinol. This protects the pharmaceutical companies from having to compete with cheaper, safer, more effective natural cures; that is the beauty of having a medical monopoly where the FDA, pharmaceutical companies, and medical professionals do what's best for them. Unfortunately, it's often what's worse for the American people.

The median annual profit margin for an American pharmaceutical company is more than three times higher than the median annual profit margin for the average Fortune 500 company. If cannabis were approved for all of its medical uses, it could possibly bankrupt the entire pharmaceutical industry by replacing numerous drugs. Since 1964, at least sixty therapeutic compounds have been isolated from cannabis. According to Dr. Mecholam, the Israeli doctor who first isolated THC in 1964, marijuana is still the world's best medicine. Dr. Mecholam said that if cannabis were legal, it would immediately replace 20 percent of all prescription drugs, and up to 50 percent of all medicines could contain some extract from the cannabis plant.

When it became clear that the U.S. government could not halt cannabis research worldwide, the government made an agreement with the pharmaceutical companies that allows them to finance and judge 100 percent of cannabis research. The end game is to find a way for them to patent every compound in cannabis that they possibly can with their own synthetic versions. So far, the drug companies have had a hard time trying to copy cannabis.

Nearly a hundred years ago, we discovered that vitamin B3 prevents pellagra, vitamin D prevents rickets, and vitamin B1 prevents beriberi. You would think that in the last hundred years, we would have advanced to the point that we would understand exactly which vitamins and minerals are needed to prevent every disease and would simply add foods that contain those vitamins and minerals to our diet. A hundred years ago, however, we were not yet in the "Medical Dark Ages." Since these discoveries, the FDA took charge of all health information, and now it is illegal to make any health claims without the FDA's approval. Although vitamin and supplement manufacturers are supposed to be free to make truthful scientific health claims, the FDA has gone to extreme degrees to censure free speech in the United States.

The FDA's Dietary Supplement Task Force published a report in 1993 that sought to determine what steps needed to be taken "to ensure that the existence of dietary supplements on the market does not act as a disincentive for drug development." At least, the FDA admits what I have been saying. The FDA is actively seeking ways to keep vitamins and supplements from preventing disease to protect the medical monopoly. Why else would the FDA allow GMOs and soy protein isolates and other allegedly unhealthy substances to enter the food supply? The FDA serves the medial monopoly and GMO companies, not the American people.

Red Rice Yeast versus Lipitor

Statin drugs such as Lipitor were originally derived from red rice yeast. You can still legally buy red rice yeast at the health food store, as of the writing of this book. Red rice yeast has been shown to reduce cholesterol levels at least as well as statin drugs do, without the side effects. It does not cost $60 million to prove red rice yeast is as effective as statin drugs; it simply costs that much to do the testing the FDA requires. Smaller studies have been done on red rice yeast and other natural cures, most of them in other countries. One such study, titled "Efficacy and Safety of Monascus Purpureus Went Rice in Subjects with Hyperlipidemia," was published in the *European Journal of Endocrinology*. In this eight-week study conducted on 70 patients, red rice yeast lowered the bad LDL cholesterol by nearly 28 percent and triglycerides by nearly 22 percent. Another study conducted on 324 people found similar results, with a drop in bad cholesterol of nearly 31percent and a drop in triglycerides of nearly 34 percent. Because red rice yeast is a natural product, the only side effects experienced by about 2 percent of the people was slight heartburn or flatulence.

Most people are not aware that patented pharmaceutical statin drugs can cause a form of memory loss called transient global amnesia, along with other types of cognitive damage. According to the FDA's own *MedWatch*, at least two thousand cases of transient global amnesia have been associated with the use of statin drugs. In addition, statin drugs can cause personality changes, muscle weakness, sexual dysfunction, liver dysfunction, suppression of the immune system, nerve damage in the hands and the feet, and cataracts.

According to a March 14, 2012, *New York Times* article titled "Do Statins Make it Tough to Exercise?" statins can wreak havoc on our ability to exercise. The article references a study in which rats given statins could not run as far and became exhausted much earlier than rats that had not been given statins. When researchers examined the rats at the cellular level, "they found that oxidative stress, a measure of possible cell damage, was increased by 60 percent in sedentary animals receiving statins compared with the unmedicated control group. The effect was magnified in the runners, whose cells showed 226 percent more oxidative stress than exercising animals that had not been given statins." In addition, the article cites the fact that animals given statins had lower levels of stored sugar in their muscles, their mitochondria (the cells' power stations) showed signs of dysfunction, and the mitochondrial respiratory rate was about 25 percent lower when compared to unmedicated runners.

Lipitor, a commonly prescribed statin, costs up to $110 per month, compared to red rice yeast, which is around $20 per month. They both reduce cholesterol and triglycerides. Red rice yeast may give you a little gas, but patented statin drugs can cause a host of dangerous side effects. Yet when your doctor discovers that you have high cholesterol, he or she will prescribe the statin drugs. Most doctors don't even know what red rice yeast extract is, and if they do know, odds are they would not prescribe it to you. In fact, they could not legally prescribe it because the FDA does not allow them to do so.

The Case for and against Ephedra

Efforts are currently under way to effectively ban all vitamins and natural herbal supplements in the United States that do not have a doctor's prescription. Whenever a natural supplement causes an adverse reaction, it is quickly banned. Earlier, I explained how genetically modified l-tryptophan had caused many deaths, and because natural tryptophan was doing a better job than drugs such as Prozac, Paxil, and Zoloft, this was used as a pretext to ban all natural tryptophan in the United States.

A Chinese herb called ma huang (ephedra) was far superior to many prescription drugs for alleviating allergies, hay fever, and asthma and was extremely beneficial at promoting quick weight loss. Ephedra is also a stimulant similar to caffeine, and some people died from abusing it by taking dosages far in excess of the amount recommended. The FDA used this as a pretext to ban ephedra several times, even though it would have been very easy to instead require a warning label and limit the dosage to a single ephedra pill. Makers went to court each time and, after a lengthy legal fight, had the ban removed by a judge. One judge rightfully stated that the FDA actually needed to show that ephedra was dangerous when the recommended dose was taken, as opposed to dangerous only when someone took an extremely excessive dose.

The FDA's Double Standard Regarding Side Effects

The FDA is the gatekeeper that determines which drugs and herbs can make a health claim, and it costs $60 million to get through the gate. Because natural herbs and plants cannot be patented, there is no incentive to spend $60 million to prove they work. If a company spent $60 million to prove to the FDA that vitamin C helps cure colds, that company would not get an exclusive patent to the vitamin. Other companies that did not spend $60 million would also be able to make a health claim. Along with its bias favoring patent medicines, the FDA downplays many severe side effects caused by patented drugs, whereas natural herbs are held to a stricter standard regarding side effects. The FDA acts to protect this pharmaceutical monopoly by helping to exclude safe, cheap, natural cures from the marketplace. It is the police force that makes this whole system legally possible.

The Gardisil Controversy

Compare what happens when a few people die from taking an excessive dose of a natural herb to what happens when children die from taking the proper dose of a patented vaccine. The vaccine Gardisil is given to teenage girls and is alleged to help prevent cervical cancer. According to the CDC's own website, Gardisil has been linked to 71 deaths (other sources put the number of deaths at more than 100), and other reports have documented thousands of permanent debilitating adverse reactions. Despite the deaths and the permanent disabilities, the CDC states that "based on all the information we have today, the CDC recommends HPV vaccination for the prevention of most types of cervical cancer." Meanwhile, there are questions about whether Gardisil actually prevents cervical cancer at all. An article titled "A Pap Smear Never Harmed Anyone" quotes Dr. Diane Harper, the lead developer of Gardisil. According to the article, Harper stated that "Pap screening with vaccination does NOT lower your chances of cervical cancer—Pap screening and vaccination lowers your chances of an abnormal Pap test." Furthermore, the article states that Gardisil is proved to last at least five years, meaning if there is any benefit, it appears to be only temporary.

According to a July 7, 2012, article in *Natural Health 365* titled "HPV Vaccine Is a Danger to Girls (and Boys)," "as of May 12, 2012, the Vaccine Adverse Event Reporting System (VAERS) showed that there have been 28,050 adverse events" post-HPV vaccination. Given that the National Vaccine Information Center estimates that only between 1 and 10 percent of those injured by vaccines report the event to VAERS, the true number of children harmed by the HPV vaccine could be much higher. According to the article, "a Gardasil vaccine is only good on four types of HPV virus and there 150 types with at least 40 of them capable of being passed from person to person." The article also claims that in one study, in a sub group of 12,852 women who had been vaccinated, HPV-16 infections were reduced by only 0.6 percent. The article concludes that "clearly, the vaccine has a high health risk with little reward."

If a natural supplement company marketed a product claiming to prevent cervical cancer, and that natural product prevented only an abnormal Pap test and killed even a few girls, that supplement would have been taken off the market after the first few deaths, and the owners of the company would be in jail and sued out of existence. In the world of the current medical monopoly, however, 71 to 100-plus dead teenage girls and more than 28,000 documented adverse eventsis simply considered business as usual. The good thing for the makers of vaccines is that they get special liability protection, so when a vaccine kills or disables a child, they do not really have to worry about a huge lawsuit. Remember that the drug Vioxx was linked to at least 27,000 cardiac deaths, and the drug Avandia was found to increase heart attacks 43 percent.

Dangerous Side Effects from Patented Drugs
Most natural herbs are safe to use because they do not cause adverse reactions in the human body. Natural herbs cannot be patented, however, so there is only a fair profit to be made from selling them. In contrast, many patented pharmaceutical drugs are sold for more than twenty times what it costs to make them. In addition, like many artificial substances, most pharmaceutical drugs are highly toxic. When scientists analyzed more than 5,600 pharmaceutical drug labels, they found that the average pharmaceutical drug comes with a list of 70 potential adverse reactions. The most commonly prescribed drugs average around 100 potential adverse side effects.

The drugs prescribed by your doctor are responsible for approximately 700,000 emergency visits per year, due to adverse reactions. There are approximately 106,000 deaths per year due to people taking pharmaceutical drugs that are both properly prescribed and properly administered. Those 70-plus side effects are often deadly.

Natural herbs are usually nontoxic and more effective than pharmaceutical drugs. For example, valerian root is claimed to be more effective than valium, 1-tryptophan is said more effective than Prozac, and cannabis is more effective than Marinol. The reason they are not prescribed is because they do not have FDA approval. The reason they do not have FDA approval is because it costs around $60 million to do the testing the FDA requires before a doctor can prescribe a drug or an herb to treat disease.

The Cure for Cancer
In the United States, we spend more than $210 billion a year on cancer treatment. When you consider that there are 5,754 hospitals in the United States, $210 billion equates to more than $36 million spent on cancer treatment per U.S. hospital each

year. If we reduced cancer by 77 percent, or nearly $28 million per hospital, many hospitals would surely close, some pharmaceutical companies would be out of business, oncologists would see their incomes plummet, and the cancer charities might even lose much of their income, because with a 77 percent reduction in cancer, many people might say that we won the "war on cancer." The day that people realize that 80 to 90 percent of cancer is preventable and that their doctors and the cancer charities are not informing them about the facts is the day the cancer charities are out of business. We do not need to "find the cure"; we simply need to avoid getting cancer in the first place, and we already know how to achieve this.

If we eliminate artificial foods and follow the recommendations suggested in the Four Seasons Diet, it will reduce not only cancer rates, but also the incidence of all other major diseases. If we then allow for the fair use of natural herbs to treat the few remaining diseases, the entire health-care system as we know it will collapse. Most doctors would be out of business, along with most pharmaceutical companies, especially if cannabis were allowed to be used to its full potential.

Vitamin D3 to Prevent Cancer

Other vitamins and minerals have the ability to stop disease from developing in the first place. More than eight hundred studies show that vitamin D has the potential to prevent cancer. A study conducted at Creighton University School of Medicine found that supplementing your diet with 1,400 to 1,500 mg per day of calcium plus 1,100 IU of vitamin D3 (it's important to take D3 and not D2) per day reduces a women's cancer risk by 77 percent! Odds are, your doctor is not going to tell you to make sure to get calcium and vitamin D3 as a way to prevent cancer, yet if there was an expensive patented pill on the market that had numerous side effects but prevented 77 percent of cancers, every doctor would probably prescribe it to his or her patients.

You would think that all of the cancer charities that collect hundreds of millions of dollars a year in donations and grants to help "find the cure" would be excited and would spend some of that money on getting the word out that we should take our vitamin D3 and have our vitamin D levels tested. Sadly, this is about the last thing you can ever expect them to do. The cancer charities are a huge business in America, and the day "the cure" is actually found is the day they are out of business. Just as doctors rely on disease to get rich, the cancer charities need cancer to keep the donations rolling in. Note that 80 to 90 percent of cancer is completely preventable if we make diet and lifestyle changes. The most important steps you can to take prevent cancer are to eat only natural foods and avoid processed foods and foods grown with artificial chemicals, along with getting out in the sun or taking vitamin D3 supplements.

The media repeatedly warn woman to get their mammograms. This puts money into the pockets of the medical establishment, so doctors and hospitals advocate regular mammograms. Yet instead, there should be a national campaign to make sure all Americans get adequate levels of vitamin D, with a special emphasis on people living in the more northern areas of the United States or those with darker skin who do not produce as much vitamin D naturally.

The FDA Targets Dr. Burzynski and His Cancer Treatment

The FDA works as the police force for the medical cartel, which helps ensure that any cheap and effective cures that could hurt the cartel are quickly put out of business. A good illustration of this is what happened to a doctor in Texas named Dr. Burzynski. I recommend that you look up a movie on the Internet that covers the details of his ordeal. Dr. Burzynski has a cancer treatment that is highly effective and completely nontoxic. The treatment he invented, called antineoplastons, is so effective that it often cures brain tumors that are normally 100 percent fatal. Even though his treatment was far more effective than anything conventional medicine had to offer, mainstream doctors claimed he was a "quack" and told their patients not to see him. Burzynski is anything but a quack. One FDA-supervised clinical trial for a deadly form of childhood brain cancer called brainstem glioma found that in children treated with "conventional" radiation and chemotherapy, only 1 out of 107 (.9 percent) was cancer free after the initial treatment, and none lived more than five years. All 107 of those poor children had to endure the horrors of chemotherapy and radiation, yet died anyway. In contrast, 40 children were treated with Burzynski's antineoplastons, and 11 were cancer free after treatment (27.5 percent); those same 11 children (27.5 percent) were still alive after five years.

Conventional medicine offered a 0.9 percent success rate after initial treatment and a zero percent success rate after five years, compared to Burzynski's 27.5 percent initial success rate and 27.5 percent success rate after five years. In addition, his treatments are completely nontoxic, so the children who did not survive did not have to suffer, as did the children who received conventional chemotherapy and radiation.   You would almost expect to see him on the cover of a magazine, being proclaimed a miracle cancer doctor who cured children of incurable cancer. A National Cancer Institute scientist who reviewed Burzynski's work stated that he had never seen anything as amazing at shrinking brain tumors. To have a documented success rate of 27.5% percent for a type of cancer that is normally fatal 100 percent of the time really is quite miraculous.

Yet instead of ending up on a magazine cover, Dr. Burzynski was relentlessly harassed by the government for more than fifteen years. The State of Texas and the U.S. government spent more than $60 million of the taxpayers' money during a fifteen-year period trying to take away his medical license and throw him in jail. Initially, the Texas Medical Board, allegedly under pressure from the FDA, spent five years filing complaint after complaint against the doctor. The board approached many of his patients, trying to get them to file a complaint, but his patients knew that Burzynski was a saint, and not one gave in to government pressure to file a complaint. Sixty of them did sign a petition against the government, stating that they wanted the government to stop harassing the doctor who had cured their children of a type of cancer that is not supposed to be curable. The Texas Medical Board filed several actions against Burzynski but lost every time, because it did not provide any evidence that Dr. Burzynski's treatments were not safe and effective. After losing its case in front of the medical board, the State of Texas next took him to district court and even to the Texas Supreme Court. The FDA was putting pressure on Texas to take away Burzynski's license. This is a common tactic of the FDA when it comes to going after doctors who threaten the current medical monopoly. When the State of Texas lost, the FDA decided to take him to court next, but now it was trying to put him in jail, not simply take away his license. When the FDA lost that fight, it informed Dr. Burzynski that it had "other ways" to get him.

The FDA then began to convene grand jury investigations, trying to find a way to destroy Burzynski. We know that at least four grand juries were convened, but the number could be as high as six, because a few of them may have been called in secret without Dr. Burzynski's knowledge. For the government to convene even three grand jury investigations against one person without filing charges is unheard of, but to convene four to six goes beyond anything considered reasonable in the legal world. While this was happening, Dr. Burzynski was still curing children of incurable cancer, but the government was trying to stop him from treating those children, even as their tumors were shrinking. The parents of these children were beyond livid. They had been told by conventional doctors that their children had a zero percent survival rate, yet Dr. Burzynski was curing their children's cancer, and the FDA was trying to pull the plug on those kids in mid-treatment, effectively signing their death warrants.

When parents scream, Congress sometimes listens, and this time it did. In 1996, congressional hearings were held to review the way that the FDA was harassing Dr. Burzynski. Yet even though Congress came down hard on the FDA during the hearings, this did not stop the FDA. A week after the hearings, the FDA charged Dr. Burzynski with seventy-five counts of violating federal law, as well as fraud. If found guilty, Dr. Burzynski would face up to 290 years in prison and more than $18 million in fines. His only crime was that his treatment threatened the $210 billion a year cancer industry. When the FDA can't throw people in jail or take away their licenses, another tactic it often uses is to attempt to bankrupt them. In this case, the FDA spent $60 million in taxpayer money trying to throw Dr. Burzynski in jail for the rest of his life. Although Dr. Burzynski was found innocent of all charges, he still had to spend $2.2 million defending himself.

Next, the National Cancer Institute claimed that it was going to test his therapy and came up with what are called "protocols" for the testing. Protocols are the agreements that describe how the experiments are to be conducted. Because Dr. Burzynski was the one who invented the treatment and refined it during a twenty-year period, he was the only one who knew how to effectively treat patients with his drugs. He was adamant that the NCI follow his protocol, and the NCI agreed. The NCI claimed for more than a year, however, that it was unable to find patients to sign up for the study. Then the NCI changed the protocol without consulting with Dr. Burzynski or even telling him. The NCI changed it in such a way that it was doomed to fail. This is another common tactic the government uses to claim that alternative medical treatments and natural herbal cures are not effective. It designs the studies in such a way that the alternative treatments are guaranteed to fail, and this is done on purpose. In fact, Li-Chuan Chen, an NCI scientist who had worked on the Burzynski study, admitted that in the past whenever the NCI studied alternative cancer therapies, it always altered the protocols in such a way to ensure that they would fail. According to Chen, the NCI did this in order to discredit the therapy.

When Dr. Burzynski found out that the agreed-on protocols had been changed, he was naturally upset. When he reviewed the study data, he found that the NCI had severely diluted the medicines in their study to the point that blood levels of one of the therapeutic ingredients called phenylacetate was 2.7 times lower than in patients who had received the treatment from Dr. Burzynski. Another of the therapeutic ingredients called phenylacetylglutamine was 36 times lower than in patients receiving treatment from Dr. Burzynski, and a third ingredient called phenylacetylisoglutamine was 169 times lower in two of the nine NCI study patients, while 7 of 9 patients had no detectable levels of this critical component of Dr. Burzynski's treatment in their system. Dr. Burzynski knew that based on the low level of medication being given, the treatments were doomed to fail. The NCI then declared that Dr. Burzynski's treatments did not work.

The government's next actions were perhaps the most shameful part of its fifteen-year crusade against him. The U.S. Department of Health and Human Services proceeded to file eleven patents for Dr. Burzynski's treatments. They were all copycat patents, because Dr. Burzynski already held the patents for his treatments. The U.S. Department of Health and Human Services was obviously trying to steal his cancer therapy and knew that if it could throw him in jail or bankrupt him, he would not be able to fight the department for stealing his life's work. Once HHS stole his patents, its plan was probably to turn them over to a pharmaceutical company, as it had done in the case of Taxol, the government-funded cancer therapy. The FDA really works for the pharmaceutical companies, and former FDA director of drugs Dr. Richard Crout stated that "I never have and never will approve a new drug to an individual but only to a large pharmaceutical firm with unlimited finances." America is supposed to be the place where the little guy has a fair chance to beat the big guys, but when it comes to pharmaceutical drugs, the little guy will never be allowed to succeed as long as the FDA gets its way. The reward for the little guy who makes a better treatment in the United States is jail time or bankruptcy.

Sadly, there are many stories such as Dr. Burzynski's in the United States. The unique thing about his story is that he did not end up in jail. Usually, the FDA ends up bankrupting these doctors, and once they are bankrupt, they are easy to throw into jail because they cannot afford to adequately defend themselves.

There are numerous cases of companies selling natural herbs and vitamin supplements being raided by SWAT teams of more than fifteen officers, with their automatic weapons drawn. As they storm the small mom-and-pop businesses, they act as if they are raiding a major illegal drug cartel headquarters that is selling cocaine or another illegal drug, instead of natural herbs that are completely legal to sell. In most cases, the raids occur because the small businesses simply stated that a certain herb has been shown to help with a particular condition, or they linked their websites to other websites that displayed a scientific study showing that the herb has been proved to cure a certain disease.

Earlier, I mentioned that red rice yeast extract has been shown to reduce cholesterol and is far less expensive and much safer than pharmaceutical statin drugs. Yet even though multiple research studies have demonstrated this health benefit, if you look online at the companies selling red rice yeast extract, you'll be hard-pressed to find any of them claiming that it lowers cholesterol. If a company made this health claim, its place of business would likely be raided by a SWAT team; its supplements, files, computers, and furniture would be confiscated; and the owners would be thrown in jail, while the FDA proceeded to use its deep pockets to bankrupt the owners to the point that they could not hope to ever defend themselves. For simply daring to link their website to a valid study or make truthful statements about a natural herb or plant, their lives could quickly be ruined.

Crime and Fraud in Big Pharma
Meanwhile, pharmaceutical companies that have engaged in fraud, illegal kickbacks, price-setting, bribery, and other such activities have not been subject to such Gestapo-style raids. Pharmaceutical companies have been found guilty of defrauding the government under the False Claims Act more than any other industry has. According to a recent *New York Times* article titled "Glaxo Settles Cases with U.S. for $3 Billion," the pharmaceutical company GlaxoSmithKline (GSK) settled litigation brought against it by the U.S. government for $3 billion. While this is a large fine, it is one that the extremely profitable pharmaceutical companies are capable of paying. GSK was charged for illegally marketing its diabetes drug Avandia, giving kickbacks to doctors, and manipulating the medical research about its drug. Recall that Avandia is the drug

shown in one analysis to increase a patient's chance of having a heart attack by 43 percent and of cardiac-related death by 64 percent. One report has linked as many as 83,000 heart attacks to this drug.

This is why I believe we are living in the "Medical Dark Ages." If you sell a natural product such as red rice yeast extract that lowers cholesterol and you dare to mention its health benefits, you will incur the full wrath of the FDA. Yet if you sell a pharmaceutical drug linked to 83,000 deaths, while allegedly engaging in multiple illegal business activities, no worries—just pay a fine you can easily afford and go off to market your next drug.

GSK is not the only pharmaceutical company accused of these types of business practices. A study done by the Public Citizen's Health Research Group reported its findings in a December 16, 2010, article titled "Rapidly Increasing Criminal and Civil Monetary Penalties against the Pharmaceutical Industry: 1991 to 2010." The study found that "of the 165 settlements comprising $19.8 billion in penalties during this 20-year interval, 73% of the settlements (121) and 75% of the penalties ($14.8 billion)" were levied against the pharmaceutical companies. Four of those companies (GSK, Pfizer, Eli Lily, and Schering-Plough) accounted for more than half of those penalties. The study also found that "deliberately overcharging state health programs, mainly Medicaid fraud, has been the most common violation against state governments and is responsible for the largest amount of financial penalties levied by these governments."

The pharmaceutical companies have been accused of just about every type of crime and fraud you could imagine. The short list includes bribery, fraud, obstruction of justice, illegally promoting a drug for a use that it has not been approved for, illegal kickbacks, covering up data that showed their drugs to be harmful, price setting, bribery, and more. Although any of these activities would throw you or me in jail, these executives are often "punished" in a way that would not seem like punishment to us. For example, when Omnicare was accused of receiving kickbacks from Johnson and Johnson for recommending Johnson and Johnson drugs, Omnicare became the subject of both a federal lawsuit and a suit by eighteen states. Omnicare was also accused by a former executive of defrauding Medicare and Medicaid. The CEO of Omnicare resigned and was paid $130 million on parting ways with the company. Compare this "punishment" to what the FDA did to Dr. Burzynski for curing children who had incurable brain cancer; the FDA spent $60 million of taxpayer money trying to bankrupt him and put him in jail for 290 years.

Although I could list numerous mom-and-pop vitamin and natural food business owners who were threatened with jail time for simply conveying truthful information about their products or linking to a website that conveyed truthful information, I am not aware of any executive at GSK, Pfizer, Eli Lily, or Schering-Plough who was sentenced to jail, despite his or her part in the reported $19.8 billion fraud against the U.S. government and the American people. Many of these pharmaceutical executives actually end up running various governmental agencies that are in charge of overseeing pharmaceutical companies. Conversely, many government officials who help these executives avoid jail time often end up trading their government jobs for extremely lucrative jobs at one of the various pharmaceutical companies.

In 1999, the FDA lost a landmark Supreme Court case called Pearson v Shalala, which was supposed to allow dietary supplement companies to make health claims that have been supported by credible science. The FDA has almost completely ignored that ruling, however, and continues to target supplement companies that make claims they are supposed to be allowed to make. The new tactic is to throw the owners in jail and take away their inventory of supplements, which effectively puts them out of business so that they cannot pay their legal bills. Most companies are now simply too afraid to make any health claims, even though the Supreme Court has said it is protected speech.

What Happened in Europe: A Cautionary Tale
The FDA and the pharmaceutical companies consider it a problem that the public currently has the freedom to buy herbs, vitamins, and other supplements without a doctor's prescription. Plans are currently underway to legally prevent you from buying these natural products unless you have a doctor's permission. It may sound crazy that such a thing would even be possible in America, but these people are smart and shrewd. They have all of the power (unless the people finally say, "Enough!") and will stop at nothing to outlaw natural supplements. To grasp how the FDA plans to outlaw all herbs, you need to understand what has been happening in Europe.

In 2004, Europe passed the "Traditional Herbal Medicinal Products Directive." Under this directive, which took effect in 2011, each and every herbal product must have prior authorization (that is, a license) before it can be sold in the European Union. The cost for each license is between $127,000 and $190,000 for each and every herbal product. Let's say, you sell peppermint tea. Natural peppermint is now considered a controllable herb, so if you want to sell natural peppermint tea or any other type of natural peppermint, you will have to pay up to $190,000 for a license. If you are a tea company or an herbal company selling other herbs, you will need to pay the same licensing fee for those herbs as well. For instance, if you sell ten types of natural herbs, you will have to pay up to $1.9 million for the right to sell those natural products. If you grow peppermint in your yard, you may now be breaking the law in Europe.

The other thing the European law does is make it illegal to sell any herbs that may be of benefit for a "serious disease." The law does not define what a "serious disease" is, so odds are, down the road, all diseases will be classified as "serious," and all herbal products taken off the market. The law also allows herbs to be sold only for a purpose for which they have been used for at least thirty years, effectively eliminating the ability to bring new herbs into the European market as new uses are discovered for them. If you make an artificial peppermint flavoring that uses artificial dyes and coloring, however, you are exempt from paying the license fee; only natural products need to pay the fee.

As ridiculous as it sounds to think of natural peppermint as a potential drug that could be outlawed if it is found to treat a "serious disease," in fact studies show that natural peppermint has many medicinal properties, such as helping in the treatment of cancer and providing relief to those who suffer from irritable bowel syndrome. The patent drug companies know this, of course, and they stand to make billions by outlawing natural peppermint and coming up with their own synthetic versions of peppermint's healing components.

As usual, when the government takes away a fundamental right, it does so under the pretext of protecting the public. In the case of the Traditional Herbal Medicinal Products Directive, the European Union claims that "the simplified registration procedure aims to safeguard public health"; however, there has not been a problem caused by herbs that is affecting public health, and there is no explanation for why a seller of natural herbs needs to pay a $190,000 licensing agreement per herb. If you make pesticides, herbicides, or other potentially dangerous chemicals, there is no need to pay a license fee, and no new regulations were established to protect the public. The real danger appears to be only those plants and herbs that have been used medicinally for thousands of years without incident. This is clearly an attempt by the pharmaceutical industry to rid Europe of safe, cheap, and effective natural herbs, once and for all.

The FDA's Ongoing Attempts to Outlaw Natural Cures

The pharmaceutical companies love this European law and are looking to do the same thing here in the United States. This is the reason corporations have been spearheading the effort to create governments that are not truly elected by the people. Although members of Congress are elected by the people, FDA bureaucrats are effectively appointed by industry. The FDA operates as a "revolving door," where pharmaceutical and GMO executives often go to work for the FDA, making regulatory decisions that directly affect their industries and even their former companies. When they have served their time at the FDA, they may return to work for those same pharmaceutical companies, sometimes earning millions in the process.

FDA Wants Prescriptions Required for High Doses of Vitamins

Most Americans are not aware that the FDA has already tried several times to effectively outlaw most vitamins. In 1973, the FDA attempted to pass regulations requiring a doctor's prescription to purchase vitamins whose dosage was more than 1.5 times the U.S. recommended daily allowance (RDA). The U.S. RDA for vitamins and minerals is extremely low; for example, the RDA for vitamin C is only 60 mg, so 90 mg would have been the maximum dosage that could have been sold under the new FDA rule without a doctor's prescription. Vitamin C is usually sold in at least 1,000 mg dosages, because studies show that low doses of vitamin C (below 250 mg) do not prevent or help cure colds. Even if you take vitamin C after you get a cold or the flu, a study titled "The Effectiveness of Vitamin C in Preventing and Relieving the Symptoms of Virus-Induced Respiratory Infections" found that taking mega doses of vitamin decreased cold and flu symptoms by 85 percent. Yet if a manufacturer of vitamin C tried to cite the study in its advertising or even link to the website that displayed the study, the manufacturer would probably end up in jail. Meanwhile, many doctors cite the studies done on only very low doses (250 mg and less) of vitamin C, which show no cold or flu benefits from vitamin C.

A study published in the *Lancet* titled "Relation between

Plasma Ascorbic Acid and Mortality in Men and Women in EPIC-Norfolk Prospective Study: A Prospective Population Study. European Prospective Investigation into Cancer and Nutrition" looked at the effect vitamin C has on several chronic diseases. The study examined 19,496 men and women between the ages of forty-five and seventy-nine during a four-year period in relation to plasma vitamin C levels and mortality from diseases such as cancer and heart disease. The study found that those with the highest quintile of plasma vitamin C levels had half the risk of mortality when compared to those with the lowest quintile during the four-year study period. Those who had plasma vitamin C levels equivalent to consuming an extra 50 grams of fruits and vegetables per day had a 20 percent reduction in all causes of mortality. As much as the patent medicine companies would love to invent a pill that could reduce cancer and heart disease mortality by 50 percent, nature has already done that, and those vitamin C pills are very affordable precisely because nature invented them and they cannot be patented. The pharmaceutical companies simply cannot compete against the healing power of Mother Nature, so they instead try to make it illegal for us to purchase those high-dose vitamin C pills.

In addition, it's been known for many years that 1,000 mg of vitamin C per day can help keep your cholesterol levels healthy and can even reduce high cholesterol. A research article titled "Effect of Ascorbic Acid on Plasma Cholesterol in Humans in a Long-Term Experiment" found that three months of vitamin C supplementation lowered high cholesterol levels. The truth is that large doses of vitamin C are extremely effective in preventing and treating the common cold and keeping cholesterol levels in a healthy range, which is the reason the FDA and pharmaceutical industries want vitamins, or at least large doses of vitamins, outlawed. Imagine a world where you could simply buy your vitamin C at the health food store, you rarely caught a cold, your cholesterol levels stayed healthy, and you reduced your risk of cancer and heart disease by 50 percent. You would require no more trips to the doctor, no more prescription drugs to reduce your cholesterol, and no more antibiotics to treat your cold; all of these expenses could be replaced by the low cost of taking high doses of vitamin C. By the way, if you supplement with vitamin C, make sure to buy a better brand that contains "bioflavonoids," because vitamin C is far more effective when it is consumed with these important cofactors. This ability of large doses of natural herbs and supplements to prevent and treat disease is the reason the FDA tried to make it illegal to sell them without a doctor's prescription.

Heavy-Handed Tactics of FDA Commissioner Kessler

There was a huge public outcry against these efforts, and the FDA was forced to back down. In 1990, Congress passed the Nutrition Labeling and Education Act (NLEA), which gave the FDA authority to approve disease prevention claims for all food and dietary supplements. Then FDA commissioner David Kessler began to implement plans that appeared to attack nutritional supplements on the grounds that they were illegal food additives that must be removed from the market. It really seemed as if the FDA was getting ready to ban vitamin and nutritional supplements, and the public reacted with outrage in 1994. Congress listened and passed the Dietary Supplement Health and Education Act of 1994 (DSHEA), which took away much of the FDA's ability to regulate supplements.

A lot of the public outrage was aimed at what were called extremely heavy-handed and arrogant tactics on the part of Commissioner Kessler. The FDA and the pharmaceutical industries usually learn from their mistakes, so now they are taking a more European-style approach to banning all supplements, by simply regulating them out of existence. In the United States, there is a huge difference between the laws passed by Congress, which answers to the people, and how those laws are implemented by the FDA, which is run by the pharmaceutical and GMO companies and answers to them.

For example, the Dietary Supplement Health and Education Act (DSHEA), which was passed by Congress when the FDA tried to outlaw vitamins in the 1990s, states some "findings" of Congress. It reads like something I would have written. For example, the DSHEA stated that

> "The importance of nutrition and the benefits of dietary supplements to health promotion and disease prevention have been documented increasingly in scientific studies."

> "There is a link between the ingestion of certain nutrients or dietary supplements and the prevention of chronic diseases such as cancer, heart disease, and osteoporosis."

"Clinical research has shown that several chronic diseases can be prevented simply with a healthful diet."

"Healthful diets may mitigate the need for expensive medical procedures, such as coronary bypass surgery or angioplasty."

"There is a growing need for emphasis on the dissemination of information linking nutrition and long-term health."

"The nutritional supplement industry is an integral part of the economy of the United States."

"Although the Federal Government should take swift action against products that are unsafe or adulterated, the Federal Government should not take any actions to impose unreasonable regulatory barriers limiting or slowing the flow of safe products and accurate information to consumers."

"Dietary supplements are safe within a broad range of intake, and safety problems with the supplements are relatively rare."

So far, I agree 100 percent with everything Congress has to say in the DSHEA. When Congress passed this law in 1994, the commissioner of the FDA was reported to have been furious. The FDA thought it was just about to outlaw all natural supplements, but when the American people revolted, Congress passed the very fair and reasonable DSHEA. The next part of the law recognizes the fact that natural ingredients currently in use should be allowed to be used, and that if a new ingredient is added to a natural supplement, the FDA should be "notified." Specifically, the DSHEA says the following:

"A dietary supplement which contains a new dietary ingredient shall be deemed adulterated under section 402(f) unless it meets one of the following requirements."

A "new dietary ingredient" (NDI) is defined as

"a dietary ingredient that was not marketed in the United States before October 15, 1994 and does not include any dietary ingredient which was marketed in the United States before October 15, 1994."

Furthermore, a "new dietary ingredient" shall be considered adulterated unless it meets one of the following requirements:

"The dietary supplement contains only dietary ingredients which have been present in the food supply as an article used for food in a form in which the food has not been chemically altered."

"There is a history of use or other evidence of safety establishing that the dietary ingredient when used under the conditions recommended or suggested in the labeling of the dietary supplement will reasonably be expected to be safe and, at least 75 days before being introduced or delivered for introduction into interstate commerce, the manufacturer or distributor of the dietary ingredient or dietary supplement provides the Secretary with information, including any citation to published articles, which is the basis on which the manufacturer or distributor has concluded that a dietary supplement containing such ingredient will reasonably be expected to be safe."

Recall that the original finding of fact stated that "the Federal Government should not take any actions to impose unreasonable regulatory barriers limiting or slowing the flow of safe products and accurate information to consumers." When you read the law and the language contained the "New Dietary Ingredient" (NDI) disclosure section, the intent is very clear. If a manufacturer is going to introduce a completely new ingredient into the market, it needs to disclose that information, along with any studies or other information it has that shows that the product is safe. It is quite clear that the manufacturer is simply to "disclose" information about a new product, and that this is not an "approval" process.

The FDA Redefines "New Ingredient"

Since this bill was passed in 1994, the FDA has been looking for a new way to outlaw natural supplements. It appears that the FDA is attempting to twist this plain language, which simply requires that the secretary of Health and Human Services be notified of new ingredients. The FDA has recently published its "draft" guidelines for the New Dietary Ingredient disclosure and has turned it into an "approval process," with the FDA acting as the gatekeeper, rather than a simple "disclosure process." Furthermore, the FDA has expanded the definition of what a "new ingredient" is, far beyond what any reasonable person would deem to be a new ingredient. The intent of the FDA is once again to outlaw all natural supplements, by declaring all supplements "new ingredients."

For example, if you increase the dose of a certain nutrient beyond the levels you used in 1994, the FDA could consider that a new ingredient. Many new techniques have been invented since 1994 that are superior at extracting nutrients from natural herbs. Even though they are extracting the same herbal compounds as before, and there has not been a single safety concern, the FDA now considers this to be a new ingredient. Simply cooking or baking a natural herb in a new way means it's now a new ingredient, according to the FDA, and requires a manufacturer to go through the NDI process. Even changing the agricultural methods used to grow a plant can mean it's now an NDI, according to the FDA. Sprouting a seed or naturally fermenting a plant product will also mean the FDA may consider it an NDI. Furthermore, if a manufacturer finds that an herb is more potent during a different stage of its life cycle, the FDA will say it's an NDI. If a manufacturer used to pick a certain herb after it flowered but now picks the same herb before it flowers, it's now a NDI. Also, using a different part of an herb means it's now an NDI. If a manufacturer once used the leaves but now uses both the leaves and the stems of an herb, it's now considered an NDI.

Consider how ludicrous this is, in light of what you learned about GMOs. A GMO company can insert new genes into a plant so that it produces toxins, which many studies show to have potentially very serious health effects, but when it comes to GMOs, the FDA claims,

> *"The agency is not aware of any information showing that foods derived by these new methods differ in any meaningful or uniform way."*

Yet if someone finds that a certain herb grows better through the use of new farming practices, the FDA now considers it an NDI, and the herb will be considered "adulterated" and illegal, unless the manufacturer conducts expensive testing or produces other evidence to the FDA's liking, even though Congress specifically intended the NDI process to be a "notification" process and not an "approval" process. The purpose of the "notification" was simply to inform the government of any new ingredients, and if the government felt there was a concern, the burden was supposed to be on the government to prove there was an issue. The assumption was supposed to be that natural plants were usually considered safe. In a world ruled by the FDA, however, if a GMO company inserts fish genes into a tomato, it is considered safe and no testing is required by the FDA. Yet if an herbal farmer finds a new and better way to grow an herb, say by using fish fertilizer (a fertilizer made from the remains of processed fish), the herb is considered an NDI and will be deemed "adulterated" by the FDA, unless expensive safety testing is done. This is the world Rockefeller created, and this is the insanity under which we all live.

The FDA's New Testing Requirements
The information that the FDA will now require will simply force many companies producing natural supplements out of business, which is the whole purpose of the FDA requiring this new testing in the first place. According to the FDA's own website, following are some of the studies the FDA may now require to prove natural herbs that are grown or processed in a new way are safe.

For natural herbs, the FDA may now require a two-study genetic toxicity battery, a three-study genetic toxicity battery, a 14-day range-finding oral study in animals, a 90-day sub-chronic oral study in animals, a one-generation rodent reproductive study, a multigeneration rodent reproductive study, a teratology study in animals, a one-year chronic toxicity or a two-year carcinogenesis study in animals, a single-dose tolerability and/or an ADME study in animals and/or humans, a repeat-dose tolerability and/or an ADME study in animals and/or humans.

So let's say you have been producing an herbal supplement with 500 mg of a certain herb since 1980. If you suddenly decide to increase the dose of that herb to 600 mg, the FDA may now consider it an NDI and may require one or many of these expensive tests to prove it's safe. If you're a GMO company, however, and you produce a whole new genetic species of a plant that contains DNA from viruses, bacteria, fish, or some other animal, you are exempt from any and all testing because the FDA states that

> *"The agency is not aware of any information showing that foods derived by these new methods differ in any meaningful or uniform way."*

As long as the FDA, which is essentially run by the pharmaceutical and GMO companies, has any oversight over natural herbal supplements, it will continue to perversely manipulate the system in order to get rid of as many natural herbs and supplements as possible.

The FDA claims on its website that "the purpose of the reproductive toxicity studies is to provide information regarding the effects of a dietary ingredient on all aspects of reproduction, including sexual behavior, spermatogenic and estrus cycles, gonadal function, fertility, parturition, lactation, and pre-natal development." So the FDA feels that if you grow an herb that's been shown to be safe for thousands of years in a new way or increase the dose from 500 mg to a new higher dosage, there is reason to be concerned about the effects on reproduction, yet if you create a new GMO species that has never existed, there is no need to conduct studies to see whether the GMO might affect reproduction. Meanwhile, a mountain of evidence has demonstrated that GMOs cause potential serious adverse reproductive effects, such as pigs being fed GMOs giving birth to "bags of water" or cows being fed GMOs becoming infertile. Yet there has never been a single case of a farmer growing an herb in some new way that has resulted in that herb causing even the slightest adverse health effect.

The FDA looks after the GMO companies and the pharmaceutical companies, and getting rid of natural herbal products helps these large businesses. The FDA has rigged the system once again by defining what constitutes a "grandfathered" supplement as narrowly as possible, while defining what constitutes a "new ingredient" as liberally as possible. The result is that almost all new supplements will be claimed to have "new ingredients" in them, which could require the companies to conduct expensive testing that simply is not warranted. The FDA turned what was supposed to be a simple "notification" process into an elaborate and expensive "approval" process, even though this is clearly not the way Congress wrote the law. Growing an herb in a new way has never harmed nature, whereas GM corn has been accused of killing off Monarch butterflies.

Suggestions for the U.S. Congress
One simple thing Congress could do in the public interest would be to require the GMO and pharmaceutical companies to disclose that they are about to conduct a study prior to beginning it and then require those companies to disclose the results of the studies, even if the results are not favorable. Lately, in the news, there have been so many cases of pharmaceutical drugs that have been on the market for years and that were later found to be harmful; they were then pulled from the market after causing serious injury and numerous deaths. In many of these cases, the drugs probably never would have been allowed on the market had the companies not been able to hide studies that were unfavorable to their products.

Placebos and the Art of Deception
Another way industry often rigs its studies is by using a placebo, which may help companies gain the results they want. Although most people think of a placebo as a "sugar pill," in actuality there are no standards for what constitutes a placebo. Companies are free to choose any placebo they want, and they are not required to disclose what placebo they used in their study. A study conducted at the University of California titled "What's in Placebos: Who Knows? Analysis of Randomized, Controlled Trials," found that only around 8 percent of the studies that were analyzed actually disclosed what the placebo used in a study was composed of. This means that a drug company can pick a placebo that may alter the experiment in its favor. Once again, this problem would be easy to solve if Congress simply passed a law requiring studies to disclose what placebo was used.

According to new research done at Harvard Medical School and published in an article titled "Placebos without Deception: A Randomized Controlled Trial in Irritable Bowel Syndrome," placebos may actually be as effective at treating irritable bowel disease as the most powerful patented medicines peddled by the pharmaceutical companies, even when the patients are told they are being given a placebo. Doctors know that placebos are often more effective than any drug the pharmaceutical companies have to offer, and according to one study ("Prescribing 'Placebo Treatments': Results of a National Survey of US Internists and Rheumatologists"), an estimated 50 percent of doctors secretly give placebos to their patients. In the Harvard experiment, patients with irritable bowel syndrome were given either no treatment or sugar pills that were honestly labeled "placebos," with no active ingredients. After three weeks, nearly twice as many patients who had received the placebo sugar pills reported adequate symptom relief, when compared to the patients who did not receive the placebos. In fact, the placebo pills improved the patients' symptoms by roughly the same degree as the most powerful medications currently available for irritable bowel syndrome.

The chapter on GMOs contains much of the research that shows that GMOs can potentially punch holes in your gut, so perhaps GMOs are contributing to irritable bowel syndrome. When people get irritable bowel disease, they go their doctors, who prescribe a patented medicine, which is as effective as if the doctors had prescribed a sugar pill and told the patients they were getting a sugar pill. Of course, the average pharmaceutical drug has more than seventy side effects, so the sugar pill is probably a much better choice.

Given how powerful the mind is at treating disease and what is known about the "placebo effect," some experts even speculate that drugs may outperform placebos in many studies simply because of all of the drugs' toxic side effects (an average of seventy per drug). Their logic is that because most people know that pharmaceutical drugs have many adverse side effects, when people in an experiment are told they are being given either a placebo or the actual drug, and when those who are given the actual drug begin to feel its toxic effects, they rightly assume they have been given the drug. Then, in a similar fashion to the way "the placebo effect" works, those who realize from all of the side effects that they got the drug actually report benefits because, in the same way that the mind can heal the body due to the placebo effect, the mind may actually heal the body if it knows it got "the drug" and believes in the drug. The real benefit of many pharmaceutical drugs may simply lie in people's belief that they work.

One recent study titled "The Effect of Treatment Expectation on Drug Efficacy: Imaging the Analgesic Benefit of the Opioid Remifentanil" examined what would happen to a patient receiving pain medication through an IV drip who was told the pain medication had been stopped, when in fact it had not. In the experiment, heat was applied to patients' legs to cause pain, and then a painkiller was added to an IV drip while the patients' level of pain was assessed. Patients were told that the pain medication was added to the IV drip, and, as expected, their level of pain dropped significantly. Next, the subjects were told that the pain medication had been stopped, when in fact it had not been stopped, and the effect was that the patients' pain returned to the original level.

So giving patients a sugar pill and telling them it's a sugar pill can cure disease, while giving patients pain medication and falsely telling them the medication has been taken away causes the pain to return. Clearly, the mind seems to be having a greater effect than the actual pharmaceutical drugs, in many cases, and the pharmaceutical industry clearly understands this fact. This is one reason why, in the current "Medical Dark Ages" under which we live, we are told that herbal cures are worthless and that only patented chemicals can cure us. In many cases, the mind is causing the healing, not the drug, so if you believe the lie about patented drugs, you may in fact be healed due to your belief in the lie.

Depression

A *60 Minutes* segment titled "Treating Depression" interviewed Irving Kirsch, who is the associate director of the placebo study at Harvard. Dr. Kirsch has been studying placebos for thirty-six years and stated that sugar pills can work miracles for many diseases, such as irritable bowel syndrome, ulcers, and Parkinson's disease. Dr. Kirsch found that the pharmaceutical companies had been publishing their research on antidepressants that showed only favorable results for their drugs, and they were not publishing studies that showed their drugs to be ineffective. Using the Freedom of Information Act, Dr. Kirsch requested the FDA to provide him with the studies done on antidepressants that had not been published. When he compared both the published and the newly acquired unpublished studies, it turned out that the antidepressants were no better at treating mild to moderate depression than a placebo is.

I would argue that the placebo is better, because it treats mild to moderate depression as well as the pharmaceutical drug, without all of the toxic side effects.

The Ineffectiveness of Most Prescription Drugs

According to an article in the *Independent* titled "Glaxo Chief: Our Drugs Do Not Work on Most Patients," a senior executive with GlaxoSmithKline (GSK) named Allen Roses stated that most prescription drugs do not work on most people who take them. Dr. Roses said that "the vast majority of drugs—more than 90%—only work in 30 or 50 percent of the people." Yet drug companies sell $11.3 billion' worth of antidepressants a year, and they are taken by 17 million Americans, most of whom believe they are effective at treating depression. The truth appears to be that they are effective for mild to moderate depression, but only to the same extent that sugar pills are effective. This $11.3 billion a year potential health fraud scheme, much of it taxpayer funded, is allowed to occur, thanks in large part to FDA policies. The FDA requires a drug company to show that its drug is more effective than a placebo in only two clinical trials. So if eight studies show that it is not as effective as a placebo, and two studies show it is more effective (a 20 percent success rate), according to the FDA the drug is effective. The drug companies then publish the two successful clinical trials but do not publish the eight that were complete failures. The result is that even though the scientific evidence shows that antidepressants are only as effective as sugar pills, the FDA claims that because two of ten studies showed that they work, then they work. Because only those two studies are published, doctors and the American public are led to believe the drugs are effective.

Saint-John's-Wort for Depression
Meanwhile, safe, cheap, and effective herbal remedies, such as Saint-John's-wort, are not allowed to advertise the fact that multiple studies prove that they are an effective treatment for depression. For example, a meta-analysis titled "St. John's Wort for Depression—An Overview and Meta-Analysis of Randomized Clinical Trials," in the August 3. 1996, *BMJ* (formerly, *British Journal of Medicine*), reviewed twenty-three randomized trials done on extracts of Saint-John's-wort as a treatment for depression. Remember that expensive and potentially toxic pharmaceutical antidepressants were found to be only as effective as sugar pills (placebos). According to this meta-analysis, however, Saint-John's-wort was found to be "significantly superior to placebo."

A study titled "Comparison of St. John's wort and Imipramine for Treating Depression: Randomized Controlled Trial," which was conducted in Germany, looked at the difference between treating depression with Saint-John's-wort and imipramine, a common antidepressant. The study found that Saint-John's-wort treated depression just as well as the imipramine; however, the Saint-John's-wort was "tolerated" better by patients. One of the biggest advantages of natural herbs is that they are much less toxic and cause far fewer negative reactions in people than patented drugs do. In this study, only 3 percent of the patients taking Saint-John's-wort had to discontinue its use due to adverse events, while 16 percent of those taking the patented drug had to stop taking it, due to adverse events. The adverse events from the patented drug included dry mouth, dizziness, nausea, headaches, and asthenia (weakness).

A review of clinical studies on Saint-John's-wort conducted at the University of Vienna, titled "Hypericum Perforatum—A Review of Clinical Studies," reached similar conclusions. It stated that Saint-John's-wort "has undergone rigorous scientific investigation, and its effectiveness has been shown in studies comparing it with placebo and preference antidepressants. Safety and tolerability studies have revealed that St. Johns wort (SJW) preparations have better safety and tolerability profiles than synthetic antidepressants."

A study conducted in Germany titled "Equivalence of St. John's Wort Extract (Ze 117) and Fluoxetine: A Randomized, Controlled Study in Mild-Moderate Depression" compared Saint-John's-wort to the patented drug fluoxetine in the treatment of mild to moderate depression. The study found that "hypericum (St. Johns wort) safety was substantially superior to fluoxetine, with the incidence of adverse events being 23% on fluoxetine and 8% on hypericum." The adverse events for the patented drug were also far more serious than those for the natural Saint-John's-wort. For example, the only negative reaction to Saint-John's-wort, which occurred in more than 2 percent of users, was GI (gastrointestinal) disturbances. Conversely, the patented drug caused far more serious reactions in more than 2 percent of the users, such as dizziness (4%), tiredness (3%), anxiety (3%), erectile dysfunction (3%), GI disturbances (6%), and vomiting (4%). The study also found that Saint-John's-wort was superior at treating depression. The study concluded that "although hypericum (St. Johns wort) may be superior in improving responder rate, the main difference between the two treatments is safety. Hypericum was superior to fluoxetine in overall incidence of side-effects, number of patients with side-effects and the type of side-effect reported."

The Dangers of Pharmaceutical Antidepressants

Although Saint-John's-wort has been found to be superior to placebos, pharmaceuticals are only as good as placebos at treating mild to moderate depression and have a host of potentially deadly side effects. A study done at Emory University found that patented pharmaceutical antidepressants caused a thickening of the main arteries in the neck that feed blood to the brain. It's not surprising that many studies have determined that certain antidepressants can increase your risk of death from both heart attack and stroke. A study titled "Antidepressant Use and Risk of Incident Cardiovascular Morbidity and Mortality among Postmenopausal Women in the Women's Health Initiative Study" found that the class of antidepressants called serotonin reuptake inhibitors was associated with an almost 40 percent increased risk of stroke and a 64 percent higher risk of death from stroke.

A study published on January 15, 2009, in the *New England Journal of Medicine* titled "Atypical Antipsychotic Drugs and the Risk of Sudden Death" analyzed the risk of sudden cardiac death among users of antipsychotic drugs. It found that "current users of typical antipsychotic drugs had an adjusted rate of sudden cardiac death that was twice that for nonusers." Other risks commonly associated with antidepressants are a doubling of the risk of suicide, a doubling to tripling of the risk of diabetes, a 20 percent higher risk of bone fracture, and a 30 percent higher risk for spinal fracture. An April 7, 2006, BBC article titled "Anti-Depressant Stillbirth Link" reported on a study done in Canada on five thousand mothers who had used antidepressants. It found that mothers who used antidepressants were twice as likely to have stillbirths, twice as likely to have low-birth-weight babies, and nearly twice as likely to have premature births. The same article also referenced a Danish study that "found the use of the drugs in the first three months of pregnancy was linked to a 40% increase in risk of birth defects such as cleft palate."

Evidence-Based Medicine?
Most doctors believe they are practicing what is called "evidence-based" medicine and that the evidence shows that patented drugs are superior to herbs, because this is the lie they are told in medical school, thanks to Rockefeller and the FDA.

Saint-John's-Wort versus Prescription Antidepressants
Let's recap the "evidence" when it comes to patented antidepressants vs. herbal Saint-John's-wort. The evidence shows that

1. The most popular antidepressant patented drugs prescribed by

most doctors in the United States work only as well as sugar pills at treating mild to moderate depression.

2. Saint-John's-wort was found in a meta-analysis of twenty-three randomized trials and published in the *BMJ* to be "significantly superior to placebo."

3. Studies that compare natural Saint-John's-wort to unnatural patented antidepressants show that Saint-John's-wort is more effective at treating depression, with many fewer side effects, and the side effects from Saint-John's-wort are also far less severe. One study concluded that "St. Johns wort preparations have better safety and tolerability profiles than synthetic anti-depressants," while another stated that the main difference between the patented drug and the natural herb was safety; the natural herb is far safer.

4. Patented antidepressants have been shown to significantly increase the risk of stroke, sudden heart attacks, birth defects, and still births. In comparison, natural Saint-John's-wort has been found to cause mild GI disturbances in about 2 percent of users.

Here is how "evidence-based" medicine in the United States works, thanks to Rockefeller and the FDA. You go to your doctor because you are depressed, and your doctor prescribes one of the common patented antidepressants to you. Your doctor most likely believes the patented drug works, because the FDA says it does. In many ways, your doctor is a victim just as you are, because he or she has been taught untruths in medical school and lied to by the FDA. So you get your prescription filled for an antidepressant, many of the most popular of which cost around $225 per month. Meanwhile, you could have bought a bottle of Saint-John's-wort for about $10, and the evidence clearly shows Saint-John's-wort is more effective than the expensive patented drugs and doesn't have all of the adverse side effects. The drug companies are making billions of dollars in profit for a product that is only as effective as a cheap sugar pill.

Fake Surgery and the Power of the Mind
Americans are not only paying for these expensive and relatively ineffective drugs, but they are also paying for costly surgeries that seem to be no more useful than a "fake surgery" or a "placebo surgery." A study published in the *New England Journal of Medicine* titled "A Controlled Trial of Arthroscopic Surgery for

Osteoarthritis of the Knee" reported on an experiment in which patients with osteoarthritis of the knee were given either real arthroscopic surgery or a fake placebo surgery. Those who received the fake surgery simply had an incision made on their knees, while a simulated fake surgery was performed without the arthroscope being inserted, and then the incision was closed up. Patients were kept on the operating table for the same amount of time a real surgery would have taken, to fool them into believing they had received the real surgery. It turns out that people who received the real surgery had about the same improvement rate as those receiving the fake surgery. The results of the study showed that both groups improved, but that the improvement appears to have been a result of the power of the mind and not due to the surgery. The "evidence" in this case clearly shows that it's the power of the mind that causes the healing, not the surgery, yet surgeons rake in hundreds of millions of dollars a year on real surgeries, which appear to be no more effective than fake surgeries.

Although most doctors believe they are practicing a type of medicine that has been validated by science, the truth appears to be that many of the drugs they prescribe do not even work. In addition, patients who knowingly get a sugar pill often experience superior results, compared to those who receive pharmaceutical drugs, because placebos and patented drugs have similar success rates at treating certain diseases, and at least sugar pills do not cause the toxic side effects that pharmaceutical drugs do. Unfortunately, a drug company can have its drug fail thirty studies, but as long as it can pass two, the FDA will consider it a success and will allow the company to market the drug as such.

It appears as though many doctors do not treat disease much differently than the "witch doctors" of long ago did. If the mind is really responsible for the healing, rather than the drugs, as the evidence suggests, modern doctors are much more like witch doctors than they are likely to admit. When you consider that people who get "fake surgery" and sugar pills have the same success rates as people who get real surgery and real pills, you may begin to question the validity of Western medicine. There really is not much difference between ancient people who were healed by their belief in witch doctors and modern people who are healed by their belief in modern doctors, when they are given treatments that are no more effective than a sugar pill. If I were to give Western medicine a report card, I would give it an A grade for trauma medicine, a C or a D in cases where pharmaceutical drugs are used to treat disease, and an F for preventing disease.

False and Misleading Research Studies

Many doctors still believe that the type of medicine they practice is "evidence-based"; however, new research suggests that the conclusions of most research studies are actually false and misleading because researchers frequently manipulate data in a way that enhances their careers. Studies on this topic were conducted by a team led by John Ioannidis, who is considered one of the world's top experts on the credibility of medical research. Two of his research papers that address this issue are "Why Most Published Research Findings Are False" and "Contradicted and Initially Stronger Effects in Highly Cited Clinical Research."

According to the mathematical research done by Ioannidis, 80 percent of nonrandomized studies (the most common type) and 25 percent of what are called "gold standard" randomized trials are dead wrong in their findings. This is usually the result of bias on the part of the researchers, as well as manipulation of the data. According to an article in *Atlantic Magazine* titled "Lies, Damned Lies, and Medical Science,"

> researchers headed into their studies wanting certain results—and lo and behold they were getting them. We think of the scientific process as being objective, rigorous, and even ruthless in separating out what is true from what we merely wish to be true, but in fact it's easy to manipulate the results, even unintentionally or unconsciously. At every step in the process, there is room to distort results, a way to make a stronger claim or to select what is going to be concluded. . . . There is an intellectual conflict of interest that pressures researchers to find whatever it is that is most likely to get them funded.

Although doctors often claim the "peer review" process will prevent this from happening, Ioannidis found that the peer review process frequently serves to help suppress opposing views. The article quoted above states that "Scientists understand that peer review per se provides only minimal assurance of quality, and that the public perception of peer review as a stamp of authentication is far from the truth."

The article rightly points out that "Vioxx, Zelnorm, and

Baycol were among the widely prescribed drugs found to be safe and effective in large randomized controlled trials before the drugs were yanked from the market as unsafe or not so effective, or both." In addition to the majority of studies actually being flawed and "dead wrong" in their findings, Ioannidis also found that even when studies thought to be valid are later refuted and proven incorrect, "researchers continued to cite the original results as correct more often than as flawed—in one case for at least 12 years after the results were discredited." While a number of medical professionals reading this may shrug off Ioannidis's findings, many doctors are taking notice of the impeccable nature of his research. "His PLoS Medicine paper is the most downloaded in the journal's history. . . . he has published 1,328 papers with different co-authors at 538 institutions in 43 countries" and receives an estimated 1,000 invitations a year to speak at conferences and institutions around the world. I mention this because many of the doctors I know like to stick their heads in the sand when any scientific research questions the supposedly "infallible" nature of the current medical establishment. The truth is that the best studies actually now show that most medical science is fatally flawed and needs to be seriously fixed. Hopefully, the day is coming where people will look back on our current "Medical Dark Ages" and equate the era with something akin to the "bloodletting" and the use of "leeches" practiced by doctors for nearly two thousand years.

In addition to the "soft fraud" of researcher bias and manipulation of data, there have been many scandals lately concerning "hard fraud" in medical research. According to a 2010 article published in the Wall Street Journal titled "Mistakes in Scientific Studies Surge," since 2001 the number of research articles that have been retracted has "leapt more than 15-fold." In 2001, there were just 22 retraction notices, but by 2009, the number had increased to 339, with approximately 73 percent being retracted for simple errors, but nearly 27 percent being retracted for outright fraud. The article stated that "at the Mayo Clinic, a decade of cancer research, partly taxpayer-funded, went down the drain when the prestigious Minnesota institution concluded that intriguing data about harnessing the immune system to fight cancer had been fabricated." The article goes on to state, "'The stakes are so high,' said the Lancet's editor, Richard Horton. 'A single paper in Lancet and you get your chair and you get your money. It's all your passport to success.'"

The extent of the problem with medical research is further

highlighted in a January 5, 2012, article in the *BMJ* (formerly, the *British Medical Journal*) titled "Missing Trial Data Threatens the Integrity of Medicine." According to that article, "a large portion of evidence from human trials is unreported, and much of what is reported is done so inadequately." Not surprising, it was found that "including this unpublished data in published meta-analyses of drug trials often changes their results."

In a March 28, 2012, article in Reuters titled "In Cancer Science, Many 'Discoveries' Don't Hold Up," nearly 90 percent of cancer studies may not withstand scientific scrutiny. The article references a former researcher at Amgen Inc. named C. Glen Begley, whose lab replication team of about a hundred scientists decided to double-check the validity of certain cancer studies before Amgen invested potentially millions of dollars producing cancer treatments based on those studies. When Begley's team attempted to replicate fifty-three separate cancer studies, it found that forty-seven of them could not be replicated. The article quotes Ferric Fang of the University of Washington, who said he "blamed a hypercompetitive academic environment that fosters poor science and even fraud, as too many researchers compete for diminishing funding. . . . the surest ticket to getting a grant or job is getting published in a high profile journal. . . . this is an unhealthy belief that can lead a scientist to engage in sensationalism and sometimes even dishonest behavior."

We live under a medical system where doctors committing research fraud are rewarded with "chairs and money," while FDA officials who do the bidding of the pharmaceutical and GMO companies are often rewarded with huge paychecks by working for those industries when they leave government, and pharmaceutical executives who commit billions of dollars' worth of fraud are not prosecuted for their crimes and often receive multimillion-dollar golden parachutes when they are forced to resign.

Summary

Let's look at some of the "evidence" in this chapter, to determine whether we are living in a world where medicine is truly "evidence-based."

1. Up to one-third of all patented pharmaceutical drugs on the market were originally derived from natural plant sources that

cannot be patented. One example is statin drugs, which were originally taken from red rice yeast extract and then changed so that they could be patented.

2. When a patented drug is compared to the natural plant as a cure, the natural plant is most often as effective as, or more effective than, the patented drug at treating the same disease, is much less expensive, and, most important, usually does not have the same toxic side effects as the unnatural drugs that can be patented. The average artificial patented drug has an average of seventy potentially adverse side effects. If medicine were truly "evidence-based," you would expect doctors to look for safe natural herbs to treat their patients, rather than toxic pharmaceutical drugs. For example, in the case of red rice yeast extract, the evidence shows that it is as effective as statin drugs, without all of the toxic side effects, and at a fraction of the cost. In the case of Saint-John's-wort, the "evidence" shows it's actually more effective at treating depression than the patented antidepressants and much safer at the same time, yet costs less than 5 percent of what the patented drug costs. So if medicine were truly "evidence based," potentially toxic patented statin drugs and antidepressants would be illegal, and doctors would prescribe or recommend red rice yeast extract and Saint-John's-wort, because they do not require a prescription. Usually, only toxic patented drugs need a prescription, precisely because of their potentially toxic and harmful side effects. The fact that doctors prescribe expensive statin drugs and antidepressants, which have a huge range of potential side effects, while never mentioning the safer, cheaper red rice yeast extract or Saint-John's-wort, are just two out of many examples that modern Western medicine is not "evidence based." Because red rice yeast extract does not require a prescription, people could simply and cheaply have their cholesterol level tested without a doctor, and if their levels were high, they could buy some of the extract at the supplement shop. This is one of the real reasons doctors often oppose natural cures; they cannot be the gatekeepers of natural cures, because people can buy them without a prescription. Imagine a world where, if you're mildly depressed, you simply spend $10 a month on Saint-John's-wort, which has been proved to be more effective than sugar pills, rather than $250 a month on patented drugs that work only as well as sugar pills, not to mention possibly thousands of dollars visiting doctors, while you suffer the potentially toxic effects from taking the patented drugs.

3. Despite the fact that thousands of patented artificial drugs are derived from natural plant sources, and those plants usually work better at treating disease, due to their lower cost and lower toxicity when compared to the patented artificial drugs, natural herbs and drugs are not approved by the FDA to treat disease. In fact, at the turn of the century, cannabis was listed in the *United States Pharmacopeia* for more than a hundred medical uses, and even though it has more healing potential than any other drug or herb, it cannot be legally used to "treat" disease, because the FDA has never approved cannabis as a drug. The FDA has been waiting for pharmaceutical companies to find a way to patent various medicinal compounds in cannabis, which, as history predicts, will produce a far less effective, more expensive, and more toxic treatment than the cheap natural version.

4. The FDA is essentially run by pharmaceutical and GMO company insiders, and the system was designed to ensure that only expensive and potentially toxic artificial patented drugs can be claimed to treat disease, while affordable, nontoxic, natural herbal cures cannot be claimed to treat disease.

5. The FDA requires expensive clinical trials that cost an average of $60 million before it gives its approval to any herb or drug that is used to treat disease. It would makes sense to require this extensive testing for artificial patented drugs, because they are new compounds and are usually inherently toxic, in that they each averages seventy potentially adverse effects. It makes no sense to require this level of testing for natural herbal cures, because they have been used throughout history without causing serious side effects. In fact, humankind has spent thousands of years discovering which plants and herbs were toxic and which herbs cured disease.

6. Because herbs cannot be patented, no company will spend $60 million for the required FDA testing. This is because when the testing does prove that a natural herb cures disease, the company that spent the $60 million to prove it will not have an exclusive patent. Other companies that did not spend the $60 million would also be able to market the herbal cure, and the company that proved it works would probably go bankrupt, while the ones that did not spend the money to prove it works would make all of the profit. The

system has been rigged this way on purpose. The FDA knows no one will spend $60 million to prove an herbal cure is effective if he or she cannot get an exclusive patent in the process. This allows a great fraud to be perpetuated on the American taxpayer. Americans spend $11.3 billion a year on patented antidepressants that are only as effective as sugar pills, much of it paid for by taxpayers through Medicare and Medicaid. Rather than spend $11.3 billion on worthless patented antidepressants, the taxpayer could spend $565 million on Saint-John's-wort, which is actually effective at treating depression, for a savings of more than $10.7 billion a year. Given the tremendous cost savings to the U.S. government from just this one herb, you would expect the government to spend the $60 million to prove the effectiveness of Saint-John's-wort. It would be money well spent, given that every year the American taxpayer would save more than $10 billion. This is the beauty and the genius of Rockefeller's scheme, however; the drug companies get rich, while you get expensive, ineffective, and toxic treatments in the process.

7. This system enriches pharmaceutical companies at the expense of the consumer. FDA policies prevent people from making truthful health claims about affordable natural herbs, and doctors cannot legally prescribe them, which means consumers are kept in the dark about better alternatives, unless they do their own research.

8. Doctors make money only when people are sick and would be very poor if not for disease. The evidence shows that 80 to 90 percent of all disease is preventable with dietary and lifestyle choices, yet doctors receive only about four hours of education in medical school about what is essentially the most powerful medicine for keeping us healthy: affordable natural foods, free of unnatural chemicals and preservatives.

9. The American Medical Association worked with Rockefeller to close the medical schools that taught how to cure disease with natural herbal remedies. The Rockefeller Foundation and the FDA both serve the pharmaceutical industry, and their common enemy has always been natural plant products that cure disease safely, affordably, and effectively.

10. The number of students allowed to attend medical school each year is kept low, so that there are not enough doctors, which helps

increase the salaries of doctors by limiting competition. This was how Rockefeller got the AMA to buy into his scheme, according to many historians.

Although I have picked on doctors quite a bit in this chapter, I truly believe that most doctors are good people who care about their patients. Yet the truth is that many of the changes that are necessary to fix health care in the United States would drastically lower the salary of the average doctor, and I am just not convinced most doctors can honestly look at how fraudulent our current system of medicine is. It's hard for people or companies to admit that the product or the service they are selling might not be good for the consumer, especially if the truth jeopardizes their livelihood.

Many of the other changes that are necessary to fix our medical system would mean that the FDA and doctors would lose much of their "power," because they would give up their stranglehold on the truth. As the first Dark Ages taught us, those who control a corrupt system do not let go of their power easily.

A Medical Reformation

What is really needed in this country is a "Medical Reformation," in which natural cures are given preference over patented drugs and not the other way around. Remember that natural cures are better for most Americans because they are more effective, safer, and more affordable than patented cures. The problem is that the system is controlled by a small minority, who have a vested interest in promoting the patented cures, and they are not going to do what's best for most Americans, but what's best for themselves.

If the government allowed the truth to be told about Saint-John's-wort, and it could be used as a "treatment" for depression, the pharmaceutical companies would lose more than $11 billion a year in business, and they are not going to give up that money without a fight. If cannabis were legalized for all of its medical uses, the pharmaceutical companies could see a 25 percent reduction in business as many of their drugs immediately became obsolete. If medicine was based on prevention, and people eliminated processed and unnatural food from their diet, 80 to 90 percent of disease would disappear, and most doctors and hospitals would go bankrupt.

Imagine if most Americans adopted a diet similar to that of the older generation of Okinawans, the "primitive" people studied by Weston Price, or the people living in the Blue Zones. Obesity would disappear, along with most forms of cancer, diabetes, heart disease, and dementia, and people would live much higher-quality lives as they aged.

Some of the money we currently spend on doctors and drugs would instead go to pay for more nutritious natural food, free of chemical additives; however, there would be an overall huge cost savings. Billions of dollars currently spent on programs such as Medicare could instead be spent on other programs like education. The answer to our current problems does not require a government solution, however; it requires an individual solution.

We are all free to choose the foods we eat, and as more and more people begin to demand natural food, more companies will begin to produce natural food. If 100 percent of the public refused to buy foods containing GMOs, the GMO companies would be out of business overnight. We are also free to vote for politicians who oppose the FDA's stranglehold on health care. What is really needed is a new government agency whose purpose is to find a way to bring more natural medicine into the U.S. marketplace. This agency would have to be completely separate from the FDA. In fact, we would have to take away any oversight the FDA has over natural foods and supplements. The FDA was created to serve the pharmaceutical industry, and we cannot hope to reform the FDA because it is simply in bed with industry.

This new government agency would approve health claims for natural cures such as Saint-John's-wort and red rice yeast extract, and those natural cures would be free to compete with patented cures in the treatment of disease. As many people adopted a natural diet, and their diseases began to disappear, other people would soon follow and choose a similar diet.

America is at a cross-roads. The most likely outcome is that many people will wake up and realize that true health lies in natural foods and natural cures, while others remain asleep and eat toxic food and use toxic patented medicines to treat the diseases that result. Tanchou's doctrine states that cancer increases in direct proportion to the "civilization" of a people, and Weston Price traveled the globe to study "primitive" people and found that they were free of disease until they adopted a "civilized" diet. The current study of areas known as Blue Zones affirms what Weston Price discovered, which is that people who adhere to a natural diet, free of processed foods, have far superior health and much lower disease rates than do those who have a diet high in processed and artificial foods. Edmund Szekely conducted what he called "The Great Experiment" during a thirty-three-year period, which consisted of placing more than 123,000 people on a natural, unprocessed, "primitive"-style diet of mainly live foods. Even though approximately 17 percent of the participants in the Great Experiment had diseases that were considered incurable by medicine, the Great Experiment resulted in a 90 percent recovery rate from various diseases, simply by people eating natural foods.

A Call to Action

In the spirit of the Great Experiment, this book is the beginning of "The Natural Project," which can be found at TheNaturalProject. com. The Natural Project is an effort to document the amazing health transformations that can take place by simply adopting a natural diet, eliminating artificial and processed foods, and following the proper diet for your season-type. The hope is to develop local chapters of the Natural Project, to help people transform their diet and, in the process, transform their health.

Rather than spend time and money fighting the FDA, the medical establishment, and the rigged system of medicine set up by Rockefeller, the Natural Project will simply gather enough evidence to show that modern so-called evidence-based medicine is far inferior to simply eating natural foods and herbs. Medicine is the science or practice of diagnosing, treating, or preventing disease, and one way the FDA has rigged the system is to make it illegal for anyone to claim that a food or a natural product can "treat" or "prevent" anything. Even though evidence shows that eating natural foods and eliminating processed and artificial foods can both treat disease and prevent more than 90 percent of all diseases, it is against the law for anyone to make this claim without the FDA declaring it is so. Just as the Vatican controlled the truth in the first Dark Ages, the FDA controls the truth in the current Medical Dark Ages.

One purpose behind the Natural Project is simply to gather overwhelming evidence that documents, with pictures and historical accounts, the amazing transformations that can take place when you eliminate the artificial and replace it with the natural. We will not claim to treat or prevent disease, because if we did so, we would likely be raided by an armed SWAT team and have our computers and records confiscated. Rather, we will simply document the before-and-after transformations that take place when you adopt a natural diet, and we will leave it up to people viewing the evidence to come to their own conclusions about the ability of natural foods to treat and prevent disease.

I invite you to visit TheNaturalProject.com and learn more about this historic effort to transform the planet. If everyone chose to eat only natural foods and rejected artificial foods and chemicals, we would no longer have artificial pesticides and herbicides poisoning the environment we all share. The FDA, the pharmaceutical companies, and the GMO companies have been the proverbial tail wagging the dog for long enough. If enough people say yes to natural foods, it will mean the end of most diseases and an end to GMOs. You all have more power than you realize, and as a group, we have all the power—not the FDA and not the pharmaceutical and GMO companies.

It truly is time for a "Medical Reformation." I know that a world is possible where most disease is a thing of the past, and people live happy and productive lives. If you believe this is possible, too, please join us in our effort to transform the planet.

Visit TheNaturalProject.com.

Glossary

Term Used in Book	**Scientific Term**
Belly fat	Intra-abdominal fat or visceral fat
Blood fat	Free fatty acids
Blood recyclable sugar	Plasma lactate
Blood sugar	Blood glucose
Body fat	Adipose tissue
Carbohydrate/fat fuel ratio	Respiratory quotient
Energy currency	Two phosphate molecules
Energy debit card	Adenosine triphosphate
Fast sugar energy	Anaerobic glycolysis
Fat-burning muscles	Slow twitch muscles
Feel full hormone	Leptin
Hunger hormone	Ghrelin
Liver sugar	Liver glycogen
Low blood sugar	Hypoglycemia
Muscle fat	Intramuscular triglycerides
Muscle sugar	Muscle glycogen
Protein building blocks	Amino acids
Regular carbohydrates	Amylopectin
Resistant-carbohydrates	Amylose; resistant starch

Slow sugar energy	Aerobic glycolysis
Stored sugar	Glycogen, both liver anmuscle
Sugar building blocks	Monosaccharides
Sugar	Usually refers to glucose
Sugar-burning muscles	Fast twitch muscles
Turbo mode	Creatine-phosphate

Bibliography

Trademark acknowledgments:
StarLink® is a registered trademark of Aventis Crop Science.
Roundup® and Roundup Ready ® are registered trademarks of Monsanto Company.
NutraSweet® is a registered trademark of NutraSweet Property Holding Inc.
Splenda® is a registered trademark of McNeil Nutritionals, LLC.

BOOKS

American Academy of Orthopaedic Surgeons, Baltimore County UMBC. *Critical Care Transport.* Burlington, MA: Jones and Bartlett Publishers, 2001.

Anwar-Saad A, Abd-Elfattah, Wechsler AS. *Purines and Mycardial Protection.* New York: Springer, 1996.

Baynes J, Dominiczak MB. *Medical Biochemistry.* Philadelphia: Mosby, 1999.

Brown ER. *Rockefeller Medicine Men: Medicine and Capitalism in America.* Berkeley: University of California Press, 1981.

Bryson C. *The Fluoride Deception.* New York: Seven Stories Press, 2004.

Buettner D. *The Blue Zone.* Margate, FL: National Geographic Society, 2008.

Calbom C, Calbom J. *The Coconut Diet.* Boston: Wellness Central, 2006.

Campbell TC, Campbell II T. *The China Study.* Dallas: Benbella Books 2006.

Connett P. *The Case against Fluoride.* White River Junction, VT: Chelsea Green Publishing, 2010.

Daniel KT. *The Whole Soy Story: The Dark Side of America's Favorite Health Food.* Lanham, MD: New Trends Publishing, 2005.

Doll R, Peto R. *The Causes of Cancer: Quantitative Estimates of Avoidable Risks of Cancer in the United States Today.* New York: Oxford Press, 1981.

Eades MR, Eades MD. *Protein Power Life Plan.* New York: Grand Central Publishing, 2001.

Eades MR, Eades MD. *Protein Power.* New York: Bantam Books, 1999.

Emord J. *Global Censorship of Health Information.* New York: Sentinel Press, 2010.

Feder D, Bonom D. *The Skinny Carbs Diet.* Emmaus, PA: Rodale Books, 2010.

Frankel EN. *Lipid Oxidation,* 2nd ed. High Wycombe: Oily Press Ltd, 2005.

Garrett RH, Grisham CM. *Biochemistry*, 2nd ed. Independence, KY Brooks and Cole, 1999.

Gravenstein JS, Jaffe MB. *Capnography: Clinical Aspects: Carbon Dioxide over Time and Volume.* Cambridge, UK: Cambridge University Press, 2004.

Griesmacher, Chiba, Muller. *Purine and Pyrimidine Metabolism in Man,* IX. New York: Plenum Press, 1998.

Gunstone FD, Harwood JL, Padley FB. *The Lipid Handbook,* 2nd ed. London: Padley, Chapman & Hall, 1994.

Hargreaves M, Spriet L. *Exercise Metabolism,* 2nd ed. Champaign, IL: Human Kinetics, 2006.

Hauser MA, Baird NM. *The Hauser Diet.* Oak Park, IL: Beulah Land Press, 2007.

Herer J. *The Emperor Wears No Clothes.* Austin, TX: Ah Ha Publishing, 2006.

Hyman M. *Ultra-Metabolism.* New York: Simon and Schuster, 2006.

Ivy J, Portman R. *Nutrient Timing.* Laguna Beach, CA: Basic Health Publications, 2004.

Ivy J, Portman R. *The Performance Zone: Your Nutrition and Action Plan for Greater Endurance and Sports Performance.* Laguna Beach, CA: Basic Health Publications, 2004.

Johnson RJ, Gover T, Gollub E. *The Sugar Fix: The High Fructose Fallout That Is Making You Sick.* New York: Pocket Books, 2008.

Kunes E, Largeman-Roth F. *The Carb Lovers Diet.* Tampa, FL: Oxmoor House, 2010.

Larsson K, Quinn P, Sato K, Tiberg F. *Lipids: Structure, Physical Properties and Functionality.* High Wycombe, UK: Oily Press Ltd, 2006.

McArdle WD, Katch FI, Katch V. *Exercise Physiology: Energy, Nutrition and Human Performance.* Philadelphia: Lippincott Williams and Wilkins, 2007.

McKeown P. *Close Your Mouth.* Dublin: Asthma Care Ireland, 2004.

Nicolaou A, Kokotos G. *Bioactive Lipids.* High Wycombe, UK: Oily Press Ltd, 2004.

Pasupuleti VK, Anderson JW. *Nutraceuticals, Glycemic Health and Type 2 Diabetes.* Hoboken, NJ: Wiley-Blackwell, 2008.

Pennington JAT, Sprungen J. *Bowes & Church's Food Values.* Philadelphia: Lippincott Williams and Wilkins, 2009.

Phillis JA. *Adenosine and Adenine Nucleotides as Regulators of Cellular Function.* Boca Raton, FL: CRC Press, 1991.

Price WA. *Nutrition and Physical Degeneration.* La Mesa, CA: Price-Pottenger Nutrition Foundation, 2003.

Rakhimov Artour. *Dr. Buteyko Lecture "Moscow State University 1969."* Self-published e-book, www.normalbreathing.com.

Rakhimov Artour. *Normal Breathing.* Self-published e-book, www.normalbreathing.com.

Revici E. *Research in Physiopathology as a Basis of Guided Chemotherapy.* Princeton, NJ: D. Van Nostrand Company, 1961.

Robbins J. *Diet for a New America.* Tiburon, CA: H. J. Kramer, 1998.

Robbins J. *Healthy at 100.* New York: Random House, 2006.

Robbins J. *The Food Revolution.* Newburyport, MA: Conari Press, 2001.

Sanhita S. *The Esoteric Philosophy of the Tantras.* Calcutta: Heeralal Dhole, 1887.

Schenker G. *An Analytical System of Clinical Nutrition,* 5th ed. Mifflintown, PA: Nutri-Spec, 2010.

Smith JM. *Genetic Roulette.* Fairfield, IA: Yes Books, 2007.

Smith JM. *Seeds of Deception.* Fairfield, IA: Yes Books, 2003.

Spurway N, Wackerhage H. *Genetics and Molecular Biology of Muscle Adaptation.* Amsterdam: Elsevier, 2006.

Stalmatski A. *Freedom from Asthma.* New York: Three Rivers Press, 1997.

Stone TW, Simmonds HA. *Purines: Basics and Clinical Aspects.* Boston: Academic Publishers, 1991.

Taubes G. *Good Calories, Bad Calories.* New York: Anchor, 2008.

Taubes G. *Why We Get Fat.* New York: Alfred A. Knopf, 2001.

Vance DA, Vance JE. *Biochemistry of Lipids, Lipoproteins and Membranes,* 4th ed. Amsterdam: Elsevier, 2002.

Watson G. *Nutrition and Your Mind.* New York: Harper Row, 1972.

Whyte G. *The Physiology of Training.* Amsterdam: Elsevier, 2006.

Wiley R. *Biobalance 2.* Orem, UT: Essential Science Publishing, 2002.

Wiley R. *Biobalance.* Orem, UT: Essential Science Publishing, 1989.

Willey W. *Better Than Steroids.* Bloomington, IN: Trafford Publishing, 2007.

Wolcott W, Fahey T. *The Metabolic Typing Diet.* New York: Broadway Books, 2000.

JOURNAL ARTICLES

Abbott WG, Howard BV, Christin L, Freymond D, Lillioja S, Boyce VL, Anderson TE, Bogardus C, Ravussin E. Short-term energy balance: relationship with protein, carbohydrate, and fat balances. *American Journal of Physiology* 255(3 Pt. 1) (September 1988): E332–E337.

Abou-Donia MB, El-Masry EM, Abdel-Rahman AA, McLendon RE, Schiffman SS. Splenda alters gut microflora and increases intestinal p-glycoprotein and cytochrome p-450 in male rats. *Journal of Toxicology and Environmental Health* 71(21) (2008): 1415–1429.

Acheson KJ, Schutz Y, Bessard T, Anatharaman K, Flatt JP, Jequier E. Glycogen storage capacity and de novo lipogenesis during massive carbohydrate overfeeding in man. *American Journal of Clinical Nutrition* 48 (August 1998): 240–247.

Acheson KJ, Schutz Y, Bessard T, Ravussin E, Jequier E, Flatt JP. Nutritional influences on lipogenesis and thermogenesis after a carbohydrate meal. *American Journal of Physiology* 246(1 Pt. 1) (January 1984): E62–E70.

Achten J, Jeukendrup AE. Maximal fat oxidation during exercise in trained men. *International Journal of Sports Medicine* 24(8) (2003); 603–608.

Acka O, Doufas AG, Morioka N, Iscoe S, Fisher J, Sessler DI. Hypercapnia improves tissue oxygenation. *Anesthesiology* 97(4) (October 2002): 801–806.

Agrawal R, Gomez-Pinilla F. "Metabolic syndrome" in the brain: deficiency in omega-3 fatty acid exacerbates dysfunctions in insulin receptor signaling and cognition. *Journal of Physiology* 590 (May 2010): 2485–2499.

Ahlborg G, Felig P. Influence of glucose ingestion on fuel-hormone response during prolonged exercise. *Journal of Applied Physiology* 41 (November 1976): 5683–5688.

Air Pollutants Affecting the Performance of Domestic Animals. U.S. Department of Agriculture Handbook no. 380, August 1970, p. 41.

Akca O, Liem E, Suleman MI, Doufas AG, Galadiuk S, Sessler DI. Effect of intra-operative end-tidal carbon dioxide partial pressure on tissue oxygenation. *Anaesthesia* 58(6) (June 2003): 536–542.

Akhavan Tina, Anderson GH. Effects of glucose-to-fructose ratios in solutions on subjective satiety, food intake, and satiety hormones in young men. *American Journal of Clinical Nutrition* 86(5) (November 2007): 1354–1363.

Akiniwa K. Re-examination of acute toxicity of fluoride. *Fluoride* 30(2) (1997): 89–104.

Alanen P, Isokangas P, Gutmann K. Xylitol candies in caries prevention: results of a field study in Estonian children. *Community Dentistry and Oral Epidemiology* 28(3) (June 2000): 218–224.

Albertazzi P, Pansini F, Bonaccorsi G, Zanotti L, Forini E, De Aloysio D. The effect of dietary soy supplementation on hot flushes. *Obstetrics and Gynecology* 91(1) (January 1998): 6–11.

Alberti E, Hoyer S, Hamer J, Stoeckel H, Packschiess P, Weinhardt F. The effect of carbon dioxide on cerebral blood flow and cerebral metabolism in dogs. *British Journal of Anesthesiology* 47(9) (1975): 941–948.

Alexander JC, Valli VE, Chanin BE. Biological observations from feeding heated corn oil and heated peanut oil to rats. *Journal of Toxicology and Environmental Health* 21(3) (1987): 295–309.

Allain P, Gauchard F, Krari N. Enhancement of aluminum digestive absorption by fluoride in rats. *Res Commun Mol Pathol Pharmacol* 91(2) (February1996): 225–231.

Allred CD, Ju YH, Allred KF, Chang J, Helferich WG. Dietary genistein stimulates growth of estrogen-dependent breast cancer tumors similar to that observed with genistein. *Carcinogenesis* 22(10) (October 2001): 1667–1673.

Almashat S, Preston C, Waterman T, Wolfe S. *Rapidly Increasing Criminal and Civil Monetary Penalties against the Pharmaceutical Industry: 1991 to 2010.* Public Citizen's Health Research Group, December 16, 2010.

Anderson GH, Cho CE, Akhavan T, Mollard RC, Luhovyy BL, Finocchiaro ET. Relation between estimates of cornstarch digestibility by the Englyst in vitro method and glycemic response, subjective appetite, and short-term food intake in young men. *American Journal of Clinical Nutrition* 91(4) (April 2010): 932–939.

Anderson GH, Woodend D. Effect of glycemic carbohydrates on short-term satiety and food intake. *Nutrition Reviews* 61(5 Pt. 2) (May 2003): s17–s26.

Anderson JW, Bridges SR. Short-chain fatty acid fermentation products of plant fiber affect glucose metabolism of isolated rat hepatocytes. *Proceedings of the Society for Experimental Biology and Medicine* 177(2) (November 1984): 372–376.

Anderson RL, Wolf WJ. Compositional changes in trypsin inhibitors, phytic acid, saponins and isoflavones related to soybean processing. *Journal of Nutrition* 125(3 Suppl) (March 1995): 581S–588S.

Aris A, Leblanc S. Maternal and fetal exposure to pesticides associated to genetically modified foods in Eastern townships in Quebec, Canada. *Reproductive Toxicology* 31(4) May 2001): 528533.

Armandi BH, Birnbaum R, Goyal NV, Getlinger MJ, Juma S, Alekel L, Hasler CM, Drum ML, Hollis BW, Kukreja SC. Bone-sparing effect of soy protein in ovarian hormone-deficient rats is related to its isoflavone content. *American Journal of Clinical Nutrition* 68(6 Suppl) (December 1998): 1364S–1368S.

Assuncao ML, Ferreira HS, dos Santos AF, Cabral CR, Florencio TM. Effects of dietary coconut oil on the biochemical and anthropometric profiles of women presenting abdominal obesity. *Lipids* 44(7) (July 2009): 593–601.

Astrup A, Meinert LT, Harper A. Atkins and other low-carbohydrate diets: hoax or an effective tool for weight loss? *Lancet* 364(9437) (September 4–10, 2004): 897–899.

Babraj JA, Vollaard NBJ, Keast C, Guppy FM, Cottrell G, Timmons JA. Extremely short duration high intensity interval training substantially improves insulin action in young healthy males. *BMC Endocrine Disorders* 28(9) (January 2009): 3.

Bachinskii PP, Gutsalenko OA, Naryzhniuk ND, Sidora VD, Shliakhta AI. Action of the body fluorine of healthy persons and thyroidopathy patients on the function of hypophyseal-thyroid the system. *Probl Endokrinol* (Mosk) 31(6) (November–December 1985): 25–29.

Bahr R, Hansson P, Sejersted OM. Triglyceride/fatty acid cycling is increased after exercise. *Metabolism* 39(9) (September 1990): 993–999.

Barrett S, et al. Elements of Precaution: *Recommendations for the Regulation of Food Biotechnoloby in Canada. An Expert Panel Report on the Future of Food Biotechnology,* prepared by the Royal Society of Canada, January 2001.

Bartsch H, Nair J, Owen RW. Dietary polyunsaturated fatty acids and cancers of the breast and colorectum: emerging evidence for their role as risk modifiers. *Carcinogenesis* 20(12) (1999): 2209–2218.

Bassin EB, Wypij D, Davis RB, Mittleman MA. Age-specific fluoride in drinking water and osteosarcoma (United States) *Cancer Causes Control* 17(4) (May

2006): 421–428.

Basta G, Schmidt AM, De Caterina R.   Advanced glycation end products and vascular inflammation: implications for accelerated atherosclerosis in diabetes. *Cardiovascular Research* 63(4) (September 1, 2004): 582–592.

Baum JA, Teng H, Erdman JW, Weigel RM, Klein BP, Persky VW, Freels S, Surya P, Bakhit RM, Ramos E, Shay NF, Potter SM.   Long-term intake of soy protein improves blood lipid profiles and increases mononuclear cell low-density-lipoprotein receptor messenger RNA in hypercholesterolemic, postmenopausal women.   *American Journal of Clinical Nutrition* 69 (September 1998): 545–551.

Begley S.   "In Cancer Science, Many 'Discoveries' Don't Hold Up."   Reuters, Wednesday, March 28, 2012.

Behall KM, Howe JC. Effect of long-term consumption of amylose vs amylopectin starch on metabolic variables in human subjects. *American Journal of Clinical Nutrition* 61 (February 1995): 334–340.

Behall KM, Howee JC. Resistant starch as energy. *Journal of the American College of Nutrition* 15(3) (1996): 248–254.

Behall KM, Scholfield DJ, Yuhaniak I, Canary J.   Diets containing high amylose vs amylopectin starch: effects on metabolic variables in human subjects. *American Journal of Clinical Nutrition* 49(2) (February 1989): 337–244.

Belfort R, Mandarina L, Kashyap S, Wirefel K, Pratipanawartr T, Berria R, Defronzo RA, Cusi K.   Dose-response effect of elevated plasma free fatty acid on insulin signaling. *Diabetes* 54(6) (June 2005): 1640–1648.

Bentley EM, Ellwood RP, Davies RM.   Fluoride ingestion from toothpaste by young children. *British Dental Journal* 186(9) (May 8, 1999): 460–462.

Bergholm R, Westerbacka J, Vehkavaara S, Seppala-Lindroos A, Goto T, Yki-Jarvinen H.   Insulin sensitivity regulates autonomic control of heart rate variation independent of body weight in normal subjects. *Journal of Clinical Endocrinology & Metabolism* 86(3) (March 1, 2001): 1403–1409.

Bergstrom J, Hermansen L, Hultman E, Saltin B.   Diet, muscle glycogen and physical performance. *Acta Physiologica Scandinavica* 71(2) (October–November 1967): 140–150.

Berry EM.   Who's afraid of n-6 polyunsaturated fatty acids?   Methodological considerations for assessing whether they are harmful.   *Nutrition, Metabolism, and Cardiovascular Disease* 11(3) (June 2001): 181–188.

Berry MN.   The effects of adenine nucleotides on pyruvate metabolism in rat liver. *Biochemistry Journal* 95 (1965): 587.

Bingel U, Wanigasekera V, Wiech K, Mhuircheartaigh RN, Lee MC, Plonger M, Tracey I.   The effect of treatment expectation on drug efficacy: imagining the analgesic benefit of the opioid remifentanil. *Science Translational Medicine* 3(70) (February 16, 2011): 70ra14.

Bjornholt JV, Erikssen G, Aaser E, Sandvik L, Nitter-Hauge S, Jervell J, Erikssen J, Thaulow E.   Fasting blood glucose: an underestimated risk factor for cardiovascular death. *Diabetes Care* 22(1) (January 1999): 45–49.

Blom PC, Hostmark AT, Vaage O, Kardel KR, Maehlum S.   Effect of different post-exercise sugar diets on the rate of muscle glycogen synthesis. *Med Sci Sports Exerc* 19(5) (October 1987): 491–496.

Bocarsly ME, Powell ES, Avena NM, Hoebel BG.   High fructose corn syrup causes characteristic of obesity in rats: increased body weight, body fat and triglyceride levels. *Pharmacology Biochemistry and Behavior* (2010): doi:10.1016/j.pbb.2010.02.012.

Boden G, Chen X, Ruiz J, White JV, Rossetti L. Mechanisms of fatty acid–induced inhibition of glucose uptake. *Journal of Clinical Investigation* 93(6) (June 1994): 2438–2446.

Boden G, Jadali F, White J, Liang Y, Mozzoli M, Chen X, Coleman E, Smith C. Effects of fat on insulin-stimulated carbohydrate metabolism in normal men. *Journal of Clinical Investigation* 88(3) (September 1991): 960–966.

Boden G. Free fatty acids, insulin resistance, and type 2 diabetes mellitus. *Proceedings of the Association of American Physicians* 111(3) (May–June 1999): 241–248.

Boden G. Free fatty acids—the link between obesity and insulin resistance. *Endocrine Practice* 7(1) (January–February 2001): 44–51.

Bodinham CL, Frost GS, Robertson MD. Acute ingestion of resistant starch reduces food intake in healthy adults. *British Journal of Nutrition.* Epub ahead of print, October 27, 2009, doi: 10.1017/ S0007114509992534.

Bodinham CL, Frost GS, Robertson MD. The acute effects of resistant starch on appetite and satiety. *Proceedings of the Nutrition Society* 67(OCE) (2008): E157.

Brofman JD, Leff AR, Munoz NM, Kirchhoff C, White SR. Sympathetic secretory response to hypercapnic acidosis in swine. *Journal of Applied Physiology* 69(2) (August 1990): 710–717.

Bronfort G, Evans R, Anderson AV, Syendsen KH, Bracha Y, Grimm RH. Spinal manipulation, medication, or home exercise with advice for acute and subacute neck pain: a randomized trial. *Annuals of Internal Medicine* 156 (1 Pt. 1) (January 3, 2012): 1–10.

Brooks, Mercier. Balance of carbohydrates and lipid utilization during exercise: the crossover concept. *Journal of Applied Physiology* 76(6) (June 1994): 2253–2261.

Brown NF, Salter AM, Fears R, Brindley DN. Glucagon, cyclic AMP and adrenaline stimulate the degradation of low-density lipoprotein by cultured rat hepatocytes. *Biochemistry Journal* 262(2) (September 1, 1989): 425–429.

Burke LM, Collier GR, Davis PG, Fricker PA, Sanigorski AJ, Hargreaves M. Muscle glycogen storage after prolonged exercise: effect of the frequency of carbohydrate feedings. *American Journal of Clinical Nutrition* 64 (July 1996): 115–119.

Burnett AL. The role of nitric oxide in erectile dysfunction: implications for medical therapy. *Journal of Clinical Hypertension* 8(12 Suppl 4) (December 2006): 53–62.

Burzynski, the Movie: Cancer Is Serious Business, www.burzynskimovie.com.

Butler LM, Sinha R, Millikan RC, Martin CF, Newman B, Gammon MD, Ammerman AS, Sandler RS. Heterocyclic amines, meat intake, and association with colon cancer in a population-based study. *American Journal of Epidemiology* 157(5) (2003): 434–445.

Calderon J, et al. Influence of fluoride exposure on reaction time and visuospatial organization in children. *Epidemiology* 11(4) (July 2000): S153.

Carrithers JA, Williamson DL, Gallagher PM, Godard MP, Schulze KE, Trappe SW. Effects of postexercise carbohydrate-protein feedings on muscle glycogen restoration. *Journal of Applied Physiology* 88(6) (June 2000): 1976–1982.

Carroll KK, Kurowska EM. Soy consumption and cholesterol reduction: review of animal and human studies. *Journal of Nutrition* 125(3 Suppl) (March 1995): 594S–597S.

Chang HC, Doerge DR. Dietary genistein inactivated rat thyroid peroxides in vivo without an apparent hypothyroid effect. *Toxicology and Applied Pharmacology* 168(3) (November 1, 2000): 244–252.

Chang-Claude J, Frentzel-Beyme R, Eiber U.   Mortality pattern of German vegetarians after 11 years of follow-up. *Epidemiology* 3(5) (September 1992): 395–401.

Chavarro JE, Toth TL, Sadio SM, Hauser R.   Soy food and isoflavone intake in relation to semen quality parameters among men from an infertility clinic. *Human Reproduction* 23(11) (November 2008): 2584–2590.

Choi HK, Willett W, Curhan G.   Fructose-rich beverages and risk of gout in women. *Journal of the American Medical Association* (November 10, 2010): doi;10.1001/jama.2010.1638.

Christensen K, Smith A. *Does the Use of Cannabis Species for the Production of Biodiesel and Ethanol Result in Higher Yields of Ethanol Than Competing Cellulotic Crops, including Zea Mays? The Case of Hemp as a Biofuel.* Undergraduate students of the University of Washington, Department of Biology, 2008.

Cinader B, Clandinin MT, Hosokawa T, Robblee NM. Dietary fat alters the fatty acid composition of lymphocyte membranes and the rate at which suppressor capacity is lost. *Immunology Letters* 6(6) (June 1983): 331–337.

Civitarese AE, Hesselink MKC, Russell AP, Ravussin E, Schrauwen P.   Glucose ingestion during exercise blunts exercise-induced gene expression of skeletal muscle fat oxidative genes. *AJP Endocrinology* 289(6) (December 2005): E1023–E1029.

Clandinin MT, Cheema S, Field CJ, Garg ML, Venkatraman J, Clandinin TR. Dietary fat: exogenous determination of membrane structure and cell function. *FASEB Journal* 5(13) (October 1991): 2761–2769.

Clifford AJ, Story DL. Levels of purines in foods and their metabolic effects in rats. *Journal of Nutrition* 106 (1976): 435–442.

Cocco T, Di Paola M, Papa S, Lorusso M. Arachidonic acid interaction with the mitochondrial electron transport chain promotes reactive oxygen species generation. *Free Radical Biology and Medicine* 27(1–2) (July 1999): 51–59.

Cohn PD. *Fluoride and Osteosarcoma in New Jersey. An Epidemiologic Report on Drinking Water Fluoridation.* New Jersey Department of Health, November 1992.

Colomb BA, Erickson LC, Koperski S, Sack D, Enkin M, Howick J.   What's in placebos: who knows? Analysis of randomized, controlled trials. *Annals of Internal Medicine* 153(8) (October 19, 2010): 532–535.

Connor S. "Glaxo Chief: Our Drugs Do Not Work on Most Patients." *Independent,* December 8, 2003.

Cook JD, Reddy MB, Burri J, Juillerat MA, Hurrell RF. The influence of different cereal grains on iron absorption from infant cereal foods.   *American Journal of Clinical Nutrition* 65 (1997): 964–969.

Corps AN, Pozzan T, Hesketh TR, Metcalfe JC. cis-unsaturated fatty acids inhibit cap formation on lymphocytes by depleting cellular ATP. *Journal of Biological Chemistry* 255(22) (November 25, 1980): 10566–10568 .

Coyle EF, Coggan AR, Hemmert MK, Ivy JL. Muscle glycogen utilization during prolonged strenuous exercise when fed carbohydrate. *Journal of Applied Physiology* 61(1) (1986).

Coyle EF, Jeukendrup AE, Wagenmakers AJ, Saris WH. Fatty acid oxidation is directly regulated by carbohydrate metabolism during exercise.   *AJP Endocrinology* 273(2) (August 1997): E268–E275.

Crapo PA, Insel J, Sperling M, Kolterman OG. Comparison of serum glucose, insulin, and glucagon responses to different types of complex carbohydrates in noninsulin-dependent diabetic patients. *American Journal of Clinical*

Nutrition 34(2) (February 1981): 184–190.

Crouse JR, Morgan T, Terry JG, Ellis J, Vitolins M, Burke GL. A randomized trial comparing the effect of casein with that of soy protein containing varying amounts of isoflavones on plasma concentrations of lipids and lipoproteins. *Archives of Internal Medicine* 159(17) (September 27, 1999): 2070–2076.

Cumming RG, Klineberg RJ. Case-control study of risk factors for hip fractures in the elderly. *American Journal of Epidemiology* 139(5) (1994): 493–503.

Cummings SR, Rubin SM, Black D. The future of hip fractures in the United States, numbers, costs, and potential effects of postmenopausal estrogen. *Clinical Orthopaedics and Related Research* (252) (March 1990): 163–166.

Cybulska B, Naruszewicz M. The effect of short-term and prolonged fructose intake on VLDL-TG and relative properties of apo CIII1 and apo CII in the VLDL fraction in type IV hyperlipoproteinaemia. *Nahrung* 26(3) (1982): 253–261.

D'Urzo AD, Jhirad R, Jenne H, Avendano MA, Rubinstein I, D'Costa MD, Goldstein RD, Rubenstein I. Effect of caffeine on ventilatory responses to hypercapnia, hypoxia, and exercise in humans. *Journal of Applied Physiology* 68(1) (January 1990): 322–328.

Davidson TL, Swithers SE. A Pavolvian approach to the problem of obesity. *International Journal of Obesity and Related Metabolic Disorders* 28(7) (July 2004): 933–935.

Davidsson L. Approaches to improve iron bioavailability from complementary foods. *Journal of Nutrition* 133(5 Suppl 1) (May 2003): 1560S–1562S.

De Glisenzinski I, Harant I, Crampes F, Trudeay F, Felez A, Cottet-Emard JM, Garrigues M, Riviere D. Effect of carbohydrate ingestion on adipose tissue lipolysis during long-lasting exercise in trained men. *Journal of Applied Physiology* 84(5) (May 1998): 1627–1632.

Deivanayagam S, Mohammed BS, Vitola BE, Naguib GH, Keshen TH, Kirk EP, Klein S. Nonalcoholic fatty liver disease is associated with hepatic and skeletal muscle insulin resistance in overweight adolescents. *American Journal of Clinical Nutrition* 88(2) (August 2008): 257–262.

Dickinson KM, Keogh JB, Clifton PM. Effects of a low-salt diet on flow-mediated dilation in humans. *American Journal of Clinical Nutrition* 89(2) (2009): 485–490.

Diesendorf M, Colquhoun J, Spittle BJ, Everingham DN, Clutterbuck FW. New evidence on fluoridation. *Australian and New Zealand Journal of Public Health* 21(2) (1997).

Dillin A, Crawford D, Kenyon C. Timing requirements for insulin/IGF-1 signaling in C. elegans. *Science* 298(5594) (2002): 830–834.

DiMasi JA, Hansen RW, Grabowski HG. The price of innovation: new estimates of drug development costs. *Journal of Health Economics* 22(2) (March 2003): 151–185.

Disendorf M. Have the benefits of water fluoridation been overestimated? *International Clinical Nutrition Review* 10 (1990): 292–303.

Doerge DR, Chang HC. Inactivation of thyroid peroxidases by soy isoflavones, in vitro and in vivo. *Journal of Chromatography B* 777(1–2) (September 2002): 269–279.

Domino KB, Lu Y, Eisenstein BL, Hlastala BP. Hypocapnia worsens arterial blood oxygenation and increases VA/Q heterogeneity in canine pulmonary edema. *Anesthesiology* 78(1) (January 1993): 91–99.

Dorman JB, Albinder B, Shroyer T, Kenyon C. The age-1 and daf-2 genes function in a common pathway to control the lifespan of Caenorhabditis elegans. *Genetics* 141(4) (1995): 1399–1406.

Du L. The effect of fluorine on the developing human brain. *Zhonghua Bing Li Xue Za Zhi* 21(4) (August 1992): 218–220.

Duke J, Friedlin J, Ryan P. A quantitative analysis of adverse events and "overwarning" in drug labeling. *Archives of Internal Medicine* 171(10) (May 23, 2011): 944–946.

Editorial. Chronic fluorine intoxication. *Journal of the American Medical Association* 123(3) (1943):150-151.

Elliorr SS, Keim NL, Stern JS, Teff K, Havel PJ. Fructose, weight gain, and the insulin resistance syndrome. *American Journal of Clinical Nutrition* 76(5) (November 2002): 911–922.

Emdin M, Gastaldelli A, Muscelli E, Macerata A, Natali A, Camastra S, Ferrannini E. Hyperinsulinemia and autonomic nervous system dysfunction in obesity. *Circulation* 103 (2001): 513.

Epstein SS. Unlabeled milk from cows treated with biosynthetic growth hormones: a case of regulatory abdication. *International Journal of Health Services* 26(1) 1996): 173–185.

Espinal J, Dohm G, Newsholme E. Sensitivity to insulin of glycolysis and glycogen syntheses of isolated soleus-muscle strips from sedentary, exercised and exercise-trained rats. *Biochemistry Journal* 212 (1983): 453–458.

Evaluation of the Health Aspects of Soy Protein Isolates as Food Ingredients, 1979 SCOGS-101. Prepared for Bureau of Foods, Food and Drug Administration by Life Sciences Research Office, FASEB.

Fabbrine, et al. Alterations in fatty acid kinetics in obese adolescents with increased intrahepatic triglyceride content. *Obesity* (2008): doi:10.1038/oby.2008.494.

Fabricant DS, Farnsworth NR. The value of plants used in traditional medicine for drug discovery. *Environmental Health Perspectives* 109(Suppl 1) (March 2001): 69–75.

Farah V, Elased KM, Chen Y, Key M, Cunha TS, Aguiar JP, Pazzine M, Irigoyen MC, Morris M. High fructose diet in mice activates brainstem angiotensin AT1a and catecholaminergic systems. *FASEB Journal* 20 (2006): A300.

Felber JP, Golay A, Felley C, Jequier E. Regulation of glucose storage in obesity and diabetes: metabolic aspects. *Diabetes Metabolism Reviews* 4(7) (June 2009): 691–700.

Felton CV, Crook D, Davies MJ, Oliver MF. Dietary polyunsaturated fatty acids and composition of human aortic plaques. *Lancet* 344 (1994): 1195.

Fernstrom JD, Fernstrom MH. Tyrosine, phenylalanine, and catecholamine synthesis and function in the brain. *Journal of Nutrition* 137 (June 2007): 1539S–1547S.

Ferrannini E, Barrett EJ, Bevilacqua S, DeFronzo RA. Effect of fatty acids on glucose production and utilization in man. *Journal of Clinical Investigation* 72(5) (November 1983): 1737–1747.

Feskanich D, Willerr WC, Stampfer MJ, Colditz GA. Milk, dietary calcium, and bone fractures in women: a 12-year prospective study. *American Journal of Public Health* 87(6) (June 1997): 992–997.

File SE, Hartley DE, Elsabagh S, Duffy R, Wiseman H. Cognitive improvement after 6 weeks of soy supplements in postmenopausal women is limited to frontal lobe function. *Menopause* 12(2) (March 2005): 193–201.

Fischer K, Colomgani PC, Langhans W, Wenk C. Carbohydrate to protein ratio in food and cognitive performance in the morning. *Physiology and Behavior*

75(3) (March 2002): 411–423.

Flatt JP, Ravussin E, Acheson KJ, Jequier E. Effects of dietary fat on postprandial substrate oxidation and on carbohydrate and fat balances. *Journal of Clinical Investigation* 76(3) (September 1985): 1019–1024.

Fluoride Action Network. "Cities That Voted against Water Fluoridation," http://www.fluoridealert.org/breaking_news.aspx, accessed on 2/7/201.

Folsom AR, Ma J, McGovern P, Eckfeld J. Relation between plasma phospholipid saturated fatty acids and hyperinsulinemia. *Metabolism* 45(2) (February 1996): 223–228.

Ford ES, Bergmann MM, Kroger J, Schienkiewitz A, Weikert C, Boeing H. Healthy living is the best revenge: findings from the European prospective investigation into cancer and nutrition-Potsdam study. *Archives of Internal Medicine* 169(15) (August 10, 2009): 1355–1362.

Foster-Powell K, Holt SHA, Brand-Miller JC. International table of glycemic index and glycemic load values. *American Journal of Clinical Nutrition* 76(1) (2002): 5–56.

Frangioudakis G, Garrard J, Raddatz K, Nadler JL, Mitchell TW, Schmitz-Peiffer C. Saturated and n-6 polyunsaturated-fat diets each induce ceramide accumulation in mouse skeletal muscle: reversal and improvement of glucose tolerance by lipid metabolism inhibitors. *Endocrinology* 151(9) (September 2010): 4187–4196.

Freedman D. "Lies, Damned Lies, and Medical Science." *Atlantic Magazine*, November 2010.

Friedlander BP. Toxic pollen from widely planted, genetically modified corn can kill monarch butterflies, Cornel study shows. *Cornell University Science News*, August 7, 1997.

Friedman M. Lysinoalanine in food and in antimicrobial proteins. *Advances in Experimental Medicine and Biology* 459 (1999): 145–159.

Friedman MI, Harris RB, Ji H, Ramirez I, Tordoff MG. Fatty acid oxidation affects food intake by altering hepatic energy status. *American Journal of Physiology—Regulatory, Integrative, and Comparative Physiology* 276 (4) (April 1999): R1046–R1053.

Friedman MI, Ramirez I. Relationship of fat metabolism to food intake. *American Journal of Clinical Nutrition* 42 (November 1985): 1093–1098.

Friedman MI, Tordoff MG. Fatty acid oxidation and glucose utilization interact to control food intake in rats. *American Journal of Physiology* 251(5 Pt. 2) (November 1986): R840–R845.

Friedman MI. An energy sensor for control of energy intake. *Proceedings of the Nutrition Society* 56(1Λ) (March 1997): 41–50.

Fulgoni V. High-fructose corn syrup: everything you wanted to know, but were afraid to ask. *American Journal of Clinical Nutrition* 88(6) December 2008): 1715S.

Gaiva MH, Couto RC, Oyama LM, Couto GE, Silveira VL, Riberio EB, Nascimento CM. Polyunsaturated fatty acid-rich diets: effect on adipose tissue metabolism in rats. *British Journal of Nutrition* 86(3) (September 2001): 371–377.

Galgani J, Ravussin E. Energy metabolism, fuel selection and body weight regulation. *International Journal of Obesity* 32(Suppl 7) (December 2008): S109–S119.

Gann PH, Hennekens CH, Sacks FM, Grodstein F, Giovannucci EL, Stampfer MJ. Prospective study of plasma fatty acids and risk of prostate cancer. *Journal of the National Cancer Institute* 86(4) (February 16, 1994): 281–286.

Gannon MC, Nuttall FQ. Effects of a high-protein, low-carbohydrate diet on blood glucose control in people with type 2 diabetes. *Diabetes* 53 (9) September 2004): 2375–2382.

Gannot MC, Nutall JA, Damberg G, Gupta C, Nuttall FQ. Effect of protein ingestion on the glucose appearance in people with type 2 diabetes. *Journal of Clinical Endocrinology and Metabolism* 86(3) (March 2001): 1040–1047.

Gibala MJ, Little JP, van Essen M, Wilkin GP, Burgomaster KA, Safdar A, Raha S, Tarnopolsky MA. Short-term sprint interval versus traditional endurance training: similar initial adaptations in human skeletal muscle and exercise performance. *Journal of Physiology* 575 (September 2006): 901–911.

Ginter E, Cerna O, Budlovsky J, Balaz V, Hruba F, Rock V, Sasko E. Effect of ascorbic acid on plasma cholesterol in humans in a long-term experiment. *International Journal for Vitamin and Nutrition Research* 47(2) (1977): 123–134.

Giovannucci E, Rimm EB, Stampfer MJ, Colditz GA, Ascherio A, Willett WC. Intake of fat, meat, and fiber in relation to risk of colon cancer in men. *Cancer Research* 54 (May 1, 1994): 2390.

Girion L, Glover S, Smith D. "Drug Deaths Now Outnumber Traffic Fatalities in U.S., Data Shows." *Los Angeles Times*, September 17, 2011.

Glisezinski ID, Harant I, Crampes F, Trudeau F, Felez A, Cottet-Emard JM, Garrigues M, Riviere D. Effect of carbohydrate ingestion on adipose tissue lipolysis during long-lasting exercise in trained men. *Journal of Applied Physiology* 84(5) (May 1998): 1627–1632.

GM-feed may harm the reproductive system of animals. *All About Feed* (June 19, 2012).

Goedecke JH, St. Clair GA, Grobler L, Collins M, Noakes TD, Lambert EV. Determinants of the variability in respiratory exchange ratio at rest and during exercise in trained athletes. *American Journal of Physiology Endocrinology and Metabolism* 279(6) (December 2000): E1325–1334.

Goedeke, Havermann. The emphasis in exercise is usually on carbohydrates, but fats are also important. *CME* 26 (7) July 2008): 347–349.

Golay A, Felber JP, Meyer HU, Curchod B, Maeder E, Jequier E. Study on lipid metabolism in obesity diabetes. *Metabolism* 33 (2) (February 1984): 111–116.

Goldstein R. "Jack LaLanne, Father of Fitness Movement, Dies at 96." *New York Times*, January 24, 2011.

Gordon SL, Corbin SB. Summary of workshop on drinking water fluoride influence on hip fracture on bone health (National Institutes of Health, April 10, 1991). *Osteoporosis International* 2(3) (May 1992): 109–117.

Gorteon HC, Jarvis K. The effectiveness of vitamin C in preventing and relieving the symptoms of virus-induced respiratory infections. *Journal of Manipulative Physiological Therapeutics* 22(8) (October 1999): 530–533.

Gould DC. The male menopause: does it exist? *Western Journal of Medicine* 173(2) (August 2000): 76–78.

Gouras GK, Xu H, Gross RS, Grenfield JP, Hai B, Wang R, Greendard P. Testosterone reduces neuronal secretion of Alzheimer's □-amyloid peptides. *PNAS* 97(3) (February 1, 2000): 1202–1205.

Gravolt CH, Moller N, Jensen MD, Christiansen JS, Schmitz O. Physiological levels of glucagon do not influence lipolysis in abdominal adipose tissue as assessed by microdialysis. *Journal of Clinical Endocrinology and Metabolism* 86(5) (May 2001): 2085–2089.

Gray AS. Fluoridation: time for a new base line? *Journal of the Canadian Dental Association* 53 (1987): 763–765.

Grene M. "Gardisil Developer Claims Vaccine Prevents Abnormal Pap Tests, Not Cervical Cancer." Free-Press-Release.com, February 14, 2011.

Griffin SO, Beltran ED, Lockwood SA, Barker LK. Esthetically objectionable fluorosis attributable to water fluoridation. *Community Dentistry and Oral Epidemiology* 30(3) (June 2002): 199–209.

Guo Z, Burguera B, Jensen M. Kinetics of intramuscular triglyceride fatty acids in exercising humans. *Journal of Applied Physiology* 89 (2000): 2057–2064.

Gustin G. "Pests Damaging Biotech Corn, Getting an Early Start." *STLtoday*, June 15, 2012.

Habito RC, Montalto J, Leslie E, Ball MJ. Effects of replacing meat with soybean in the diet on sex hormone concentrations in healthy adult males. *British Journal of Nutrition* 84(4) (October 2000): 557–563.

Haddad LS, Kelbert L, Hulbert AJ. Extended longevity of queen honey bees compared to workers is associated with peroxidation-resistant membranes. *Experimental Gerontology* 42(7) (July 2007): 601–609. Epub March 3, 2007.

Hak AE, Witteman JCM, Jong FH, Geerlings MI, Hofman A, Pois HAP. Low levels of endogenous androgens increase the risk of atherosclerosis in elderly men: the Rotterdam study. *Journal of Clinical Endocrinology and Metabolism* 87(8) (August 1, 2002): 3632–3639.

Haman F, Peronnet F, Kenny GP, Doucet E, Massicotte D, Lavoie C, Weber JM. Effects of carbohydrate availability on sustained shivering I. Oxidation of plasma glucose, muscle glycogen, and proteins. *Journal of Applied Physiology* 96(1) (January 2004): 32–40.

Hankinson SE, Willett W, Colditz GA, Hunter DJ, Michaud DS, Deroo B, Rosner B, Speizer FE, Pollak M. Circulation concentrations of insulin-like growth factor I and risk of breast cancer. *Lancet* 351 (9113) May 1998): 1393–1396.

Hare G, Kavanagh BP, Mazer CD, Hum KM, Kim SY, Coackley C, Barr A, Baker A. Hypercapnia increases cerebral tissue oxygen tension in anesthetized rats. *Canadian Journal of Anesthesia* 50(1) (December 2003): 1061–1068.

He FJ, MacGregor GA. A comprehensive review on salt and health and current experience of worldwide salt reduction programs. *Journal of Human Hypertension* 23(6) (June 2009): 363–384.

He J, Watkins S, Kelley D. Skeletal muscle lipid content and oxidative enzyme activity in relation to muscle fiber type in type 2 diabetes and obesity. *Diabetes* 50(4) (April 2001): 817–823.

Heaney RP, Weaver CM, Fitzsimmons ML. Soybean phytate content: effect on calcium absorption. *American Journal of Clinical Nutrition* 53(3) (March 1991): 745–747.

Helferich WG, Andrade JE, Hoadland MS. Phytoestrogens and breast cancer: a complex story. *Inflammopharmacology* 16(5) (October 2008): 219–226.

Helge JW, Watt PW, Richter EA, Rennie MJ, Kiens B. Fat utilization during exercise: adaptation to a fat-rich diet increases utilization of plasma fatty acids and very low density lipoprotein-triacylglycerol in humans. *Journal of Physiology* 537(Pt. 3) (December 15, 2001): 1009–1020.

Henkel J. Sugar substitutes: Americans opt for sweetness and lite. *FDA Consumer* (November–December 1999).

Henriksson J, Reitman JS. Quantitative measures of enzyme activities in type I and type II muscle fibres of man after training. *Acta Physiologica Scandinavica* 97(3) (July 1976): 392–397.

Hermanowski-Vosatka A, Balkovec JM, Cheng K, Chen HY, Hernandez M, Koo GC,

Le Grand CB, Li Z, Metzger JM, Mundt SS, Noonan H, Nunes CN, Olson SH, Pikounis B, Ren N, Robertson N, Schaeffer JM, Shah K, Springer MS, Strack AM, Strowski M, Wu K, Wu T, Ziao J, Zhang BB, Wright SD, Thieringer R. 11□-HSD1 inhibition ameliorates metabolic syndrome and prevents progression of atherosclerosis in mice. *Journal of Experimental Medicine* 202(4) (August 15, 2005): 517–527.

Herrero A, Portero-Otin M, Bellmunt MJ, Pamplona R, Barja G. Effect of the degree of fatty acid unsaturation of rat heart mitochondria on their rates of H2O2 production and lipid and protein oxidative damage. *Mechanisms of Aging and Development* 122(4) (April 2001): 427–443.

Herskind AM, McGue M, Holm NV, Sorensen TIA, Harvald B, Vaupel JW. The heritability of human longevity: A population-based study of 2872 Danish twin pairs born 1870–1900. *Human Genetics* 97(3) (March 1996): 319–323.

Higgins JA, Higbee DR, Donahoo WT, Brown IL, Bell ML, Bessessen DH. Resistant starch consumption promotes lipid oxidation. *Nutrition and Metabolism* 1 (2004): 8.

Hildebolt CF, Elvin-Lewis M, Molnar S, McKee JK, Perkins MD, Young KL. Caries prevalences among geochemical regions of Missouri. *American Journal of Physical Anthropology* 78(1) January 1989): 79–92.

Hileman B. Bisphenol A on trial. *Chemical Engineering News* 85(15) (April 16, 2007): 38.

Ho Mae-Wan. "Mass Deaths in Sheep Grazing on Bt Cotton." ISIS Press Release, April 25, 2006.

Hoffman JR, Falvo MJ. Protein—which is best? *Journal of Sports Science and Medicine* 3(3) (September 2004): 118–130.

Hogervorst E, Sadjimim T, Kreager P, Rahardjo TB. High tofu intake is associated with worse memory in elderly Indonesian men and women. *Dementia and Geriatric Cognitive Disorders* 26(1) (2008): 50–57.

Hogstrom M, Nordstrom P, Nordstrom A. N-3 fatty acids are positively associated with peak bone mineral density and bone accrual in healthy men: the NO2 study. *American Journal of Clinical Nutrition* 85(3) March 2007): 803–807.

Holland WL, Brozinick JT, Want LP, Hawkins ED, Sargent KM, Liu Y, Narra K, Hoehn KL, Knotts TA, Siesky A, Nelson DH, Karathanasis SK, Fontenot GK, Birnbaum MJ, Summers SA. Inhibition of ceramide synthesis ameliorates glucocorticoid-, saturated fat-, and obesity-induced insulin resistance. *Cell Metabolism* 5(3) (March 2007): 167–179.

Holt SH, Miller JC, Petocz P, Farmakalidis E. A satiety index of common foods. European *Journal of Clinical Nutrition* 49(9) (September 1995): 675–690.

Holt SH, Miller JC, Petocz P. An insulin index of foods: the insulin demand generated by 1000-kJ portions of common foods. *American Journal of Clinical Nutrition* 66(5) (November 1997): 1264–1276.

Holzer RG, Park EJ, Li N, Tran H, Chen M, Choi C, Solinas G, Karin M. Saturated fatty acids induce c-Src clustering within membrane subdomains, leading to JNK activation. *Cell* 147(1) (September 30, 2011): 173–184.

Honkala S, Honkala E, Tynjala J, Kannas L. Use of xylitol chewing gum among Finnish schoolchildren. *Acta Odontol Scand* 57(6) (December 1999): 306–309.

Horowitz BZ. Bromism from excessive cola consumption. *Journal of Toxicology—Clinical Toxicology* 35(3) (1997): 315–320.

Horowitz JF, Mora-Rodriguez R, Byerley LO, Coyle EF. Lipolytic suppression following carbohydrate ingestion limits fat oxidation during exercise.

American Journal of Physiology 273(4 Pt. 1) (October 1997): E768–E775.

Hostmark AT, Spydevold O, Eilertsen E. Plasma lipid concentration and liver output of lipoproteins in rats fed coconut fat or sunflower oil. *Artery* 7(5) (1980): 367–383.

Houlihan LM, Wyatt ND, Harris SE, Hayward C, Gowl AJ, Marioni RE, Strachan MWJ, Price JF, Starr JM, Wright AF, Deary IJ. Variation in the uric acid transporter gene (SLC2A9) and memory performance. *Human Molecular Genetics* 19(11) (2010): 2321–2330.

Hulbert AJ, Faulks SC, Harper JM, Miller RA. Extended longevity of wild-derived mice is associated with peroxidation-resistant membranes. *Mechanisms of Ageing and Development* 127(8) (August 2006): 653–657.

Hulbert AJ. On the importance of fatty acid composition of membranes for aging. *Journal of Theoretical Biology* 234(2) (May 21, 2005): 277–288.

Hurni M, Burnand B, Pittet P, Jequier E. Metabolic effects of a mixed and a high-carbohydrate low-fat diet in man, measured over 24 h in a respiration chamber. *British Journal of Nutrition* 47(1) (January 1982): 33–34.

Hurrell RF, Juillerate MA, Reddy MB, Lyncy SR, Dassenka SA, Cook JD. Soy protein, phytate, and iron absorption in humans. *American Journal of Clinical Nutrition* 56 (September 1992): 573–578.

Hurrell RF, Reddy MB, Juillerat MA, Cook JD. Degradation of phytic acid in cereal porridges improves iron absorption by human subjects. *American Journal of Clinical Nutrition* 77(5) (May 2003): 1213–1219.

Hurrell RF. Influence of vegetable protein sources on trace element and mineral bioavailability. *Journal of Nutrition* 133 (September 2003): 2973S–2977S.

Hyon K, Choi MD, Atkinson K, Karlson E, Willett W, Curhan G. Purine-rich foods, dairy and protein intake, and the risk of gout in men. *New England Journal of Medicine* 350 (2004): 1093–1103.

Ikemoto A, Thompson KS, Takahashi M, Itakura H, Lane MD, Ezaki O. High fat diet–induced hyperglycemia: prevention by low level expression of a glucose transporter (GLUT4) minigene in transgenic mice. *PNAS* 92(8) April 11, 1995): 3096–3099.

Inouye K, Shum K, Chan O, Mathoo J, Matthews S, Vranic M. Effects of recurrent hyperinsulinemia with and without hypoglycemia on counterregulation in diabetic rats. *American Journal of Physiology Endocrinology and Metabolism* 282 (June 2002): E1369–E1379.

Ioannidis JP. Contradicted and initially stronger effects in highly cited clinical research. *Journal of the American Medical Association* 294(2) (July 13, 2005): 218–228.

Ioannidis JP. Why most published research findings are false. *PLoS Medicine* 2(8) (August 2005): e124.

Isaacson RA, Varner JA, Jensen KF. Toxin-induced blood vessel inclusions caused by the chronic administration of aluminum and sodium fluoride and their implications for dementia. *Fluoride* 31(2) (1998): 96–99; abstracted from *Annals of the New York Academy of Sciences* 825 (1997): 152–166.

Ishizuki Y, Hirooka Y, Murata Y, Togashi K. The effects on the thyroid gland of soybeans administered experimentally in healthy subjects. *Nippon Naibunpi Gakkai Zasshi* 67(5) (May 20, 1991): 622–629.

Ismail M. "Syngenta Charged for Covering up Livestock Deaths from GM Corn." *QW Magazine*, June 14, 2010.

Israel B. "Brominated Battle: Soda Chemical Has Cloudy Health History." *Environmental Health News*, December 12, 2011.

Ivy JL, Withers RT, Van Handel PJ, Elger DH, Costill DL. Muscle respiratory capacity and fiber type as determinants of the lactate threshold. *Journal of Applied Physiology* 48(3) (March 1980): 523–527.

Jacobsen SJ, Goldberg J, Cooper C, Lockwood SA. The association between water fluoridation and hip fracture among white women and men aged 65 years and older. A national ecologic study. *Annals of Epidemiology* 2(5) (September 1992): 617–626.

Jalal DI, Smits G, Johnson RJ, Chonchol M. Increased fructose associates with elevated blood pressure. *Journal of the American Society of Nephrology* 21(9) (September 2010): 1543–1549.

Janowsky JS, Chavez B, Orwoll E. Sex steroids modify working memory. *Journal of Cognitive Neuroscience* 12(3) (May 2000): 407–414.

Jefferson W, Newbold R, Padilla-Banks E, Pepling M. Neonatal genistein treatment alters ovarian differentiations in the mouse: inhibition of oocyte nest breakdown and increased oocyte survival. *Biology of Reproduction* 74(1) (January 2006): 161–168.

Jefferson WN, Padilla-Banks E, Newbold RR. Adverse effects on female development and reproduction in CD-1 mice following neonatal exposure to the phytoestrogen genistein at environmentally relevant doses. *Biology of Reproduction* 73(4) (October 2005): 798–806.

Jefferson WN, Padilla-Banks E, Phelps JY, Cantor AM, Williams CJ. Neonatal phytoestrogen exposure alters oviduct mucosal immune response to pregnancy and affects preimplantation embryo development in the mouse. *Biology of Reproduction* (May 2, 2010).

Jenkins DJ, Kendall CW, Augustin LS, Franceschi S, Hamidi M, Marchie A, Jenkins AL, Axelsen M. Glycemic index: overview of implications in health and disease. *American Journal of Clinical Nutrition* 76 (July 2002): 266S–273S.

Jiang X, Patterson NM, Ling Y, Xie J, Helferich WG, Shapiro DJ. Low concentrations of the soy phytoestrogen genistein induce proteinase inhibitor 9 and block killing of breast cancer cells by immune cells. *Endocrinology* 149(11) November 2008): 5366–5373.

Jimenez R, Torres H, Duran T, Gonzalez R, Mascher, Romero P, Oropeza J. The respiratory exchange ratio is associated with fitness indicators both in trained and untrained men: a possible application for people with reduced exercise tolerance. *Clinical Medicine: Circulatory, Respiratory and Pulmonary* 2 (2008): 1–9.

Johnson F, Mavrogianni A, Ucci M, Vidal-Puig A, Wardle J. Could increased time spent in thermal comfort zone contribute to population increases in obesity? *Obesity Reviews* 12(7) (July 2011): 543–551,.

Johnson PM, Kenny P. Dopamine D2 receptors in addiction-like reward dysfunction and compulsive eating in obese rats. *Nature Neuroscience* 13 (2010): 635–641.

Johnson RJ, Nakagawa T. The effect of fructose on renal biology and disease. *Journal of the American Society of Nephrology* (November 29, 2010): doi:10.1681/ASN.2010050506.

Johnston KL, Thomas EL, Bell JD, Frost GS, Robertson MD. Resistant starch improves insulin sensitivity in metabolic syndrome. *Diabetic Medicine* 27(4) (April 2010): 391–397.

Jones JM, Anderson JW. Grain foods and health; a primer for clinicians. *Physician and Sportsmedicine* 36(1) (December 2008): 18–33.

Jones T, Steelink C, Sierka J. Analysis of the causes of tooth decay in children in Tucson, Arizona. Paper presented at annual meeting of the American Association for the Advancement of Science, San Francisco, February

1994. Abstract in *Fluoride* 27(4) (1994): 238.

Ju YH, Allred CD, Allred KF, Karko KL, Doerge DR, Helferich WG. Physiological concentrations of dietary genistein dose-dependently stimulate growth of estrogen-dependent human breast cancer (MCF-7) tumors implanted in athymic nude mice. *Journal of Nutrition* 131(11) (November 2001): 2957–2962.

Juel C. Regulation of cellular pH in skeletal muscle fiber types, studied with sacrolemmal giant vesicles obtained from rat muscles. *Biochim Biophys Acta* 1265(2–3) (March 16, 1995): 127–132.

Jump DB, Thelen A, Mater M. Dietary polyunsaturated fatty acids and hepatic gene expression. *Lipids* 34(Suppl) (1999): s209–s212.

Kaptchuk TJ, Friedlander E, Kelley JM, Sanchez MN, Kokkotou E, Singer JP, Kowalczykowski M, Miller FG, Kirsch I, Lemo AJ. Placebos without deception: a randomized controlled trial in irritable bowel syndrome. *PLoS One* 5(12) (December 22, 2010): e15591.

Karjalainen J, Tikkanen H, Hernelahti M, Kujala U. Muscle fiber-type distribution predicts weight gain and unfavorable left ventricular geometry: a 19 year follow-up study. *BMC Cardiovascular Disorders* 6(2) (2006).

Kasper S. Hypericum perforatum—a review of clinical studies. *Pharmacopsychiatry* 34(Suppl 1) (2001): 51–55.

Kastorini CM, Milionis HJ, Esposito K, Giugliano D, Goudevenos JA, Panagiotakos DB. The effect of Mediterranean diet on metabolic syndrome and its components: a meta-analysis of 50 studies and 534,906 individuals. *Journal of the American College of Cardiology* 57 (2001): 1299–1313.

Kawamata I, Harada M, Kobayashi M, Fujii R, Fukusumi S, Ogi K, Hosoya M, Tanaka Y, Uejima H, Tanaka H, Maruyama M, Satoh R, Okubo S, Kizawa H, Komatsu H, Matusmura F, Noguchi Y, Shinohara T, Hinuma S, Fujisawa Y, Fujino M. Free fatty acids regulate insulin secretion from pancreatic beta cells through GPR40. *Nature* 422(6928) (March 13, 2003): 173–176.

Kazarinov VA. Buteyko Method: the experience of implementation in medical practice. The biochemical basis of KP Buteyko's theory of the diseases of deep respiration. *Patriot Press Moscow* (1990): 198–218; translation from http://www.wt.com.au/~pkolb/biochem.htm, May 22, 2010.

Keller U, Shulman G. Effect of glucagon on hepatic fatty acid oxidation and ketogenesis in conscious dogs. *American Journal of Physiology* 237(2) (August 1979): E121–E129.

Kelley DE, Goodpaster B, Wing R, Simoneau JA. Skeletal muscle fatty acid metabolism in association with insulin resistance, obesity, and weight loss. *American Journal of Physiology, Endocrinology, and Metabolism* 277(6) (December 1999): E1130–E1141.

Kelley DE, Mokan M, Simoneau JA, Mandarino LJ. Interaction between glucose and free fatty acid metabolism in human skeletal muscle. *Journal of Clinical Investigation* 92(1) July 1993): 91–98.

Kenfield I. "Michael Taylor: Monsanto's Man in the Obama Administration." Organic Consumers Association, *Counterpunch*, August 14, 2009.

Kennedy AR. The Bowman-Birk inhibitor from soybeans as an anticarcinogenic agent. *American Journal of Clinical Nutrition* 68 (December 1998): 1406S–1412S.

Kestin S, Knowles T. The Chardon LL Hearing: *An Analysis of "the Chicken Study." The Effect of Glufosinate Resistant Corn on Growth of Male Broiler Chickens.* Department of Animal Poultry Sciences, University of Guelph, report no. A56379, July 12, 1996.

Khaw KT, Bingham S, Welch A, Luben R, Warenham N, Oakes S, Day N. Relation between plasma ascorbic acid and mortality in men and women in EPIC-Norfolk prospective study: a prospective population study. European prospective investigation into cancer and nutrition. *Lancet* 357(9257) (March 3, 2001): 657–663.

Kiens B, Richter EA. Types of carbohydrate in an ordinary diet affect insulin action and muscle substrates in humans. *American Journal of Clinical Nutrition* 63(1) (January 1996): 47–53.

Knopp R, Retzlaff BM. Saturated fat prevents coronary artery disease? An American paradox. *American Journal of Clinical Nutrition* 80(5) (November 2004): 1102–1103.

Kobayashi R, Nagano M, Nakamura F, Higaki J, Fujioka Y, Ikegami H, Mikami H, Kawaguchi N, Onishi S, Ogihara T. Role of angiotensin II in high fructose-induced left ventricular hypertrophy in rats. *Hypertension* 21(6 Pt. 2) (June 1993): 1051–1055.

Kobylewski S, Jacobson M. "Food Dyes a Rainbow of Risks." Center for Science in the Public Interest, 2010, http://cspinet.org/new/pdf/food-dyes-rainbow-of-risks.pdf.

Komarek A, Lesaffre E. A Bayesian analysis of multivariate doubly-interval-censored dental data. *Biostat* 6 (1) (2005): 145–155.

Kopp W. Chronically increased activity of the sympathetic nervous system: Our diet-related "evolutionary" inheritance. *Journal of Nutrition, Health, and Aging* 13(1) (January 2009): 27–29.

Krajcovicova-Kudlachova M, Sebekova K, Schinezel R, Klvanova J. Advanced glycation end products and nutrition. *Physiology Research* 51(3) (2002): 313–316.

Kumar JV, Swango PA, Lininger LL, Leske GS, Green EL, Haley VB. Changes in dental fluorosis and dental caries in Newburgh and Kingston, New York. *American Journal of Public Health* 88(12) (December 1998): 1866–1870.

Laforgia J, Withers RT, Shipp NJ, Core CJ. Comparison of energy expenditure elevations after submaximal and supramaximal running. *Journal of Applied Physiology* 82(2) (February 1997): 661–666.

Lambert, Goedecke. You are what you eat. *CME* 23(11) (November–December 2005).

Landsberg L. Feast or Famine: The sympathetic nervous system response to nutrient intake. *Cellular and Molecular Neurobiology* 26(4–6) (July–August 2006): 495–506.

Lappe JM, Travers-Gustafson D, Davies KM, Recker RR, Heaney RP. Vitamin D and calcium supplementation reduces cancer risk: results of a randomized trial. *American Journal of Clinical Nutrition* 85(6) (June 2007: 1586–1591.

Layton L. "Strategy Is Being Devised to Protect Use of Bisphenol A and Block U.S. Ban." *Washington Post*, Sunday, May 31, 2009.

Le KA, Ith M, Kreis R, Faeh D, Bortolottie M, Tran C, Boesch C, Tappy L. Fructose overconsumption causes dyslipidemia and ectopic lipid deposition in healthy subjects with and without family history of type 2 diabetes. *American Journal of Clinical Nutrition* 89(6) (June 2009): 1760–1765.

Levine, B. HPV vaccine is a danger to girls (and boys). *Natural Health 365*. July 8, 2012, http://www.naturalhealth365.com/big_pharma/hpv-vaccine.html.

Lee SA, Shu XO, Li H, Yang G, Cai H, Wen W, Ji BT, Gao J, Gao YT, Zheng W. Adolescent and adult soy food intake and breast cancer risk: results from the Shanghai women's health study. *American Journal of Clinical Nutrition* 89(6) (June 2009): 1920–1926.

Lee SJ, Murphy CT, Kenyon C. Glucose shortens the lifespan of Caenorhabditis elegans by down-regulating DAF-16/FOXO activity and aquaporin gene expression. *Cell Metabolism* 10(5) (2009): 379–391.

Lee YS, Ha MS, Lee YJ. The effects of various intensities and durations of exercise with and without glucose in milk ingestion on postexercise oxygen consumption. *Journal of Sports Medicine and Physical Fitness* 39(4) (December 1999): 341–347.

Lenzen S. The mechanisms of alloxan– and streptozotocin–induced diabetes. *Diabetologia* 51(2) (February 2008): 216–226.

Li XS, Zhi JL, Ro G. Effect of fluoride exposure on intelligence in children. *Fluoride* 28(4) (1995): 189–192.

Li Y, Li X, Wei S. Effect of excessive fluoride intake on mental work capacity of children and a preliminary study of its mechanism. *Hua Xi Yi Ke Da Xue Xue Bao* 25(2) (June 1994): 188–191.

Lidbeck WL, Hill IB, Beehman JA. Acute sodium fluoride poisoning. *Journal of the American Medical Association* 121(11) (1943): 826–827.

Liddle RA, Goldfine ID, Rosen MS, Taplitz RA, Williams JA. Chlecystokinin bioactivity in human plasma. Molecular forms, responses to feeding, and relationship to gallbladder contraction. *Journal of Clinical Investigation* 75(4) (April 1985): 1144–1152.

Liener IE, Goodale RL, Deshmukh A, Satterberg TL, Ward G, DiPietro CM, Bankey PE, Borner JW. Effect of a trypsin inhibitor from soybeans (Bowman-Birk) on the secretory activity of the human pancreas. *Gastroenterology* 94(2) (February 1998): 419–427.

Liener IE. Letter to Dockets Management Branch, Food and Drug Administration, December 31, 1998.

Liener IE. Trypsin inhibitors: concern for human nutrition or not? *Journal of Nutrition* 116(5) (May 1986): 920–923.

Liljenquist JE, Bomboy JD, Lewis SB, Sinclair-Smith BC, Felts PW, Lacy WW, Crofford OB, Liddle GW. Effects of glucagon on lipolysis and ketogenesis in normal and diabetic men. *Journal of Clinical Investigation* 53(1) (January 1974): 190–197.

Lillioja S, Bogardus C, Mott DM, Kennedy AL, Knowler WC, Howard BV. Relationship between insulin-mediated glucose disposal and lipid metabolism in man. *Journal of Clinical Investigation* 75(4) (April 1985): 1106–1115.

Lillioja S, Young AA, Culter CL, Ivy JL, Abbott WG, Zawadzki JK, Yki-Jarvinen H, Christin L, Secomb TW, Bogardus C. Skeletal muscle capillary density and fiber type are possible determinants of in vivo insulin resistance in man. *Journal of Clinical Investigation* 80(2) (August 1987): 415–424.

Lin CC, Li TC, Lai MM. Efficacy and safety of Monascus purpures Went rice in subjects with hyperlipidemia. *European Journal of Endocrinology* 153(5) (November 2005): 679–686.

Lin YH, Tsu BS. Some factors affecting levels of trypsin inhibitor activity of sweet potato roots. *Botanical Studies—Academia Sinica* 28 (1987): 139–149.

Linde K, Ramirez G, Murlow C, Pauls A, Weidenhammer W, Melchart D. St. John's wort for depression—an overview and meta-analysis of randomized clinical trials. *BMJ* (1996): 313 doi: 10.

Lindinger MI, Kowalchuk JM, Heigenhauser JF. Applying physicochemical principles to skeletal muscle acid-base status. *American Journal of Physiology—Regulatory, Integrative, and Comparative Physiology* 289(3) (September 2005): R891–R894.

Lo CY, Li S, Wang Y, Tan D, Pan MH, Sang S, Ho CT. Reactive dicarbonyl compounds are 5-(hydroxymethyl)-2-furfural in carbonated beverages containing high fructose corn syrup. *Food Chemistry* 107(3) (April 2008): 1099–1105.

Loder E. Missing trial data threatens the integrity of medicine. *BMJ* (January 5, 2012).

Lu Y, Sun ZR, Wu LN, Wang X, Lu W, Liu SS. Effect of high-fluoride water on intelligence in children. *Fluoride* 33(2) (May 2000): 74–78.

Luke J. Fluoride deposition in the aged human pineal gland. *Caries Research* 35 (March–April 2001): 125–128.

Lum LC. Hyperventilation: the tip and the iceberg. *Journal of Psychosomatic Research* 19(5–6) (1975): 375–383.

Luo J, Rizkalla SW, Boillot J, Alamowitch C, Chaib H, Bruzzo F, Desplanque N, Dalix AM, Durand G, Slama G. Dietary (n-3) polyunsaturated fatty acids improve adipocyte insulin action and glucose metabolism in insulin-resistant rats: relation to membrane fatty acids. *Journal of Nutrition* 126(8) (August 1996): 1951–1958.

Lustig RH. Childhood obesity: behavioral aberration or biochemical drive? Reinterpreting the First Law of Thermodynamics. *Nature Clinical Practice Endocrinology and Metabolism* 2 (2006): 447–458.

Lustig RH. "The Trouble with Fructose." YouTube presentation. University of California, San Francisco.

Madison LL, Seyffert WA, Unger RH, Barker B. Effect of plasma free fatty acids on plasma glucagon and serum insulin concentrations. *Metabolism* 17(4) (April 1968): 301–304.

Malatesta M, Caporaloni C, Gavaudan S, Rocchi MB, Serafini S, Tiberi C, Gazzanelli G. Ultrastructural morphometrical and immunocytochemical analysis of hepatocyte nuclei from mice fed on genetically modified soybean. *Cell Struct Funct* 27(4) (August 2002): 173–180.

Malenfant P, JoanisseDR, Thériault R, Goodpaster BH, Kelley DE, Simoneau JA. Fat content in individual muscle fibers of lean and obese subjects. *International Journal of Obesity* 25(10) (September 2001): 1316–1321.

Manninen AH. Metabolic effects of the very-low-carbohydrate diets: misunderstood "villains" of human metabolism. *Journal of the International Society of Sports Nutrition* 1(2) (2004): 7–11.

Marmot M, Atinmo T, Byers T, Chen J, Hirohata T, Jackson A, James W, Kolonel L, Kumanyika S, Leitamann C, Mann J, Powers H, Reddy K, Riboli E, Rivera JA, Schatzkin A, Seidell J, Shuker D, Uauy RW, Zeisel W. *Food, Nutrition, Physical Activity, and the Prevention of Cancer, a Global Perspective,* 2007, University College London: American Institute for Cancer Research.

Marsh AG, Sanchez TV, Chaffee FL, Mayor GH, Mickelson O. Bone mineral mass in adult lacto-ovo-vegetarian and omnivorous males. *American Journal of Clinical Nutrition* 37 (March 1983): 453–456.

Martin-Dominguez IR, Trejo-Vazquez R, Rodriguez-Dozal S. Well water fluoride, dental fluorosis, and bone fractures in the Guadiana Valley of Mexico. *Fluoride* 34(2) (2001): 139-149.

Masini E, Palmerani B, Gambassi F, Pistelli A, Giannella E, Occupati B, Ciuffi M, Sacchi TB, Mannaioni PF. Histamine release from rat mast cells induced by metabolic activation of polyunsaturated fatty acids into free radicals. *Biochemical Pharmacology* 39(5) (March 1, 1990): 879–889.

Masters RD, Coplan MJ. Water treatment with silicofluorides and lead toxicity. *International Journal of Environmental Studies* 56 (1999): 435–449.

Mattson FH, Grundy SM. Comparison of effects of dietary saturated, monounsaturated, and polyunsaturated fatty acids on plasma lipids and lipoproteins in man. *Journal of Lipid Research* 26 (February 1, 1985): 194–202.

Maughan RJ. Effects of prior exercise on the performance of intense isometric exercise. *British Journal of Sports Medicine* 22(1) March 1988): 12–15.

Mccay CM, Ramseyer WF, Smith CA. Effect of sodium fluoride administration on body changes in old rats. *Journal of Gerontology* 12(1) (January 1957):14–19.

McCollum EV, Simmonds N, Becker JE, Buntikg RTV. *The Effect of Additions of Fluorine to the Diet of the Rat on the Quality of the Teeth.* Department of Chemical Hygiene, School of Hygiene and Public Health, the Johns Hopkins University and the College of Dental Surgery, University of Michigan, February 18, 1925.

McDonagh MS, Whiting PF, Wilson PM, Sutton AJ, Chestnut I, Cooper J, Misso K, Bradley M, Treasure E, Kleijnen J. Systematic reviews of water fluoridation. *BMJ* 321(7265) (October 7, 2000): 855–859.

McGowan J. Health education: does the Buteyko Institute method make a difference? *Thorax* 58 (Suppl III) (December 2003): 28.

McKeown NM, Troy LM, Jacques PF. Whole- and refined-grain intakes are differentially associated with abdominal visceral and subcutaneous adiposity in healthy adults: the Framingham Heart Study. *American Journal of Clinical Nutrition* 92(5) (November 2010): 1165–1171.

McKnight CB, Levy SM, Cooper SE, Jakobesen JR. A pilot study of esthetic perceptions of dental fluorosis vs. selected other dental conditions. *ASDC J Dent Child* 65(4) (July–August 1998): 233–238.

McMichael-Phillips DF, Harding C, Morton M, Roberts SA, Howell A, Potten CS, Bundred NJ. Effects of soy-protein supplementation on epithelial proliferation in the histologically normal human breast. *American Journal of Clinical Nutrition* 68(6 Suppl) (December 1998): 1431S-1435S.

Melanson K, Zukley L, Lowndes J, Hguyen V, Angelopoulos TJ, Rippe J. Effects of high-fructose corn syrup and sucrose consumption on circulating glucose, insulin, leptin, and ghrelin and on appetite in normal weight women. *Nutrition* 23(2) (February 2007): 103–112.

Mendis GS, Wissler RW, Bridenstein RT, Prodbielski FJ. The effects of replacing coconut oil with corn oil on human lipid profiles and platelet derived factors active in atherogenesis. *Nutri Reports International* 40(4) (October 1998): 773–782.

Mepham TB, Schofield PN, Zumkeller W, Cotterill AM. Safety of milk from cows treated with bovine somatotropin. *Lancet* 344(8934) (November 19, 1994: 1445–1446.

Merchant AT. Carbohydrate intake and overweight and obesity among healthy adults. *Journal of the American Dietetic Association* 109 (2009): 1165–1172.

Mercola, Dr. "Caution: The 'Best Route' to Good Health Is Causing 106,000 Deaths/Year." Posted by Dr. Mercola, December 31, 2011.

Mercola, Dr. "Organic Pesticides Not Always Best Choice." Posted by Dr. Mercola, July 17, 2010.

Mercola, Dr. "The Major Cause of Breast Cancer Almost Everyone Ignores." Posted by Dr. Mercola, February 14, 2012.

Mercola, Dr. "The Potential Dangers of Sucralose." Mercola.com, retrieved December 31, 2011.

Meropol NJ, Schulman KA. Cost of cancer care: issues and implications. *Journal of Clinical Oncology* 25(2) (January 10, 2007).Migrennel S, Cruciani-

Guglielmaccil C, Kang L, Wang R, Rouch C, Lefevrel A, Ktorzal A, Routh V, Levin B, Magnan C. Fatty acid signaling in the hypothalamus and the neural control of insulin secretion. *Diabetes* 55(Suppl 2) (December 2006): S139–S144.

Milton K. Nutritional characteristics of wild primate foods: do the diets of our closest living relatives have lessons for us? *Nutrition* 15(6) (June 1999): 488–498.

Miyata T, Inagi R, Asahi K, Yamada Y, Horie K, Sakai H, Uchida K, Kurokawa K. Generation of protein carbonyls by glycoxidation and lipoxidation reactions with autoxidation products of ascorbic acid and polyunsaturated fatty acids. *FEBS Letters* 437(1–2) (October 16, 1998: 24–28.

Moffat SD, Zonderman AB, Metter EJ, Blackman MR, Harman SM, Resnick SM. Longitudinal assessment of serum free testosterone concentration predicts memory performance and cognitive status in elderly men. *Journal of Clinical Endocrinology and Metabolism* 87(11) (November 1, 2002): 5001–5007.

Monsivais P, Perrigue MM, Drewnowski A. Sugars and satiety: does the type of sweetener make a difference? *American Journal of Clinical Nutrition* 86(1) (July 2007): 116–123.

Morgan K, Obici S, Rossetti L. Hypothalamic responses to long-chain fatty acids are nutritionally regulated. *Journal of Biological Chemistry* 279(30) (July 23, 2004): 31139–31148.

Mortality in Sheep Flocks after Grazing on Bt Cotton Fields—Warangal District, Andhra Pradesh. Report of the Preliminary Assessment, April 2006, http://www.gmwatch.org/archive2.asp?arcid=6494.

Mosley JB, O'Malley K, Peterson NJ, Menke TJ, Brody BA, Kuykendall DH, Hollingsworth JC, Ashton CM, Wray MP. A controlled trial of arthroscopic surgery for osteoarthritis of the knee. *New England Journal of Medicine* 347 (July 2002): 81–88.

Mourot J, Thouvenot P, Couet C, Antoine JM, Krobicka A, Derby G. Relationship between the rate of gastric emptying and glucose and insulin responses to starchy foods in young healthy adults. *American Journal of Clinical Nutrition* 48(4) (October 1988): 1035–1034.

Mozaffarian D, Stein PK, Prineas RJ, Siscovick DS. Dietary fish and [omega]-3 fatty acid consumption and heart rate variability in US adults. *Circulation* 177 (2008): 1130–1137.

Mullenix PJ, Debesten PK, Schunior A, Kernan WJ. Neurotoxicity of sodium fluoride in rats. *Neurotoxicology and Teratology* 17(2) (March–April 1995): 169–177.

Munto IC, Hand B, Middleton EJ, Heggtveit HA, Grice HC. Toxic effects of brominated vegetable oils in rats. *Toxicology and Applied Pharmacology* 22(3) (July 1972): 423–429.

Murphy M, Spungen Douglas J, Birkett A. Resistant starch intakes in the United States. *Journal of the American Dietetic Association* 108 (2008): 67–78.

Murry R. "How Aspartame Became Legal—The Timeline." Rense.com, retrieved December 20, 2011.

Muscelli E, Emdin M, Natali A, Pratali L, Camastra S, Gastaldelli A, Baldi S, Carpeggiani C, Ferrannini E. Autonomic and hemodynamic responses to insulin in lean and obese humans. *Journal of Clinical Endocrinology and Metabolism* 83(6) (June 1998): 2084–2090.

Nagao T, Yoshimura S, Saito Y, Nakagomi M, Usumi K, Ono H. Reproductive effects in male and female rats of neonatal exposure to genistein. *Reproductive*

572

Toxicology 15(4) (July–August 2001): 399–411.

Naik G. "Mistakes in Scientific Studies Surge." *Wall Street Journal*, August 10, 2011.

Nakai M, Cook L, Pyter LM, Black M, Sibona J, Turner RT, Jeffrey EH, Bahr JM. Dietary soy protein and isoflavones have no significant effect on bone and a potentially negative effect on the uterus of sexually mature intact Sprague-Dawley female rats. *Menopause* 12(3) (May–June 2005): 291–298.

Nakashima E, Rein L. "FDA Staffers Sue Agency over Surveillance of Personal E-Mail." *Washington Post*, January 29, 2012.

National Academies Press. *Fluoride in Drinking Water: A Scientific Review of EPA's Standards*. National Research Council (2006).

National Fluoridation News (Fall 1983). 14 Nobel Prize winners who object to fluoridation.

Newbold RR, Banks EP, Bullock B, Jefferson W. Uterine adenocarcinoma in mice treated neonatally with genistein. *Cancer Research* 61(11) (June 1, 2001): 4325–4328.

Newsholme EA. Mechanisms for starvation suppression and refeeding activation of infection. *Lancet* 309(8012) (March 19, 1977): 654.

Nilsson AC, Ostman EM, Holst JJ, Bjorck IME. Including indigestible carbohydrates in the evening meal of healthy subjects improves glucose tolerance, lowers inflammatory markers, and increases satiety after a subsequent standardized breakfast. *Journal of Nutrition* 138 (April 2008): 732–739.

Nixon PGF. Hyperventilation and cardiac symptoms. *Internal Medicine* 10(12) (December 1989): 67–84.

Nordlee JA, Tayor SL, Townsend JA, Thomas LA, Bush RK. Identification of a Brazil-nut allergen in transgenic soybeans. *New England Journal of Medicine* 334(11) (March 14, 1996).

Nuutila P, Koivisto VA, Knuuti J, Ruotsalainen U, Teras M, Haaparanta M, Bergman J, Solin O, Voipio-Pulkki LM, Wegelius. Glucose-free fatty acid cycle operates in human heart and skeletal muscle in vivo. *Journal of Clinical Investigation* 89(6) (June1992): 1767–1774.

O'Dea K, Esler M, Leonard P, Stockigt JR, Nestel P. Noradrenaline turnover during under- and over-eating in normal weight subjects. *Metabolism* 31(9) (September 1982): 896–899.

O'Dell TJ, Kandel ER, Grant SGN. Long-term potentiation in the hippocampus is blocked by tyrosine kinase inhibitors. *Nature* 353 (October 10, 1991): 558–560.

Offner B, Czachurski J, Konig SA, Seller H. Different effects of respiratory and metabolic acidosis on preganglionic sympathetic nerve activity. *Journal of Applied Physiology* 77(1) (July 1994): 173–178.

Osteosarcoma Legal Help. "Fluoride in Water," http://www.fluoride-osteosarcoma law.com/fluoride_water.htm, accessed on January 25, 2012.

Ostman EM, Liljeberg EHG, Bjork IM. Inconsistency between glycemic and insulinemic responses to regular and fermented milk products. *American Journal of Clinical Nutrition* 74(1) (July 2001): 96–100.

Painter J. Comparing theories, meal plans and macronutrient compositions of popular high protein diets. *Journal of Foodservice* 13(2) (June 2006): 111–117.

Pamplona R, Barja G, Portero-Otin M. Membrane fatty acid unsaturation, protection against oxidative stress and maximum life span. *Annals of the New York Academy of Sciences* 959 (April 2002): 475–490.

Pamplona R, Portero-Otin M, Requena JR, Thorpe SR, Herro A, Barja G. A low degree of fatty acid unsaturation leads to lower lipid peroxidation and lipoxidation-derived protein modification in heart mitochondria of the longevous pigeon than in the short-lived rat. *Mechanism of Ageing and Development* 106(3) (January 15, 1999: 283–296.

Pamplona R, Portero-Otin M, Sanz A, Requena J, Barja G. Modification of the longevity-related degree of fatty acid unsaturation modulates oxidative damage to proteins and mitochondria DNA in liver and brain. *Experimental Gerontology* 39(5) (May 2004): 725–733.

Paolisso G, Di Maro G, Cozzolino D, Salvatore T, D'Amore A, Lama D, Varricchio M, D'Onofrio F. Chronic magnesium administration enhances oxidative glucose metabolism in thiazide treated hypertensive patients. *American Journal of Hypertension* 5(10) (October 1992): 681–686.

Paolisso G, Scheen A, Cozzolino D, Di Maro G, Varrichio M, D'Onofrio F, Lefebvre PJ. Changes in glucose turnover parameters and improvement of glucose oxidation after 4-week magnesium administration in elderly noninsulin-dependent (type II) diabetic patients. *Journal of Clinical Endocrinology and Metabolism* 78(6) (June 1994): 1510–1514.

Paolisso Giuseppe, Manzella D, Rizzo M, Ragno E, Barbieri M, Varricchio G, Varricchio M. Elevated plasma fatty acid concentrations stimulates cardiac autonomic nervous system in healthy subjects. *American Journal of Clinical Nutrition* 72(3) (September 2000): 723–730.

Paschenko S. Study of application of the reduced breathing method in a combined treatment of breast cancer. *Ukrainian National Journal of Oncology* (Kiev, 2001) 3(1): 77–78, English translation from http://www.normalbreathing.com/diseases-cancer-1-clinical-trial.php, May 22, 2012.

Pawlak DB, Kushere JA, Ludwig DS. Effects of dietary glycaemic index on adiposity, glucose homeostasis, and plasma lipids in animals. *Lancet* 364 (2004): 778–785.

Pearce ML, Dayton S. Incidence of cancer in men on a diet high in polyunsaturated fat. *Lancet* 297(7697) March 6, 1971): 464–467.

Pearson PN, Palmer MR. Atmospheric carbon dioxide concentrations over the past 60 million years. *Nature* 406 (August 17, 2000): 695–699.

Pellizzer AM, Stranznicky NE, Lim S, Kamen PW, Krum H. Reduced dietary fat intake increases parasympathetic activity in healthy premenopausal women. *Clinical and Experimental Pharmacology and Physiology* 26(8) (August 1999): 656–660.

Peppa M, Uribarri J, Vlassara H. Glucose, advanced glycation end products, and diabetes complications: what is new and what works. *Clinical Diabetes* 21(4) (October 2003): 186–187.

Perciaccante A, Fiorentini A, Paris A, Serra P, Tubani L. Circadian rhythm of the autonomic nervous system in insulin resistant subjects with normoglycemia, impaired fasting glycemia, impaired glucose tolerance, type 2 diabetes mellitus. *BMC Cardiovascular Disorders* 6(19) (2006), doi:10.1186/1471-2261-6-19.

Pereira JN, Holland GF. The effect of nicotinamide adenine dinucleotide on lipolysis in adipose tissue in vitro. *Cellular and Molecular Life Sciences* 22(10) (October 1966): 658–659.

Perera FP, Li Z, Whyatt R, Hoepner L, Wang S, Camann D. Prenatal airborne polycyclic aromatic hydrocarbon exposure and child IQ at age 5 years. i 124(2) (August 1, 2009).

Perry IJ, Beevers DG. Salt intake and stroke: a possible direct effect. *Journal of*

Human Hypertension 6(1) (February 1992): 23–25.

Peterson HR, Rothschild M, Weinberg CR, Fell RD, McLeish KR, Pfeifer MA. Body fat and the activity of the autonomic nervous system. *New England Journal of Medicine* 318(17) (April 28, 1988): 1077–1083.

Pette. Metabolic heterogeneity of muscle fibers. *Journal of Experimental Biology* 115 (1985): 179–189.

Phillips DIW, Caddy S, Ilic V, Fielding BA, Frayn KN, Borthwick AC, Taylor R. Intramuscular triglyceride and muscle insulin sensitivity: evidence for a relationship in nondiabetic subjects. *Metabolism* 45(8) (August 1996): 947–950.

Pitteloud N, Mootha VK, Dwyer AA, Hardin M, Lee H, Eriksson KF, Tripathy D, Yialamas M, Groop L, Elahi D, Hayes FJ. Relationships between testosterone levels, insulin sensitivity, and mitochondrial function in men. *Care* 28(7) (July 2005): 1636–1642.

Poirier P, Hernandez TL, Weil KM, Shepard TJ, Eckel RH. Impact of diet-induced weight loss on the cardiac autonomic nervous system in severe obesity. *Obesity Research* 11 (2003): 1040–1047.

Poole DC, Gaesser GA. Response of ventilatory and lactate thresholds to continuous and interval training. *Journal of Applied Physiology* 58(4) (April 1985): 1115–1121.

Potter SM, Baum JA, Teng H, Stillman RJ, Shay NF. Soy protein and isoflavones: their effects on blood lipids and bone density in postmenopausal women. *American Journal of Clinical Nutrition* 68(6 Suppl) (December 1998): 1375S–1379S.

Pritchard PJ, Lee DJW. The effect of dietary citrate on glycolysis in the intestinal mucosa and liver of the chicken. *International Journal of Biochemistry* 3(15) (June 1972): 322–328.

Purnell JQ, Klopfenstein AA, Stevens PJ, Havel SH, Adams SH, Dunn TN, Krisky C, Rooney WD. Brain functional magnetic resonance imaging response to glucose and fructose infusions in humans. *Diabetes, Obesity and Metabolism* 13(3) (2001): 229.

Qin X. What made Canada become a country with the highest incidence of inflammatory bowel disease: could sucralose be the culprit? *Canadian Journal of Gastroenterology* 25(9) (September 2011): 511.

Rahmatulla AH. Clinical evaluation of two different techniques for the removal of fluorosis stains. *Egyptian Dental Journal* 41(3) (July 1995): 1287–1294.

Ramasamy R, Vannucci SJ, Yan SS, Herold K, Yan SF, Schmidt AM. Advanced glycation end products and RAGE: a common thread in aging, diabetes, neurodegeneration, and inflammation. *Glycobiology* 15(7) (July 2005): 16R–28R.

Ravussin E, Bogardus C, Scheidegger K, LaGrange B, Horton ED, Horton ES. Effect of elevated FFA on carbohydrate and lipid oxidation during prolonged exercise in humans. *Journal of Applied Physiology* 60(3) (March 1986): 893–900.

Ray WA, Murray KT, Hall K, Stein CM. Atypical antipsychotic drugs and the risk of sudden cardiac death. *New England Journal of Medicine* 360(3) (January 15, 2009): 225–235.

Reinhold JG, Lahimgarzadeh A, Nasr K, Hedayati H. Effects of purified phytate and phytate-rich bread upon metabolism of zinc, calcium, phosphorus, and nitrogen in man. *Lancet* 301(7798) (February 10, 1973): 283–288.

Relyea R. The lethal impact of Roundup on aquatic and terrestrial amphibians. *Ecological Applications* 15 (August 2005): 1118–1124.

Reynolds G. "Do Statins Make It Tough to Exercise?" *New York Times*, March 14, 2012.

Riggs BL, Hodgson SF, O'Fallon WM, Chao EY, Wahner HW, Muhs JM, Cedel SL, Melton LJ.   Effect of fluoride treatment on the fracture rate in postmenopausal women with osteoporosis.   *New England Journal of Medicine* 322(12) (March 22, 1990): 802–809.

Ritz P, Krempf M, Cloarec D, Champ M, Charbonnel B.   Comparative continuous-indirect-calorimetry study of two carbohydrates with different glycemic indices.   *American Journal of Clinical Nutrition* 54(5) (November 1991): 855–859.

Robergs RA, Ghiasvand F, Parker D.   Biochemistry of exercise-induced metabolic acidosis.   *American Journal of Physiology—Regulatory, Integrative, and Comparative Physiology* 287(3) (September 2004): R502–R516.

Robert H. Lustig, MD: UCSF Faculty Bio Page, and YouTube presentation, "Sugar: The Bitter Truth" and "The Fructose Epidemic." *The Bariatrician* 24(1) (2009): 10).

Robertson MD, Bickertson AS, Dennis AL, Vidal H, Frayn KN.   Insulin-sensitizing effects of dietary resistant starch and effects on skeletal muscle and adipose tissue metabolism.   *American Journal of Clinical Nutrition* 82(3) (September 2005): 559–567.

Roden M, Price TB, Perseghin G, Petersen KF, Rothman DL, Cline GW, Shulman GI.   Mechanism of free fatty acid–induced insulin resistance in humans.   *Journal of Clinical Investigation* 97(12) (June 15, 1996): 2859–2865.

Romijn JA, Coyle EF, Sidossis LS, Gastaldelli A, Horowitz JF, Endert E, Wolfe RR.   Regulation of endogenous fat and carbohydrate metabolism in relation to exercise intensity and duration.   *AJP Endocrinology* 265(3) (September 1993): E380–E391.

Romon M, Lebel P, Velly C, Marecaux N, Fruchart JC, Dallongeville J.   Leptin response to carbohydrate or fat meal and association with subsequent satiety and energy intake.   *American Journal of Physiology* 277(5 Pt. 1) (November 1999): E855–E861.

Rose CE, Althaus JA, Kaiser DL, Miller ED, Carey RM.   Acute hypoxemia and hypercapnia: increase in plasma catecholamines in conscious dogs.   *American Journal of Physiology* 245(6) (December 1983): H924–H929.

Rose DP, Connolly JM, Meschter CL. Effect of dietary fat on human breast cancer growth and lung metastasis in nude mice.   *Journal of the National Cancer Institute* 83(20) (Oct 16, 1991): 1491–1495.

Rosenkilde M, Nordby P, Nielsen LB, Stallknecht BM, Helge JW.   Fat oxidation at rest predicts peak fat oxidation during exercise and metabolic phenotype in overweight men.   *International Journal of Obesity* 34 (May 2010): 871–877.

Safar ME, Thuilliez C, Richard V, Benetos A. Pressure-independent contribution of sodium to large artery structure and function in hypertension.   *Cardiovascular Research* 46(2) (2000): 269–276.

Saloranta C, Koivisto V, Widen E, Falholt K, DeFronza RA, Harkonen M, Groop L.   Contribution of muscle and liver glucose-fatty acid cycle in humans.   *American Journal of Physiology* 264(4 Pt. 1) (April 1993): E599–E605.

Samuel D.   A review of the effects of plant estrogenic substances on animal reproduction. *Ohio Journal of Science* 67(5) (September 1967): 308–312.

Samuelsson RG, Nagy G. Effects of respiratory alkalosis and acidosis on myocardial excitation. *Acta Physiologica Scandinavica* 97(2) (June 1976): 158–165.

Sanders PW.   Vascular consequences of dietary salt intake. *American Journal of*

Physiology—Renal Physiology 297(2) (2009): pF237–F243.

Sarwar G. The protein digestibility-corrected amino acid score method overestimates quality of proteins containing antinutritional factors and of poorly digestible proteins supplemented with limiting amino acids in rats. *Journal of Nutrition* 127(5) (May 1997): 758–764.

Schaafsma G. The protein digestibility-corrected amino acid score. *Journal of Nutrition* 130(7) (July 2000): 1865S–1867S.

Scheinin A, Pienihakkinen K, Tiekso J, Banoczy J, Szoke J, Esztan I, Zimmerman P, Hadas E. Collaborative WHO xylitol field studies in Hungary. VII. Two-year caries incidence in 976 institutionalized children. *Acta Odontol Scand* 43(6) (December 1985): 381–387.

Scherrer U, Randin D, Tappy L, Vollenweider P, Jequier E, Nicod P. Body fat and sympathetic nerve activity in healthy subjects. *Circulation* 89(6) (June 1994): 2634–2640.

Schrader E. Equivalence of St. Johns wort extract (Ze 117) and fluoxetine: a randomized, controlled study in mild-moderate depression. *International Clinical Psychopharmacology* 15(2) (March 2000): 61–68.

Schribner KB, Pawlak DB, Aubin CM, Majzoub JA, Ludwig DS. Long-term effects of dietary glycemic index on adiposity, energy metabolism and physical activity in mice. *American Journal of Physiology, Endocrinology and Metabolism*, (Epub ahead of print) doi: 10.1152/ajpendo.90487.2008.

Schroder S, Fischer A, Vock C, Bohme M, Schmelzer C, Dopner M, Hulsmann O, Doring F. Nutrition concepts for elite distance runners based on macronutrient and energy expenditure. *Journal of Athletic Training* 43(5) (September–October 2008): 489–504.

Schulze MB, Manson JE, Ludwig DS, Colditz GA, Stampfer MJ, Willett WC, Hu FB. Sugar-sweetened beverages, weight gain, and incidence of type 2 diabetes in young and middle-aged women. *Journal of the American Medical Association* 292 (2004): 927–934.

Seralini GE, Mesnage R, Clair E, Gress S, de Vendomois JS, Cellier D. Genetically modified crops safety assessments: present limits and possible improvements. *Environmental Sciences Europe* 23 (2001): 10.

Sheehan DM, Doerge DR. Letter to docket # 98P-0683; Food labeling: health claims: soy protein and coronary heart disease. February 18, 1999.

Sherman WM, Brodowicz G, Wright DA, Allen WK, Simonsen J, Dernbach A. Effects of 4 h preexercise carbohydrate feedings on cycling performance. *Med Sci Sports Exerc* 21(5) (October 1989): 598–604.

Shu X, Jia L, Ye H, Li C, Wu D. Slow digestion properties of rice different in resistant starch. *Journal of Agriculture and Food Chemistry* 57(16) (August 26, 2009):7552–7559.

Sidossis LS, Stuart CA, Shulman GI, Lopaschuk GD, Wolfe RR. Glucose plus insulin regulate fat oxidation by controlling the rate of fatty acid entry into the mitochondria. *Journal of Clinical Investigation* 98(10) (November 15, 1996): 2244–2250.

Siener R, Hesse A. The effects of a vegetarian and different omnivorous diets: urinary risk factors for uric acid stone formation. *European Journal of Nutrition* 42(6) (December 2003): 332–337.

Simon G. Experimental evidence for blood pressure-independent vascular effects of high sodium diet. *American Journal of Hypertension* 16(12) (2003): 1074–1078.

Simoneau JA, Bouchard C. Human variation in skeletal muscle fiber-type proportion and enzyme activities. *American Journal of Physiology* 257(4

Pt. 1) (October 1989): E567–E572.

Simoneau JA, Colberg SR, Thaete FL, Kelley DE. Skeletal muscle glycolytic and oxidative enzyme capacities are determinants of insulin sensitivity and muscle composition in obese women. *FASEB Journal* 9(2) (February 1995): 273–278.

Simoneau JA, Kelley DE. Altered glycolytic and oxidative capacities of skeletal muscle contribute to insulin resistance in NIDDM. *Journal of Applied Physiology* 83(1) (July 1997): 166-171.

Simopoulos AP. The importance of the ratio of omega-6/omega-3 essential fatty acids. *Biomedicine and Pharmacotherapy* 66(3) (October 2002): 161–236.

Singh AK, Amlal H, Haas P, Dringenberg U, Fussell S, Barone S, Engelhardt R, Zuo J, Seidler U, Soleimani M. Fructose-induced hypertension: essential role of chloride and fructose absorbing transporters PAT1 and Glut 5. *Kidney International* 74 (2008): 438–447.

Singh PN, Sabate J, Fraser GE. Does low meat consumption increase life expectancy in humans? *American Journal of Clinical Nutrition* 78(3) (September 2003): 526S–532S.

Smoller JW, Allison M, Cochrane BB, Curb DC, Perlis RH, Robinson JG, Rosal MC, Wenger NK, Wasserheil-Smoller S. Antidepressant use and risk of incident cardiovascular morbidity and mortality among postmenopausal women in the women's health initiative study. *Archives of Internal Medicine* 169(22) (2009): 2128–2139.

Soenen Stijn, Westerterp-Plantenga MS. No difference in satiety or energy intake after high-fructose corn syrup, sucrose, or milk preloads. *American Journal of Clinical Nutrition* 86(6) (December 2007): 1586–1594.

Soffritti M, Belpoggi F, Cevolani D, Guarino M, Padovani M, Maltoni C. Results of long-term experimental studies on the carcinogenicity of methyl alcohol and ethyl alcohol in rats. *Annals of the New York Academy of Sciences* 982 (December 2002): 46–69.

Soffritti M, Belpoggi F, Esposti DD, Lambertini L, Tibaldi E, Rigano A. First experimental demonstration of the multipotential carcinogenic effects of aspartame administered in the feed of Sprague-Dawley rats. *Environmental Health Perspectives* 114(3) (March 2006): 379–385.

Soffritti M, Belpoggi F, Esposti DD, Lambertini L. Aspartame induces lymphomas and leukemias in rats. *European Journal of Oncology* 10(2) (2005): (in press).

Song XM, Ryder JW, Kawano Y, Chibalin AV, Krook A, Zierath JR. Muscle fiber type specificity in insulin signal transduction. *American Journal of Physiology* 277(6 Pt. 2) (December 1999): R1690–R1696.

Spiller GA, Jensen CD, Pattison TS, Chuck CD, Whittam JH, Scala J. Effect of protein dose on serum glucose and insulin response to sugars. *American Journal of Clinical Nutrition* 46 (September 1987): 474–480.

Stattin P, Bylund A, Rinaldi S, Biessy C, Bechaud H, Stenman UH, Egevad L, Riboli E, Hallmans G, Kaaks R. Plasma insulin-like growth factor-I, insulin like growth factor-binding proteins, and prostate cancer risk: a prospective study. *Journal of the National Cancer Institute* 92(23) (December 6, 2000): 1910–1917.

Stauffer BL, Konhilas JP, Luczak ED, Leinwand LA. Soy diet worsens heart disease in mice. *Journal of Clinical Investigation* 116(1) (2006): 209–216.

Steelink C. Fluoridation controversy. *Chemical & Engineering News*: Letters, July 27, 1992.

Sun ZR, Lie FZ, Wu LN, et al. Effects of high fluoride drinking water on the cerebral functions of mice. *Chinese Journal of Endemiology* 19(4) (2000): 262–263, as cited and abstracted in *Fluoride* 34(1) (2001): 80.

Susheela AK, Jethanandani P. Circulating testosterone levels in skeletal fluorosis patients. *Journal of Toxicology—Clinical Toxicology* 34(2) (1996): 183–189.

Takahashi K, Akiniwa K, Narita K. Regression analysis of cancer incidence rates and water fluoride in the U.S.A., based on IACR/IARC (WHO) data (1978–1992). International Agency for Research on Cancer. *Journal of Epidemiology* 11(4) (July 2001): 170–179.

Takahashi K. Fluoride-linked Down syndrome births and their estimated occurrence due to water fluoridation. *Fluoride* 31(2) (1998): 61–73.

Tanner CJ, Barakat HA, Dohm GL, Pories WJ, MacDonald KG, Cunningham PR, Swanson MS, Houmard JA. Muscle fiber type is associated with obesity and weight loss. *American Journal of Physiology Endocrinology and Metabolism* 282(6) (June 2002): E1191–E1196.

Tarnopolsky LJ, MacDougall JD, Atkinson SA, Tarnopolsky MA, Sutton JR. Gender differences in substrate for endurance exercises. *Journal of Applied Physiology* 68(1) (January 1990): 302–308.

Tarnopolsky M, Ruby B. Sex differences in carbohydrate metabolism. *Clinical Nutrition and Metabolic Care* 4(6) (November 2001): 521–526.

Teff KL, Elliott SS, Tschop M, Kieffer TJ, Rader D, Heiman M, Townsend RR, Keim NL, D'Alessio DD, Havel PJ. Dietary fructose reduces circulation insulin and leptin, attenuates postprandial suppression of ghrelin, and increases triglycerides in women. *Journal of Clinical Endocrinology and Metabolism* 89(6) (June 1, 2004): 2963–2972.

Teixeira SR, Potter SM, Weigel R, Hannum S, Erdman JW, Hasler CM. Effects of feeding 4 levels of soy protein for 3 and 6 wk on blood lipids and apolipoproteins in moderately hypercholesterolemic men. *American Journal of Clinical Nutrition* 71(5) (May 2000): 1077–1084.

Tentolouris N, Argyrakopoulou G, Katsilambros N. Perturbed autonomic nervous system function in metabolic syndrome. *Neuromolecular Medicine* 10(3) (2008): 169–178.

Tentolouris N, Tsigos C, Perea D, Koukou E, Kyriaki D, Kitsou E, Daskas S, Daifotis Z, Makrilakis K, Raptis SA, Katsilambros N. Differential effects of high-fat and high-carbohydrate isoenergetic meals on cardiac autonomic nervous system activity in lean and obese women. *Metabolism* 52(11) (November 2003): 1426–1432.

Teotia SPS, Teotia M. Dental caries: a disorder of high fluoride and low dietary calcium interactions (30 years of personal research). *Fluoride* 27(2) (1994): 59–66.

Tilburt JC, Emanuel EJ, Kaptchuk TJ, Curlin FA, Miller FG. Prescribing "placebo treatments": results of a national survey of US internists and rheumatologists. *BMJ* 337 (October 2008): a1938.

Tohyama E. Relationship between fluoride concentration in drinking water and mortality rate for uterine cancer in Okinawa prefecture, Japan. *Journal of Epidemiology* 6(4) (December 1996): 184–191.

Tokita Y, Hirayama Y, Sekikawa A, Kotake H, Toyota T, Miyazawa T, Sawai T, Oikawa S. Fructose ingestion enhances atherosclerosis and deposition of advanced glycated end-products in cholesterol-fed rabbits. *Journal of Atherosclerosis and Thrombosis* 12(5) (2005): 260–267.

Tornheim K. Oscillations of the glycolytic pathway and the purine nucleotide cycle. *Journal of Theoretical Biology* 79 (1979): 491–541.

Tornroth-Horsefield S. Opening and closing the metabolic gate. *Proceedings of the National Academy of Sciences of the United States of America* 105(50) (December 2008): 19565–19566.

Trabelsi M, et al. Effect of fluoride on thyroid function and cerebellar development in mice. *Fluoride* 34 (2001): 165–173.

Travison TG, Araujo AB, Kupelian V, O'Donnell AB, McKinlay JB. The relative contributions of aging, health, and lifestyle factors to serum testosterone decline in men. *Journal of Clinical Endocrinology and Metabolism* 92(2) (February 1, 2007): 549–555.

Tremblay A, Simoneau JA, Bouchard C. Impact of exercise intensity on body fatness and skeletal muscle metabolism. *Metabolism* 43 (7) (July 1994): 814–818.

Treuth MS, Hunter GR, Williams M. Effects of exercise intensity on 24-h energy expenditure and substrate oxidation. *Med Sci Sports Exerc* 28(9) (September 1996): 1138–1143.

Troisi RJ, Weiss ST, Parker DR, Sparrow D, Young JB, Landsberg L. Relation of obesity and diet to sympathetic nervous system activity. *Hypertension* 17 (May 1991): 669–677.

Tucker KL, Hannan MT, Chen H, Cupples LA, Wilson PWF, Kiel DP. Potassium, magnesium, and fruit and vegetable intakes are associated with greater bone mineral density in elderly and women. *American Journal of Clinical Nutrition* 69(4) (April 1999): 727–736.

Turner CH, Owan I, Brizendine EJ, Zhang W, Wilson ME, Dunpace AJ. High fluoride intakes cause osteomalacia and diminished bone strength in rats with renal deficiency. *Bone* 19(6) (December 1996): 595–601.

Unfer V, Casini ML, Costabilt L, Mignosa M, Geril S, Di Renzo GC. Endometrial effects of long-term treatment with phytoestrogens: a randomized, double-blind, placebo-controlled study. *Fertility and Sterility* 82(1) (July 2004): 145–148.

Van Amelsvoort JM, Westrate JA. Amylose-amylopectin ratio in a meal affects postprandial variables in male volunteers. *American Journal of Clinical Nutrition* 55(3) (March 1992): 712–718.

Van Hall G, Steensberg A, Sacchetti M, Fischer C, Keller C, Schjerling P, Hiscock N, Moller K, Saltin B, Febbraio MA, Pedersen BK. Interleukin-6 stimulates lipolysis and fat oxidation in humans. *Journal of Clinical Endocrinology and Metabolism* 88(7) (July 2003): 3005–3010.

Vanden Bussche J, Kiebooms JAL, De Clercq N, Deceuninck Y, Le Bizec B, De Bradander HF, Vanhaecke L. Feed or food responsible for the presence of low-level thiouracil in urine of livestock and humans. *Journal of Agriculture and Food Chemistry* 59(10) (2011): 5786–5792 .

Varner JA, Jensen KF, Horvath W, Isaacson RL. Chronic administration of aluminum-fluoride or sodium-fluoride to rats in drinking water: alterations in neuronal and cerebrovascular integrity. *Brain Research* 784 (1998): 284–298.

Varol E, Akcay S, Ersoy IH, Koroglu BK, Varol S. Impact of chronic fluorosis on left ventricular diastolic and global functions. *Science of the Total Environment* 408(11) (May 1, 2010): 2295–2298.

Vatanparast H, Barlas S, Denghan M, Ali Shah SM, De Koning L, Steck SE. Carbohydrate intake and overweight and obesity amoung healthy adults. *Journal of the American Dietetic Association* 109(7) (July 2009): 1165–1172.

Vergauwen L, Hespel P, Richter EA. Adenosine receptors mediate synergistic stimulation of glucose uptake and transport by insulin and by contractions in rat skeletal muscle. *Journal of Clinical Investigation* 93(3) (March 1994): 974–981.

Vorhees CV, Butcher RE, Wooten V, Brunner RL. Behavioral and reproductive effects of chronic developmental exposure to brominated vegetable oil in rats. *Teratology* 28(3) (December 1983): 309–318.

Wade AJ, Marbut MM, Round JM. Muscle fibre type and aetiology of obesity. *Lancet* 335(8693) (April 7, 1990): 805–808.

Walker BR. Cortisol–cause and cure for metabolic syndrome? *Diabetes Medicine* 23(12) (December 2006): 1281–1288.

Wallie GA, Dawson R, Achgen J, Webber J, Jeukendrup AE. Metabolic response to carbohydrate ingestion during exercise in males and females. *AJP Endocrinology* 290(4) (April 2006): E708–E715.

Wamil M, Battle JH, Turban S, Kipari T, Seguret D, de Sousa Peixoto R, Nelson YB, Nowakowska D, Ferenbach D, Ramage L, Chapman KE, Hughes J, Dunbar DR, Seckl JR, Morton NM. Novel fat depot-specific mechanisms underlie resistance to visceral obesity and inflammation in 11-hydroxysteroid dehydrogenase type 1-deficient mice. *Diabetes* (February 24, 2001).

Wang C, Kurzer M. Phytoestrogen concentration determines effects on DNA synthesis in human breast cancer cells. *Nutrition and Cancer* 28(3) (1997): 236–237.

Wang Y, Oram JF. Unsaturated fatty acids inhibit cholesterol efflux from macrophages by increasing degradation of ATP-binding cassette transporter A1. *Journal of Biological Chemistry* 227(7) (February 15, 2002): 5692–5697.

Wang Z, Su F, Bruhn A, Yang X, Vincent JL. Acute hypercapnia improves indices of tissue oxygenation more than dobutamine in septic shock. *American Journal of Critical Care Medicine* 177(2) (January 15, 2008): 178–183.

Weber KS, Setchell KD, Stocco DM, Lephart ED. Dietary soy-phytoestrogens decrease testosterone levels and prostate weight without altering LH, prostate 5alpha-reductase or testicular steroidogenic acute regulatory peptide levels in adult male Sprague-Dawley rats. *Journal of Endocrinology* 170(3) (September 2001): 591–599.

Weiss LA, Barrett-Connor E, von Muhlen D. Ratio of n-6 to n-3 fatty acids and bone mineral density in older adults: the Rancho Bernardo study. *American Journal of Clinical Nutrition* 81(4) (April 2005): 934–936.

Weltan S, Bosch A, Dennis S, Noakes T. Influence of muscle glycogen content on metabolic regulation. *American Journal of Physiology Endocrinology and Metabolism* 274(1) (January 1, 1998): E72–E82.

Wen H, Gris D, Lei Y, Jha S, Zhang L, Huand MTH, Brickey WJ, Ting JPY. Fatty acid–induced NLRP3-ASC inflammasome activation interferes with insulin signaling. *Nature Immunology* 12 (2001): 408–415.

Westphal SA, Gannon MC, Nuttal FQ. Metabolic response to glucose ingested with various amounts of protein. *American Journal of Clinical Nutrition* 52 (August 1990): 267–272.

White LR, Petrovitch H, Ross GW, Masaki K, Hardman J, Nelson J, Davis D, Markesbery W. Brain aging and midlife tofu consumption. *Journal of the American College of Nutrition* 19(2) (April 2000): 242–255.

Wiley RA. The effect of acid/alkaline nutrition on psychophysiological function. *International Journal of Biosocial Research* 9(2) (1987): 182–202.

Willis H, Eldridge A, Beiseigel J, Thomas W, Slavin J. Greater satiety response with resistant starch and corn bran in human subjects. *Nutrition Research Journal* 29(2) (February 2009): 100–105.

Wilson D. "Glaxo Settles Cases with U.S. for $3 Billion." *New York Times*, November 3, 2011.

Wiseman CE, Higgins JA, Denyer GS, Miller JC. Amylopectin starch induces nonreversible insulin resistance in rats. *Journal of Nutrition* 126(2) (February 1996): 410–415.

Woelk H. Comparison of St. Johns wort and imipramine for treating depression: randomized controlled trial. *BMJ* 321(7260) (September 2, 2000): 536–539.

Wojtaszewsji JF, MacDonald C, Nielsen JN, Hellsten Y, Hardie DG, Kemp BE, Kiens B, Richter EA. Regulation of 5'AMP-activated protein kinase activity and substrate utilization in exercising human skeletal muscle. *American Journal of Physiology, Endocrinology and Metabolism* 284(4) (April 2003): E813–E822.

Wolever TM, Campbell JE, Geleva D, Anderson GH. High-fiber cereal reduces postprandial insulin responses in hyperinsulinemic but not normoinsulinemic subjects. *Diabetes Care* 27(6) (June 2004): 1281–1285.

Wolfe RR, Peters EJ. Lipolytic response to glucose infusion in human subjects. *American Journal of Physiology* 252(2 Pt. 1) (February 1987): E218–E223.

Wolk A, Bergstrom R, Hunter D, Willett W, Ljung H, Holmberg L, Bergkvist L, Bruce A, Adami HO. A prospective study of association of monounsaturated fat and other types of fat with risk of breast cancer. *Archives of Internal Medicine* 158 (1998): 41–45.

Wolstenholme JT, Edwards M, Shetty SRJ, Gatewood JD, Taylow JA, Rissman EF, Connelly JJ. Gestational exposure to bisphenol A produces transgenerational changes in behaviors and gene expression. *Neuroendocrinology* (June 15, 2012).

Wu DQ, Wu Y. Micronucleus and sister chromatid exchange frequency in endemic fluorosis. *Fluoride* 28(3) (August 1995): 125–127.

Xiang Q, Liang Y, Chen L, Wang C, Chen B, Chen X, Zhou M. Effect of fluoride in drinking water on children's intelligence. *Fluoride* 36(2) (2003): 84–94.

Xiong X, Liu J, He W, Xia T, He P, Chen X, Yang K, Wang A. Dose-effect relationship between drinking water fluoride levels and damage to liver and kidney functions in children. *Environmental Research* 103(1) (January 2007): 112–116.

Yam D, Eliraz A, Berry EM. Diet and disease—the Israeli paradox: possible dangers of a high omega-6 polyunsaturated fatty acid diet. *Israel Journal of Medical Sciences* 32(11) (November 1996): 1134–1143.

Yang Y, Wang X, Guo X. Effects of high iodine and high fluorine on children's intelligence and the metabolism of iodine and fluorine. *Zhonghua Liu Xing Bing Xue Za Zhi* 15(5) (October 1994): 296–298.

Yellayi S, Naaz A, Szewczykowski MA, Sato T, Woods JA, Chang J, Segre M, Allred CD, Helferich WG, Cooke PS. The phytoestrogen genistein induces thymic and immune changes: a human health concern? *PNAS* 1 99(11) (May 28, 2002).

Yeo SE, Jentjens R, Wallis GA, Jeukendrup AE. Caffeine increases exogenous carbohydrate oxidation during exercise. *Journal of Applied Physiology* 99(3) (2005): 844–850

Yiamouyiannis JA. *Water Fluoridation and Tooth Decay: Results from the 1966–1987 National Survey of U.S. Schoolchildren.* Delaware, Ohio, http://www.fluorideresearch.org/232/files/FJ1990_v23_n2_p055-067.pdf.

Yoshioka M, Doucet E, St. Pierre S, Almeras N, Richard D, Labrie A, Despres JP, Bouchard C, Tremblay A. Impact of high-intensity exercise on energy expenditure, lipid oxidation and body fatness. *International Journal of Obesity* 25(3) (2001): 332–339.

Zawadzki KM, Yaspelkis BB, Ivy JL. Carbohydrate-protein complex increases the rate of muscle glycogen storage after exercise. *Journal of Applied Physiology* 72(5) (1992 May): 1854–1859.

Zderic, Davidson, Schenk, Byerley, Coyle. High-fat diet elevates resting intramuscular triglyceride concentration and whole body lipolysis during exercise. *American Journal of Physiology Endocrinology and Metabolism* 286 (2004): E217–E225.

Zhou J, Martin RJ, Tulley RT, Raggio AM, McCutheon KL, Shen L, Danna SC, Tripathy S, Hegsted M, Kennan MJ. Dietary resistant starch up-regulates total GLP-1 and PYY in sustained daylong manner through fermentation in rodents. *American Journal of Physiology, Endocrinology and Metabolism* (Epub ahead of print) doi: 10.1152/ajpendo.90637.2008.

Zhou JR, Erdman JW. Phytic acid in health and disease. *Critical Reviews in Food Science and Nutrition* 35(6) (November 1995): 495–508.

Zhou X, Kaplan ML. Soluble amylose cornstarch is more digestible than soluble amylopectin potato starch in rats. *Journal of Nutrition* 127(7) (July 1997): 1349–1356.

Ziegelbecker R, Ziegelbecker RC. WHO data on dental caries and natural fluoride levels. *Fluoride: Journal of the International Society for Fluoride Research (ISFR)* 26 (1993): 263–266.

Zierath J, Hawley J. Skeletal muscle fiber type: influence on contractile and metabolic properties. *PLoS Biology* 2(10) (October 2004): e348.

Zurlo F, Larson K, Bogardus C, Ravussin E. Skeletal muscle metabolism is a major determinant of resting energy expenditure. *Journal of Clinical Investigation* 86(5) (November 1990): 1423–1427.

Zurlo F, Lillioja S, Esposito-Del Puente A, Nyomba BL, Raz I, Saad MF, Swinburn BA, Knowler WC, Bogardus C, Ravussin E. Low ratio of fat to carbohydrate oxidation as predictor of weight gain: study of 24-h RQ. *American Journal of Physiology* 249(5 Pt. 1) (November 1990): E650–E657.

Zurlo F, Nemeth PM, Choksi RM, Sesodia S, Ravussin E. Whole-body energy metabolism and skeletal muscle biochemical characteristics. *Metabolism* 43(4) (April 1994): 481–486.

CHART 6.1 MACRONUTRIENT PERCENTAGES FOR EACH SEASON-TYPE

	Winter	Autumn	Spring	Summer
Protein	35-45%	30-35%	25-30%	20-25%
Carbohydrates	25-35%	35-50%	50-60%	60-70%
Fat	25-35%	20-30%	15-20%	10-15%

CHART 6.2 A WINTER'S CALORIES/GRAMS OF PROTEIN, CARBOHYDRATES, AND FAT BASED ON TOTAL CALORIES IN A MEAL

Total Calories	Winter Calorie and Gram Counts											
	PROTEIN				CARBOHYDRATES				FAT			
	Calories		Grams		Calories		Grams		Calories		Grams	
	Low	High	Low	High	Low	High	Low	High	Low	High	Low	High
350	123	158	31	39	88	123	22	31	88	123	10	14
400	140	180	35	45	100	140	25	35	100	140	11	16
450	158	203	39	51	113	158	28	39	113	158	13	18
500	175	225	44	56	125	175	31	44	125	175	14	19
550	193	248	48	62	138	193	34	48	138	193	15	21
600	210	270	53	68	150	210	38	53	150	210	17	23
650	228	293	57	73	163	228	41	57	163	228	18	25
700	245	315	61	79	175	245	44	61	175	245	19	27
750	263	338	66	84	188	263	47	66	188	263	21	29
800	280	360	70	90	200	280	50	70	200	280	22	31
850	298	383	74	96	213	298	53	74	213	298	24	33
900	315	405	79	101	225	315	56	79	225	315	25	35

CHART 6.3 AN AUTUMN'S CALORIES/GRAMS OFPROTEIN, CARBOHYDRATES, AND FAT BASED ON TOTAL CALORIES IN A MEAL

Total Calories	An Autumn's Calorie and Gram Counts											
	PROTEIN				CARBOHYDRATES				FAT			
	Calories		Grams		Calories		Grams		Calories		Grams	
	Low	High	Low	High	Low	High	Low	High	Low	High	Low	High
350	105	123	26	31	123	175	31	44	70	105	8	12
400	120	140	30	35	140	200	35	50	80	120	9	13
450	135	158	34	39	158	225	39	56	90	135	10	15
500	150	175	38	44	175	250	44	63	100	150	11	17
550	165	193	41	48	193	275	48	69	110	165	12	18
600	180	210	45	53	210	300	53	75	120	180	13	20
650	195	228	49	57	228	325	57	81	130	195	14	22
700	210	245	53	61	245	350	61	88	140	210	16	23
750	225	263	56	66	263	375	66	94	150	225	17	25
800	240	280	60	70	280	400	70	100	160	240	18	27
850	255	298	64	74	298	425	74	106	170	255	19	28
900	270	315	68	79	315	450	79	113	180	270	20	30

CHART 6.4 A SPRING'S CALORIES/GRAMS OF PROTEIN, CARBOHYDRATES, AND FAT BASED ON TOTAL CALORIES IN A MEAL

Total Calories	A Spring's Calorie and Gram Counts											
	PROTEIN				CARBOHYDRATES				FAT			
	Calories		Grams		Calories		Grams		Calories		Grams	
	Low	High	Low	High	Low	High	Low	High	Low	High	Low	High
350	88	105	22	26	175	210	44	53	53	70	6	8
400	100	120	25	30	200	240	50	60	60	80	7	9
450	113	135	28	34	225	270	56	68	68	90	8	10
500	125	150	31	38	250	300	63	75	75	100	8	11
550	138	165	34	41	275	330	69	83	83	110	9	12
600	150	180	38	45	300	360	75	90	90	120	10	13
650	163	195	41	49	325	390	81	98	98	130	11	14
700	175	210	44	53	350	420	88	105	105	140	12	16
750	188	225	47	56	375	450	94	113	113	150	13	17
800	200	240	50	60	400	480	100	120	120	160	13	18
850	213	255	53	64	425	510	106	128	128	170	14	19
900	225	270	56	68	450	540	113	135	135	180	15	20

CHART 6.5 A SUMMER'S CALORIES/GRAMS OF PROTEIN, CARBOHYDRATES, AND FAT BASED ON TOTAL CALORIES IN A MEAL

Total Calories	A Summer's Calorie and Gram Counts											
	PROTEIN				CARBOHYDRATES				FAT			
	Calories		Grams		Calories		Grams		Calories		Grams	
	Low	High	Low	High	Low	High	Low	High	Low	High	Low	High
350	70	88	18	22	210	245	53	61	35	53	4	6
400	80	100	20	25	240	280	60	70	40	60	4	7
450	90	113	23	28	270	315	68	79	45	68	5	8
500	100	125	25	31	300	350	75	88	50	75	6	8
550	110	138	28	34	330	385	83	96	55	83	6	9
600	120	150	30	38	360	420	90	105	60	90	7	10
650	130	163	33	41	390	455	98	114	65	98	7	11
700	140	175	35	44	420	490	105	123	70	105	8	12
750	150	188	38	47	450	525	113	131	75	113	8	13
800	160	200	40	50	480	560	120	140	80	120	9	13
850	170	213	43	53	510	595	128	149	85	128	9	14
900	180	225	45	56	540	630	135	158	90	135	10	15

CHART 6.7 PROTEIN FOOD CHART

Calories per Serving							Recommended % of Calories			
							Winter	Autumn	Spring	Summer
	Protein					Protein:	35-45%	30-35%	25-30%	20-25%
		Carbohydrates				Carbohydrates:	25-35%	35-50%	50-60%	60-70%
			Fat			Fat:	25-35%	20-30%	15-20%	10-15%
Serving Size	Total Cal	P Cal	C Cal	F Cal	Pur=Purines* Pur	Purines*:	High Winter	Medium Autumn	Low Spring	Very Low Summer
						PROTEIN				
						MEAT				
4 oz.	302	122	0	180	+	Beef, 70% lean	:-)	:-|	:-(	:-(
4 oz.	304	129	0	175	+	Beef, 80% lean	:-)	:-|	:-(	:-(
4 oz.	228	122	0	108	+	Beef, 90% lean	:-)	:-)	:-(	:-(
4 oz.	183	123	0	60	+	Beef, 95% lean	:-)	:-)	:-|	:-(
4 oz.	286	116	0	170	+	Lamb	:-)	:-|	:-(	:-(
4 oz.	153	97.2	17	36.8	++	Liver	:-):-)	:-)	:-(	:-(:-(
1 slice	41	13	0	28	+	Pork, bacon	:-)	:-|	:-(	:-(
6 oz.	252	136	8	108	+	Pork, Canadian bacon	:-)	:-)	:-|	:-(
4 oz.	187	84	6	97	+	Pork, chop	:-)	:-)	:-(	:-(
4 oz.	123	77	8	38	+	Pork, tenderloin	:-)	:-)	:-|	:-(
1 oz.	34	22	0	12	+	Pork, extra lean ham	:-)	:-)	:-|	:-(
						POULTRY				
4 oz.	266	81	0	185	+	Chicken, dark with skin	:-)	:-|	:-(	:-(
4 oz.	123	111	0	12	+	Chicken, light no skin	:-|	:-|	:-)	:-|
4 oz.	224	82	0	142	+	Cornish hen	:-)	:-|	:-(	:-(
4 oz.	148	88	0	60	+	Duck	:-)	:-)	:-(	:-(
4 oz.	180	108	0	72	+	Goose	:-)	:-)	:-(	:-(
4 oz.	248	132	0	116	+	Turkey, dark with skin	:-)	:-)	:-(	:-(
4 oz.	128	112	0	16	+	Turkey, light, no skin	:-|	:-)	:-)	:-|
						SEAFOOD				
1 oz.	37	25	0	12	+++	Anchovies	:-):-)	:-)	:-(	:-(:-(
4 oz.	109	85	0	23.6		Bass	:-(	:-|	:-)	:-|
4 oz.	143	85	0	56	+	Carp	:-)	:-)	:-(	:-(
4 oz.	151	76	0	77		Catfish	:-(	:-|	:-(	:-|
4 oz.	83	61	12	10	+	Clams	:-)	:-)	:-(	:-(
4 oz.	92	86	0	6	+	Cod	:-|	:-|	:-)	:-|
4 oz.	94	88	0	6	+	Crab	:-)	:-)	:-(	:-(
4 oz.	103	91	0	12		Flounder	:-(	:-(	:-)	:-|
4 oz.	103	93	0	10		Grouper	:-(	:-(	:-)	:-|
4 oz.	123	100	0	23		Halibut	:-(	:-(	:-)	:-|
4 oz.	101	90	2	9	+	Lobster	:-)	:-)	:-|	:-(
4 oz.	230	89	0	141	++	Mackerel	:-):-)	:-|	:-(	:-(:-(
4 oz.	100	57	17	23	+	Mussels	:-)	:-)	:-)	:-(
4 oz.	91	45	23	23	+	Oysters	:-)	:-)	:-(	:-(
4 oz.	106	91	0	17	++	Perch	:-)	:-)	:-|	:-(

* + = medium, ++ = high, +++ = very high

CHART 6.7 PROTEIN FOOD CHART

Calories per Serving							Recommended % of Calories			
							Winter	Autumn	Spring	Summer
	Protein					Protein:	35-45%	30-35%	25-30%	20-25%
		Carbohydrates				Carbohydrates:	25-35%	35-50%	50-60%	60-70%
			Fat			Fat:	25-35%	20-30%	15-20%	10-15%
Serving	Total	P	C	F	Pur=Purines*	Purines*:	High	Medium	Low	Very Low
Size	Cal	Cal	Cal	Cal	Pur		Winter	Autumn	Spring	Summer
						PROTEIN				
						SEAFOOD CONT.				
4 oz.	85	78	0	7		Roughy	:-(	:-(	:-)	:-|
4 oz.	201	95	0	106	++	Salmon	:-):-)	:-)	:-(	:-(:-(
4 oz.	209	100	3	106	+++	Sardines	:-):-)	:-)	:-(	:-(:-(
4 oz.	98	80	11	7.6	++	Scallops	:-)	:-)	:-(	:-(
4 oz.	119	97	4	18	++	Shrimp	:-)	:-)	:-|	:-(
4 oz.	112	98	0	14		Snapper	:-(	:-(	:-)	:-|
4 oz.	104	75	15	14	+	Squid	:-|	:-|	:-)	:-(
4 oz.	136	95	0	41		Swordfish	:-(	:-|	:-(	:-(
4 oz.	166	99	0	67	+++	Trout	:-)	:-)	:-(	:-(
4 oz.	122	112	0	10	+	Tuna, yellowfin	:-|	:-)	:-)	:-|
4 oz.	150	91	0	59	+	Whitefish	:-)	:-)	:-(	:-(
						MISC. PROTEIN				
1 white	16	15	0	1		Egg whites	:-(	:-(	:-|	:-)
Per individual product						Whey protein	:-|	:-|	:-(	:-(
Per individual product						Milk (casein protein)	:-|	:-|	:-(	:-(
Per individual product						Soy protein	:-(	:-(	:-(	:-(
Per individual product					+++	Brewer's yeast	:-)	:-)	:-(	:-(
Per individual product					+++	Chlorella/blue-green algae	:-)	:-)	:-(	:-(

* + = medium, ++ = high, +++ = very high

CHART 6.8 DAIRY BEAN FOOD CHART

	Calories per Serving						Recommended % of Calories			
							Winter	Autumn	Spring	Summer
	Protein					Protein:	35-45%	30-35%	25-30%	20-25%
		Carbohydrates				Carbohydrates:	25-35%	35-50%	50-60%	60-70%
			Fat			Fat:	25-35%	20-30%	15-20%	10-15%
Serving Size	Total Cal	P Cal	C Cal	F Cal	Pur =Purines*	Purines*:	High	Medium	Low	Very Low
					Pur		Winter	Autumn	Spring	Summer
						DAIRY				
						DAIRY				
1 oz.	99	26	3	70		Blue cheese	:-|	:-|	:-(	:-(
1 oz.	94	25	1	68		Brie	:-|	:-|	:-(	:-(
1 oz.	113	30	2	81		Cheddar cheese	:-|	:-|	:-(	:-(
1 oz.	110	28	3	79		Colby cheese	:-|	:-|	:-(	:-(
4 oz.	111	54	14	43		Cottage cheese/whole	:-|	:-|	:-(	:-(
4 oz.	81	60	11	10		Cottage cheese, 1%	:-(	:-(	:-|	:-(
1 tbsp.	50	4	2	44		Cream cheese	:-|	:-|	:-(	:-(
1 egg	71	25	1	45		Eggs, chicken	:-|	:-|	:-(	:-(
1 oz.	74	17	5	52		Feta	:-|	:-|	:-(	:-(
1 oz.	100	30	2	68		Gouda	:-|	:-|	:-(	:-(
1 cup	118	41	51	26		Milk, low fat	:-(	:-|	:-|	:-(
1 cup	101	42	54	5		Milk, nonfat	:-(	:-(	:-|	:-|
1 cup	146	31	44	71		Milk, whole	:-|	:-|	:-(	:-(
1 oz.	104	29	1	74		Monterey jack	:-|	:-|	:-(	:-(
1 oz.	71	29	3	39		Mozzarella, part skim	:-|	:-|	:-|	:-|
1 oz.	84	27	2	55		Mozzarella, whole	:-|	:-|	:-(	:-(
1 oz.	110	43	3	64		Parmesan	:-|	:-|	:-(	:-(
1 oz.	98	31	2	65		Provolone	:-|	:-|	:-(	:-(
1 oz.	39	14	6	19		Ricotta, part skim	:-|	:-|	:-(	:-(
1 oz.	49	14	3	32		Ricotta, whole	:-|	:-|	:-(	:-(
1 oz.	108	38	4	66		Romano	:-|	:-|	:-(	:-(
1 tbsp.	20	2	3	16		Sour cream, low fat	:-|	:-|	:-(	:-(
2 tbsp.	24	8	16	0		Sour cream, nonfat	:-|	:-|	:-|	:-|
1 tbsp.	23	1	1	21		Sour cream, whole	:-|	:-|	:-(	:-(
1 oz.	106	32	6	68		Swiss	:-|	:-|	:-(	:-(
1 cup	149	36	43	70		Yogurt, whole	:-|	:-|	:-(	:-(
1 cup	154	55	66	33		Yogurt, low fat	:-(	:-|	:-|	:-(

Calories per Serving							Recommended % of Calories			
							Winter	Autumn	Spring	Summer
	Protein					Protein:	35-45%	30-35%	25-30%	20-25%
		Carbohydrates				Carbohydrates:	25-35%	35-50%	50-60%	60-70%
			Fat			Fat:	25-35%	20-30%	15-20%	10-15%
Serving Size	Total Cal	P Cal	C Cal	F Cal	Pur=Purines* Pur	Purines*:	High Winter	Medium Autumn	Low Spring	Very Low Summer
						BEANS				
						LEGUMES*				
1 cup	294	60	232	2	+*	Aduki beans, cooked	:-)	:-)	:-|	:-(
1 cup	227	53	166	8	+*	Black beans, cooked	:-)	:-)	:-(	:-(
1 cup	198	46	145	8	++	Black-eyed peas, cooked	:-):-)	:-)	:-(	:-(:-(
1 cup	241	57	177	7	+	Cranberry beans, cooked	:-)	:-)	:-)	:-|
1 cup	187	45	136	6	+*	Fava beans, cooked	:-)	:-)	:-|	:-(
1 cup	269	50	183	36		Garbanzo beans, cooked	:-|	:-|	:-)	:-)
1 cup	209	51	151	7	++	Great northern, cooked	:-):-)	:-)	:-(	:-(:-(
1 cup	44	6	35	3	+	Green beans	:-):-)	:-)	:-|	:-(
1 cup	225	54	164	7	+*	Kidney beans, cooked	:-)	:-)	:-|	:-(
1 cup	230	62	161	7	++	Lentils, cooked	:-):-)	:-)	:-(	:-(:-(
1 cup	216	51	159	6	+	Lima beans, cooked	:-)	:-)	:-|	:-(
1 cup	212	49	156	7	++	Mung beans, cooked	:-):-)	:-)	:-(	:-(:-(
1 cup	255	52	193	10	+*	Navy beans, cooked	:-)	:-)	:-|	:-(
1 oz.	164	23	25	116	+*	Peanuts, dry roasted	:-)	:-)	:-|	:-(
2 tbsp.	188	28	25	135	+*	Peanut butter	:-)	:-)	:-|	:-(
1 cup	252	53	192	7	+*	Pink beans, cooked	:-)	:-)	:-|	:-(
1 cup	245	54	182	9	++	Pinto beans, cooked	:-)	:-)	:-(	:-(
1 cup	219	56	162	1	+	Red beans, cooked	:-)	:-)	:-(	:-(
1 cup	231	57	168	6	++	Split peas, cooked	:-):-)	:-)	:-(	:-(:-(
1 cup	298	100	69	129	++	Soybeans, cooked	:-(	:-(	:-(	:-(
1 oz.	54	18	11	25	++	Tempeh	:-|	:-|	:-|	:-(
1 oz.	20	8	2	10	++	Tofu	:-(	:-(	:-(	:-(
1 cup	254	56	189	9	++	White beans, cooked	:-)	:-)	:-(	:-(

If the purine value of a bean was unknown, it was assumed to have a + value. Unknown beans marked +

* + = medium, ++ = high, +++ = very high

CHART 6.9 CARBOHYDRATES FOOD CHART

									Winter	Autumn	Spring	Summer
Calories per Serving								Recommended % of Calories				
		Protein					Protein:		35-45%	30-35%	25-30%	20-25%
		Carbohydrates					Carbohydrates:		25-35%	35-50%	50-60%	60-70%
			Fat				Fat:		25-35%	20-30%	15-20%	10-15%
Serving	Total	P	C	F	Pur=Purines*		Purines*:		High	Medium	Low	Very Low
Size	Cal	Cal	**Cal**	Cal	Pur	GI	GI=Glycemic Index		Winter	Autumn	Spring	Summer
							CARBS					
							GRAINS					
1 cup	251	32	186	33		High	Amaranth, cooked		:-)	:-)	:-|	:-|
1 cup	193	13	175	5	+	Low	Barley, cooked		:-):-)	:-)	:-(	:-(
1 cup	155	19	127	9		Low	Buckwheat, cooked		:-|	:-|	:-)	:-)
1 cup	176	24	150	2		Medium	Couscous, cooked		:-|	:-|	:-)	:-)
1/2 cup	208	15	175	18		Medium	Corn meal, uncooked		:-|	:-|	:-)	:-)
1 cup	251	40	198	13		Low	Kamut, cooked		:-|	:-|	:-)	:-)
1 cup	207	24	169	14		High	Millet, cooked		:-|	:-|	:-|	:-|
1/4 cup	152	23	106	23	+	Low	Oats, raw		:-)	:-)	:-(	:-(
2 oz.	200	24	168	8		Low-Med	Pasta, uncooked		:-|	:-|	:-)	:-)
1 cup	222	33	157	32		Low	Quinoa, cooked		:-|	:-|	:-)	:-)
1 cup	218	15	189	14		Medium	Rice, brown, cooked		:-|	:-|	:-)	:-)
1 cup	225	15	195	15		Low	Rice, br., parboiled, cooked					
1 cup	205	16	185	4		Medium	Rice, white, cooked		:-|	:-|	:-)	:-)
1/4 cup	141	19	115	9		Low	Rye, uncooked		:-|	:-|	:-)	:-)
1 cup	220	32	177	11		Low-Med	Spaghetti, cooked		:-|	:-|	:-)	:-)
1 cup	246	38	194	14		Medium	Spelt, cooked		:-|	:-|	:-)	:-)
1 oz.	102	13	85	4		Low	Wheat flour, white		:-|	:-|	:-)	:-)
1 cup	166	23	138	5		Low	Wild rice, cooked		:-|	:-|	:-)	:-)
							VEGETABLES					
1/2 cup	45	6	36	3	+	High	Artichoke, hearts		:-):-)	:-)	:-(	:-(:-(
4 stalks	13	4	8	1	+	Low	Asparagus, boiled		:-):-)	:-)	:-(	:-(:-(
1/2	114	5	21	88		Low	Avocado, California		:-)	:-)	:-|	:-(
1 oz.	3	1	2	0		Low	Bamboo shoots, boiled		:-(	:-|	:-)	:-)
1 cup	44	6	35	3	+	Low	Beans, green, cooked		:-):-)	:-)	:-|	:-(
1/2 cup	37	4	32	1		High	Beets, boiled*		:-|	:-|	:-)	:-)
1 cup	9	3	5	1		Low	Bok choy		:-(	:-|	:-)	:-)
1/2 cup	26	7	18	1	+	Low	Broccoli, cooked		:-(	:-(	:-)	:-)
1/2 cup	28	5	20	3		Medium	Brussels sprouts, cooked		:-(	:-(	:-)	:-)
1/2 cup	17	2	15	0		Low	Cabbage, cooked		:-(	:-|	:-)	:-)
1 med.	25	2	22	1		High	Carrot, raw		:-)	:-)	:-|	:-|
1/2 cup	14	3	9	2	+	Low	Cauliflower, cooked		:-):-)	:-)	:-(	:-(
1 stalk	6	1	5	0		Low	Celery		:-)	:-)	:-|	:-|
1 ear	124	20	104	4		High	Corn, on the cob		:-)	:-)	:-|	:-(
1 cup	177	13	146	18		High	Corn, sweet, cooked		:-)	:-)	:-|	:-(
1 cup	16	3	11	2		Low	Cucumber, peeled		:-(	:-(	:-)	:-)

* + = medium, ++ = high, +++ = very high

Calories per Serving								Recommended % of Calories			
								Winter	Autumn	Spring	Summer
		Protein					Protein:	35-45%	30-35%	25-30%	20-25%
			Carbohydrates				Carbohydrates:	25-35%	35-50%	50-60%	60-70%
				Fat			Fat:	25-35%	20-30%	15-20%	10-15%
					Pur = Purines*		Purines*:	High	Medium	Low	Very Low
Serving Size	Total Cal	P Cal	C Cal	F Cal	Pur	GI	GI=Glycemic Index	Winter	Autumn	Spring	Summer
							CARBS				
							VEGETABLES CONT.				
1 cup	35	2	31	2		Low	Eggplant, cooked*	:-(	:-|	:-)	:-)
1 clove	5	1	4	0		Low	Garlic	:-(	:-(	:-)	:-):-)
1 cup	36	6	26	4		Low	Kale, cooked	:-(	:-(	:-)	:-)
1 leek	38	2	34	2		Medium	Leeks, cooked	:-(	:-(	:-)	:-)
1 cup	8	2	5	1		Low	Lettuce	:-(	:-(	:-)	:-)
1 cup	16	6	8	2	+	Low	Mushrooms, raw	:-):-)	:-)	:-(	:-(
1/2 cup	18	4	13	1		Medium	Okra, cooked	:-|	:-|	:-)	:-)
1 oz.	23	1	6	16		Low	Olives, canned	:-)	:-)	:-|	:-)
1 slice	6	1	5	0		Medium	Onion, raw	:-(	:-(	:-)	:-):-)
1/2 cup	56	51	3	2		High	Parsnip, cooked	:-(	:-(	:-)	:-)
1 cup	67	18	46	3	+	Medium	Peas, green cooked*	:-):-)	:-)	:-(	:-(
1 cup	30	3	25	2		Medium	Pepper, bell, raw*	:-(	:-(	:-)	:-)
1 pepper	18	2	15	1		Medium	Pepper, hot, raw	:-(	:-(	:-)	:-)
1 large	278	21	254	3		High	Potato, baked	:-|	:-|	:-)	:-)
1 cup	49	4	43	2		Medium	Pumpkin, cooked	:-(	:-(	:-)	:-)
1 med.	1	0	1	0		Low	Radish, raw	:-(	:-|	:-)	:-)
1 cup	66	6	57	3		High	Rutabaga, cooked	:-(	:-|	:-)	:-)
1 med.	5	1	4	0		Low	Scallion	:-(	:-(	:-)	:-):-)
1 oz.	13	2	9	2		Low	Seaweed	:-|	:-|	:-)	:-)
1 cup	41	13	24	4	+	Low	Spinach, boiled	:-):-)	:-)	:-|	:-|
1 cup	36	4	27	5		Low	Squash, summer, cooked	:-(	:-|	:-)	:-)
1 cup	115	6	107	2		High	Squash, winter, cooked	:-|	:-|	:-)	:-)
1 med.	103	7	95	1		Medium	Sweet potato, cooked*	:-|	:-|	:-)	:-)
1 med.	22	3	17	2		Low	Tomato, red, raw*	:-(	:-(	:-)	:-)
1 med.	34	3	30	1		Medium	Turnip, raw	:-|	:-|	:-)	:-)
1/2 cup	60	2	57	0		Low	Water chestnuts, raw	:-(	:-|	:-)	:-)
1 cup	158	6	151	1		Medium	Yams, cooked	:-|	:-|	:-)	:-)
1/2 cup	14	1	13	0		Low	Zucchini, sliced*	:-(	:-|	:-)	:-)

*Contains moderate amounts of fructose of approximately 2 grams, except peas, which contain approximately 4 grams.

* + = medium, ++ = high, +++ = very high

	Calories per Serving							Recommended % of Calories			
								Winter	Autumn	Spring	Summer
		Protein					Protein:	35-45%	30-35%	25-30%	20-25%
			Carbohydrates				Carbohydrates:	25-35%	35-50%	50-60%	60-70%
				Fat			Fat:	25-35%	20-30%	15-20%	10-15%
Serving Size	Total Cal	P Cal	C Cal	F Cal	Pot = Potassium,		Potassium:	Low	Medium	Medium	High
					Pot	Fru	Fru = Fructose	Winter	Autumn	Spring	Summer
							CARBS				
							FRUIT*				
1 med.	95	2	90	3	195 mg	13 g	Apple	:-|	:-|	:-)	:-|
1 med.	17	2	14	1	91 mg	1 g	Apricot	:-|	:-|	:-)	:-)
1 med.	105	4	98	3	422 mg	7 g	Banana	:-)	:-)	:-|	:-|
1 cup	62	7	49	6	233 mg	4 g	Blackberries	:-|	:-|	:-)	:-)
1 cup	84	4	76	4	114 mg	7 g	Blueberries	:-|	:-|	:-)	:-|
1/2 med.	94	8	82	5	737 mg	11 g	Cantaloupe	:-(	:-|	:-)	:-)
1 cup	87	5	80	2	306 mg	8 g	Cherries, sweet	:-|	:-|	:-)	:-)
1 oz.	99	3	17	79	100 mg	2 g	Coconut, meat, raw	:-)	:-)	:-|	:-|
1 med.	67	2	65	0	167 mg	8 g	Dates, medjool	:-(	:-(	:-)	:-)
1 med.	37	1	35	1	116 mg	4 g	Fig	:-(	:-(	:-|	:-|
1 cup	104	4	98	2	288 mg	6 g	Grapes	:-(	:-|	:-)	:-)
1/2 med.	52	3	47	1	166 mg	4 g	Grapefruit, pink/red	:-(	:-(	:-)	:-):-)
1 cup	112	14	85	13	688 mg	6 g	Guava	:-(	:-(	:-)	:-)
1/4 med.	90	5	83	3	570 mg	14 g	Honeydew	:-(	:-(	:-)	:-)
1 cup	108	7	94	7	522 mg	8 g	Kiwifruit	:-(	:-(	:-)	:-)
1 oz.	7	0	7	0	35 mg	3 g	Lemon juice	:-(:-(	:-(	:-)	:-):-)
1 oz.	7	1	6	0	33 mg	0	Lime	:-(:-(	:-(	:-)	:-):-)
1 med.	135	4	126	5	323 mg	16 g	Mango	:-(	:-(	:-)	:-)
1 med.	63	5	54	4	286 mg	5 g	Nectarine	:-|	:-|	:-)	:-|
1 med.	69	4	63	2	232 mg	6 g	Orange, navel	:-(:-(	:-(	:-)	:-):-)
1 med.	119	6	109	4	781 mg	11 g	Papaya	:-(	:-(	:-)	:-)
1 med.	59	5	51	3	285 mg	6 g	Peach	:-|	:-|	:-)	:-)
1 med.	103	2	99	2	212 mg	12 g	Pear	:-)	:-)	:-|	:-(
1 cup	83	3	78	2	180 mg	9 g	Pineapple	:-(	:-(	:-)	:-):-)
1 med.	30	2	27	1	104 mg	3 g	Plum	:-|	:-|	:-)	:-)
1 med.	234	16	191	27	666 mg	19 g	Pomegranate	:-(	:-(	:-)	:-)
1 med.	23	1	22	0	70 mg	1 g	Prune, dried	:-(	:-(	:-|	:-|
1 oz.	83	2	80	1	231 mg	10 g	Raisin	:-(	:-(	:-|	:-|
1 cup	64	5	52	7	186 mg	3 g	Raspberry	:-|	:-|	:-)	:-)
1 stalk	11	2	8	1	147 mg	1 g	Rhubarb	:-|	:-|	:-)	:-)
1 cup	46	3	39	4	220 mg	4 g	Strawberries, whole	:-|	:-|	:-)	:-)
1 med.	47	2	43	2	146 mg	5 g	Tangerine	:-(	:-(	:-)	:-)
1 cup	46	3	41	2	170 mg	6 g	Watermelon, diced	:-(	:-(	:-)	:-)

*Limit due to high fructose content. Do a two-week fructose fast twice a year.

CHART 6.95: FATS AND OILS, NUTS AND SEEDS FOOD CHART

Calories per Serving							Recommended % of Calories			
							Winter	Autumn	Spring	Summer
		Protein				Protein:	35-45%	30-35%	25-30%	20-25%
			Carbohydrates			Carbohydrates:	25-35%	35-50%	50-60%	60-70%
				Fat		Fat:	25-35%	20-30%	15-20%	10-15%
Serving Size	Total Cal	P Cal	C Cal	F Cal	Pur=Purines*	Purines*:	High	Medium	Low	Very Low
					Pur		Winter	Autumn	Spring	Summer
						FATS & OILS				
1 tbsp.	119	0	0	119		Almond oil	:-|	:-|	:-|	:-|
1 tbsp.	100	0	0	100		Butter**	:-)	:-)	:-(	:-(
1 tbsp.	124	0	0	124		Canola oil	:-(	:-(	:-(	:-(
1 tbsp.	116	0	0	116		Coconut oil**	:-)	:-)	:-)	:-)
1 tbsp.	124	0	0	124		Corn oil	:-(	:-(	:-(	:-(
1 tbsp.	119	0	0	124		Cottonseed oil	:-(	:-(	:-(	:-(
1 tbsp.	52	0	0	52		Cream, heavy**	:-)	:-)	:-(	:-(
1 tbsp.	122	0	0	122		Fish oil**	:-|	:-|	:-)	:-)
1 tbsp.	120	0	0	120		Flaxseed oil**	:-(	:-(	:-)	:-)
1 tbsp.	112	0	0	112		Ghee**	:-)	:-)	:-(	:-(
1 tbsp.	119	0	0	119		Lard**	:-)	:-)	:-(	:-(
1 tbsp.	124	0	0	124		Olive oil**	:-)	:-)	:-)	:-)
1 tbsp.	116	0	0	116		Palm oil**	:-)	:-)	:-(	:-(
1 tbsp.	116	0	0	116		Palm kernel oil**	:-)	:-)	:-)	:-)
1 tbsp.	119	0	0	119		Peanut oil	:-|	:-|	:-|	:-|
1 tbsp.	119	0	0	119		Safflower oil	see *** below			
1 tbsp.	119	0	0	119		Sesame oil	:-|	:-|	:-|	:-|
1 tbsp.	119	0	0	119		Sunflower oil	see *** below			
						NUTS & SEEDS				
1 oz.	162	21	25	117		Almonds	:-|	:-|	:-)	:-)
1 oz.	185	14	14	157		Brazil nuts	:-)	:-)	:-|	:-|
1 oz.	155	18	35	103		Cashews	:-(	:-(	:-)	:-)
1 oz.	55	2	50	3		Chestnuts	:-(	:-(	:-)	:-)
1 oz.	185	7	27	151		Coconut, meat, dried	:-)	:-)	:-|	:-|
1 oz.	177	15	19	144		Filberts	:-)	:-)	:-|	:-|
1 oz.	184	12	21	151		Hickory nuts	:-)	:-)	:-|	:-|
1 oz.	203	8	16	179		Macadamia nuts	:-)	:-)	:-|	:-|
1 oz.	164	23	25	116		Peanuts, dry roasted	:-)	:-)	:-|	:-(
1 oz.	199	9	16	174		Pecans	:-)	:-)	:-|	:-|
1 oz.	190	13	15	162		Pine nuts	:-(	:-(	:-)	:-)
1 oz.	157	20	32	105		Pistachios	:-|	:-|	:-)	:-)
1 oz.	151	24	20	107		Pumpkin seeds	:-|	:-|	:-|	:-|
1 oz.	86	10	16	60		Sesame butter, tahini	:-|	:-|	:-)	:-)
1 oz.	164	20	23	121		Sunflower seeds	:-(	:-(	:-)	:-)
1 oz.	185	15	16	154		Walnuts	:-)	:-)	:-|	:-|

* + = medium, ++ = high, +++ = very high
**These are the healthiest oils and should be the primary ones consumed.
***Cold-pressed high oleic is :-\|. Commercially processed or high linoleic is :-(.

CPSIA information can be obtained at www.ICGtesting.com
Printed in the USA
LVOW122003210912

299852LV00001B/22/P